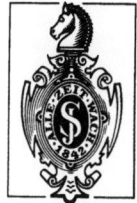

T. Tobe
H. Kameda · M. Okudaira · M. Ohto
Y. Endo · M. Mito · E. Okamoto
K. Tanikawa · M. Kojiro (Eds.)

Primary
Liver Cancer
in Japan

With 304 Illustrations, Including 2 in Color

Springer-Verlag
Tokyo Berlin Heidelberg
New York London Paris
Hong Kong Barcelona

Chief Editor
Takayoshi Tobe, M.D.
Chairman and Professor, 1st Department of Surgery, Faculty of Medicine, Kyoto University, 54-Shogoin Kawara-cho, Sakyo-ku, Kyoto, 606 Japan

Editors
Haruo Kameda
The First Department of Internal Medicine, Jikei University School of Medicine, Minato-ku, Tokyo, 105 Japan

Michio Mito
The Second Department of Surgery, Asahikawa Medical College, Nishikagura 4–5, Asahikawa, Hokkaido, 078 Japan

Masahiko Okudaira
Department of Pathology, School of Medicine, Kitasato University, Sagamihara, 228 Japan

Eizo Okamoto
The First Department of Surgery, Hyogo College of Medicine, Nishinomiya, Hyogo, 663 Japan

Masao Ohto
First Department of Medicine, School of Medicine, Chiba University, Chiba 280 Japan

Kyuichi Tanikawa
Second Department of Medicine, Kurume University School of Medicine, Kurume, 830 Japan

Yasuo Endo
Sanraku Hospital, 2–5 Kanda Surugadai, Chiyoda-ku, Tokyo 101 Japan

Masamichi Kojiro
First Department of Pathology, Kurume University School of Medicine, Fukuoka, 830 Japan

ISBN-13:978-4-431-68179-3   e-ISBN-13:978-4-431-68177-9
DOI: 10.1007/978-4-431-68177-9

Library of Congress Cataloging-in-Publication Data
Primary liver cancer in Japan / Takayoshi Tobe (ed.). p. cm. Includes bibliographical references. ISBN 4-431-70089-7. · ISBN-13:978-4-431-68179-3   1. Liver · Cancer · Japan. I. Tobe, Takayoshi. [DNLM: 1. Hepatoma · epidemiology · Japan. 2. Liver Neoplasms · epidemiology · Japan. WI 735 P9515] RC280.L5P76 1992 616.99'436'00952 · dc20 DNLM/DLC for Library of Congress. 91-5245

© Springer-Verlag Tokyo 1992
Softcover reprint of the hardcover 1st edition 1992

Typesetting: Best-set Typesetter Ltd., Hong Kong

Preface

Primary liver cancer is common in Japan, as in other Asian countries, but it is not so common in Western countries. In Japan, its incidence now ranks next to that of stomach cancer, and the number of patients with liver cancer is showing a gradual and definite increase.

The Liver Cancer Study Group of Japan has been conducting follow-up studies since 1965 with the cooperation of institutions throughout the country. Records of 38,222 patients have been collected and analyzed by computer. The pathogenesis of primary liver cancer was unknown in 1970, and its diagnosis was difficult. Patients who could be treated in the early stage were scarce. The records of these patients show that primary liver cancer in Japan has the following characteristics:

1. Over 90% of liver cancers are hepatocellular carcinomas
2. The incidence of primary liver cancer is highest in the sixth decade of life
3. Primary liver cancer is more common in men than in women
4. Many patients have a past history of hepatitis and frequently have hepatic cirrhosis; however, the number of HBs antigen carriers has been definitely decreasing

On the basis of these characteristics, examinations of high risk patients and greater use of ultrasonography and computed tomography imaging have made it possible to detect primary liver cancer in the early stage. The 9th report by the Liver Cancer Study Group of Japan showed that small liver cancers (less than 2 cm in diameter) were detected in 10% of the patients.

The number of operable cases is also showing a gradual but definite increase. Safe surgical procedures for liver cancer associated with severe hepatic cirrhosis have been safely established in Japan. Recent reports indicate that postoperative complications after hepatectomy in Japan occur in 3%–4% of cases, with 0% being recorded in a few institutes. Further advances have been made through the clarification of various backgrounds and factors that influence the survival rate after hepatic resection and the determination of important risk factors for recurrence.

This monograph contains contributions from the leaders of the Liver Cancer Study Group of Japan and is based on enormous amounts of data gathered over the years in the fields of epidemiology, molecular biology, diagnostics, and surgical and sophisticated conservative treatments. Famous specialists in other Asian countries have also contributed: Professor Tang in the People's Republic of China, Professor Kim in Korea, Professor Lai in Hong Kong and Professor Ker in Taiwan.

It is expected that this monograph will provide valuable information and various suggestions for clinicians and basic researchers throughout the world.

Takayoshi Tobe, M.D., FACS
President
27th Annual Meeting of Liver Cancer
Study Group of Japan

Contents

Part 4   Diagnosis

Part 5   Hepatic function

Part 6   Mass screening

Part 7   Treatment

Section 1   Surgical treatment

Section 2   Conservative and multidisciplinary treatment

Part 8   Recurrence

Addendum (1)

Addendum (2)

XI

Addendum (3)

Contributors

Part 1   Epidemiology

CHAPTER 1

Epidemiology of primary liver cancer

Kunio Okuda[1]

Epidemiology of Hepatocellular Carcinoma

Geographic prevalence. The incidence of hepatocellular carcinoma (HCC) varies considerably with the geographic region perhaps due to differences in the major etiologic factors. Whereas the incidence of HCC is low among Causacians in the United Kingdom, United States, and Australia, it is much higher among the black population in Mozambique, sub-Saharan Africa, and in the Far East [1–3].

It is rather difficult to grasp the exact incidence rate of HCC, because the vital statistics are based on diagnoses made by physicians which mostly lack histological confirmation, and which list HCC and cholangiocarcinoma (CCC) together as "primary liver cancer". Without histological diagnosis, secondary liver cancer may be mistaken for primary cancer or vice versa. However, liver tumors associated with cirrhosis are almost invariably HCC in areas where the incidence rate is high. In our case control study in Japan based on autopsy, 369 of 391 liver cancers associated with cirrhosis were found to be primary as contrasted by 88 out of 226 cirrhosis-associated liver cancers being primary in Trieste, Italy [4]. As far as histological diagnosis is concerned, autopsy studies are reliable, but only a relative frequency of HCC among all deaths or all malignancies can be calculated; there is certain bias at the time of hospital admission and autopsy, due to socioeconomic state of the society and changing interest on the part of physicians. A well-established cancer registry with frequent histological diagnosis may be more reliable, yet the statistics based on a cancer registry are quite different from vital statistics which depend on death certificates [5].

It was Berman [6] and later Higginson [7] who called world attention to the extremely high incidence rate of HCC among the male black population (Shangaan tribe) in Mozambique. Table 1 gives the age-adjusted incidence rates of primary liver cancer per 100,000/year in various countries, areas and ethnic groups. They may be divided into the high incidence areas/peoples (>20/100,000/yr) which include Mozambique, Zimbabwe, Rhodesia, Senegal, Singapore Chinese, South African blacks, China, Taiwan, and Japan (after 1976); intermediate incidence areas/peoples (5–20/100,000/yr) including Singapore Malay, Singapore Indian, Brazil (Recife), Nigeria, Indian in South Africa, Switzerland (Geneva), Poland, Spain, New Zealand Maori, American Indian, Jamaica, Cuba, Canadian Eskimo, etc; and low incidence areas/peoples (<5/100,000/yr) such as New Zealand white, Sweden, United Kingdom, Ireland, Mauritius, Norway, American white and black, Australian white, Algeria, Canadian white, Israel, Germany, Denmark, Yugoslavia (Slovenia), Hungary, India (Bombay), Pakistan, and so on [1–3]. The relative significance of this type of cancer among all malignancies may be appreciated from the age-standardized cancer rates shown in Tables 2 and 3, the former being taken from the paper by Munoz and Bosch [2], and the latter from the statistics compiled by the Ministry of Health and Welfare of Japan [8].

It is clear from Table 4, which compares different ethnic groups within a given region and a given race in different countries, that within the same region or city, the incidence rate varies markedly with the ethnic group. Although the African black and Chinese have high incidence rates, it is much lower among the blacks in the United States who originally came from Africa

---

[1] Department of Medicine, Chiba University Hospital, Chiba, Japan

Table 1. Age-adjusted incidence rates of liver cancer per 100,000/year population in various countries cities and ethnic groups

Country (Registry)	Incidence rate (per 100,000/yr)	
	Males	Females
Mozambique, Lourenco Marques	112.9	30.8
Zimbabwe, Bulawayo	64.6	25.4
Cape, Bantu	26.3	8.4
Colored	1.5	0.7
White	1.3	0.6
Algeria	1.6	1.4
Argentina, Tandil	9.9	5.8
Brazil, Fortaleza	3.8	3.8
Jamaica	6.1	2.1
USA, San Francisco, Chinese	19.1	3.6
Black	3.9	1.8
Japanese	3.0	0.4
White	2.9	1.1
Canada, Eskimos	6.9	3.7
Alberta	1.3	0.5
Switzerland, Geneva	9.7	1.3
Spain, Zaragoza	6.9	5.1
France, Doubs	1.9	1.1
W.Germany, Hamburg	3.6	1.6
Denmark	2.9	1.6
Yugoslavia, Slovenia	2.0	0.9
UK, Oxford	1.1	0.4
China, Shanghai	31.7	9.1
Singapore, Chinese	32.2	7.1
Malay	17.1	3.1
Indian	14.0	4.8
Korea	13.8	3.2
Japan, Nagasaki	11.9	2.9
India, Bombay	2.7	1.0
Pakistan	0.7	0.8
New Zealand, Maori	8.7	3.5
Australia, South	1.3	0.4

From Munoz and Bosch [2] with permission

Table 2. Age-standardized cancer ratio for primary liver cancer in developing countries

Country (Registry)	Males (%)	Females (%)
Uganda, West Nile	21.0	9.2
Zambia, Kuska	15.9	17.0
Kenya, National Registry	8.8	4.7
Sudan	6.4	2.6
Tunisia	0.6	0.2
Malaysia, Kuala Lumpur		
Malyasians	13.8	0.4
Chinese	12.9	3.6
Indian	6.0	0
Iraq, Bagdad	2.1	1.1
Bangladesh	1.3	1.3
Sri Lanka, Colombo	0.8	0.5
Argentina, Santa Fe	1.3	1.3
Uruguay, Montevideo	0.2	0.2

Types of registry are not the same.
(From Munoz and Bosch [2] with permission)

compared with contemporary African blacks; and a similar difference exists between the Chinese in Hawaii and those in the Far East. The Chinese in San Francisco Bay Area who still have a relatively high incidence may not have lived in the United States long enough to have had the incidence rate reduced as much as the black population in the United States shows. San Francisco Chinese are known to have a high carrier rate for the hepatitis B surface antigen (HBsAg) which may be an important etiologic factor. Even within the same ethnic group, the incidence differs because of the differences in living conditions. In Mozambique, for instance, there is a nine-fold difference between the coastal and inland regions [9]. In Japan, HCC is more prevalent in the southwest than in the northern areas (Fig. 1), probably due to the warmer and more humid climate, and a higher hepatitis B infection rate.

China has a unique history of cancer epidemiology study. After the founding of the People's Republic of China, the central government set out to determine the regional incidences of various cancers. From 1972 to 1977, 250,000 physicians and more than 600,000 assistants (bare-foot doctors) were mobilized in a mass survey on cancer incidence in 2,392 counties where 840 million people were chosen as the study population. With a special census, the causes of 18 million deaths were studied retrospectively from the medical records and by interview of the relatives. Prospectively, 71% of the cancers were diagnosed either by histology, exploratory surgery, or laboratory assay [11]. For liver cancer, the alpha-fetoprotein (AFP) tests were used [12]. Based on this survey, it became clear that the main endemic areas for liver cancer in this country are along the southeast seacost, and particularly deltas, valleys and islands. The hyperendemic areas such as Fusui and Qidong counties have standardized mortality of more than 60/100,000/yr whereas low incidence areas have mortalities of about 6/100,000/yr [13]. A mortality of 60/100,000/yr for both sexes combined may be nearly equivalent to that in Mozambique, considering an M:F ratio of 2–3:1 in China.

Time trends. Studies on time trends are subject to errors because of changing diagnostic capability and classification, as exemplified by the repeated revisions in the International Classification of Diseases (ICD) and because of registration artifacts. Statistics based on autopsy give relative frequency of histologically proven HCC among

Table 3. Frequency (%) of primary liver cancer among all malignancies and relative to other other major cancers in developed countries

Organ	Males			Females		
	Japan	United States	England·Wales	Japan	United States	England·Wales
Stomach	25.4	3.3	7.8	22.5	2.5	5.6
Lung	19.0	34.3	33.8	10.7	19.2	15.3
Liver	13.6 (3rd)	1.7	0.9	7.4 (6th)	1.3	0.8
Pancreas	5.7	4.5	4.1	6.5	5.5	4.6

Japan; Vital statistics, 1987, Japan
United States: Vital statistics of the United States, Vol II, Part A, 1987
England·Wales; Mortality statistics cause 1987

Table 4. Incidence rates of primary liver cancer in certain areas and among different ethnic groups (per 100,000 males/year)

Areas/community	Incidence rate	Ethnic group/area	Incidence rate
South Africa		Chinese	
Arican	28.4	Singapore	34.2
Indian	9.5	Hong Kong	27.6
Causasian	1.2	San Francisco Bay Area	21.1
Hawaii		Shanghai	20.6
Hawaiian	17.5	Hawaii	4.4
Filipino	8.9	Japanese	
Japanese	4.5	Japan	13.8
Chinese	4.4	Hawaii	4.5
Caucasian	3.8	Spaniard	
Singapore		Spain	7.8
Chinese	34.2	United States (New Mexico)	3.0
Malay	14.6	Black	
Indian	11.4	Lourenco Marques	98.2
United States, San Francisco		Rhodesia	64.6
Chinese	34.2	United States (Calfornia)	4.3
Black	4.2	Anglosaxon	
Caucasian	2.8	Switzerland	9.8
Israel		W. Germany	3.6
All Jews	2.5	Sweden	2.9
Jews born in Africa or Asia	4.3	United States (Michigan)	2.6
Jews born in Europe or America	2.0	Canada (Quebec)	1.9
Jews born in Israel	0.6	United Kingdom (Birmingham)	1.0
Non-Jews	3.6		

Standardized to World Standard Population. (From Nagasue [10])

all autopsies, and a comparison of various countries is given in Table 5. From this table, time trends are apparent in all the areas where old and new data are available. In the National Autopsy Registry, published annually by the Japan Pathological Society which records nearly 90% of all individual autopsy cases compiled by major hospitals throughout the country, HCC constituted 1.68% among 26,445 necropsies in 1961–62 in Japan, and this rate steadily increased in the ensuing 30 years to the current (1986–87) 7.66% demonstrating an indisputable 4-fold increase as shown in Table 6. In this table, HCC among all malignancies also rose from 4.51% to 13.01%. This same trend was verified by our study based on the Cancer Registry in the Osaka area, one of the most reliable cancer registries in Japan (Fig. 2) [14]. In this study, the incidence rate was found to have risen from 16.3/100,000/yr in 1966–68 to 40.9/100,000/yr in 1984–86 among males, but peculiarly the increase among females was much less. The time trends in other types of malignancies are given in Table 7 for comparison. The increase has been the greatest with liver cancer followed by colon cancer and rectum cancer, whereas cancers of the esophagus and

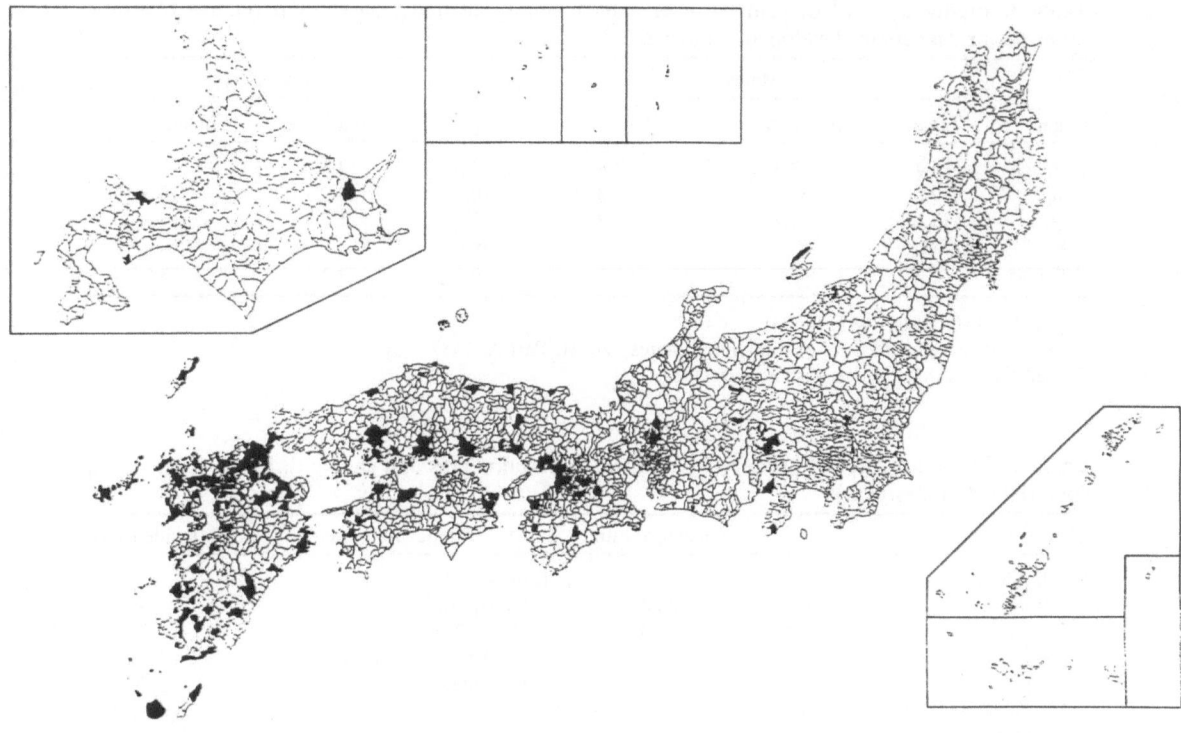

■ Incidence higher than national average

Fig. 1. Areas of high incidence for hepatocellular carcinoma in Japan. Clearly, HCC is more common in the south-west regions. (From [9] with permission)

stomach have been reduced in incidence. This recent remarkable increase in HCC incidence is most likely due to chronic hepatitis C disease. Thus, there is a distinct sex difference not only in the incidence rate but also in the time trends. In Los Angeles, the rate of HCC among all autopsies was 0.15% in 1918–53, and it rose to 1.48% in 1964–83 [15], again the increase being remarkable. In the Florence area, Italy, an eight fold increase has been reported [16]. A less dramatic but significant increase was also noted in west Scotland [17]. According to the study of Saracci and Repeto [18] in 1980 based on cancer registries, there was an increase in incidence rate among males in 24 out of 37 countries, and among females in 26 of 37 countries. Analysis of more recent data is needed. Liver cancer mortality increased about two fold from 1959 to 1976 in Shanghai, China [13].

Sex and age. Without regard to geography, HCC is nearly always more common in males than in females, but the male:female ratio (M:F) differs with the country, as well as with the year of the survey because of changing time trends. It

appears that the M:F ratio of incidence is greater in the high prevalence regions such as Africa, China, Hong Kong, Singapore and Japan, and lower in the low-incidence regions such as Latin America and Europe. This ratio rises as the incidence rate increases, as is the case in Japan, because the increase occurs mainly in males [14]. The greater susceptibility of males may be hormonal or genetic, or due to a greater exposure to carcinogenic environmental factors. The incidence rate of cancer generally increases in proportion to age with a tendency to level off in the old age. In the high-incidence areas such as Mozambique and Zimbabwe, the age curve shifts toward the younger age groups. The crude incidence among Mozambican males aged 25 to 34 years is more than 500 times that of the equivalent white population of the United Kingdom or the United States because HCC under age 40 years is very rare in the latter. The difference becomes smaller (15 times) in the aged populations above 65 years [1, 3]. HCC can occur in childhood and adolescence, but primary liver cancer in the young is often fibrolamellar carcinoma [38], a variant HCC, and under age 5 years it is mostly

Table 5. Relative frequencies of primary liver cancer in autopsy series

Country	Period	No. of autopsies	No. of primary liver cancer	%
Europe				
Denmark [19]	1938–59	14,881	50	0.34
Finland [20]	1952–62	15,545	93	0.60
Sweden [21]	1957–64	8,837	121	1.47
France [22]	1959–66	2,540	42	1.65
Federal Republic of Germany [23]	1961–70	4,411	47	1.06
Scotland [17]	1949–58	26,158	96	0.38
	1959–65	29,160	178	0.61
Switzerland [24]	1901–66	86,549	300[a]	0.35
Bulgaria [25]	1901–67	50,361	306	0.60
Italy-Trieste [26]	1980–84	12,340	205[a]	1.66
Italy-Florence [16]	1958–62	8,514	113	0.30
	1978–82			2.56
Africa				
Lagos [27]	1957	2,000	26	1.30
Uganda [28]	?	5,728	108	1.90
Asia				
Japan (Autopsy Registry of Japan)	1958–59	19,356	369	1.92
	1968–69	49,128	1,278[a]	2.60
	1978–79	62,565	3,113[a]	4.98
	1986–87	79,420	6,081[a]	7.66
Thailand [29]	1954–66	1,480	100	6.76
Pakistan [30]	1960–65	5,450	11	0.20
India—Bombay [31]	1947–68	12,616	45	0.36
China [32]	?	3,498	107	3.06
North America				
Boston [33]	1917–68	14,000	84[a]	0.60
Los Angeles [15]	1918–53	49,915	75[a]	0.15
	1954–63	23,476	79[a]	0.34
	1964–83	6,427	95[a]	1.48
Latin America				
Mexico [34]	1935–66	6,558	37	0.56
Costa Rica [35]	?	3,000	25	0.83
Chile [36]	1960–70	4,140	25	0.60
Argentina [37]	1905–67	22,170	64	0.28

[a] HCC only, not including CCC

Table 6. Relative frequency of hepatocellular carcinoma among all autopsies and all autopsied malignancies in Japan (National Autopsy Registry)

Year	All autopsies	All malignancies	HCC	Percent in	
				All autopsies	Malignancies
1961,62	26,445	9,821	443	1.68	4.51
1963,64	30,479	12,359	610	2.00	4.94
1965,66	35,342	17,695	779	2.20	4.40
1967,69	44,806	24,203	1,115	2.49	4.61
1970,71	43,728	22,250	1,376	3.15	6.18
1972,73	46,201	24,748	1,516	3.28	6.13
1974,75	45,744	23,960	1,758	3.84	7.34
1976,77	49,965	27,389	2,270	4.54	8.29
1978,79	62,565	32,720	3,113	4.98	9.51
1980,81	64,821	42,045	4,131	6.37	9.83
1982,83	78,341	45,052	4,921	6.28	10.92
1984,85	80,072	48,514	5,584	6.97	11.51
1986,87	79,420	46,765	6,082	7.66	13.01

8   K. Okuda

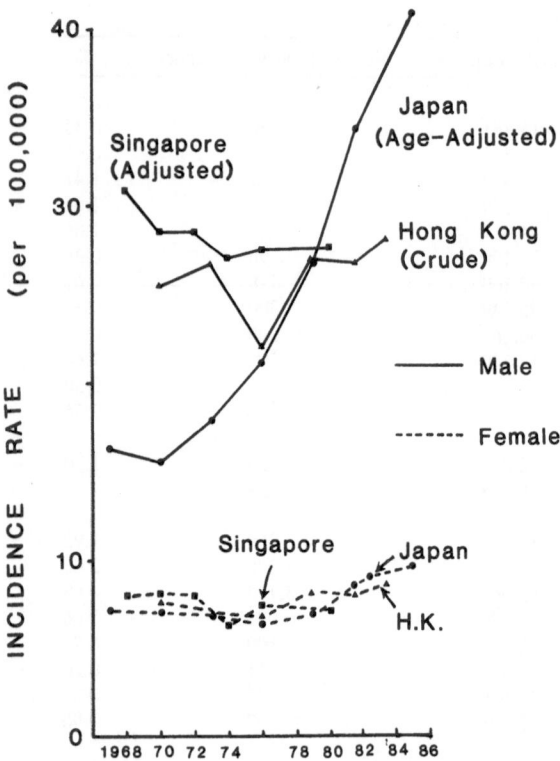

Fig. 2. Time trends in the incidence rate of primary liver cancer in Japan, Singapore, and Hong Kong. The incidence rate has been rising at a remarkable pace among men in Japan, and no parallel has been observed elsewhere. (Modified from [14] with permission)

hepatoblastoma (Table 8) [39]. The M:F ratio tends to decrease with younger ages [21, 22] and frequency of underlying cirrhosis is also low [40, 41, 42]. Our study [26] based on autopsies comparing Chiba and Trieste, Italy, demonstrated a significant difference in the age of patients. The average age of onset was nearly 20 years older in Trieste (Fig. 3). The age difference is presumably due to carcinogenic factors, posthepatic cirrhosis vs. alcoholic cirrhosis.

Relation to cirrhosis. The vast majority of patients with HCC have chronic liver disease, notably cirrhosis. It is the underlying disease in 80–90% of HCC patients in most countries, and nonalcoholic posthepatitic cirrhosis is more frequently associated with HCC than is alcoholic micronodular cirrhosis. It is known, as already discussed, that among African blacks who have a high incidence of HCC, the association of cirrhosis with HCC is weaker and cirrhosis is mild, if present, whereas in low-incidence areas cirrhosis is more frequently associated with HCC [27, 43–46]. However, if one compares young and older patients with HCC, cirrhosis is less common and HBsAg much more frequently positive in younger patients [47]. Studies of Miyaji [48] and Shikata [49] in Japan clearly showed that cirrhotic livers with large nodules and thin stromas are more commonly associated with HCC than livers with small nodules and thick stromas.

Table 7. Age-adjusted incidence rates of malignancies in the Osaka Cancer Registry (per 100,000/yr) (Cancer in Osaka, No. 48, Osaka Prefectural Health Department, 1990. Courtesy of Dr. I. Fujimoto)

Year	All sites	Esophagus	Stomach	Colon	Rectum	Liver	Gallbladder bile duct	Pancreas	Lung air way	Urinary bladder	Leukemia and malignant lymphoma
Males											
1966–68	205.6	9.6	97.9	4.8	6.0	16.2	1.5	5.5	20.1	5.3	8.1
1969–71	200.6	9.0	89.6	5.6	6.8	15.5	2.3	5.4	22.5	5.5	8.6
1972–74	201.9	9.1	82.6	6.1	7.4	17.7	2.6	5.4	26.1	5.8	9.2
1975–77	213.8	8.4	78.5	8.6	8.6	21.2	3.2	5.9	31.7	6.0	10.8
1978–80	234.9	7.8	78.3	10.6	10.1	27.3	4.2	7.2	35.0	7.2	11.1
1981–83	249.8	7.7	75.1	12.7	11.1	35.3	5.2	7.9	37.0	8.0	13.3
1984–86	263.9	8.5	72.8	14.7	11.6	40.9	5.7	8.5	41.5	7.9	13.8
Females											
1966–68	149.6	3.4	48.6	3.8	4.8	7.2	1.2	2.8	6.2	1.9	4.7
1969–71	142.7	2.8	44.5	4.6	4.6	7.0	2.1	3.1	6.7	1.5	5.6
1972–74	142.8	2.4	41.7	5.4	4.3	6.8	2.9	3.2	8.1	1.7	5.8
1975–77	142.8	2.0	38.8	6.2	5.1	6.3	3.1	3.5	8.9	1.7	6.6
1978–80	150.9	2.2	37.9	7.5	5.8	7.0	4.0	4.1	10.0	2.1	6.8
1981–83	154.1	2.0	34.0	8.8	6.4	8.6	4.7	4.8	10.6	1.9	8.1
1984–86	153.9	1.8	32.8	10.0	6.0	9.6	5.9	4.7	11.7	2.0	8.0

Rates are adjusted to world population

Table 8. Age distrubution of patients with hepato-cellular carcinoma, cholangiocarcinoma and hepato-blastoma in Japan (1980–81)

Age (yrs)	HCC		CCC[a]	HB[b]
0–4	0		0	23
5–0	1		0	1
10–14	6		0	1
15–19	3		0	1
20–24	3		1	0
25–29	6		1	0
30–34	20		0	0
35–39	38		8	0
40–44	84		8	0
45–49	234		14	0
50–54	326		18	0
55–59	326		22	1
60–64	272		13	0
65–69	226		16	0
70–74	146		15	1
75–79	64		8	0
80–84	4		1	0
85–	0		0	0
Total	1797	(14.8:1)	125	28
Mean age Men	56.8		58.2	
Women	59.9		57.7	

[a] Cholangiocarcinoma
[b] Hepatoblastoma (From [39] with permission)

The former type is assumed to have a greater regenerative activities of hepatocytes with increased DNA synthesis, hence more frequent rearrangement of DNA sequences in the chromosomes. In a study in London, there was a higher incidence of HCC among patients with alcoholic cirrhosis who had abstained and whose micronodular cirrhosis had turned macronodular [50]. With abstinence, there is a surge of regenerative activity, transforming small nodules to large ones. Clinically, patients with alcoholic cirrhosis seldom develop HCC while they are imbibing. Alcoholic cirrhosis is the predominant type in the western countries whereas posthepatitic cirrhosis is much more common in the Far East [51], and there is a considerable difference in the frequency of HCC and age of onset for patients who develop HCC. As shown in Fig. 3, patients with alcoholic cirrhosis such as those in North italy have a weaker potential to develop HCC compared to the Japanese patients with posthepatitic cirrhosis [26].

The death rate is proportionally higher for cirrhosis observed in Chile, Mexico, Portugal, France, Puerto Rico, Italy, Ireland and Austria

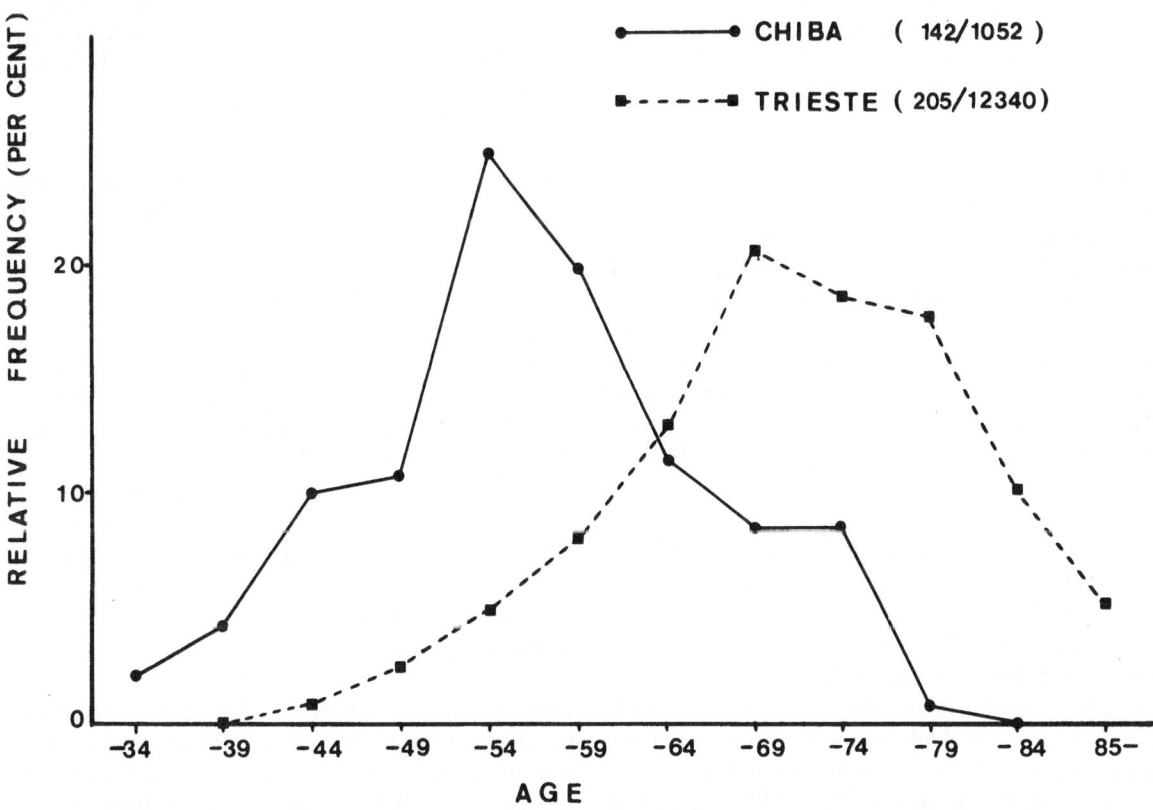

Fig. 3. The frequency of HCC among all autopsies and its relation to age—Chiba, Japan compared with Trieste, North Italy. The average age is nearly 20 years older in the latter

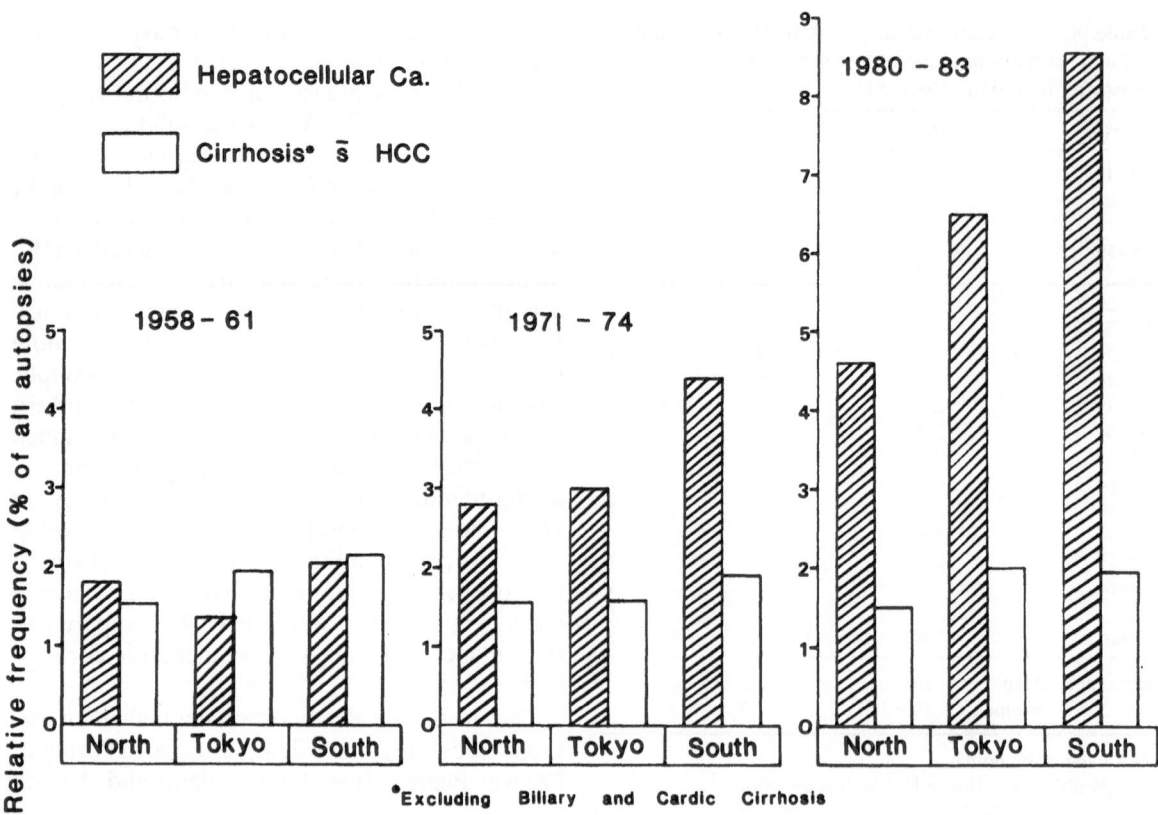

Fig. 4. Time trends and geographic differences in frequency of HCC and cirrhosis in Japan based on Autopsy Registry. The north region (Hokkaido and Tohoku), Tokyo region (Tokyo/Chiba) and south region (Kyushu) are represented by five major medical Schools in the region. In 1958–61, the numbers of autopsies for HCC and cirrhosis were about the same. Currently, the number of HCC far exceeds that of cirrhosis

which have low rates for HCC, and by contrast lower death rates for cirrhosis are reported in Thailand, Hong Kong, Greece and Switzerland which have relatively high rates for HCC [52]. It is generally thought that macronodular cirrhosis is more commonly associated with hepatitis B virus (HBV) infection and is more prone to hepatocarcinogenesis [48], but association of HBV and HCC is even stronger among young HCC patients without cirrhosis in Japan [47]. In Senegal, it was estimated that in 62% of HCC cases positive for HBsAg, cancer arose in non-cirrhotic livers and that the degree of association with HBV was similar for HCC, with or without cirrhosis [53]. In Japan, this association has been emphasized in HBV positive cirrhosis up to 1980 or so [54], but more recently this trend has disappeared with increasing C virus-associated cirrhosis [55]. In high incidence areas, cirrhosis terminates in HCC in more than half of the patients. In Japan, death due to HCC was about 30% among cirrhotics before 1970, but this rate has steadily increased to the current 80% [14].

Figure 4 compares relative frequency of cirrhosis alone and cirrhosis complicated by HCC among all autopsies during 1958–61, 1971–74 and 1980–83 in Japan. The increase in HCC is staggering. The change has been attributed to various factors, such as prolongation of survival of patients as a result of improved management and increase in hepatitis C virus-induced cirrhosis which is a slowly pregressive, mixed macro- and micronodular cirrhosis [56].

Under experimental conditions in animals, high doses of hepatocarcinogens induce cirrhosis and HCC [57], but in humans there is no evidence that aflatoxins or other hepatocarcinogens are responsible for the development of cirrhosis underlying HCC.

Hepatitis virus infections. Numerous epidemiological and biological studies have suggested an important role of HBV infection in hepatocarcinogenesis. When the close relationship between HBV infection and HCC incidence was found, it was thought that the age-old enigma of close association of cirrhosis was resolved, namely both cirrhosis and HCC were caused by HBV infection. However, HBV is not an oncovirus in a strict sense, and the exact mechanism of hepatocarcinogenesis induced by this virus is yet to be elucidated. Nevertheless, the evidence is strong that chronic HBV infection or HBsAg carriage is intimately associated with HCC. World-wide, there is a certain parallelism between the HBsAg carrier rate and the incidence rate of HCC in various populations or ethnic groups, namely, the carrier rate is high in areas of high incidence HCC and low in areas of low HCC incidence [58].

It is also established that HBsAg rate is significantly higher in patients with HCC compared to those without HCC or to control groups. All the case-control studies have demonstrated this correlation, and cohort studies showed that HBsAg carriers have a significantly higher risk of developing HCC [1, 2]. The study made in Taiwan of male government employees is of particular interest because of the large size of cohort and the long study period; it showed a relative risk greater than 100 [59]. In Taiwan, about 90% of these HCC patients were positive for HBsAg [60]. Our own study in Tokyo similarly came up with a relative risk of 30 among adult carriers compared to the control [61]. Conversely, those having anti-HBs antibody have a lower risk [58]. Hepatitis C virus infection is currently the major etiologic factor in Japan, and readers are referred to the chapter 7 on this virus for details.

Epidemiology of Cholangiocarcinoma

Incidence. The incidence of cholangiocarcinoma (CCC), the second most prevalent primary liver cancer, seems to vary less with geography than does HCC except for several areas where liver fluke infestation is endemic, such as Thailand and Hong Kong. CCC constituted 0.49% of 136,475 autopsies during the period 1958 to 1969 [62] and 0.44% of 39,399 autopsies in the Japan Autopsy Registry in 1987. In the Liverpool region, primary liver cancer was seen in 0.145% of 60,600 necropsies in 1947–1959, and CCC accounted for about one fifth of them [63]. In the Edmondson-Steiner series of 48,900 necropsies in the United States, CCC occurred in only 0.05% [64]. Thus, it seems that CCC is nearly ten times more common in Japan than in the United States or the United Kingdom. The average age of CCC patients is

generally older compared to HCC [27, 65–67], and the ratio of male predominance is much less, ranging from 1 to 2.2 [64, 65, 67–69]. The relative frequency of CCC among all primary liver cancers varies from 2.6% in Africa [27] to 35.5% in the United States [70] as shown in Table 9. In western countries it has been around 20% in most studies, whereas it is less than 10% in the areas where HCC is prevalent, such as South Africa and Singapore [63, 71]. In other words, this ratio indirectly reflects the prevalence of HCC. In Japan, where HCC has been increasing at a rapid pace, this ratio has been reduced from 9.5% in 1968–1977 [72] to 5.4% in 1982–1985 under the same conditions for the national survey [73].

For the same reason, the ratio of CCC to HCC is an indicator, albeit indirect, of prevalence of CCC among the areas where the incidence of HCC is about the same. According to Hou in Hong Kong [74] and Liang and Tung in Southern China [75], it is about 1:5; and both areas are known for liver fluke endemicity. By contrast, it is 1:56 in Java and Indonesia [76], and 1:38 [27] to 1:20 [77] in Africa where liver flukes are uncommon but where HCC is common. These statistics seem to strongly suggest that the prevalence of liver fluke infection is associated with the increased incidence of CCC.

Etiologic factors. According to Hou, 58% of autopsies for CCC had *Clonorchis sinensis* in Hong Kong [71]. The northeastern part of Thailand is known for high prevalence of *Opisthorchis vivarrini* infection. In one study in Tailand, 11 of 14 autopsy cases of CCC had *O. Vivarrini* worms whereas this fluke was found in none of 33 cases of HCC [78], and in another hospital-based case-controlled study, patients with *O. Vivarrini* infection had a significantly higher incidence of CCC. According to Sonakul et al. [79], the incidence of primary liver cancer among 154 patients with opisthorchiasis was 56.6%, and 77% of them were CCC. In a Hong Kong study by Belamaric [80], 18 of 19 autopsy cases of CCC had severe infection of *C. sinensis* but none had cirrhosis. The tumor was located in close relationship to parasitized ducts deep in liver parenchyma. Adenomatous hyperplasia was often seen in the ductal wall around the flukes.

A number of recent studies in Japan suggest an etiologic relationship between intrahepatic gallstones and CCC: 5.7% to 11.7% of CCC cases had associated hepatolithiasis [71, 81–83]. In the presence of intrahepatic stones, adenomatous (sometimes atypical) hyperplasia of the bile duct

Table 9. Relative frequency of cholangiocarcinoma among primary liver cancers, histologically confirmed

Author	Country	Year	Primary liver cancer, total	Cholangiocarcinoma	
				Number	Percent
Hoyne [70]	USA	1947	31	11	35.5
Edmondson [64]	USA	1954	100	25	25.0
MacDonald [69]	USA	1956	108	24	22.2
Steiner [27]	Africa[a]	1960	860	22[b]	2.6
Cruckshank [63]	United Kingdom	1961	108	21	20.0
Patton [66]	United States	1964	60	13	21.7
Lopez-Corella [34]	Mexico	1968	37	7	18.9
Miyaji [62]	Japan	1960	410	29	7.1
Okuda [72]	Japan	1980	2829	268	9.5
Liver Cancer Study Group of Japan [73]	Japan	1990	4765	256	5.4

All but the last two studies are based on autopsies.
[a] African blacks only
[b] Including cholangiolocellular carcinoma

epithelium is frequently seen in the vicinity of stones [81, 84–86]. Repeated bouts of inflammation of the bile duct epithelium due to stones may be a contributory factor. For the same reason, extrahepatic gallstones could have a similar role. In our study of 57 cases of CCC, 17.5% of them had stone disease [65] and in a series of 102 autopsy cases in Japan, stones were found in 21% [87]. Recently, a group of pathologists at Kanazawa University described glandular tissues in the large intrahepatic bile ducts [88], and found atypical hyperplasia in 0.1% of 799 livers not bearing malignancies, suggesting that some CCC could arise from these peribiliary glands [89].

Association of bile duct carcinoma with ulcerative colitis and primary sclerosing cholangitis is now well established. According to Ritchie [90], the incidence of bile duct carcinoma in ulcerative colitis patients is one in 256 and one-third of these tumors occur within the liver. The entire colon is usually affected and the average duration of colitis before cancer evolves is 5 (0–30) years. In the case of primary sclerosing cholangitis, cancer occurs at a relatively young age [91]. Chronic inflammation and glandular regeneration may predispose to carcinogenesis [15]. There are a number of reports on the association of cystic liver diseases and CCC. They include von Meyenburg complexes, congenital hepatic fibrosis, hepatic cysts, Caroli's diseases and choledochal cysts. These are biliary system diseases and perhaps share a similar etiologic mechanism with stones and cholangitis.

Of the other known etiological factors, Thorotrast (ThO_2) is the best documented. In one study in Japan, hepatic malignancies accounted for two-thirds of deaths due to hepatic thorotrastosis, and CCC was the most frequent among them [92].

References

1. Munoz N, Lincell A (1982) Epidemiology of primary liver cancer. In: Correa P, Haenszel W (eds) Epidemiology of cancer of the digestive tract. Martinus Nijhoff, Hague, 161–195
2. Munoz N, Bosch X (1987) Epidemiology of hepatocellular carcinoma. In: Okuda K, Ishak KG (eds) Neoplasms of the liver. Springer, Tokyo. 3–19
3. Waterhouse JAH, Nuir CS, Correa P, Powell J (1976) Cancer incidence in five continents, Vol III. Internatiuonal Agency for Research on Cancer, Lyon
4. Melato M, Laurino L, Mucli E, Valente M, Okuda K (1989) Relationship between cirrhosis, liver cancer, and hepatic metastases. An autopsy study. Cancer 64:455–459
5. Okuda K, Beasley RP (1982) Epidemiology. In: Okuda K, Mackay I (eds) Hepatocellular carcinoma. UICC, Geneva, 9–30
6. Berman C (1951) Primary carcinoma of the liver. Lewis, London, 5–14
7. Higginson J (1963) The geographic pathology of primary liver cancer. Cancer Res 23:1624–1633
8. Health and Welfare Statistics Assocation (1990) Trends in the health of nation (in Japanese). Kosei no Shihyo 35:5962
9. Hirayama T (1988) Epidemiology. In: Oda T (ed) Cancer of the liver. Diagnosis and treatment (in Japanese). Kodansha, Tokyo, 11–30
10. Nagasue N (1982) The epidemiology and etiology of primary liver cancer: A current trend. Fukuoka Acta Med 7:281–295

11. Li EP, Shiang EL (1980) Cancer mortality in China. JCNI 65:217–221

12. Tang ZY (1985) Subclinical hepatocellular carcinoma—historical aspects and general considerations. In: Tang ZY (ed) Subclinical hepatocellular carcinoma. China Acad Publ, Beijing, 1–11

13. Yu SZ (1985) Epidemiology of primary liver cancer. In: Tang ZY (ed) Subclincal hepatocellular carcinoma. China Acad Publ, Beijing, 189–211

14. Okuda K, Fujimoto I, Hanai A, Urano Y (1987) Changing incidence of hepatocellular carcinoma in Japan. Cancer Res 47:4967–4972

15. Craig JR, Peters RL, Edmondson HA (1989) Tumors of the liver and intrahepatic bile ducts. AFIP, Washington DC, 6–7

16. Bartoloni ST, Omer F, Giannini A, Napoli P (1984) Hepatocellular carcinoma and cirrhosis: a review of their relative incidence in a 25-year period in the Florence area. Hepato-gastro-enterology 31:215–217

17. Manderson WG, Patrick RS, Peters EE (1968) Incidence of primary carcinoma of the liver in the west of Scotland between 1949 and 1965. Gut 9: 480–484

18. Sarraci R, Repetto F (1980) Time trends of primary liver cancer: indication of increased incidence in selected cancer registry populations. J Nat Cancer Inst 65:241–247

19. Glennert J (1969) Primary carcinoma of the liver. A post-mortem study of 104 cases. Acta Pathol Microbiol Immunol Scand 53:50–60

20. Evrasti J (1964) Primary carcinoma of the liver. A pathologic and clinical study of 100 cases. Acta Chir Scand, Suppl 334:1–65

21. Ohlsson EGH, Noden JG (1965) Primary carcinoma of the liver. A study of 21 cases. Acta Pathol Microbiol Immunol Scand 64:430–440

22. Pequignot H, Ethiene JP, Delavierre P, Petite JP (1967) Cancers primitifs du foie sur cirrhose. Augmentation de frequence et observation chez des cirrhotiques connus et suivis. Presse Med 75:2595–2600

23. Sievers BU (1969) Leberzirrhose und Leberkarzinom in 10 Yahren einer Prosektur. Acta Hepatogastroenterol 20:483–490

24. Fierz L (1969) Das Hepatom in Sektionsgut des Zuricher Pathologischen Instituts der Jahre 1901–1966 (86,549 Autopsien). Acta Hepatol-Splenol 16:383–389

25. Brailski C (1978) Primary liver carcinoma in Bulgaria. In: Remmer H, Bolt HM, Bannasch P, Popper H (eds) Primary liver tumors. NTP Press, Lancaster, 137–139

26. Tiribelli C, Melato M, Croce LS, Giarelli L, Okuda K, Ohnishi K (1989) Prevalence of hepatocellular carcinoma and relation to cirrhosis: comparison of two different cities of the world—Trieste, Italy, and Chiba, Japan. Hepatology 10:998–1002

27. Steiner PE (1960) Cancer of the liver and cirrhosis in trans-Saharan Africa and the Unites States of America. Cancer 13:1085–1145

28. Davies JN (1961) Primary liver carcinoma in Uganda. Acta Un Int Cancer 17:787–792

29. Stitnimankarn T (1976) Primary hepatic carcinoma in Thailand. In: Hirayama T (ed) Cancer in Asia. Univ Park Press, Tokyo, 123–127

30. Islam AKN (1969) Primary carcinoma of the liver. E Pak Med J 13:92–96

31. Patwardhan JR, Kshirsagar VH, Gadgil PK (1970) Primary carcinoma of the liver in Bombay. Indian J Cancer 7:113–118

32. Ying UY, Ma CC, Hsu UT, Lei HH, Liang SF, Liu CH, Ku CY (1963) Primary carcinoma of the liver. Chin Med J 82:279–294

33. Purtilo DT, Gottlieb LS (1973) Cirrhosis and hepatoma occurring at Boston City Hospital (1917–1968) Cancer 32:458–462

34. Lopez-Corella E, Ridaura-Sanz C, Abares-Savedra J (1968) Primary carcinoma of the liver in Mexican adults. Cancer 22:678–685

35. Mena Solera H (1964) Freceuencia cancer en Costa Rica. Acta Med Cost 7:26–33

36. Ugarte G, Donos S (1978) Primary hepatic tumors in Chile. In: Remmer H, Bolt HM, Bannach P, Popper H (eds) Primary liver tumors. MTP, Lancaster, 165–169

37. Elsner B, Jauregui EM (1974) Autopsy study of primary liver carcinoma in Buenos Aires, Artgentina. Acta Hepato gastroenterol 21:26–34

38. Craig JR, Peters RL, Edmondson HA, Omata M (1980) Fibrolamellar carcinoma of the liver: a tumor of adolescents and young adults with distinctive clinicopathologic features. Cancer 46:372–379

39. The Liver Cancer Study Group of Japan (1987) Primary liver cancer in Japan. Sixth report. Cancer 60:1400–1411

40. Lack EE, Neave C, Vawters GF (1983) Hepatocellular carcinoma. Review of 32 cases in childhood and adolescence. Cancer 52:1510–1515

41. Farhi DC, Shikes RH, Maurari PJ, Silverberg SG (1983) Hepatocellular carcinoma in young people. Cancer 52:1516–1545

42. Okuda K, Nakashima T, Sakamoto K, Ikari T, Hidaka H, Kubo Y, Sakuma K, Motoike Y, Okuda H, Obata H (1982) Hepatocellular carcinoma arising in noncirrhotic and highly cirrhotic livers: a comparative study of histopathology and frequency of hepatitis markers. Cancer 49:450–455

43. Kew MC (1981) Clinical, pathologic, and etiologic heterogeneity in hepatocelleular carcinoma: evidence from southern Africa. Hepatology 1: 366–369

44. Kew MC, Geddes EW (1982) Hepatocellular cacinoma in rural southern African blacks. Medicine 61:98–108

45. Okuda K, Peters RL, Simson IW (1984) Gross anatomical features of hepatocellular carcinoma

from three disparate geograpahic areas. Proposal of new classification. Cancer 54:2165–2173

46. Kashala LO, Conne B, Kalengayi MMR, Kapanchi Y, Frei PC, Lambert PH (1990) Histopathologic features of hepatocellular carcinoma in Zaire. Cancer 65:130–134

47. Furuta T, Kanematsus T, Matsumata T, Shirabe K, Yamagata M, Utsunomiya T, Sugimachi K (1990) Clinicopathologic features of hepatocellular carcinoma in young patients. Cancer 66:2395–2398

48. Miyaji T (1976) Association of hepatocellular carcinoma with cirrhosis among autopsy cases in Japan during 14 years from 1958 to 1971. Gann Monogr 18:129–149

49. Shikata T (1976) Primary liver carcinoma and liver cirrhosis. In: Okuda K, Peters RL (eds) Hepatocellular carcinoma. Wiley, New York, 53–95

50. Lee FK (1966) Cirrhosis and hepatoma in alcoholics. Gut 7:77–95

51. Mori W (1867) Cirrhosis and primary cancer of the liver: comparative study in Tokyo and Cincinnati. Cancer 20:627–631

52. World Health Organization (1982) World health statistics annual, 1978–1982. Vital statistics and causes of death. WHO, Geneva

53. Prince AM, Szmuness W, Michon J, Demaille J, Dieblt G, Linhard J, Quenum C, Sankale M (1975) A case-control study of the association between primary liver cancer and hepatitis B infection in Senegal. Int J Cancer 16:376–383

54. Obata H, Hayashi N, Motoike Y, Hisamitsu T, Okuda H, Kobayashi S, Nishioka K (1980) A prospective study of the development of hepatocellular carcinoma from liver cirrhosis with persistent hepatitis B virus infection. Int J Cancer 25:741–747

55. Okuda K (1991) Hepatitis C virus and hepatocellular carcinoma. In: Tabor E, DiBiscegli A (eds) Etiology, pathology and treatment of hepatocellular carcinoma in North America. Portfolio Publ Co, Woodlands, 119–126

56. Nakashima T, Okuda K, Kojiro T, Jimi A, Yamaguchi R, Sakamoto K, Ikari T (1983) Pathology of hepatocellular carcinoma in Japan. 232 consecutive cases autopsied in ten years. Cancer 51:863–877

57. Wogan GN (1976) Aflatoxins and their relationship to hepatocellular carcinoma. In: Okuda K, Peters RL (eds) Hepatocellular carcinoma. Wiley, New York, 25–42

58. Szmuness W (1978) Hepatocellular carcinoma and the hepatitis B virus: evidence for a causal association. Prog Med Virol 24:40–69

59. Beasley RP (1982) Hepatitis B virus as the etiologic agent in hepatocellular carcinoma—epidemiologic considerations. Hepatology 2:21S–26S

60. Sung JL (1981) Hepatitis B virus infection and its sequelae in Taiwan Proc Natl Sci Counc Repub China 5:385–399

61. Sakuma K, Saitoh N, Kasai M, Jitsukawa H, Yoshino I, Yamaguchi M, Nobutomo K, Mayumi M, Tsuda F, Komazawa T, Nakamura T, Yoshida Y, Okuda K (1988) Relative risks of death due to liver disease among Japanese male adults having various statuses for hepatitis B s and e antigen/antibody in serum: a prospective study. Hepatology 8:1642–1646

62. Miyaji T (1873) Association of hepatocellular carcinoma with cirrhosis among autopsy cases in Japan (1958–1967) In: Hirai H, Miyaji T (eds) Alpha-fetoprotein in hepatoma. Univ Tokyo Press, Tokyo, 179–198

63. Cruckshank AH (1961) The pathlogy of 111 cases of primary hepatic malignancy collected in the Liverepool region. J Clin Pathol 14:1120–130

64. Edmondson HA, Steiner PE (1954) Primary carcinoma of the liver. A study of 110 cases among 48,900 necropsies. Cancer 7:452–503

65. Okuda K, Kubo Y, Okazaki N, Arishima T, Hashimoto M, Jinnouchi S, Sawa Y, Shimokawa Y, Nakajima Y, Noguchi T, Nakano M, Kojiro M, Nakashima T (1977) Clinical aspects of intrahepatic bile duct carcinoma including hilar carcinoma. A study of 57 autopsy-proven cases. Cancer 39:232–246

66. Patton RB, Horn RC Jr (1964) Primary liver carcinoma. Atuopsy of 60 cases. Cancer 17:757–768

67. MacSween RNM (1974) A clinicopathological review of 100 cases of primary malignant tumors of the liver. J Clin Pathol 27:669–682

68. Anthony PP (1972) Primary carcinoma of the liver. A study of 282 cases in Uganda, Africa. J pathol 110:37–48

69. MacDonald RA (1957) Primary carcinoma of the liver. A clinicopathologic study of one hundred eight cases. Arch Intern Med 99:266–279

70. Hoyne RM, Kernohan JW (1947) Primary carcinoma of the liver. A study of thirty-one cases. Arch Intern Med 79:532–554

71. Sugihara S, Kojiro M (1987) Pathology of cholangiocarcinoma. In: Okuda K, Ishak KG (eds) Neoplasms of the liver. Springer, Tokyo, 143–158

72. Okuda K, Liver Cancer Study Group of Japan (1980) Primary liver cancers in Japan. Cancer 45:2663–2669

73. Liver Cancer Study Group of Japan (1990) Follow-up primary liver cancer patients. Report 9 (1986–1987). Dept Surgery II, Kyoto Univ, p 25

74. Hou PC (1856) The relationship between primary carcinoma of the liver and infestation with *Clonorchis sinensis*. J Pathol Bacteriol 87:239–246

75. Liang PC, Tung C (1959) Morphologic study and etiology of primary liver carcinoma and its incidence in China. Chin Med J 79:336–347

76. Flavell DJ (1981) Liver-fluke infection as an etiological feature in bile-duct carcinoma of man. Trans R Soc Trop Med Hyg 75:814–824

77. Higginson J (1955) Relation of carcinoma of the liver to cirrhosis, malaria, syphilis and parasitic diseases. Schweiz Ztsch allg Pathol Bacteriol 18:625–643

78. Bhamarapravati N, Viranauvatti V (1966) Liver diseases in Thailand. An analysis of liver biopsies. Am J Gastroenterol 45:267–275

79. Sonakul D, Koomprochana C, Chida K, Stitnimankarn J (1978) Hepatic carcinoma with opisthorchiasis. Southeast Asian J Trop Med Public Health 9:215–219

80. Belamaric J (1973) Intrahepatic bile duct carcinoma and *C. sinensis* infection in Hong Kong. Cancer 31:468–473

81. Kinamii Y, Noto H, Miyazaki I, Matsubara F (1984) A study of hepatolithiasis associated with cholangiocarcinoma. Acta Hepatol Jpn 19:578–583

82. Yamamoto K, Tsuchiya R, Ito T, Harada N, Yoshino T, Tsunoda T, Noda T, Izawa K, Yamaguchi T, Oribe T, Motoshima M (1984) A study of cholangiocarcinoma coexistent with hepatolithiasis. Jpn J Gastroenterol Surg 17:601–619

83. Chen PH, Lo HW, Wang CS, Tsai KR, Chen YI, Lin KY. Siauw CP, Hwang RR, Lin MH, Ko HC, Chen TY (1984) Cholangiocarcinoma in hepatolithiasis. J Clin Gastreoenterol 6:539–547

84. Falchuk KR, Leser PB, Galdabini JJ, Isselbacher KJ (1976) Cholangioma in hepatoliothiasis. Am J Pathol 18:675–678

85. Sanes S, MacCallum JD (1942) Primary carcinoma of the liver. Cholangioma in hepatolithiasis. Am J Pathol 18:675–687

86. Nakanuma Y, Terada T, Tanaka Y, Ohta G (1985) Are hepatolithiasis and cholangioma etiologically related: a morphological study of 12 cases of hepatolithiasis associated with cholangiocarcinoma. Virchows Arch (Pathol Anat) 406:45–58

87. Nakajima T, Kondo Y, Miyazaki M, Okui K (1988) A histological study of 102 cases of intrahepatic cholangiocarcinoma: histological classification and modes of spreading. Hum Pathol 19:1228–1234

88. Terada T, Nakanuma Y, Ohta G (1987) Glandular elements around the intrahepatic bile ducts in man: their morphology and distribution in normal livers. Liver 7:1–8

89. Terada T, Nakanuma Y (1990) Pathological observations of intrahepatic peribiliary glands in 1,000 consecutive autopsy livers. II. A possible source of cholangiocarcinoma. Hepatology 12:92–97

90. Ritchie JK, Allan RN, Macrtney J, Thompson H, Hawley PR, Cooke WT (1974) Biliary tract carcinoma associated with ulcerative colitis. Q J Med 43:263–279

91. Wee A, Ludwig J, Doffey RJ, LaRusso NF, Wiesner RH (1985) Hepatobiliary carcinoma associated with primary sclerosing cholangitis and chronic ulcerative colitis. Hum Pathol 16:719–726

92. Mori T (1984) Epidemiological study of late effect of Thorotrast administration. Annual report of research on thorium fuel. Ministry of Education Science and Culture, Tokyo

Part 2. Pathology.

CHAPTER 2

Pathology of primary liver cancer – Overview

Masahiko Okudaira[1]

1 Introduction

Since the beginning of this century, primary liver cancers have been extensively investigated in Japan. The terms hepatoma and cholangioma were proposed by Yamagiwa [1], and an experimental induction of hepatic cancer utilizing azo-compounds was pioneered by Sasaki and Yoshida [2]. A number of other noteworthy works on primary liver cancers have been carried out over the years by Japanese researchers.

Both macroscopic and histopathological findings of primary liver cancers have been fairly well documented in authentic monographs [3–8]. It is well known that there is a very wide geographical difference in the incidence of primary liver cancers. This is especially of hepatocellular carcinoma which is rare in Western countries, but in Africa and South East Asia, it is the most frequent cause of death from malignant disease.

2 Incidence of primary liver cancers in Japanese pathological autopsy cases

According to the Annual of the Pathological Autopsy Cases in Japan, 1964–1988 [9], autopsy cases of primary liver cancers have been increasing remarkably in recent years, as shown in Fig. 1. It should be mentioned that autopsy cases which confirmed the presence of primary liver cancer was 379 in 1964, and 3620 in 1988. This represents an increase by almost a factor of ten during the past twenty five years.

[1] Department of Pathology, School of Medicine, Kitasato University, Sagamihara, 228 Japan

In 1988, a total of 22,942 malignancies were registered in the Annual. Of these, there were 4,122 cases of pulmonary cancer with a male-to-female ratio of 3.3 : 1, 3,620 cases of primary liver cancer with a ratio of 3.6 : 1, 3,506 cases of gastric cancer with a ratio of 2.3 : 1, 1,904 cases of intestinal cancer with a ratio of 1.6 : 1, and 1,342 cases of pancreatic cancer with a ratio of 1.8 : 1. Thus, primary liver cancer is the second most frequent type of malignancy and the most remarkable malignancy of male predominance.

3 Morphological types of primary liver cancer

Primary liver cancer is usually divided into two major types: Hepatocellular carcinoma (liver cell carcinoma, hepatocarcinoma), which is composed of malignant cells somewhat resembling hepatocytes, often in the setting of cirrhosis; and cholangiocellular carcinoma (cholangiocarcinoma, intrahepatic bile duct carcinoma) which is composed of tumors cells resembling biliary epithelium. According to the national survey [10–12], the approximate incidence of hepatocellular carcinoma among primary liver cancer was about 90%, 6–7% for cholangiocelllualr carcinoma, and 2–3% for others (Table 1).

Hepatocellular carcinomas can be soft or solid, and tumors of various sizes are formed within the liver. Usually, a large number of tumors are present. These tumors have a strong tendency to cause hemorrhage and necrosis, and they can appear in various colors, such as white, yellow (as a result of fatty change), dark red (due to hemorrhage), or green (owing to bilirubin production). Subcapsular tumors protrude as hemispheres, and do not generally show a cancer

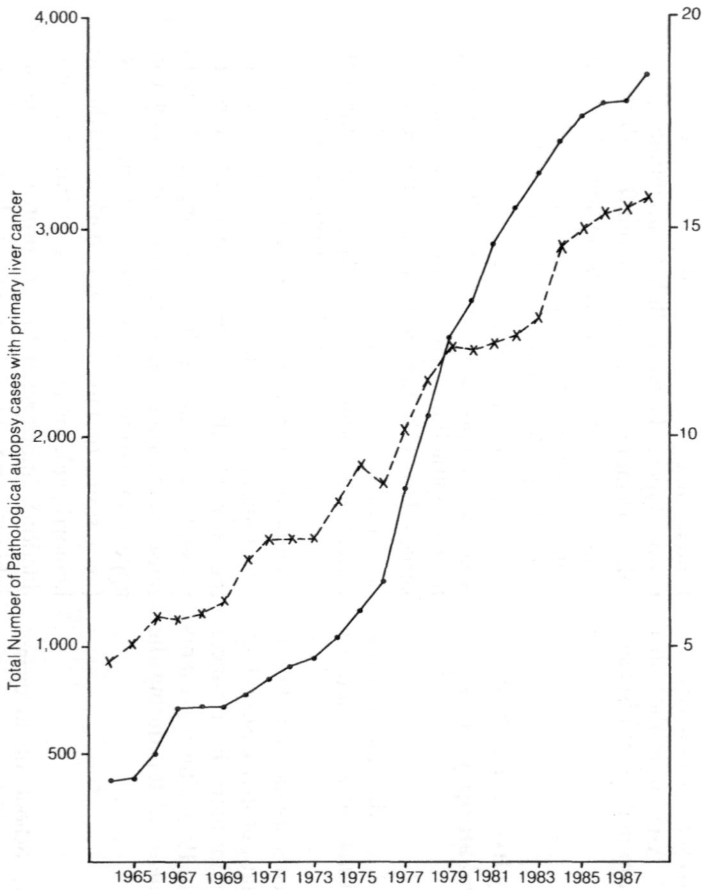

M. Okudaira

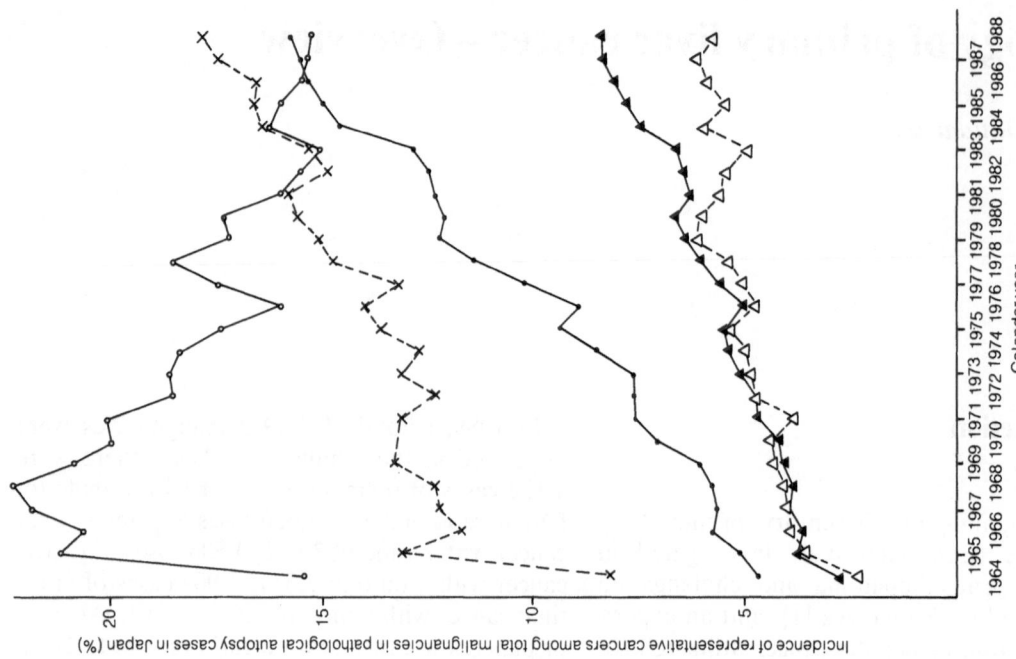

Fig. 2. Yearly incidence of five major cancers in Japan (Data from Annual of Pathological Autopsy Cases in Japan [9]) *Open circle,* gastric cancer; *closed circle,* liver cancer; *cross,* lung cancer; *open triangle,* pancreatic cancer; *closed triangle,* intestinal cancer

Incidence of representative cancers among total malignancies in pathological autopsy cases in Japan (%)

Incidence of primary liver cancer among total malignancies in pathological autopsy cases (%)

Total Number of Pathological autopsy cases with primary liver cancer

Calendar Year	1964	1966	1968	1970	1972	1974	1976	1978	1980	1982	1984	1986	1988
Number of total neoropsies	17375	17830	25224	22003	22717	22976	24125	32698	38851	39583	40154	39399	38439
Number of total malignancies	8039	8710	12399	11013	12133	12336	14856	18396	21931	24803	23302	23332	22942
No. of total liver cancers	379	504	716	786	927	1050	1320	2098	2644	3103	3408	3588	3620

Fig. 1. Yearly incidence of primary liver cancers in Japanese pathological autopsy cases (1964–1988) [9] *Solid line,* number of primary liver cancers; *dotted line,* percent incidence of primary liver cancer among total malignancies

Table 1. Histological classification and percent incidence of primary liver cancers (The Liver Cancer Study Group of Japan) [11–13]

Periods studied	1978–1979	1980–1981	1982–1985
No. of cases studied	1198	2286	4765
Histological classification			
Hepatocellular carcinoma	87.4%	89.2%	91.4%
Cholangiocellular carcinoma	7.8%	6.4%	5.4%
Mixed hepatocellular and cholangiocarcinoma	0.8%	1.4%	1.0%
Hepatoblastoma	1.3%	1.3%	0.5%
Others	2.8%	1.7%	1.8%
Total	100%	100%	100%

umbilication. There is a great tendency to vascular invasion and tumor thrombus formation in the portal and hepatic veins, both within and outside the liver. Moreover, it is not uncommon to find tumor invasion in the bile duct which can cause hemobilia. Cirrhosis is quite frequently associated with hepatocellular carcinoma as a precursor.

Cholangiocellular carcinoma is rarely accompanied by cirrhosis of the liver. In most cases, it is a hard, compact, whitish-gray massive type or nodular type tumors are formed in non-cirrhotic liver. Diffuse, invasive proliferation and metastasis sometimes take place within the liver along the portal tract, but this does not affect a very large area of the liver as a whole. Moreover, hemorrhage and necrosis are not often observed. Tumors located in the subcapsular area of the liver, like many metastatic liver cancers, form a cancer umbilication. Bile duct cystadenocarcinoma has been included in cholangiocellular carcinoma in the Japanese study group [10–13], however, the malignant cystic tumor lined by mucus-secreting epithelium will be separated in the near future from cholangiocellular carcinoma in accordance with the WHO classification [14].

Hepatocellular carcinoma and cholangiocellular carcinoma can be found together or separately within the same liver. Usually, the former component is predominant, and confirmation of the production of mucin is an important factor in the identification of the latter component.

Figure 2 demonstrates yearly incidence and recent variation of five major cancers in Japan. Decreasing tendency of the gastric cancer in recent years is remarkable, however, even at the present time, the number of gastric cancer patients is the largest in Japan. This fact indicates that the number of cured gastric cancer patients is increasing due to great advances in diagnostic methodology and therapeutic measures for gastric cancer. It has been estimated that at the beginning of the 21st Century, the incidence of primary liver cancer will surpass all others in Japan [15]. Further progress in diagnostic and therapeutic measures in hepatology is greatly anticipated.

Hepatoblastoma is frequently encountered in the postnatal period, developing in livers free of cirrhosis. The tumor is composed of either epithelial or mesenchymal elements, or of both. The epithelial type is composed of fetal and embryonal type hepatocytes. Mesenchymal components include primitive mesenchymal spindle cells, fibroblasts with collagen, osteoid tissue with focal calcification, cartilaginous tissue, rhabdomyoblastic elements, and areas of hematopoiesis.

Other types include embryonal sarcoma (rhabdomyoblastoma), malignant hemangioendothelioma (hemangiosarcoma), epithelioid hemangioendothelioma, leiomyosarcoma, fibrosarcoma, liposarcoma, osteosarcoma, chondrosarcoma, carcinosarcoma, malignant fibrous histiocytoma, malignant schwannoma, and carcinoid tumor of the liver.

4 Early primary liver cancer

Recently, various diagnostic procedures such as ultrasonography, computed tomography, single photon or positron emission CT, magnetic resonance imaging, and digital subtraction angiography are widely used for the early detection of primary liver cancers.

Based on the recent advances in imaging, in particular real-time ultrasonography, one can detect small nodular lesions less than 2 cm in diameter in the liver, and an increasing number of small hepatocellular carcinomas have been detected during the follow-up study of chronic liver diseases [16–21]. Histopathological distinction between benign lesions and malignant tumors by the earlier method of needle biopsy specimens obtained from those small nodular lesions was a difficult task for pathologists. Through recent extensive and enthusiastic studies on small hepatocellular carcinomas and related lesions [17–22], nuclear crowding, increased cytoplasmic basophilia and microacinar pattern, among others, have been recognized as important histologic findings of well-differentiated hepatocellular carcinoma. Morphometrical studies [23–24] indicated that a high nuclear cytoplasmic ratio, increased thickeness of trabecular cords, increase of the nuclear coefficient of variance, and a decrease of the nuclear form factor seemed to be reliable indicators for hepatocellular carcinoma.

Further studies are urgently required to determine unicentricity versus multicentricity of the cancer development. This factor might be essential to determine the most appropriate treatment for hepatocellular carcinoma patients.

It should be noted that little is known about the early or precancerous lesions of cholangiocellular carcinomas.

5 Etiological considerations

Approximately 75–80% of all cases of hepatocellular carcinoma are associated with liver cirrhosis, which of itself could have favored formation of the carcinoma, however, it has not been clarified whether or not additional factors are required for the development of hepatocellular carcinoma.

It is well known that a number of chemical compounds exhibit carcinogenic activity in experimental animals, especially on rodents [6]. Recently, a close relation was confirmed between longterm massive exposure to vinyl chloride monomer and the occurrence of angiosarcoma in the human liver [25, 26], however, there is no clear-cut envidence that confirms any single chemical agent as the causative factor for liver cell cancer in man. Mycotoxins (aflatoxins, sterigmatocystin, and luteoskyrin, etc.), plant poisons (cycasin and pyrrolizidin alkaloids) and many other etiological factors, such as alcohol,

malnutrition, and environmental contaminations are thought possibly to be operative in hepatocarcinogenesis [6].

A number of reports have stressed the close relation between hepatitis B virus infection and hepatocellular carcinomas. More recently, intensive studies have been focused on the more intimate relationship between hepatitis C virus infection and hepatocellular carcinoma. However, no evidence has been presented yet which suggests the mechanism by which HBV and HCV may be oncogenic.

Sophisticated molecular biological studies should be undertaken to clarify hepatocarcinogenesis. The interaction between chronic alcoholism and HBV and HCV infection in the development of hepatocellular carcinoma also needs to be elucidated.

References

1. Yamagiwa K (1911) Zur Kentnis der primären parenchymatösen Leberkarzinoms "Hepatoma". Virchows Arch Pathol Anat Physiol 206:437–476
2. Sasaki T, Yoshida T (1935) Experimentelle Erzeugung des Lebercarcinoms durch Futterung mit o-Amidazotoluol. Virchows Arch Pathol Anat Physiol 295:175–200
3. Edmondson HA (1958) Tumors of the liver and intrahepatic bile ducts. Armed Forces Institute of Pathology, Washington, pp 32–105
4. Okuda K, Peters RL (eds) (1976) Hepatocellular carcinoma. John Wiley, New York, pp 53–246
5. Leevy CM, Popper H, Sherlock S (eds) (1979) Disease of the liver and biliary tract. Standardization of nomenclature, diagnostic criteria, and diagnostic methodology. Castle House, London
6. Okuda K, Ishak KG (eds) (1978) Neoplasms of the liver. Springer-Verlag, Tokyo
7. Nakashima T, Kojiro M (1986) Hepatocellular carcinoma: An atlas of its pathology. Springer-Verlag, Tokyo
8. Craig K, Peters RL, Edmondson HA (1989) Tumors of the liver and intrahepatic bile ducts, 2nd Series. Armed Forces Institute of Pathology, Washington, pp 123–222
9. The Japanese Pathological Society (1965–1988) Annual of the Pathological Autopsy Cases in Japan. The Japanese Pathological Society, Tokyo
10. The Liver Cancer Study Group of Japan (1984) Primary liver cancer in Japan. Cancer 54: 1747–1755
11. The Liver Cancer Study Group of Japan (1987) Primary liver cancer in Japan, sixth report. Cancer 60:1400–1411

12. The Liver Cancer Study Group of Japan (1990) Primary liver cancer in Japan. Clinicopathologic features and results of surgical treatment. Annals of Surg 211:277–287

13. The Liver Cancer Study Group of Japan (1989) The general rules for the clinical and pathological study of primary liver cancer. Jpn J Surg 19:98–129

14. Gibson JB, Sobin LH (1978) Histological typing of tumours of the liver, biliary tract and pancreas, WHO, Geneva

15. Hirayama T (1987) Preventive oncology (in Japanese) Medical Science, Tokyo, pp 122–130

16. Okuda K (1986) Early recognition of hepatocellular carcinoma. Hepatology 6:729–738

17. Arakawa, M, Kage M, Sugihara S, Nakashima T, Suenaga M, Okuda, K (1986) Emergence of malignant lesions within and adenomatous hyperplastic nodule in a cirrhotic liver: Observation in five cases. Gastroenterology 91:198–208

18. Kanai T, Hirohashi S, Noguchi M, Kishi K, Makuuchi M, Yamazaki S, Hasegawa H, Shimosato Y (1986) Pathological features of small hepatocellular carcinoma (in Japanese). Pathol and Clin Med 4:396–405

19. Kenmochi K, Sugihara S, Kojiro M (1987) Relationship of histologic grade of hepatocellular carcinoma (HCC) to tumor size, and demonstration of tumor cells of multiple different grades in single small HCC. Liver 7:18–26

20. Kondo F, Wada K, Nagato Y, Nakajima T, Kondo Y, Hirooka N, Ebara M, Ohto M, Okuda K (1989) Biopsy diagnosis of well-differentiated hepatocellular carcinoma based on new morphologic criteria. Hepatology 9:751–755

21. Takayama T, Makuuchi M, Hirohashi S, Sakamoto M, Okazaki N, Takayasu K, Kosuge T, Motoo Y, Yamazaki S, Hasegawa H (1990) Malignant transformation of adenomatous hyperplasia to hepatocellular carcinoma. Lancet 10:1150–1153

22. Nakano, M, Saito A, Takasaki K, Obata H, Kobayashi S (1990) A histopathologic study of early hepatocellular carcinoma (HCC): Portal tract invasion and progression to advanced HCC (in Japanese with English abstract). Acta Hepatol Jpn 31:754–762

23. Motohashi I (1990) A morphometrical study on hepatocellular carcinoma (HCC) and HCC-like tumors of the liver by means of image analyzer (in Japanese with English abstract). Acta Hepatol Jpn 31:625–635

24. Motohashi I, Okudaira M, Takai T, Kaneko S, Futagami R (1990) Micromorphometric investigations of hepatocellular carcinomas (HCC) and HCC-like liver lesions with particular emphasis on nuclear and cellular pleomorphism (in Japanese with English abstract). Acta Hepatol Jpn 31: 1274–1281

25. Creech JL, Johnson MN (1974) Angiosarcoma of the liver in the manufacture of polyvinyl chloride. J Occup Med 16:150–151

26. Okudaira M (1982) Hepatic fibrosis and hemangiosarcoma induced by vinyl chloride monomer. J Univ Occup Environ Health 4 (suppl):135–146

CHAPTER 3

Hepatocellular carcinoma in the early stage

Setsuo Hirohashi and Michiie Sakamoto[1]

1 Introduction

Progress in imaging diagnosis has made it possible to detect an increasing number of minute hepatocellular carcinomas (HCCs), some of which can be removed successfully by surgery. In addition, lesions intermediate between regenerative nodules and minute HCCs, i.e. borderline lesions, can also be detected. Through analysis of these lesions, we have learned the natural course of human hepatocarcinogenesis. Long after infection with hepatitis viruses, small nodular lesions (adenomatous hyperplasia), which do not destroy substantially the underlying liver structure, develop in liver showing chronic hepatitis or cirrhosis. Some of these nodules show structural abnormalities and are diagnosed as well-differentiated HCC (early HCC). Nodule-in-nodule lesions composed of a peripheral area of early HCC and a central area of less well differentiated HCC are also observed. Clinico-pathologically, it is very important to establish criteria for differentiating between adenomatous hyperplasia and early HCC. The presence of structural abnormalities such as small acinar structures or an abnormal cord structure, an increase in cell density to more than twice that of the surrounding liver, and infiltration into the stroma are now considered useful as criteria for HCC among pathologists working in this field. Although adenomatous hyperplasia is not considered to be cancer on the basis of these pathological criteria, clinical follow-up study has revealed its precancerous nature. Additionally, a gross classification of HCC has been established by studies of large numbers of relatively small

HCCs, and the subtypes have been shown to be correlated with the clinical behavior of HCCs. The detailed results of these studies have already been reported [1–9], and are summarized in this article.

2 Pathology of minute HCCs and borderline lesions

2.1 Adenomatous hyperplasia and early HCC [1]

Fifty-eight small but sizeable nodular lesions, not substantially destroying the underlying liver structure, were collected from materials surgically resected because of the presence of HCC. Metastatic lesions of HCC and large regenerative nodules were excluded from the study. The mean age of the affected patients was 59.0 years and 85.4% were male. All cases were associated with chronic liver disease, chronic active hepatitis or cirrhosis. Within the small nodular lesions, Glisson's sheath or connective tissue between pseudolobules were recognized. From the level of atypia, these lesions were classified into three groups: Adenomatous hyperplasia (AH), atypical adenomatous hyperplasia (AAH), and early HCC (Figs. 1–4). In AH, hepatocytes in nodules were smaller and more cellular than those in the surrounding liver tissue, but no structural abnormalities were detected. The cytoplasm of hepatocytes in AH was often more eosinophilic. In AAH, cell density was much higher than in AH, and the cord structure was prominent. Structural abnormalities were recognizable focally. In early HCC, areas showing structural abnormalities, such as small acinar structures and abnormal cord structures, were detected in addition to increased cell density. Cellular

[1] Pathology Division, National Cancer Center Research Institute, Tsukiji, Chuo-ku, Tokyo, 104 Japan

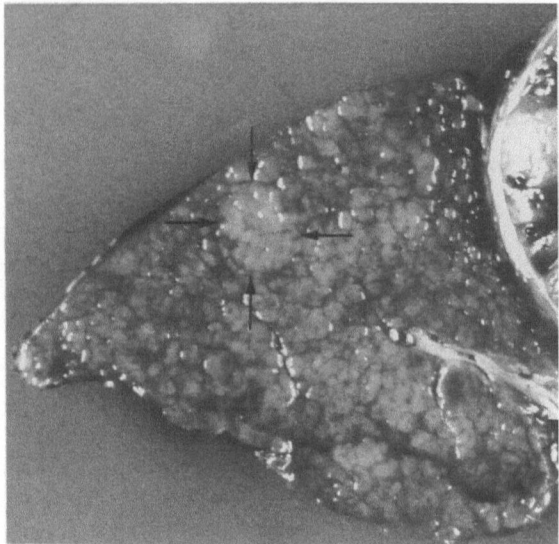

Fig. 1. Macroscopic view of adenomatous hyperplasia (AH) in liver with chronic hepatitis. A yellowish lesion indicated by *arrows* shows preserved underlying liver structures

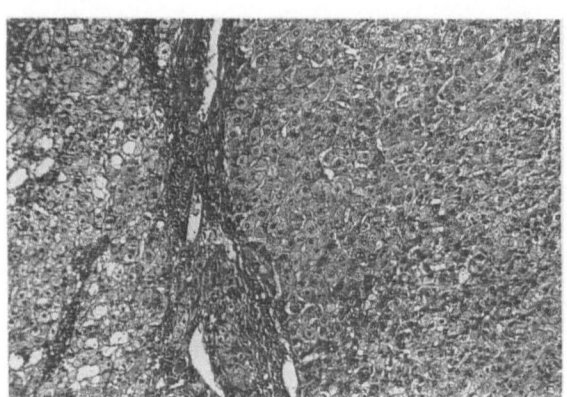

Fig. 2. Histology of AH. Cell density is slightly increased and cytoplasm is more eosinophilic compared with the surrounding liver on the left. (H&E stain)

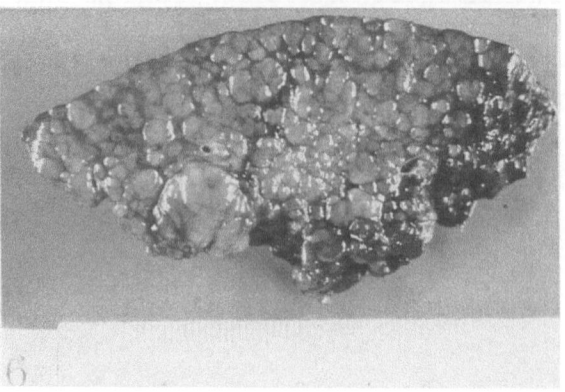

Fig. 3. Macroscopic view of an early HCC in a cirrhotic liver. The lesion bulges slightly from the cut surface and is partly yellowish due to fatty change

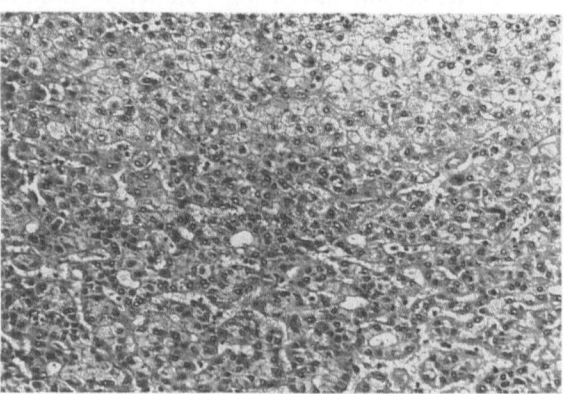

Fig. 4. Histology of an early HCC. Small hepatocytes are arranged in thin trabeculae with small acinar structures. Upper part is a component resembling AH. (H&E stain)

atypia of tumor cells was unremarkable and corresponded to grade 1 HCC by Edmondson and Steiner's classification [10]. Focal areas of grade 2 HCC were sometimes present in early HCC. Areas showing the histology of AH or AAH often co-existed in nodules of early HCC. The largest diameter of these small nodular lesions ranged from 0.4–2 cm. With the increase of atypia from AH and AAH to early HCC, the lesions showed a tendency to become larger. Cell nuclear density also increased in the order regenerative nodule, AH, AAH, early HCC. Early HCC showed increased cell nuclear density to more than twice that in the surrounding liver and in regenerative nodules (Fig. 5).

2.2 Transition from early HCC to advanced HCC [1, 2]

Nodule-in-nodule lesions, each composed of an area of early HCC and an area of advanced HCC, were detected, and these were considered to be a transitional state between early and advanced HCC (Figs. 6–7). Surgically resected HCCs with a diameter of less than 3 cm were carefully examined, and one fourth of them grossly showed nodule-in-nodule lesions. When the tumor diam-

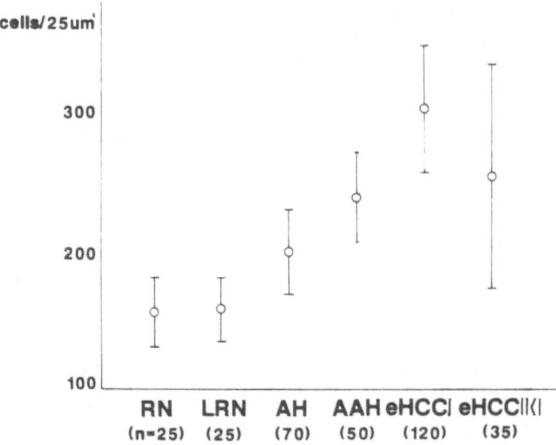

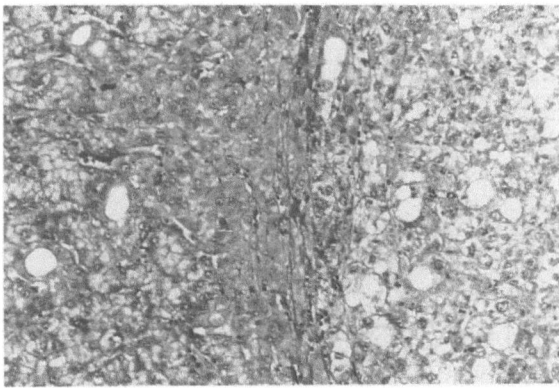

Fig. 5. Cell density in small nodular lesions. *RN*, Regenerative nodule; *LRN*, Large RN; *AH*, Adenomatous hyperplasia; *AAH*, Atypical AH; *eHCC*, Early HCC; *eHCC* (II < 1), Early HCC with a focal component of grade II HCC

Fig. 7. Histology of the border between an early HCC component and an advanced HCC component in a nodule-in-nodule lesion. Early HCC on the left shows a trabecular structure with a shift of nuclei to the sinusoidal side. (Azan-Mallory stain)

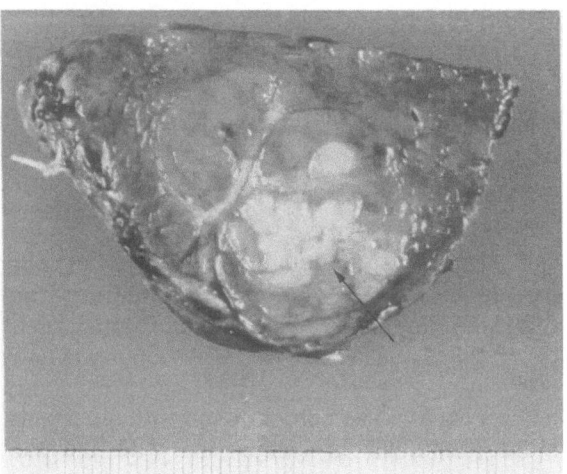

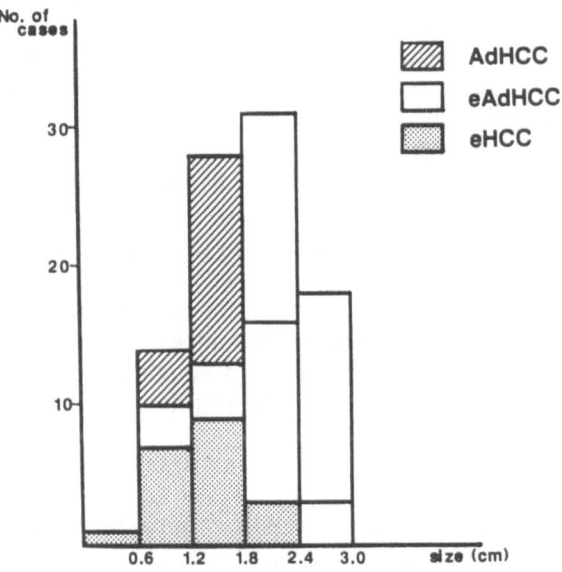

Fig. 6. Microscopic view of a nodule-in-nodule lesion. Central yellowish area (*arrow*) corresponds to an advanced carcinoma component that has emerged from early HCC

Fig. 8. Macroscopic types of small HCCs and tumor sizes. *AdHCC*, Advanced HCC; *eHCC*, Early HCC; *eAdHCC*, Nodule-in-nodule lesion with components of early HCC and advanced HCC

eter was smaller, the majority of the lesions were diagnosed as early HCC. The incidence of nodule-in-nodule lesions indicating transition from early HCC to advanced HCC increased as the tumor diameter became larger (Fig. 8). These results suggest that some HCCs progress from the early to advanced stage through nodule-in-nodule lesions. Histologically, early HCCs were always very well differentiated, corresponding to grade I carcinoma according to Edmondson and Steiner's classification. In some of these HCCs (about

30%), a focal area of moderately differentiated HCC was also detected. In contrast, advanced HCCs and the advanced HCC component in nodule-in-nodule lesions were moderately or poorly differentiated, corresponding to grade II or III. Portal vein tumor thrombi and intrahepatic metastasis were rarely detected in early HCCs, whereas they became more frequent in nodule-in-nodule lesions and advanced HCCs as the tumor diameter increased. These results indicate that early HCCs are different from usual HCCs of high-grade malignancy, and early HCCs are the lesions which correspond to the early stage of hepatocarcinogenesis, being precursors of advanced HCCs.

2.3 Clonal origin of small nodular lesions in liver with chronic hepatitis or cirrhosis [3, 4]

Viral DNA is a useful market of cell origin when the virus is integrated randomly into the cellular DNA of host cells. Hepatitis B virus fulfills this requirement, but no information on the integration of hepatitis C virus has so far been reported. We analyzed a few AHs, early HCCs, nodule-in-nodule lesions and advanced HCCs. The DNA was extracted and integration patterns of hepatitis B virus were analyzed by Southern blotting using several restriction enzymes. A clonal integration pattern indicating the clonal origin of the lesion was detected not only in advanced HCCs but also in AHs, early HCCs and nodule-in-nodule lesions. Most interestingly, the early HCC and advanced HCC components of one nodule-in-nodule lesion showed an identical pattern of integration, indicating that the same cell within an early HCC had progressed to advanced HCC. When multiple lesions, suggested morphologically to be independent in origin, were analyzed by the same technique, the integration patterns of hepatitis B virus differed among the lesions clearly indicating their multicentric origin.

3 Proposal of diagnostic criteria for early HCC and borderline lesions

Small but sizeable nodules, which do not substantially destroy the underlying liver structure, often develop in liver with chronic hepatitis or cirrhosis. In these nodular lesions, Glisson's sheaths or connective tissue between pseudolobules are frequently recognized. The lesions are usually less than 2 cm in diameter, and are classified into the following three groups.

3.1 Early hepatocellular carcinoma (early HCC)

In addition to an increase in cell density, areas showing structural abnormality such as small acinar structures or an abnormal cord structure, are detected in this group. Alternatively, obvious invasion into the stromal tissue is present. Cellular atypia of tumor cells is unremarkable, but the nuclear cytoplasmic ratio is increased due to the decrease in cell size. The cytoplasm shows increased eosinophilia or basophilia.

Comments:
1. In some cases, an area showing the histological features of AH co-exists in the same nodule.
2. Fatty change or clear cell change is often observed in this type of lesion, and cell density becomes lower where the tumor cells show this type of change. Interpretation of cell density should be performed carefully in areas where these changes are less prominent.
3. In some cases, a very small area showing the histology of moderately differentiated HCC may be present. However, if such an area is large enough to be detected grossly as a nodule-in-nodule lesion, the lesion should be excluded from the category of early HCC.
4. The term "early" is used to indicate that the lesion corresponds to the early stage of hepatocarcinogenesis.

3.2 Adenomatous hyperplasia (AH)

Cell density is moderately increased in comparison with the surrounding liver, but no structural abnormality is evident. Due to the slight decrease in cell size, the nuclear cytoplasmic ratio is slightly increased. Nuclear size often shows heterogeneity. The cord structure often becomes more prominent in comparison with the surrounding liver.

Comments:
1. There are some lesions which show very focal areas containing structural abnormalities, or which show a marked increase in cell density without structural abnormalities. At present, it is difficult to judge whether these lesions are malignant, and they are diagnosed as borderline lesions or atypical adenomatous hyperplasia.

3.3 Large regenerative nodule (LRN)

Histologically, no significant difference is detected between the lesion and the surrounding cirrhotic liver. An area showing liver cell dysplasia (Anthony) is often detected [11].

Table 1. Gross classification of HCC (National Cancer Center)

Type	Description
Early HCC	(early hepatocellular carcinoma): a lesion that does not substantially destroy the pre-existing architecture of the liver lobule or pseudolobule.

Nodular type
1 *single nodular type*: a roughly spherical and well-demarcated nodular tumor.
2 *single nodular type with extranodular growth*: a tumor resembling Type 1, but with extranodular tumor growth.
3 *contiguous multinodular type*: a unifocal but multinodular and well demarcated tumor, without any identifiable large tumor nodule suggesting a primary focus.
4 *poorly demarcated nodular type*: a nodular tumor entirely with a poorly demarcated boundary.
Massive type
Diffuse type

4 Pathology of small HCC [5]

4.1 Gross findings and gross classification

It has been reported that the main characteristics of small HCC are expansive growth and the presence of a capsule. However, we have observed small tumors with extracapsular growth and small tumors composed of aggregates of small nodules in addition to typical encapsulated tumors. Therefore, we have added these two subtypes to the gross classification of HCC proposed by Eggel, as shown in Table 1. The majority of small HCCs less than 3 cm in diameter were easily classified into types 1 to 3. The boundaries of these lesions were mostly clear. However, there was a special form of HCC which showed markedly invasive growth and an ill-demarcated boundary, which was classified as type 4.

4.2 Histological findings

Variation in gross findings is based on differences in the behavior of tumor cells, especially their growth and invasion. HCCs show both expansive growth and replacement growth. Expansive growth predominated in type 1 tumors and replacement growth was more pronounced in type 3 tumors which are composed of aggregates of small nodules. When the tumor cells show invasive growth similar to that of adenocarcinoma, the tumor becomes ill-demarcated

and is classified as type 4. Many combined hepatocellular and cholangiocellular carcinomas are classified as type 4. Portal vein tumor thrombi and intrahepatic metastases are very important markers for the advanced nature of HCC and the poor prognosis of patients. The incidence of these markers was highest (71.4%) for type 2 tumors, whereas they were detected in only 7.7% of type 1 tumors. The incidence of intrahepatic metastasis was also closely correlated with tumor size. When the tumor diameter was less than 1 cm, intrahepatic metastasis was not detected at all, but it was detected in 15% of tumors 1.1–2.0 cm in diameter and in 39% of tumors 2.1–3.0 cm in diameter.

4.3 Clinical findings

Gross findings showed a close correlation with clinical findings. The prognosis of patients with type 2 or type 3 tumors was significantly worse than that of patients with type 1 tumors. A statistically significant difference was obtained in the prognostic curves four years after surgical treatment. Type 1 tumors were more often associated with fully developed cirrhosis (87.5%) and were positive for hepatitis B surface antigen in 50% of the cases. Tumors of type 1 responded well to trans-catheter arterial embolization (TAE) whereas type 3 tumors were not treated successfully by this method.

4.4 Gross findings of advanced HCC [6]

We have applied this gross classification of nodular lesion to far-advanced HCC in autopsy material, and have found that even these lesions can be classified into subtypes.

5 Conclusion

The incidence of HCC in Japan is clearly increasing in males and the increase is associated with the spread of hepatitis C virus infection [7]. Fundamental studies including molecular biology are rapidly progressing with regard to the etiology and mechanism of multi-stage development and progression of HCCs. Multiple genetic alterations including inactivation of tumor suppressor genes have already been detected in HCCs [8]. It is expected that correlations among clinico-pathological findings, multi-factorial etiology and multiple genetic alterations will be elucidated in the near future. However, the diagnostic criteria for small nodular lesions including AH and early HCC are not identical among pathologists in different institutions and countries. It is very important to have common diagnostic criteria and to understand the clinical course or natural course of these lesions through careful clinical follow-up [9]. Genetic alterations and tumor markers specific to the early stage of hepatocarcinogenesis have not yet been found in humans. Efforts to obtain such markers are also important, and would perhaps be helpful for arriving at objective diagnostic criteria for small nodular lesions in the liver.

References

1. Sakamoto M, Hirohashi S, Shimosato Y (1991) Early stages of multistep hepatocarcinogenesis: Adenomatous hyperplasia and early hepatocellular carcinoma. Hum Pathol 22:172–178
2. Watanabe H, Hirohashi S, Sakamoto M, Hasegawa H, Yamazaki S, Makuuchi M, Moriyama N, Takayasu K (1990) New macroscopic subtype of small hepatocellular carcinoma—common type in early type—and histological consideration of the multistep progression of HCC (in Japanese). Acta Hepatol Jpn 31:1267–1273
3. Sakamoto M, Hirohashi S, Tsuda H, Shimosato Y, Makuuchi M, Hosoda Y (1989) Multicentric independent development of hepatocellular carcinoma revealed by analysis of hepatitis B virus integration pattern. Am J Surg Pathol 13:1064–1067
4. Tsuda H, Hirohashi S, Shimosato Y, Terada M, Hasegawa H (1988) Clonal origin of atypical adenomatous hyperplasia of the liver and clonal identity with hepatocellular carcinoma. Gastroenterology 95:1664–1666
5. Kanai T, Hirohashi S, Upton M, Noguchi M, Kishi K, Makuuchi M, Yamasaki S, Hasegawa H, Takayasu K, Moriyama N, Shimosato Y (1987) Pathology of small hepatocellular carcinoma: a proposal for a new gross classification. Cancer 60:810–819
6. Yuki K, Hirohashi S, Sakamoto M, Kanai T, Shimosato Y (1990) Growth and spread of hepatocellular carcinoma: A review of 240 consecutive autopsy cases. Cancer 66:2174–2179
7. Sakamoto M, Hirohashi S, Tsuda H, Ino Y, Shimosato Y, Yamasaki S, Makuuchi M, Hasegawa H, Terada M, Hosoda Y (1988) Increasing incidence of hepatocellular carcinoma possibly associated with non-A, non-B hepatitis in Japan, disclosed by hepatitis B virus DNA analysis of surgically resected cases. Cancer Res 48:7294–7297
8. Tsuda H, Zhang W, Shimosato Y, Yokota J, Terada M, Sugimura T, Miyamura T, Hirohashi S (1990) Allele loss on chromosome 16 associated with progression of human hepatocellular carcinoma. Proc Natl Acad Sci USA 87:6791–6794
9. Takayama T, Makuuchi M, Hirohashi S, Sakamoto M, Okazaki N, Takayasu K, Kosuge T, Motoo Y, Yamazaki S, Hasegawa H (1990) Malignant transformation of adenomatous hyperplasia to hepatocellular carcinoma. Lancet 336:1150–1153
10. Edmondson H, Steiner P (1954) Primary carcinoma of the liver: a study of 100 cases among 48,900 necropsies. Cancer 7:462–503
11. Anthony P, Vogel C, Barker L (1973) Liver cell dysplasia: a pre-malignant condition. J Clin Pathol 26:217–223

CHAPTER 4

Pathomorphology of advanced hepatocellular carcinoma

Masamichi Kojiro[1]

1 Introduction

After such a long hopeless period in the diagnosis and management of hepatocellular carcinoma (HCC), early detection of HCC has been made possible by advances in various diagnostic techniques, in particular the remarkable advance of diagnostic imaging in the past decade [1]. However, the majority of HCCs are still detected in the advanced stage and the curative therapies are not as effective as they are in earlier stages.

In this section, the author describes the pathomorphologic characteristics of advanced HCC based on the study of 439 autopsy cases at our institute.

2 Gross features

Although the gross features of HCC vary widely depending on the size of the tumor and the presence or absence of the association of liver cirrhosis, many advanced HCCs exhibit an expansile tumor growth with a combination of varying degrees of infiltrative tumor growth and intrahepatic metastasis.

Fibrous capsule and septa are the most frequent gross characteristic features in HCC. Capsule and septum formation can be frequently observed even in small HCCs and their presence has been determined to be the most helpful imaging diagnostic criteria of small HCC, particularly in ultrasonography [2].

The frequency of capsule and septum formation increases with tumor size. Both capsules

and septa have been found to co-exist in about 50% of tumors ranging from 1.5 cm to 2.0 cm in diameter, and this increases to about 70% in tumors larger than 2 cm. It is rare to find both of them in tumors smaller than 1.0 cm in diameter. Thus, capsule and septum formation seems to begin when the tumor size reaches around 1.5 cm in diameter.

2.2 Gross classification of advanced HCC

The gross classification proposed by Eggel [3] in 1901 has been widely employed in Japan. The author has classified advanced HCC into four major types: Expansive type (single nodular and multinodular), infiltrative type, mixed expansive and infiltrative type, and diffuse type [4].

2.2.1 Expansive type HCC
In this type, the tumor grows expansively as if it were pushing intact tissues aside. The tissue is mostly nodular and is frequently encapsulated. This type corresponds to Eggel's nodular type and is classified into single nodular and multinodular subtypes.

Single nodular type. The tumor is solitary and is mostly well-demarcated with a fibrous capsule. The single nodular HCC with a distinct fibrous capsule is also called an encapsulated HCC (Fig. 1). Single nodular HCC accounts for 10% of advanced HCCs.

Multinodular type. This type of HCC involves no fewer than two similar sized nodules with an expansile growth, regardless of intrahepatic metastasis or multicentric origin. This type accounts for 7.7% of advanced HCCs.

2.2.2 Infiltrative type HCC
In this type, the tumor-nontumor boundary is irregular and often indistinct (Fig. 1). Large

---

[1] First Department of Pathology, Kurume University School of Medicine, Kurume, 830 Japan

31

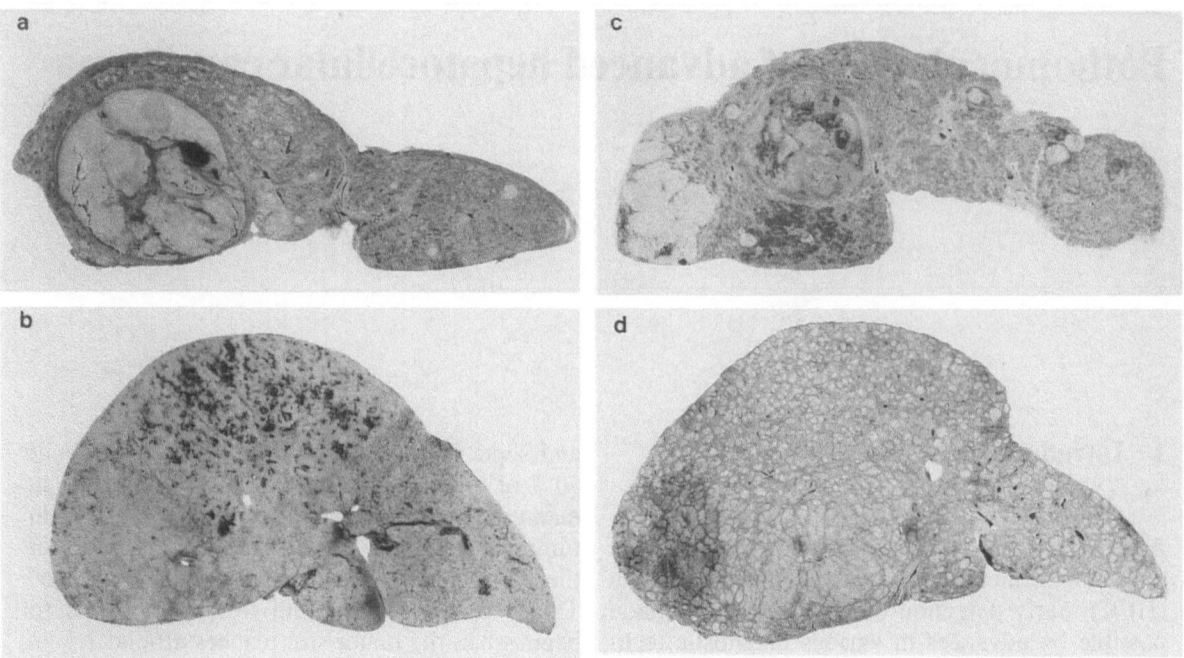

Fig. 1a–d. Gross classification of advanced HCC. **a** Expansive type, single nodular. **b** Infiltrative type. Ill-defined tumor occupies almost the entire right lobe of the non-cirrhotic liver. **c** Mixed expansive and infiltrative type. **d** Diffuse type

infiltrative type HCC corresponds to Eggel's massive type. This type accounts for 33% of advanced HCCs.

2.2.3 Mixed expansive and infiltrative type HCC

In this type, varying degrees of infiltrative tumor growth are present with an encapsulated tumor (Fig. 1). Infiltrative tumor growths are mostly an infiltration of the tumor outside the capsule and/or infiltrative tumor which has been spread from tumor thrombi of the portal vein.

2.2.4 Diffuse type HCC

In diffuse type HCC, multiple minute nodules ranging from 0.5 cm to 1.0 cm in diameter, which do not fuse with each other, are distributed throughout the liver. Liver cirrhosis is always associated with this type (Fig. 1) which accounts for 5.4% of advanced HCC.

3 Pedunculated HCC

Massive tumors proliferating extrahepatically with or without pedicles are sporadically encountered among HCC [5–8].

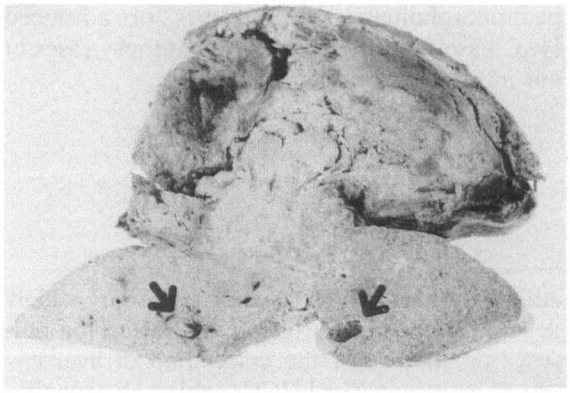

Fig. 2. Pedunculated HCC. There are little tumor growths within the liver, but main portal branches are filled with tumor thrombi (arrows)

Pedunculated HCC was found in 13 (2.9%) of the 439 autopsy cases. The pedunculated tumor growth seems to be mostly caused by the extrahepatic extension of the tumor which occured directly beneath the capsule of the liver (Fig. 2). In one case, however, it is strongly suggested that the tumor occured in the accessory hepatic lobe (Fig. 6).

Fig. 3. a Intrabile duct tumor growth with massive hemobilia. The tumor invaded into the bifurcation and the dilated bile ducts are filled with blood clot. **b** Intra-atrial tumor growth. Tumor cast extended from the vena cava to the right atrium and ventricle

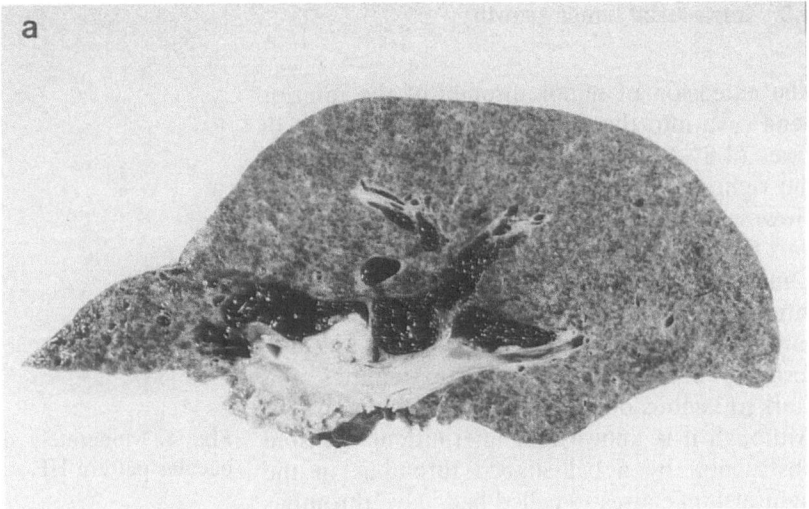

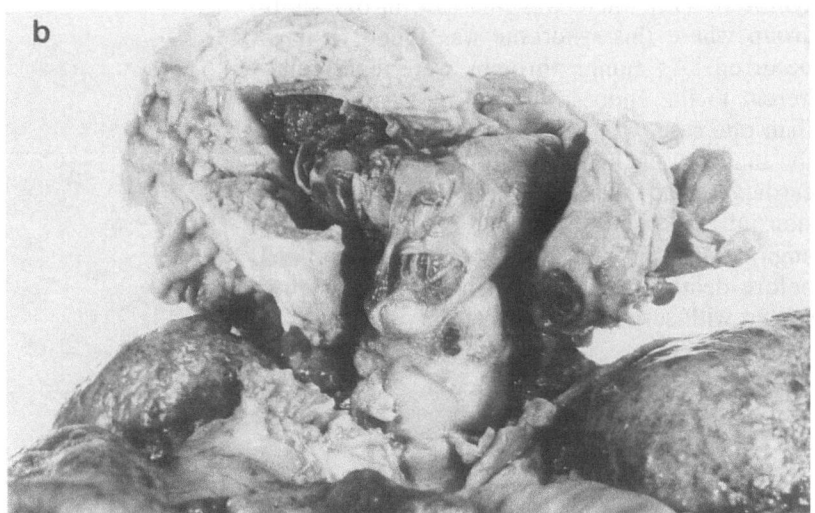

4   Unusual tumor growths in HCC

Unusual tumor growths such as intrabile duct tumors and intra-atrial tumors through the inferior vena cava have often been encountered [9, 10]. Although such unusual tumor growths had been considered as an incidental finding at autopsy, they have been clinically detected by means of imaging.

4.1   Intrabile duct tumor growth

Tumor growths into the hepatic duct and/or common bile duct are seen in 27 (6.1%) of the 439 cases and progressive obstructive jaundice was seen in all these cases. Although Lin [11] designated such cases as "icteric hepatoma" and stated that they presented difficulty in differential diagnosis, it is not so difficult at the present time because of remarkable advances in various diagnostic imaging techniques. Intrabile duct tumor growth is not merely one of the terminal signs in advanced HCC. This type of growth is mainly caused by a direct invasion of an infiltrative tumor located near the major bile duct, regardless of tumor size.

The extension of massive tumor thrombi of the portal vein into the neighboring hepatic duct and massive hemorrhage in the bile duct (hemobilia) due to intrabile duct tumor growth were encountered in one case (Fig. 3).

4.2 Intra-atrial tumor growth

The extension of tumor thrombi of the inferior vena cava into the right atrium was found in 18 cases (4.8%) and the tumor further extended to the right ventricle in 5 of the 18 cases (Fig. 3). However, direct tumor invasion from tumor bolus into the myocardium was found only in 2 cases. Clinically, the majority of the patients with intra-atrial tumor growth did not present serious cardiovascular symptoms other than diuretic-resistant edema in the lower extremities and marked venous dilatation in the abdominal wall. Although it is known that intermittent tricuspid obstruction by a ball-shaped thrombus in the right atrium causes so-called ball-valve thrombus syndrome [12], there was one case in our study group where this syndrome was found to have occurred. As tumor thrombi were lightly adherent to the endocardium in most cases, other than one case with ball-shaped tumor thrombus, the majority of the cases did not present serious cardiovascular signs. Clinically, tumor extension into the right atrium had been detected by angiography and ultrasonography 3–4 months before death in 5 cases, but none of them presented with serious cardiac symptoms.

5 Histologic features

Basically, HCC consists of the tumor parenchyma, comprising a liver cell cord-like (trabecular) structure, and the stroma, comprising a sinusoid-like blood space lined by a single layer of endothelial cells. The majority of the advanced HCCs studied were moderately differentiated HCC with a trabecular pattern (Fig. 4), and varying degrees of pseudoglandular pattern were also found in about 30% of the trabecular HCCs.

5.1 Histologic growth pattern of HCC

The histologic growth patterns at the tumor-nontumor boundary can be divided into two basic patterns: Replacing and sinusoidal [13]. The replacing growth pattern is considered to be the basic growth pattern of HCC and the cancer cells are seen replacing hepatocytes along the liver cell cords (Fig. 5). In the sinusoidal growth pattern, the cancer cells grow in an infiltrating fashion in

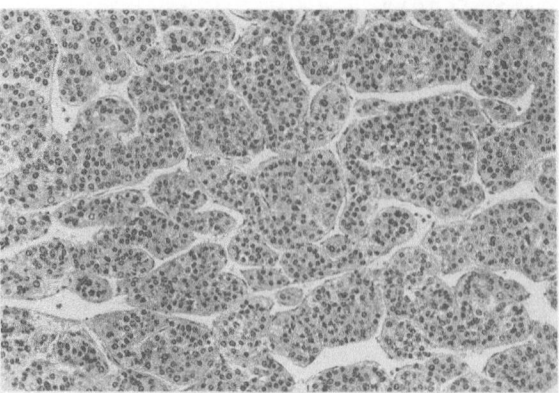

Fig. 4. Moderately differentiated HCC with a trabecular pattern HE stain ×50

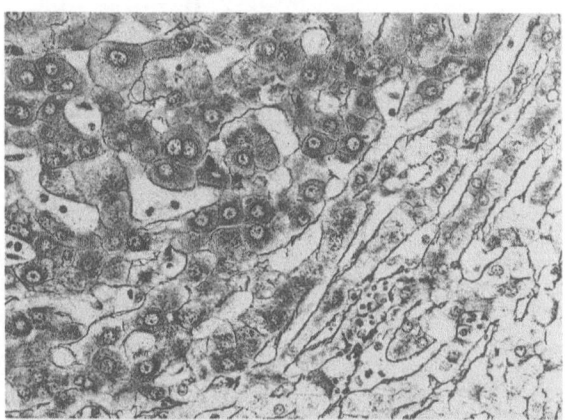

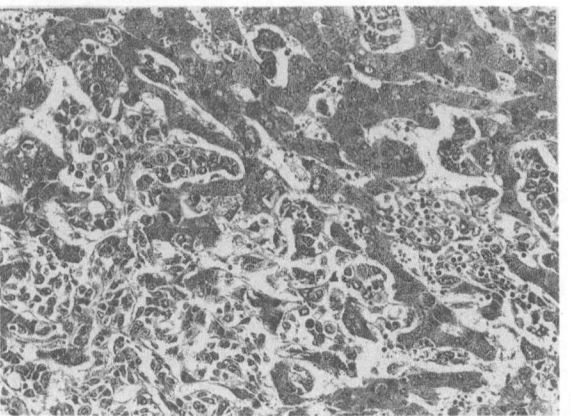

Fig. 5a,b. Histologic growth pattern of HCC. **a** Replacing growth pattern. The cancer cells are growing as if they are replacing the adjacent hepatocytes without destroying liver cell cords Retculin stain ×100. **b** Sinusoidal growth pattern. The cancer cells with poor mutual contact are proliferating along the sinusoids and liver cell cords are atrophied HE stain ×50

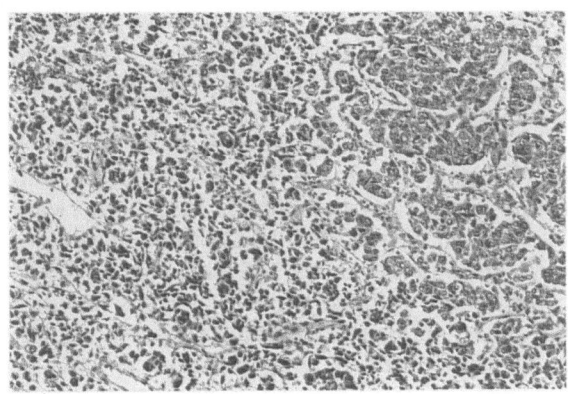

Fig. 6. HCC with sarcomatous change. Transitional feature between trabecular HCC and sarcomatous area is evident HE stain ×50

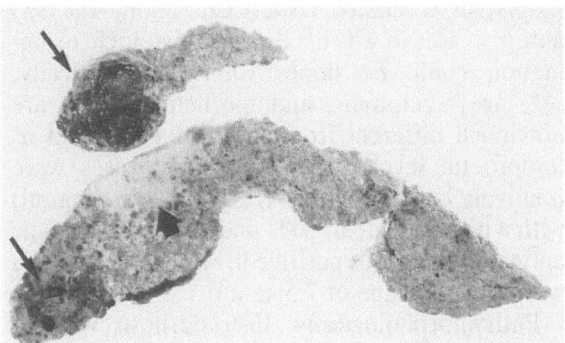

Fig. 7. Gross appearance of combined hepatocellular and cholangiocarcinoma. HCC components (*thin arrows*) and the area of cholangiocarcinoma (*thick arrow*) are clearly identified. This tumor corresponds to double cancer

the sinusoids at the boundary, compressing liver cell cords and hepatocytes (Fig. 5). In 26 autopsy cases of HCC which had not received effective anticancer therapies such as transcatheter arterial embolization (TAE) and arterial injection of anti-cancer agents, 12 of the tumors (42.3%) were of the replacing type and 7 (26.9%) were of the sinusoidal type. In the other 7 cases, the tumors were encapsulated, but the cancer cells growing beyond the capsule showed the replacing growth pattern. The incidence of extrahepatic metastasis was strongly correlated to the growth pattern. Extrahepatic metastasis was found in 6 (85.7%) of the 7 sinusoidal cases, 6 (50%) of the 12 replacing cases, and in 2 (28.6%) of the 7 encapsulated cases of non-treated HCC.

5.2 HCC with sarcomatous change

Occasionally, sarcomatous features consisting of spindle-shaped and/or pleomorphic anaplastic tumor cells are found in a portion of the HCC (Fig. 6). Sarcomatous change was found in 16 cases (3.6%) of the 439 autopsy cases, and the frequency has been increasing over the last decade. In particular, the incidence of sarcomatous change is significantly higher among the cases treated with effective anticancer therapies such as TAE and intra-arterial injection of anti-cancer agents, and it is suggested that sarcomatous change may be caused by morphological change of HCC cells due to anticancer therapy in a ceratin portion of the cases [15].

6   Association of liver cirrhosis

Liver cirrhosis was associated in 352 (80.2%) of the 439 autopsy cases. In the majority of cases with associated cirrhosis, the cirrhosis was macronodular or mixed macro- and micronodular. Serum HBs Ag was found to be positive in 81 (33.7%) of the 240 cases examined during the 8 years from 1978 to 1986, but it was positive in 20% of the 92 cases examined after 1986. Although micronodular cirrhosis, which was considered alcoholic cirrhosis, was associated in only 3 cases, long term alcohol abuse was recorded in about 10% of the 439 cases.

7   Combined hepatocellular and cholangiocarcinoma

Combined hepatocellular and cholangio-carcinoma (combined HCC-CCC) consists of both HCC and CCC in the same liver.

Allen and Lisa [16] classified combined HCC and CCC into three categories: 1) tumors in which the areas of HCC and CCC are present separately (double cancer), 2) tumors where both components are present adjacent to each other and mixed together as one mass (combined type), and 3) tumors in which both components are intimately mixed (mixed type). Alternatively, Goodman et al. [17] classified combined HCC-CCC into three types: collision type, transitional type, and fibrolamellar type. We found 10 cases

(2.5%) of combined HCC-CCC among the 393 autopsy cases in which a detailed histologic examination could be done. Clinicopathologically, sex, age, symptoms, and biochemical data are not much different from those of HCC, but α-fetoproetin levels in the combined cases were relatively low or negative (less that 10,000 ng/ml) with a positive rate of 60% and carcinoembryonic antigen (CEA) was positive in 88% of these cases with a mean value of 7.5 ng/ml.

Pathomorphologically, liver cirrhosis was associated in 50% of the combined cases. Grossly, each area of HCC and CCC could be distinguished in only 2 cases (Fig. 7). The remainder of the combined HCC-CCC cases mostly showed CCC-like appearance. There was only one case of double cancer in which both components of HCC and CCC were completely separated. Histologically, the transitional feature between HCC and CCC was found in 6 of the combined cases (60%).

Although the histogenesis of combined HCC-CCC is still obscure, the following three possibilities are conceivable: 1) double cancer 2) HCC partly differentiate to CCC, 3) the cancers arise from a common intermediate (transitional) cell type between hepatocyte and bile duct epithelium which differentiates into both components.

Yano et al. [18] reported the establishment of a cell line from HCC which transformed to adenocarcinoma after culturing.

8 Extrahepatic metastasis in HCC

Although intrahepatic metastasis through the portal vein branches occurs frequently even from a relatively early stage in HCC, extrahepatic metastasis seems more likely to occur in the late stage. Among the 439 autopsy cases, extrahepatic metastases were found in 63.3%. It was reported that the incidence of extrahepatic metastasis is slightly higher in HCC without liver cirrhosis than HCC associated with liver cirrhosis [19, 20]. In our study, extrahepatic metastases were found in 67.0% of HCCs without cirrhosis and in 46.2% of HCCs with cirrhosis. As described in the section on the growth pattern of HCC, extrahepatic metastasis is significantly higher in HCCs with the sinusoidal growth pattern. Hematogenic metastasis is much more common than lymphatic metastasis: The incidence for the former was 48.7% and it was significantly higher than 29.4% for lymphatic metastasis. The hematogenic metastasis to the lungs was the most common, followed in order by bone and adrenal gland metastasis.

Extrahepatic metastasis was found in 4 of the 10 cases of combined HCC-CCC, and both hematogenic and lymphatic metastases were found in all 4 cases. All hematogenic metastases were seen in the lungs and consisted of HCC components. Lymphatic metastasis was found in the hilar, peripancreatic, and periaortic nodes, and consisted of CCC components.

References

1. Okuda K (1986) Early recognition of hepatocellular carcinoma. Hepatology 6:729–738
2. Majima Y, Tanaka M, Fujimoto T, Iwai I, Sasaki T, Abe M, Tanikawa K, Sugihara S, Kojiro M, Nakayama T (1987) Ultrasonographical features and its pathological findings of hepatocellular carcinomas smaller than 2 cm in diameter. Acta Hepatol Jpn 28:1188–1195
3. Eggel H (1901) Über das primare Carcinoma der Leber. Beitr. Pathol Anat Allg Pathol 30:506–604
4. Nakashima T, Kojiro M (1987) Hepatocellular carcinoma: An atlas of its pathology Springer-Verlag, Tokyo
5. Arakawa M, Kage M, Isomura T, Motoyama F, Kubo Y, Nakayama T (1982) Pathomorphological studies on hepatocellular carcinoma (HCC): Seven cases of HCC with an extrahepatic tumor growth—"pedunculated hepatoma" Acta Hepatol Jpn 23:942–948
6. Horie Y, Kato S, Yoshida H, Imaoka T, Suou T, Hirayama C (1983) Pedunculated hepatocellular carcinoma: Report of three cases and review of literature. Cancer 51:746–751
7. Horiuchi N, Kitamura T, Tateishi R, Wada A (1973) Hepatoma originated in the retroperitoneal space. Oncology 27:235–243
8. Nonomiya F, Kawahara T, Yamaguchi G, Maruyama N, Motoori H, Tanikawa K, Arakawa M (1980) A case of pedunculated hepatoma. Acta Hepatol Jpn 21:1581–1586
9. Kojiro M, Nakahara H, Sugihara S, Murakami T, Nakashima T (1984) Hepatocellular carcinoma with intra-atrial tumor growth. A clinicopathologic study of 18 autopsy cases. Arch Pathol Lab Med 108:989–992
10. Kojiro M, Kawabata K, Kawano Y, Shirai F, Takemoto N, Nakashima T (1982) Hepatocellular carcinoma presenting as intrabile duct tumor growth. A clinicopathologic study of 24 cases. Cancer 49:2144–2147

11. Lin T (1972) Tumor of the liver. Part I: Primary malignant tumors. In: Bockus, H, Berk, J, Haubrich, W, et al. (eds) Gastroenterology Sanders, Philadelphia p 522

12. Hahne O, Climie A (1962) Right atrial thrombi with ball-valve action. Am J Med 32:942–946

13. Nakashima T, Kojiro M, Kawano Y, Shirai F, Takemoto N, Tomimatsu H, Kawasaki H, Okuda K (1982) Histologic growth pattern of hepatocellular carcinoma. Relationship to orcein (hepatitis B surface-antigen) positive cells in cancer tissue. Hum Pathol 13:563–568

14. Kakizoe S, Kojiro M, Nakashima T (1987) Pathomorphological study of hepatocellular carcinoma with sarcomatous change. Cancer 59:310–316

15. Kojiro M, Sugihara S, Kakizoe S, Nakashima O, Kiyomatsu K (1989) Hepatocellular carcinoma with sarcomatous change: A special reference to the relationship with anticancer therapy. Cancer Chemother Pharmacol 23 (Suppl):4–8

16. Allen R, Lisa J (1949) Combined liver cell and bile duct carcinoma. Am J Pathol 25:647–655

17. Goodman Z, Ishak K, Langloss JM, Sesterhenn IA, Rabin L (1985) Combined hepatocellular-cholangioma. A histological and immuno-histological study. Cancer 55:124–135

18. Yano H, Kojiro M, Nakashima T (1986) A new human hepatocellular carcinoma cell line (KYN-1) with a transformation to adenocarcinoma. In Vitro 22:637–646

19. Peters R (1976) Pathology of hepatocellular carcinoma. In: Okuda K, Peters R (eds) Hepatocellular carcinoma Wiley, New York p 107

20. Mori W (1956) Study on extrahepatic metastasis in hematoma. A special reference to the relationship with liver cirrhosis. Tr Soc Pathol Jpn 45:224–236

CHAPTER 5

Pathology of cholangiocellular carcinoma

Yasuni Nakanuma, Hiroshi Minato, Tetsuji Kida, and Tadashi Terada[1]

1 Introduction

Cholangiocellular carcinoma (CCC) is an intrahepatic malignant tumor composed of cells resembling the biliary epithelium [1, 2]. A majority of CCC arise in the biliary lining epithelial cells, but it can also occur in the intrahepatic peribiliary glands [3] and also in Hering's ductules [4, 5]. Carcinoma arising under pre-existing pathologic conditions or anomalies of biliary epithelial cells, such as von Meyenburg's complexes or benign cysts, is also included in CCC [6–9].

CCC is the second most common type of malignant tumor found in the liver after hepatocellular carcinoma (HCC). The geographical incidence of CCC varies to a lesser degree than does HCC [1, 2, 5, 10–13] and association with cirrhosis is infrequent. Sex difference is either very small or nil with CCC, and patients aged between 50 and 60 years of age are usually affected [5, 11, 13]. The proportion of CCC among primary liver malignancies is about 8%–20% [1, 2, 5, 10–13], and some variation in incidence may be due to differences in histologic interpretation. While diagnostic modalities for detection of the tumor and therapeutic approaches have progressed considerably [11, 14], CCC still remains one of the intractable malignant tumors.

Although the etiology and pathogenesis remains unclear in a great majority of cases, preceding pathologic conditions or etiologies are known or suspected in some cases [1, 2, 5, 10–13]. Some special forms of CCC, such as those associated with liver flukes or hepatolithiasis, are endemic in

some parts of the world, particularly in East Asia [6, 8].

In this chapter, we will describe the anatomy of the intrahepatic biliary tree, then address the gross and histologic features of CCC, spread and metastases, immunohistochemistry, differential diagnosis, and etiology and preceding pathologic conditions of CCC. Special forms or related types of CCC are also described. This review is based on the observations of 118 cases of CCC experienced in our laboratory and in affiliated hospitals.

2 Anatomy of the intrahepatic biliary system and definition of cholangiocellular carcinoma

The intrahepatic biliary tree is defined as the biliary tree proximal to the hepatic duct confluence and is classified into the right and left hepatic duct, segmental duct (the first major branches of each hepatic duct), area ducts (the first major branches of each segmental duct) and their finer branches [15]. The hepatic, segmental and area ducts are collectively termed "large intrahepatic bile ducts", around which peribiliary glands consisting of the intramural and extramural glands are present [16]. Intramural glands are found within the ductal wall and extramural glands in the periductal tissue. Bile ductules are tubular structures in the peripheral zone of the portal tract with a lumen of $<20\,\mu m$, and ductules adjacent to hepatocytes are called Hering's ductules. Interlobular bile ducts are found in the peripheral zone of the portal tracts and have a lumen of $20–80\,\mu m$. Septal bile ducts are larger than the interlobular bile ducts and are seen in the central parts of portal tracts [17].

CCC is generally defined as carcinoma arising from the biliary epithelium of the bifurcation of

---

[1] Second Department of Pathology, Kanazawa University School of Medicine, Kanazawa, Ishikawa, 920 Japan

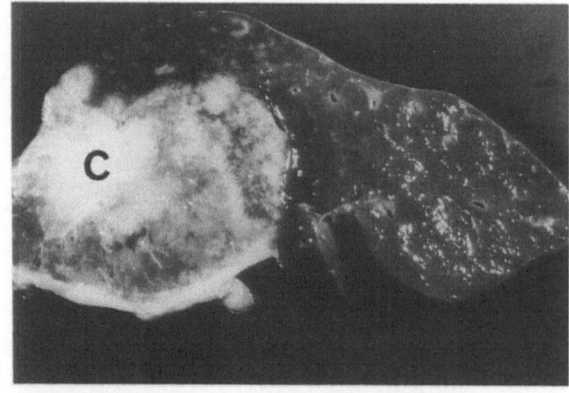

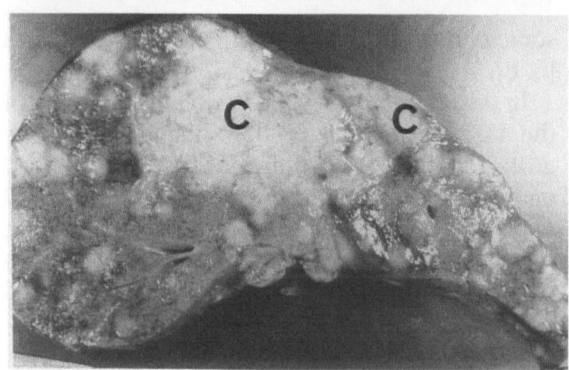

Fig. 1a,b. Gross findings of cholangiocellular carcinoma of the peripheral type. **a** The tumor mass (C) occupies a great majority of the right hepatic lobe, corresponding to the massive type described by Eggel. **b** Variable sized tumor nodules (C) are found in both hepatic lobes, corresponding to the nodular type described by Eggel

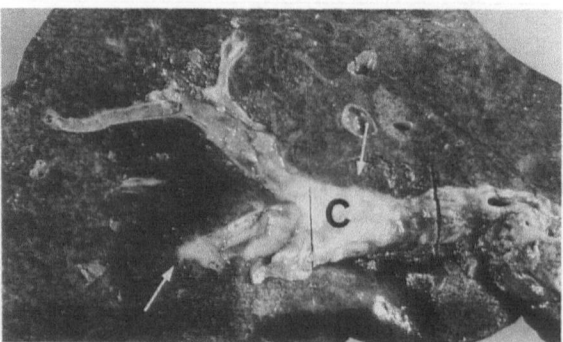

Fig. 2. Gross findings of cholangiocellular carcinoma of the hilar type. A small tumor (C) found in the hepatic hilus has spread along the portal tract and also infiltrated the surrounding hepatic parenchyma (*arrows*)

the right and left hepatic ducts and their intrahepatic branches [2]. However, the Japanese Biliary Surgical Society defines CCC as carcinoma arising from the bile duct located on the liver side of the first intrahepatic branches of the right and left hepatic ducts [18]. While the latter definition seems valuable in cholangiographic studies, the former is useful in autopsies or surgically resected specimens. In this chapter, the Japanese Biliary Surgical Society definition of CCC is used.

3 Gross features of cholangiocellular carcinoma

CCC is usually a white-gray or white colored solid tumor (Figs. 1, 2), and its consistency is either elastic, firm, or hard. Foci of coagulative necrosis are not infrequent, especially in the central por-

tions. Hemorrhage is also occasionally found, but fibrous encapsulation is not. The fact that some tumors have blurred boundaries suggests an infiltration of the carcinoma into the hepatic parenchyma. Miliary green spots are occasionally found at the border of the tumor, reflecting dilated bile ductules with microcalculi or extravasated bile [1]. In the large majority of cases, the non-tumorous liver parenchyma is greenish and shows variable biliary fibrosis or even biliary cirrhosis due to prolonged cholestasis [13]. There are several gross classifications of CCC using several parameters such as size, shape and location of the tumor [5, 13, 19–22].

Eggel [19, 22] classified CCC into massive, nodular, and diffuse types. The massive type is characterized by the tumor occupying largely the right or left lobe, or more of the liver (Fig. 1a). Major branches of portal veins and biliary elements are totally obliterated within the carcinoma mass. Hepatic lobes replaced by carcinoma are usually not enlarged. Nodular type of CCC is characterized by one or multiple nodules of the tumor (Fig. 1b). They are usually round and the sizes are variable. A majority of these nodules may correspond to the intrahepatic metastases of CCC, and the largest nodule is generally regarded as primary. A diffuse type is rare, and is characterized by numerous tumor foci with unclear borders [5]. This classification is applicable to most cases of CCC, especially advanced CCC, though an overlapping of these three types is not infrequent.

CCC is also grossly divided into 2–4 types according to the location of the main tumor [5,

13]. Okuda et al. [13] classified CCC into the hilar and peripheral types. The peripheral type is more common than the hilar type [13]. This classification is valuable in clinical evaluation and selection of therapy for CCC, although the exact site of tumor origin in the intrahepatic biliary tree is usually impossible to identify in clinically diagnosed cases.

3.1 Hilar type

The hilar type, or Klatskin type [13, 20, 21] is shown in Fig. 2. The main tumor occupies the hilar region with no indication of extrahepatic origin. This type of CCC has a tendency to cause obstruction, stenosis, or obliteration of the large biliary tree in which the primary focus is usually obliterated and its exact identification is difficult. This type has densely sclerotic connective tissue and shows infiltration into the hepatic parenchyma. Nodule formation or diffuse thickening of the major intrahepatic bile ducts is a frequent gross finding. Papillary growth into the lumen of the bile ducts is rarely encountered. The hilar type resembles the extrahepatic bile duct carcinoma clinicopathologically, and differentiation between the hilar type from carcinoma in the extrahepatic bile ducts or in the gallbladder is often difficult. The size of the hilar type is usually small compared to the peripheral type.

3.2 Peripheral type

The peripheral type of tumor is located mainly in the parenchyma remote from the hilum. Single or multiple tumors may be present (Fig. 1). There are frequently umbilications in the subcapsular tumor nodules, as seen in metastatic liver cancers.

Peripheral CCC shows continuous infiltration or metastasis via blood vessels or lymphatic vessels to the hepatic hilus, resulting in obstruction or stenosis of the intrahepatic large bile ducts. Similarly, hilar CCC can spread continuously along the portal tracts or metastasize to the hepatic peripheries. In this case, differentiation between the hilar and peripheral types is difficult, and their clinical behavior is also similar.

CCC associated with hepatolithiasis occasionally shows predominant periductal spread, and cannot be classified by either of the gross types mentioned above.

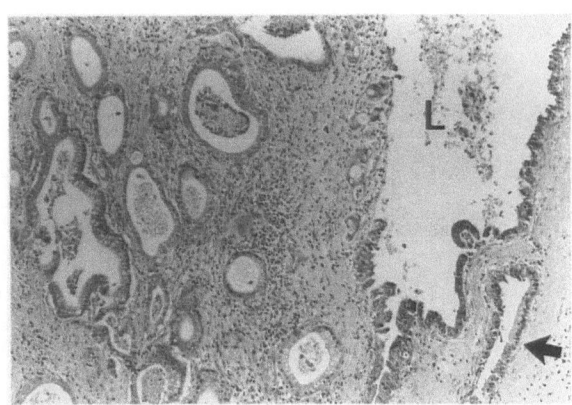

Fig. 3. Atypical biliary epithelium (carcinoma cells) with mild papillary configuration lines in the ductal surface. Some parts of the ductal surface are eroded. There are well-differentiated tubular adenocarcinoma beneath the ductal surface (*left half*). One biliary branch is being replaced by carcinoma cells (*arrow*). *L*, ductal lumen. H&E, ×150

4 Histology of cholangiocellular carcinoma

A majority of CCC, hilar or peripheral types, are adenocarcinoma of variable histologies [1, 2, 19]. The Japanese Society of Biliary Surgery [18] classifies CCC histologically into papillary, tubular (well, moderately, or poorly differentiated), mucinous, signet ring cell, adenosquamous, undifferentiated, miscellaneous, and unclassified types. Although more than one pattern may be seen in a single tumor, each case is categorized into either of these nine types according to their predominant features [2, 18, 23]. Papillary, papillotubular, and well- to moderately—differentiated adenocarcinoma are the most common [23]. Carcinoma cells with a pale or eosinophilic cytolplasm are usually cuboidal or columnar, and their cytological features more or less resemble bile duct epithelial cells [1, 2, 18, 23]. There have been, however, no standardized histologic criteria of carcinoma cells representing the exact bile duct level in which CCC arises. Carcinoma cells lining the ductal lumina, when preserved, show papillary or pseudopapillary configuration (Fig. 3), especially in the early stages. While the lumen of the bile duct with the primary focus may be present, it is erosive, compressed, or obliterated in a majority of advanced cases so that the primary focus is usually obscured. Infiltrating carcinoma near the bile duct

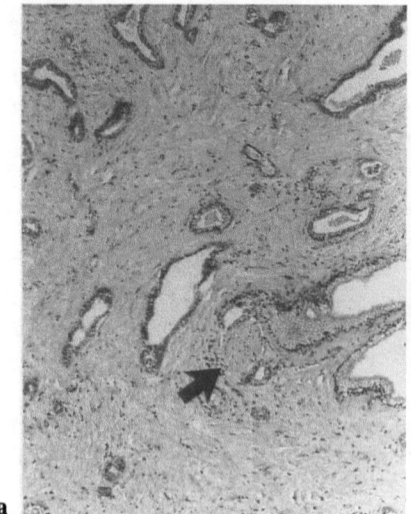
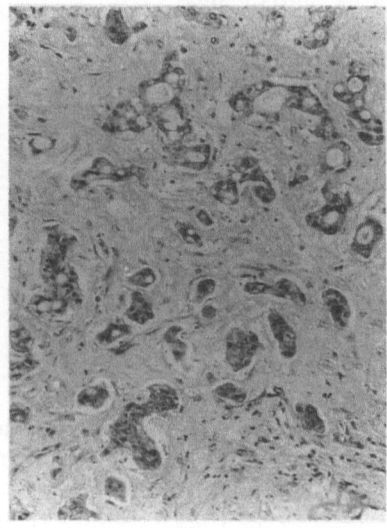

Fig. 4a,b. Histologies of cholangiocellular carcinoma. **a** Well-differentiated tubular adenocarcinoma with prominent desmoplastic reaction. There is perineural invasion of carcinoma cells (*arrow*). H&E, ×100. **b** Moderately to poorly differentiated adenocarcinoma with prominent desmoplastic reaction. Trabecular to acinar patterns are intermingled. H&E, ×200

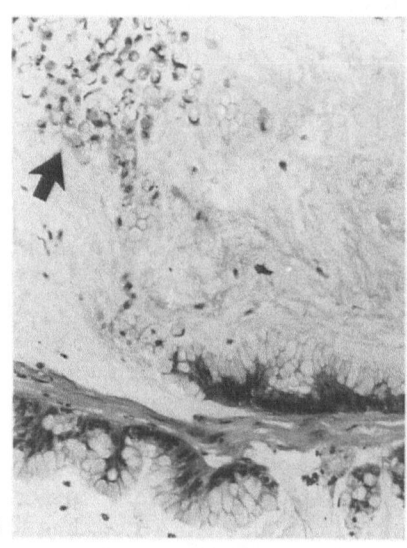
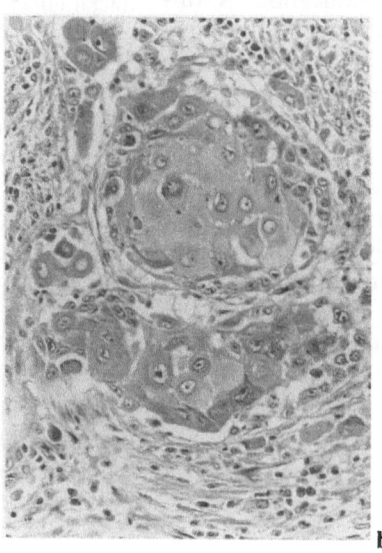

Fig. 5a,b. Unusual histologies of cholangiocellular carcinoma. **a** Mucinous carcinoma with signet ring cells (*arrow*) floating in mucus. H&E, ×300. **b** Foci of squamous cell carcinoma. H&E, ×400

lumen is usually well-differentiated (Fig. 3), and carcinoma in the portal tracts and also in the hepatic parenchyma is variably differentiated (Fig. 4). Characteristically, epithelial mucin is demonstrable in carcinoma tissue [1, 2, 5]. That is, periodic acid-Schiff and alcian blue stains can be used to confirm the presence of mucin in the glandular lumina or cytoplasm along the apical rim and in the extraglandular tissue. This characteristic is important in differentiating CCC from HCC, although a few cases of anaplastic CCC with negative mucus staining have been reported [24, 25].

There is a considerable amount of fibrous stroma (Fig. 4) with occasional hyalinization and even calcification. Vasculatures are indistinct compared to those in HCC [5]. There is frequently perineural invasion and portal venous tumor thrombi associated with CCC. In the early stages of CCC, especially at the intrahepatic large bile ducts, carcinomatous epithelial cells mainly grow and replace the non-neoplastic biliary lining epithelial cells as well as conduits of the peribiliary glands on the basement membranes with focal stromal infiltration.

Signet ring cell carcinoma, or mucinous carcinoma without cyst formation, are also encountered in the liver (Fig. 5a) [1]. We recently encountered one case of mucinous carcinoma which showed rapid growth and pseudomyxoma peritonei. Focal squamous metaplasia is not infrequent in CCC (Fig. 5b), and Nakajima et al.

reported that 11 of 117 cases of CCC revealed a component of squamous cell carcinoma (SCC) [5, 24]. The area of SCC ranged from focal to overwhelming. SCC almost never occurs in the liver by itself, while adenosquamous cell carcinoma containing equal amounts of squamous and glandular elements with transitional forms are on occasionally reported [1, 24]. There have been, however, no reports to date of squamous metaplasia in the non-neoplastic intrahepatic biliary tree in CCC cases which also contain components of SCC. Nakajima et al. [24] disclosed that despite the close similarity in age and sex ratios between CCC with and without squamous metaplasia, a component of squamous cell carcinoma was prone to develop in a rather advanced stage of CCC, as indicated by short survival time, large tumor size, aggressive modes of intrahepatic spreading, and frequent metastasis. However, several other reports failed to confirm these results [26, 27]. The occurrence of the squamous element in CCC is generally interpreted as the result of the metaplastic transformation of adenocarcinoma cells because of their intimate coexistence in the primary and metastatic lesions. Mucoepidermoid tumors, resembling the tumor in salivary glands, have also been reported to co-exist with CCC [1, 26, 27].

Anaplastic carcinoma presenting predominantly spindle, small round cell, or large pleomorphic cells is also on occasion reported with CCC. SCC can also be intermingled in some cases [5, 28]. We have recently noted such a case in which a considerable amount of sarcomatous tissue resembling malignant fibrous histiocytoma were intermingled with components of adenocarcinoma and SCC in the liver [28].

Some CCCs are speculated to arise from several specific anatomical components. That is, CCC originates as microtubular adenocarcinoma with cuboidal shapes, and histologically resembles the ductules of Hering [1, 4, 5]. However, it is still not clear whether or not this type is a special form of CCC which arises from Hering's ductules.

It is also probable that CCC arises in the intrahepatic peribiliary glands [3, 29]. Our previous study disclosed that dysplasia or papillary hyperplasia (Fig. 6a) and in situ carcinoma of the peribiliary glands and their conduits are, on occasion, found in autopsy livers [3]. This type may progress to the hilar type of CCC.

We have recently seen an advanced type of CCC, probably arising in the peribiliary glands, in which carcinoma mainly spread along the hepatic hilar connective tissue causing jaundice. Peribiliary glands adjacent to the carcinoma in this type showed extensive papillary hyperplasia with various dysplastic changes (Figs. 6b,c) [29]. It is of interest that cholangiographic findings revealed that the duct contour was smooth, and that the inner surface of the hepatic ducts was grossly smooth. It seems necessary to examine what proportion of CCC are derived from peribiliary glands or biliary lining epithelium, especially in the hilar type, though its determination is difficult and arbitrary in advanced cases of CCC.

5 Spreads and metastases of cholangiocellular carcinoma

CCC usually spreads continuously along the portal tracts including vascular and lymphatic involvement, permeation into the portal connective tissue, and perineural or intraneural invasion. Intraductal spread represented by a replacing growth pattern (abrupt transition between malignant invading cells and non-malignant biliary epithelial cells) is occasionally seen at the interlobular, septal, and intrahepatic large bile ducts. Nakajima et al. [24] reported such a replacing growth pattern in 15.8% of CCC cases examined. Such spread also involves the intrahepatic peribiliary glands (intramural and extramural glands) and their conduits. This glandular involvement and subsequent infiltration into the peribiliary connective tissue seems important regarding spread and progression of the hilar CCC.

It is widely suggested that spread of carcinoma via lymphatic and blood vessels or nerve fibers is important in the continuous infiltration or metastases of CCC [5, 23]. The presence of carcinoma thrombi in the vasculature in the hepatic parenchymal areas, either surrounding or remote from the carcinoma, support this suggestion. However, it is usually difficult to identify lymphatics in routinely stained sections. Direct invasion into the surrounding liver resembling the compressing or sinusoidal growth of HCC [30] are also seen histologically.

Extrahepatic metastases are rather frequent, especially at autopsy [5, 23]. Nakajima et al. [23] recently reported that the peripheral type is more prone to metastasize to lymph nodes and remote organs such as lung and pancreas (83% and 86%)

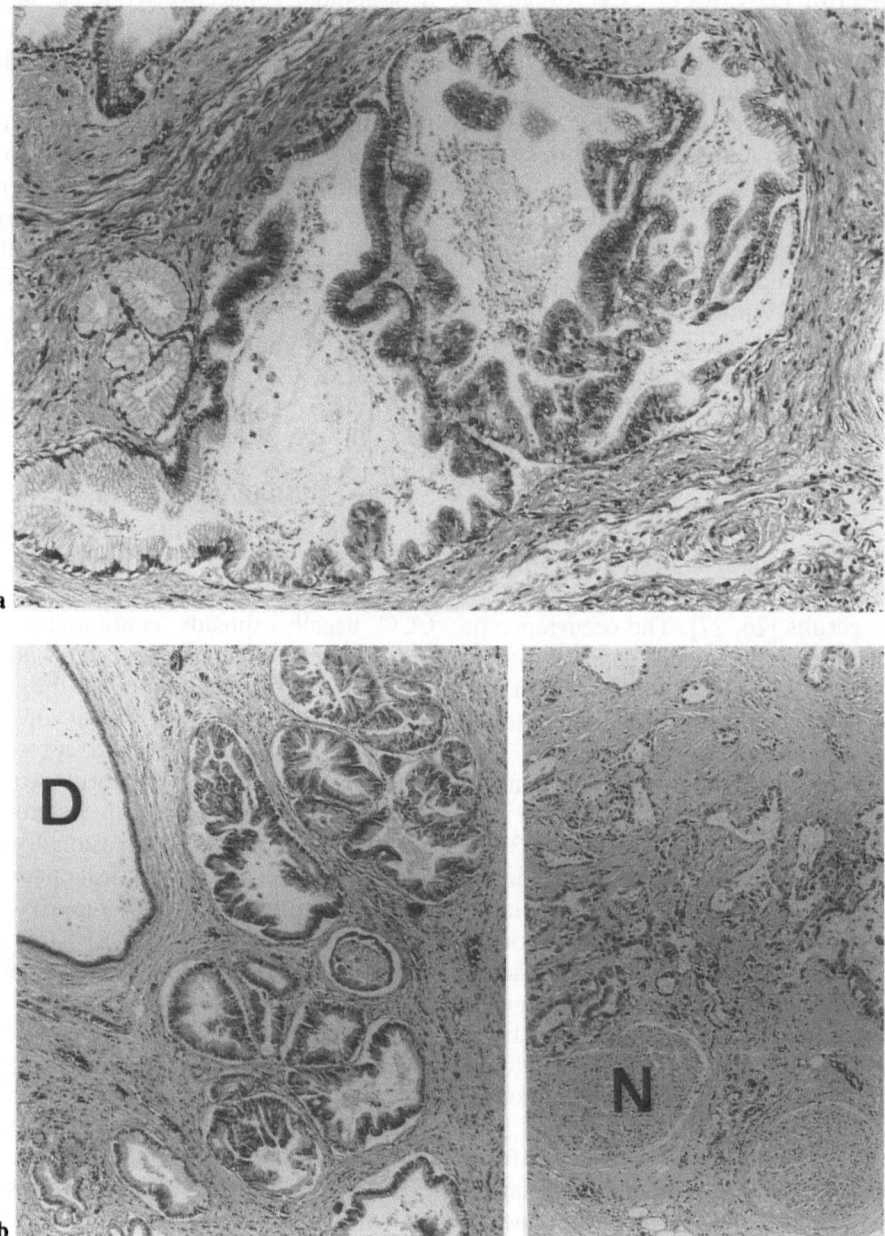

Fig. 6a–c. a Papillary hyperplasia of intrahepatic peribiliary glands is admixed with non-papillary glandular epithelium. These lesions are incidentally found in the intrahepatic peribiliary glands in an autopsy liver H&E, ×100. **b** and **c** are from an autopsy case of cholangiocellular carcinoma probably arising in the intrahepatic peribiliary glands. Atypical hyperplasia of glandular epithelium can be found here and there in the intrahepatic peribiliary glands adjacent to or intermingled with infiltrating carcinoma (**b**). One gland shows cystic dilatation (*D*) H&E, ×100. **c** Infiltrating carcinoma. *N*, nerve fibers. H&E, ×100

compared to the hilar type (33% and 41%). With relation to the histological grades, remote organ metastases were less frequent in well-differentiated CCC relative to poorly differentiated CCC [23].

Some cases of CCC show extensive portal venous involvement, or thrombosis, especially at the hepatic hilus. In such instances, congestive splenomegaly and even esophageal varices develop secondarily [31]. However, collateral vessels are likely to occur [32] and portal hypertension itself is not frequent relative to HCC [13].

6 Immunohistochemistry of cholangiocellular carcinoma

There have been a number of immunohistochemical studies of CCC [33–42], and several selected publications are reviewed here. Purified carcinoembryonic antigen (CEA), carbohydrate antigen 19-9 (CA19-9) and DU-PAN-2 are frequently detected in CCC, usually along the luminal and lateral surfaces and in the apical cytoplasm of the carcinoma cells. Some carcinoma cells show a diffuse and granular cytoplasmic staining pattern. It is also suggested that lectin receptor distribution in CCC is different from that in normal intrahepatic bile ducts and from HCC. Cytokeratin polypeptides (molecular weight: 40, 50, 54, 56.5, 56, and 66 kd) which are positive in normal bile ducts, are retained in CCC cells, though these cytokeratin profiles are negative in HCC. Human chorionic gonadotropin and alpha-fetoprotein were positive in 25% and 2% of CCC cases examined, respectively, especially in poorly differentiated adenocarcinoma or anaplastic carcinoma cells.

7 Pathologic differentiation from reactive hyperplasia or dysplasia, other primary hepatic tumors, and metastastic tumors

7.1 Reactive biliary hyperplasia or dysplasia

It is sometimes difficult to distinguish well-differentiated adenocarcinoma in situ or when there is intraductal spread from reactive hyperplasia of biliary epithelial cells with atypical features (dysplasia) or active proliferation. The latter is seen in biliary obstruction and chronic cholangitis, including hepatolithiasis and primary sclerosing cholangitis (PSC) [6, 43]. It is also of interest that biliary epithelial hyperplasia or dysplasia are found in the biliary tree in the non-neoplastic area of livers with CCC (see section 8.1 below). Nakajima et al. [34] recently reported that nuclear changes (nuclear size variation, irregular nuclear configuration, and increased

nuclear-cytoplasmic ratio), formation of a secondary gland (distended intracytoplasmic lumina or focal cribriform pattern), and positive reaction for CEA were shown to be important histologic criteria for the diagnosis of CCC. One of the three indicators was occasionally positive in non-cancerous bile ducts, but two or three indicators were only found in CCC. Increased expression of CA19-9 and/or DU-PAN-2, and also loss or reduction of sialomucin or sulfomucin in the biliary lining epithelium may be indicative of malignant changes [3, 44]. Qualman et al. emphasized the presence of overt cytological atypia, atypical prominent nucleoli, atypical mitosis, or perineural invasion in histologic diagnosis of CCC [45].

7.2 Hepatocellular carcinoma

Histologic differentiation of CCC from HCC showing glandular differentiation is sometimes difficult. Positive staining for mucin and gland formation indicate a diagnosis of CCC; bile production, Mallory body formation, and trabecular/sinusoidal pattern are suggestive of HCC [39]. The cytokeratin profile is also valuable in the differentiation (see section 6). Combined or mixed HCC and CCC will be described in detail in the section on HCC below.

7.3 Metastatic carcinoma

Because metastatic adenocarcinoma, especially carcinoma from the extrahepatic biliary tree or pancreas, mimics the histologic features of CCC, comprehensive clinicopathologic evaluations, especially autopsy, are required to confirm the diagnosis of CCC. Tumor lesions are usually more numerous in metastatic carcinoma than in CCC. Occurrence of apparently normal epithelium and carcinoma cells within the same duct and also dysplasia of bile ducts in the non-neoplastic liver (see section 8.1) are findings suggestive of a diagnosis of CCC [46, 47]. Immunohistochemical studies using several phenotypic markers of carcinoma failed to differentiate CCC from metastatic adenocarcinoma [35], with the exception that metastatic carcinoma showing characteristic and peculiar phenotypes could be differentiated from CCC. CCC is usually impossible to differentiate on biopsy specimens from metastatic carcinoma.

8   Etiology, preceding pathologic conditions and pathogenesis of cholangiocellular carcinoma

Etiology and preceding pathologic conditions or associated lesions and developmental processes of CCC remain unclear in a great majority of cases. A number of genetic and environmental factors may be involved in the initiation, promotion, or progression of CCC. It has been generally accepted that the following pathologic conditions are likely to precede the development of CCC.

8.1   Suspected etiologies and preceding pathologic conditions in cholangiocellular carcinoma

8.1.1   Gallstones

It is generally accepted that gallstones occur more frequently in patients with CCC compared to the general population [13], though the causal relationship between gallstones and CCC remains only speculative. A few cases of hepatolithiasis associated with CCC, mainly calcium bilirubinates and occasionally cholesterol stones, have been reported in Japan [6, 47–49]. The association of CCC in hepatolithiasis itself is about 10% [6, 50], although an epidemiological survey to determine the exact incidence of CCC in this disease has not yet been done. This condition is different from secondary formation of microcalculi or sludges in the dilated biliary tree in CCC or other hepatic malignancies [51]. CCC is usually found in the stone-containing bile ducts, and CCC tends either to spread along the intrahepatic large bile ducts or to form a tumor mass around the calculi itself. Histologically, adenocarcinoma of variable differentiaton is admixed with non-neoplastic chronic proliferative cholangitis with proliferation of peribiliary glands, characterizing stone-containing bile ducts. Biliary epithelial hyperplasia and dysplasia are occasionally seen in the adjoining non-neoplastic bile ducts bearing bile ducts in these cases. There are also findings of intestinal metaplasia [52]. These atypical biliary epithelia are positive for purified CEA, suggesting that chronic proliferative cholangitis and intestinal metaplasia may be forerunners of CCC [6].

8.1.2   Thorotrast deposition

This contrast medium has been associated with malignant hepatic tumors including CCC, HCC, or angiosarcoma, singly or in various combinations [5, 53]. Non-neoplastic bile ducts in the surrounding liver also show proliferation, and some of the latter show dyslasia or carcinoma in situ.

8.1.3   Liver flukes

CCC has been occasionally reported in Hong Kong and southern China in patients infected with liver flukes [8, 52, 53]. In livers infected with these parasites, the bile ducts show adenomatous proliferation of the peribiliary intramural glands. CCC is reported to develop in bile ducts showing such hyperplastic changes. An experimental model of CCC arising in the bile ducts infected with liver flukes is also known [54]. Such cases have not been reported in Japan to the best of our knowledge.

8.1.4   Bile duct anomalies (Caroli's disease, congenital hepatic fibrosis, and von Meyenburg complexes)

There have been several reports of CCC in livers showing biliary malformations [1, 5, 9, 50]. Hyperplasia of the biliary epithelia with variable atypia in the cystically dilated bile ducts and these proliferative changes may give rise to malignant transformation. Cholangitis associated with bile stasis in the dilated biliary portion may be a contributing factor in CCC development. The formation of von Meyenburg complexes (biliary microhamartoma) is known as a precursor of CCC, while bile duct adenoma is not followed by carcinoma. On occasion, it is important to distinguish small-sized, well-differentiated, peripheral CCC from von Meyenburg complexes or bile duct adenoma.

8.1.5   Carcinoma arising in benign hepatic cysts other than cystadenoma

This condition is heterogeneous. One type is a carcinoma associated with developmental multiple hepatic cysts preferentially occuring in the left hepatic lobe, and the prognosis of this type is very poor [7, 50, 55]. The etiology of this multiple cyst type with CCC is speculated as a hamartomatous cyst. In addition, polycystic liver or solitary liver cysts are also involved in malignant transformation of the lining epithelia. In the early stages, carcinomatous transformation is seen either focally in the lining epithelia of the cyst walls or adjacent to the cyst walls. Some examples of SCC arising in the wall of a hepatic cyst were considered to occur through the squamous metaplasia of the lining epithelium before malignant transformation [56].

Fig. 7a,b. **a** Atypical bile duct in the neighborhood of cholangiocellular carcinoma (*C*). H&E, ×100. **b** A higher magnification of the atypical bile duct. Over half of the circumference of bile duct shows stratification and hyperchromasia. H&E, ×250

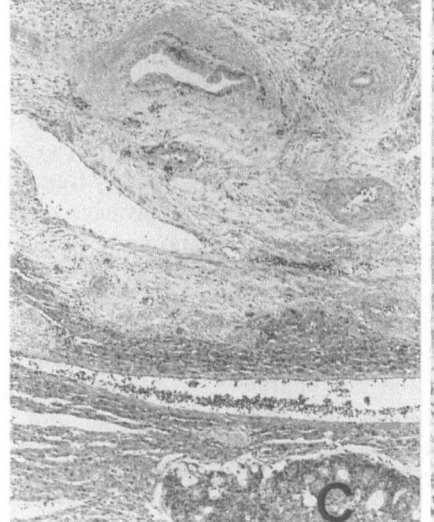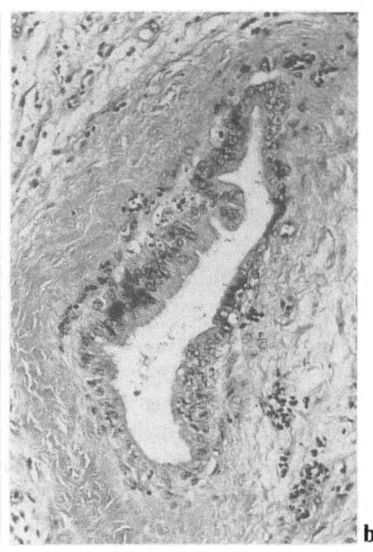

Fig. 8a,b. **a** Biliary cystadenocarcinoma with a papillary growth pattern. The stroma shows hypercellular spindle cells, resembling ovarian stroma. H&E, ×150. **b** Intrahepatic biliary papillomatosis with a villous pattern. Thin fibrous stroma are found beneath the villous tumor. H&E, ×200

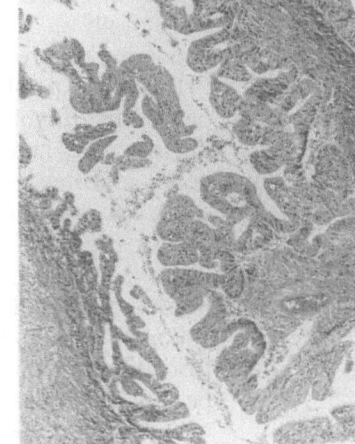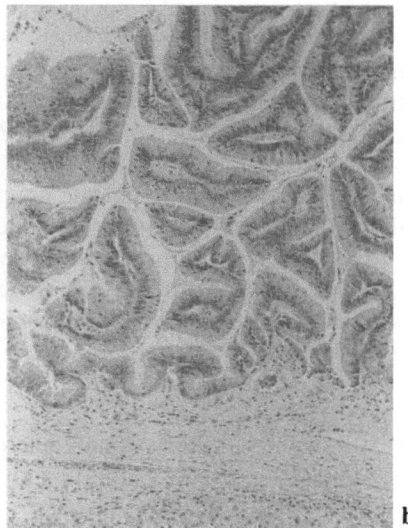

8.1.6 Primary sclerosing cholangitis (PSC) and ulcerative colitis

Some cases of CCC are known to occur in patients suffering from PSC and ulcerative colitis [57, 58]. CCC has been known to develop during clinical follow up of PSC or ulcerative colitis. However, in fully developed cases of CCC, establishing PSC as a preceding condition is frequently difficult because CCC showing biliary stenosis or obstruction frequently manifest biliary sclerosis and non-specific inflammation resembling PSC. Chronic inflammation and regeneration of the biliary lining cells are possible pre-neoplatic changes. The incidence of PSC is now increasing in Japan, suggesting that this complication may be given more attention in the near future.

8.1.7 Biliary dysplasia and/or transition to adenocarcinoma in the non-neoplastic bile ducts in cholangiocellular carcinoma

In CCC without known etiologies or preceding pathologic conditions, dysplasia of biliary epithelia is occasionally encountered in the non-carcinomatous bile ducts at any anatomical level, either remote from or adjacent to the carcinoma (Fig. 7) [10, 53]. These changes may be related to the development and progression of CCC and some could be actually involved in multicentric carcinogenesis. Some changes may be undergoing malignant transformation or may actually become carcinoma in situ. Their exact nature and final form are open to future studies.

9 Special forms or related types of choangiocellular carcinoma

9.1 Biliary Cystadenocarcinoma

Biliary cystadenocarcinoma is a malignant cystic tumor lined by mucus-secreting epithelium with papillary infoldings (Fig. 8a), which usually arises from biliary cystadenoma [1, 5, 50, 59]. This carcinoma is rare, and shows slight predominance among females. Multilocular mucinous cysts which are grossly identifiable are characteristically seen in this type of tumor. The cysts are usually well-demarcated. Histologically, a papillary or villous pattern of adenocarcinoma with high columnar neoplastic epithelia and mucinous overproduction is seen. Goblet cells and endocrine cells are also intermingled with the neoplastic epithelial cells. The presence of non-malignant epithelial neoplastic components suggests that cystadenoma coexists or is intermingled with this carcinoma, and there are abrupt transitions between these benign and malignant components in one half of the cases. Mesenchymal stroma resembing ovarian stroma and smooth muscle fibers is seen under the neoplastic epithelium in some cases. However, cystadenocarcinoma without such peculiar stroma is also well known. Biologic differences between cystadenocarcinoma with and without peculiar stromal changes remain unclarified.

9.2 Intrahepatic biliary papillomatosis

Papillomatosis is a papillary tumor of variable distribution and extent in the intrahepatic biliary tree with varying histologic atypia (Fig. 8b) [60]. The extrahepatic biliary tree, including the gallbladder, is also involved on occasion. The course is marked by recurrence and biliary tract obstruction with cholangitis. Papillary, fragile tumors are seen on the inner surface of the dilated biliary tree either mulitply or diffusely. Some cases show such papillary tumors in one confined segment of the intrahepatic biliary tree [61]. Histologically, papillary or villous tumors show fine fibrovascular stalks from which branching papillary fronds lined by columnar to cuboidal epithelial cells with basal nuclei emanate (Fig. 9). In addition to macroscopically identifiable tumors, other biliary epithelial lining cells are also neoplastic in their character histologically. This type of tumor is usually associated with overproduction of mucinous substances which fill the dilated bile ductal lumina [62]. While infiltration into the surrounding liver and also extrahepatic metastases are rare, this tumor is potentially malignant and the potential for growth and spread along and within the biliary tree is great. Some cases even progress to invasive, mucin-producing papillary carcinoma, especially at the terminal stages.

9.3 Carcinoids or endocrine tumours and pancreatic-like tumors

Carcinoid tumors [5] are rarely reported in the liver. We have seen an autopsy case of endocrine carcinoma of the liver with a rosetta formation resembling small cell carcinoma of the lung. The tissue of origin remains, however, speculative. Recently, neuroendocrine differentiation has been reported in primary neoplasm of the liver. While such differentiation was rather common in HCC, only 2 of 6 cases of CCC showed such endocrine differentiation [5, 33].

Recently, papillary cystic tumors resembling pancreatic tumors in terms of clinical, gross, microscopic, and ultrastructural features have been reported [63]. Large, well-demarcated, solid, and cystic tumors in the liver showed two basic patterns of cellular arrangement histologically: a papillary pattern with fairly prominent fibrovascular stalks with 1–3 cell layers of tall to cuboidal cells, and a solid growth with microcyst formation. Ectopic pancreatic tissue around the peribiliary glands may be related to the occurence of this type of carcinoma [64].

References

1. Gibson JB, Sobin LH (1978) Histological typing of tumours of the liver, biliary tract and pancreas. World Health Organization, Geneva
2. Sugihara S, Kojiro M (1987) Pathology of cholangiocarcinoma. In: Okuda K, Ishka K (eds) Neoplasms of the liver. Springer-Verlag, Tokyo, pp 143–158
3. Terada T, Nakanuma Y (1990) Pathological observations of intrahepatic peribiliary glands in 1,000 consecutive autopsy livers: A possible source of cholangiocarcinoma. Hepatology 12:92–97
4. Steiner PE, Higginson J (1959) Cholangiocellular carcinoma. Cancer 12:753–759

5. Craig JR, Peters RL, Edmondson HA (1989) Tumors of the liver and intrahepatic bile ducts. Armed Forces Institute of Pathology, Washington DC, vol 26 pp 197–222

6. Nakanuma Y, Terada T, Tanaka Y, Ohta G (1985) Are hepatolithiasis and cholangiocarcinoma etiologically related? A morphological study of 12 cases of hepatolithiasis with cholangiocarcinoma. Virchows Arch [A] 406:45–58

7. Imamura M, Miyashita T, Tani T, Naito A, Tobe T, Takahashi K (1984) Cholangiocellular carcinoma associated with multiple liver cysts. Am J Gastroenterol 79:790–795

8. Flavell DJ (1981) Liver-fluke infection as an etiological factor in bile-duct carcinoma of man. Trans R Soc Trop Med Hyg 75:814–824

9. Homer LW, White HJ, Read RC (1968) Neoplastic transformation of von Meyenburg complexes of the liver. J Pathol Bact 96:499–502

10. Anthony PP (1979) Hepatic neoplasms. In: RNM MacSween, PP Anthony, PJ Scheuer (eds) Pathology of the liver. Churchill Livingstone, Edinburgh, pp 387–413

11. The Liver Cancer Study Group of Japan (1980) Primary liver cancers in Japan. Cancer 45: 2663–2669

12. Mori W, Nagasako K (1976) Cholangiocarcinoma and related lesions. In: Okuda K, Peters RL (eds) Hepatocellular carcinoma. Wiley, New York, pp 227–246

13. Okuda K, Kubo Y, Okazaki N, Arishima T, Hashimoto M, Jinnouchi S, Sawa Y, Shimokawa Y, Nakajima Y, Noguchi T, Nakano M, Kojiro M, Nakashima T (1977) Clinical aspects of intrahepatic bile duct carcinoma including hilar carcinoma. A study of 57 autopsy-proven cases. Cancer 39:232–246

14. Kamiyama Y, Tobe T (1987) Treatment of primary liver cancer in Japan. In: Okuda K, and Ishak K (eds) Neoplasms of the liver. Springer-Verlag, Tokyo, pp 375–380

15. Healey JE, Schroy PC (1953) Anatomy of the biliary ducts within the human lives. Arch Surg 66:599–616

16. Terada T, Nakanuma Y, Ohta G (1987) Glandular elements around the intrahepatic bile ducts in man; their morphology and distribution in normal livers. Liver 7:1–8

17. Nakanuma Y, Ohta G (1979) Histometric and serial section observations of the intrahepatic bile ducts in primary biliary cirrhosis. Gastroenterology 76:1326–1332

18. Japanese Biliary Surgical Society (1981) General rules for surgical studies on cancer of biliary tract. Kanehara, Tokyo

19. Liver Cancer Study Group of Japan (1987) The general rules for the clinical and pathological study of primary liver cancer (2nd edn) Kanehara, Tokyo

20. Klatskin G (1965) Adenocarcinoma of the hepatic duct at its bifurcation within the porta hepatis. Am J Med 38:241–256

21. Bosma A (1990) Surgical pathology of cholangiocarcinoma of the liver hilus (Klatskin tumor). Semin Liver Dis 10:85–90

22. Eggel H (1901) Über das Carcinom der Leber. Beitr. z Path Anat u z allgem Pathol 30:506–604

23. Nakajima T, Kondo Y, Miyazaki M, Okui K (1988) A histopathologic study of 102 cases of intrahepatic cholangiocarcinoma: Histologic classification and modes of spreading. Hum Pathol 19:1228–1234

24. Nakajima T, Kondo Y (1990) A clinicopathologic study of intrahepatic cholangiocarcinoma containing a component of squamous cell carcinoma. Cancer 65:1401–1404

25. Hayashi M, Sugiura H, Ohta G, Shimazaki H, Kyoui Y, Nakanuma Y (1988) Cholangiocellular carcinoma with negative mucin staining (in Japanese). Jap J Gastroenterol 85:1555–1558

26. Ho JCI (1980) Two cases of mucoepidermoid carcinoma of the liver. Pathology 12:123–128

27. Arase Y, Endo Y, Kumada H, Ikeda K, Yoshiba A (1988) Hepatic squamous cell carcinoma with hypercalcemia in liver cirrhosis. Acta Pathol Jpn 38:643–650

28. Sasaki M, Nakanuma Y, Nagai Y, Nonomura A (1991) An autopsy case of intrahepatic cholangiocarcinoma with sarcomatous transformation. J Clin Gastroenterol 13:220–225

29. Terada T, Sasaki M, Nakanuma Y, Takeda Y, Masunaga T (in press) Hilar cholangiocarcinoma (Klatskin tumor) probably arising from intrahepatic peribiliary glands. J Clin Gastroenterol

30. Nakashima T, Kojiro M, Kawano Y, Shirai F, Takemoto N, Tomimatsu H, Kawasaki H, Okuda K (1982) Histologic growth pattern of hepatocellular carcinoma. Relationship to orcein (hepatitis B surface-antigen)-positive cells in cancer tissue. Hum Pathol 13:563–568

31. Gold JA, Sostman HD, Burrell MI (1979) Cholangiocarcinoma with portal vein obstruction. Radiology 130:15–20

32. Terada T, Hoso M, Nakanuma Y, Ohta T, Makino Y (1989) Extrahepatic portal venous obstruction of different pathogenesis in pancreatic diseases: Report of 4 autopsy cases with chronic pancreatitis and pancreatic carcinoma. Gastroenterol Jpn 24:414–420

33. Wang J, Dhillon AP, Sankey EA, Wightman AK, Lewin JF, Scheuer PJ (1990) "Neuroendocrine" differentiation in primary neoplasms of the liver. J Pathol 163:61–67

34. Nakajima T, Kondo Y (1989) Well-differentiated cholangiocarcinoma: diagnostic significance of morphologic and immunohistochemical parameters. Am J Surg Pathol 13:569–573

35. Hurlimann J, Gardiol D (1991) Immunohistochemistry in the differential diagnosis of liver carcinomas. Am J Surg Pathol 15:280–288

35. Zhang S, Wu W, Chen H, Zhang X, Cong W, Sho H (1989) Characteristics of the distribution of

lectin receptors in intrahepatic cholangiocellular carcinoma. Histochem J 21:296–300

37. Nakanuma Y, Unoura M, Noto H, Ohta G (1986) Human chorionic gonadotropin in primary liver carcinoma in adults: An immunohistochemical study. Virchows Arch [A] 409:365–373

38. Nonomura A, Mizukami Y, Matsubara F, Izumi R, Nakanuma Y, Hayashi M, Watanabe K, Takayanagi N (1989) Human chorionic gonadotropin and alpha-fetoprotein in cholangiocarcinoma in relation to expression of p21: An immunohistochemical study. Liver 9:205–215

39. Goodman ZD, Ishak KG, Longloss JM, Sesterhenn IA, Rabin LL (1985) Combined hepatocellular-cholangiocarcinoma. A histologic and immunohistochemical study. Cancer 55: 124–135

40. Nakanuma Y, Sasaki M (1989) Expression of blood group-related antigens in the intrahepatic biliary tree and hepatocytes in normal livers and various hepatobiliary diseases. Hepatology 10:174–178.

41. Hurliman J, Gardiol D (1991) Immunohistochemistry in the differential diagnosis of liver carcinomas. Am J Surg Pathol 15:280–288

42. Lai YS, Thung SN, Gerber MA, Chen ML, Schaffner F (1989) Expression of cytokeratins in normal and diseased livers and primary liver carcinoma. Arch Pathol Lab Med 113:134–138

43. Nakanuma Y, Yamaguchi K, Ohta G, Terada T, Japanese Study Group of Hepatolithiasis (1988) Pathologic features of hepatolithiasis in Japan. Hum Pathol 19:1181–1186

44. Chou ST, Chan CW, Ng WL (1976) Mucin histochemistry of human cholangiocarcinoma. J Pathol 118:165–170

45. Qualman SJ, Haupt HM, Bauer TW, Taxy JB (1984) Adenocarcinoma of the hepatic duct junction: A reappraisal of the histologic criteria of malingancy. Cancer 53:1545–1551

46. Scheuer PJ (1988) Liver biopsy interpretation. 4th ed., Bailliere Tindall, London, Philadelphia, Toronto, Sydney, Tokyo

47. Weibern K, Mutum SS (1983) Pathological aspects of cholangiocarcinoma. J Pathol 139:217–238

48. Koga A, Ichimiya H, Yamaguchi K, Miyazaki K, Nakayama F (1985) Hepatolithiasis associated with cholangiocarcinoma. Possible etiologic signifiance. Cancer 55:2826–2829

49. Terada T, Ishida F, Nakanuma Y (1989) Intrahepatic cholesterol stones associated with peripheral cholangiocellular carcinoma: An autopsy case. Am J Gastroenterol 84:1434–1436

50. Mizumoto R, Kawarada Y (1987) Diagnosis and treatment of cholangiocarcinoma and cystic adenocarcinoma of the liver. In: Okuda K, and Ishka K (eds) Neoplasms of the liver. Springer-Verlag, Tokyo, pp 381–396

51. Terada T, Nakanuma Y, Saito K, Kono N (1990) Biliary sludge and microcalculi in intrahepatic bile ducts. Morphologic and X-ray microanalytical observations in 18 among 1,179 consecutively autopsied livers. Acta Pathol Jpn 40:894–901

52. Kurumaya H, Terada T, Nakanuma Y (1990) 'Metaplastic lesions' in intrahepatic bile ducts in hepatolithiasis: A histochemical and immuno-histochemical study. J Gastroenterol Hepatol 5:532–538

53. Rubel LR, Ishak KM (1982) Thorotrast-associated cholangiocarcinoma. An epidemiologic and clinicopathologic study. Cancer 50:1408–1415

54. Kim YI, Yu ES, Kim ST (1989) Intraductal variant of peripheral cholangiocarcinoma of the liver with Clonorchis sinensis infection. Cancer 63:187–197

55. Azizah N, Oaradubas FJ (1980) Cholangiocarcinoma coexisting with developmental liver cysts: A distinct entity different from liver cystadenocarcinoma. Histopathology 4:391–400

56. Bloustein PA, Silverberg SG (1976) Squamous cell carcinoma originating in a hepatic cyst: Case report with a review of the hepatic cyst-carcinoma association. Cancer 38:2002–2005

57. Wee A, Ludwig J, Coffey RJ, LaRusso NF, Wiesner RH (1985) Hepatobiliary carcinoma associated with primary sclerosing cholangitis and chronic ulcerative colitis. Hum Pathol 16:719–726

58. Haworth AC, Manely PN, Groll A, Pace R (1989) Bile duct carcinoma and biliary tract dysplasia in chronic ulcerative colitis. Arch Pathol Lab Med 113:434–436

59. Wheeler DA, Edmondson HA (1985) Cystadenoma with mesenchymal stroma (CMS) in the liver and bile ducts. A clinicopathological study of 17 cases, 4 with malignant change. Cancer 56:1434–1445

60. Okulski EG, Dolin BJ, Kandawalla NM (1979) Intrahepatic biliary papillomatosis. Arch Pathol Lab Med 103:647–649

61. Terada T, Mitsui T, Nakanuma Y, Miura S, Toya D (in press) Intrahepatic papillomatosis in non-obstructive intrahepatic biliary dilatations confined to the hepatic left lobe. Am J Gastroenterol

62. Ohta T, Konishi K, Higashino Y, Asano A, Izumi R, Nagakawa T, Kinami Y, Miyazaki I, Okada Y (1983) A case of mucinous biliary obstruction associated with multiple cholangiocarcinoma (in Japanese). Tan To Sui 4:687–692

63. Kim YI, Kim ST, Lee GK, Choi BI (1990) Papillary cystic tumor of the liver. A case report with ultrastructural observation. Cancer 65: 2740–2746

64. Terada T, Nakanuma Y, Kakita A (1990) Pathologic observations of intrahepatic peribiliary glands in 1,000 consecutive autopsy livers: Heterotropic pancreas in the liver. Gastroenterology 98: 1333–1337

CHAPTER 6

Historical overview of research into the etiology of hepatocellular carcinoma

Toshitsugu Oda[1]

1 Introduction

Whether hepatocellular carcinoma (HCC) can be induced by viruses or not is a recent area of study in the field of molecular biomedicine and also a medical issue of worldwide concern. In Japan, cancer claims the life of 190,000 people a year and now ranks as the number one cause of death. Deaths from the disease have recently exceeded the figures for circulatory diseases, which kill more than 140,000 annually. We have overcome diseases caused by bacteria one after the other, with tuberculosis as a most recent example, and as a result during these past decades, our average life span has been extended significantly. In parallel with this extended longevity, cancer and circulatory diseases have begun to draw general attention today.

Of all the kinds of cancers, lung cancer and liver cancer are on the increase; slightly fewer than 30,000 people die of lung cancer and approximately 20,000 of liver cancer every year. On the other hand, stomach cancer is somehow on the decrease; fewer than 50,000 people now die of this disease annually. If things continue like this, before long, HCC will exceed stomach cancer in terms of the claim on lives, at least as far as men are concerned. HCC should receive serious consideration when planning measures for adult diseases. Of all adult diseases, Liver-related diseases rank in fourth place as the most common cause of death, after circulatory diseases, lung cancer, and stomach cancer. About 16,000 people die of liver cirrhosis, 18,000 of HCC, and 3,000 of fulminant hepatitis every year. All together, about 40,000 people die of liver-related diseases annually.

The main causes of liver-related diseases include alcohol and toxins of chemical and bacterial origin. A range of viruses are also responsible, including those causing latent infection and those with vertical transmission. In Japan, since January 1, 1986, initiatives have been taken to prevent mother to child transmission of hepatitis B virus (HBV). Under this scheme, new babies born to mothers positive HBe for antigens are treated using funds from the national and local government. About 4,500 newborn babies a year are administered 1,000 IU of HBs antibody γ-globulin. This is followed with HB vaccine (HBs antigen 10 μg) 2 months after birth and additional vaccine treatment 3 months and 5 months after birth. We think this treatment will be able to prevent about 95% of the vertical transmission. If so, it is expected that hepatitis B will be eradicated in Japan after about 50 years. The World Health Organization (WHO) is showing a strong interest in the program because at present there are 280 million HBV carriers worldwide. It should be noted that three-fourths of the carriers are concentrated in the Asia-Pacific region. The former Director of WHO, Dr. Mahler, emphasizes that the HB vaccine trials are the first ever to focus on an immunological measure for the prevention of human cancer. It goes without saying that other measures for cancer will follow suit.

Liver cancer serves as evidence confirming that human cancer can be caused by a virus. At present, cancers of known viral origin in humans include nasopharynginoma caused by the EB virus, adult T cell leukemia caused by HTLV-1, and cancer of the uterus, probably caused by a papilloma virus. Hopefully, vaccines to treat these diseases will be developed in the near future.

The direct relationship between cancer and viruses has been confirmed only recently. This

[1] Japanese Red Cross Medical Center, Hiroo, Shibuya-ku, Tokyo, 150 Japan

development is attributable to the progress of genetic engineering and of the cloning of human viruses. From a recent discovery, it is now thought that HBV-DNA integrates into the chromosomal DNA of HCC cells or its cultured cells derived from HBV carriers. This is considered as requisite for viral carcinogenesis. In light of this research, carcinogenesis can now be interpreted on the gene level, and progress can be made towards determining the relationship between the transformation by oncogenic viruses in animals and the integration of viral DNA. Our knowledge of the process of carcinogenesis has developed from studies into celluar multiplication, and with the progress to interpretation at the gene level, much attention is currently being paid to human oncogenes. In addition, recent interesting research has shown that other viruses, such as hepatitis C virus (HCV) and the RNA virus Flavi, can induce HCC more easily, as they are not integrated in the host hepatocyte DNA.

The study of human hepatitis, especially in Asia where it is most common, is coincidentally triggering great interest and is contributing to the study of HCC and related liver diseases.

2 Background of liver cancer research in Japan

Miura first recorded primary liver cancer in 1889. Until then, most of the papers that appeared in Europe and the United States described metastatic one and they could not easily distinguish these two types of liver cancers. In 1911, Yamagiwa, named the two types of primary liver cancer "hepatoma" and "cholangioma." In 1914, Nagayo classified liver cirrhosis into types A and B, and in 1929, Kiya claimed the annexation of liver cancer into type B. The high incidence in Japan was thought to be something to do with the nature and circumstances of the country, and in fact there were many patients with liver diseases due to hepatitis viruses.

Of all industrialized nations, the Soviet Union, Eastern European countries, and Japan are cited as countries where HBV carriers account for more than 2% of the population. This result may be related to the fact that the immunoadherence hemagglutination (IAHA) method was developed by Nishioka et al. in 1971 while the reverse passive hemagglutination (RPHA) method was invented by Juji et al. in 1975. The development of RPHA followed the discovery of Australia antigen by Blumberg in 1964, and the clarification of its significance as a certain antigen related to post-transfusion hepatitis by Okochi in 1970. Because of this, epidemiological research into hepatitis B made rapid progress in Japan. Serum hepatitis was also a kind of social problem in those days. Since many people suffered jaundice after blood transfusions, we launched a nationwide drive, the so-called yellow blood campaign. Our research group played a leading role in promoting the study of viral hepatitis and its sequelae. We began to work on a vaccine in 1975, and the type B vaccine was developed in 1979, as mentioned earlier. The development of the vaccine led to the government's full understanding of measures required concerning the disease; many Japanese suffering from liver cirrhosis and liver cancer had carried the viruses from generation to generation.

Another reason for the progress of liver cancer research in Japan is that the country was the site of study into experimental chemical carcinogenesis in the liver. In 1915, Yamagiwa released his study on coal tar-induced cancer in the rabbit ear; in 1932, Sasaki and Yoshida described the use of orthoaminoazotoluol; in 1936, Kinoshita described butter yellow. It is to be noted that the studies of viral carcinogenesis in Rous sarcoma in 1911 and Fujinami sarcoma in 1913 were made almost at the same time. Today, the theories of chemical and viral carcinogenesis go hand in hand through the elucidation of the role of the oncogene in the body.

The high incidence of HCC in Japan and neighboring countries was initially attributed to red pepper, and curry and rice were suspected as enhancing the probability of jaundice, and so on. Today, however, HCC is seen as a typical cancer induced by viruses. We came to know that hepatitis is caused by viruses through a report by Hiro (1941) of the successful transmission of jaundice to human volunteers by coating the pharyngeal mucous membrane with the ultrafiltrate of the serum from other patients with acute hepatitis. In addition Voegt (1942) achieved similar results by the oral administration of duodenal juice or by the subcutaneous and intramuscular injection of blood or serum from jaundiced patients. Following this, researchers all over the world eagerly looked for other such viruses. For infection experiments, Kitaoka used Japanese monkeys (*Macaca fuscata*) during World War II.

3 Past search of causes of HCC

The search for the cause of liver cancer, especially HCC, began with experiments on chemical carcinogenesis. The experiment on coal tar-induced cancer was derived from the clinical theory that there might be a relation between chimney cleaning and scrotal carcinoma. Yamagiwa used rabbit ears for experiments on carcinogenesis, although we now know they do not become cancerous easily, and Sasaki and Yoshida studied orthoaminoazotoluol from the viewpoint of its affinity with organ tissues. Fortunately, this proved to be a good combination of easily carcinogenic liver cells and azo pigments.

The supposition that HCC is of viral origin comes from epidemiological studies as an infectious disease. The study of liver diseases started at the same time as the search for the cause of jaundice and liver cirrhosis, and these diseases were also found to be infectious. As ever most, obvious phenomena are looked at first.

In 1819 Laennec adopted the name "cirrhose" after "kirrhos," which is a Greek yellow bird. In his writing he pointed out that it was not "skirrhos." It was translated into "kankohen" in Japanese, literally liver hardening, and not "kan ohen" which literally means liver yellowing. However, the reason for the original emphasis on liver yellowing regardless of liver hardening by Laennec may have been that cirrhosis is softer than cancer. It was known that the word "skirrhos" was used by Hippocrates for a hard tumor. Being aware of this, perhaps, Laennec intentionally avoided words which meant hardness.

Research into liver diseases consisted of the search for the cause of the above-mentioned yellow hardening and yellowing. It is the same with the search for the causes of HCC. Comparatively, carcinogenesis draws as much attention today, with liver cells being considered as a suitable target to approach.

4 Relationship between HBV, cirrhosis, and cancer of the liver

It is quite often the case that HCC accompanies liver cirrhosis (LC), but the frequency of this combination largely varies from place to place.

Explaining this fact is one of the most important aspects in research into the causes of LC. Alcohol poisoning and chemical or bacterial toxins were regarded as the main causes. Amano [1], suggested vaguely that viral hepatitis might develop into cirrhosis and then into cancer, a great insight for those early days.

In Europe and the United States, in general, LC does not accompany HCC, where as in Japan and Asian countries LC often accompanies HCC. As it was considered attributable to alcohol in Europe and the US, it was thought there was no common ground for the LC seen there and in Japan. Alcohol is not the cause in ours, and the inference is that a virus may be the cause. When this assumption was introduced in the Congress of geological pathology in north European countries there was strong opposition from many researchers of the world. The evidence was requested, so that alcohol might be ruled out in patients with LC in our country.

There were, on the other hand, case reports on the combination of viral hepatitis and HCC at that time, but they were very few in number; only a few reports by Sheldon and James [2], Walsche and Wolff [3] and some others. In Japan, a long-term follow-up study of viral hepatitis conducted by Kosaka et al. revealed some cases of HCC, but it has since been found that they were neither hepatitis A nor B. The statistics of the National Cancer Center of Japan (Arima, 1968) showed that of 238 cases of hepatitis accompanied by cirrhosis, 39 cases had HCC and that of these 39 cases, 16 cases had had transfusion and 21 cases had hepatitis patients within their families. These facts gradually drew the attention of investigators concerned.

At this stage in the research, Australian antigen, or HBs antigen (HBs Ag), was discovered. This matter was raised in the hepatitis symposium for the WHO report on viral hepatitis [4], especially in Nishioka's seroepidemiological work [5-7] and Obayashi's work [8] concerning LC and families with Australia antigen. A 1975 WHO report also revealed that HBs Ag was very often detected in the serum of HCC patients in Africa, Japan, and other parts of Asia where there are many HCC patients. Further research by Shikata [9] showed HBs Ag inclusion bodies by orcein. As a matter of fact, Japanese researchers have participated in and contributed to the research of hepatitis viruses since the early days (Table 1).

As already mentioned, there are 280 million HBV carriers over the world and three quarters

Table 1. Hepatitis virus research, related to HCC

Author	Year	Discovery
McDonald	1908	Virus suggested as the cause of epidemic hepatitis
Hiro	1941	Human innoculations with hepatitis virus
Voegt	1942	Human innoculations with hepatitis virus
MacCallum	1944	Human innoculations with types A and B hepatitis virus
Amano	1952	Virus-induced liver cirrhosis suggested
Blumberg	1964	Australia antigen
Krugman	1967	MS1, MS2
Okochi	1967	Unidentified antigen in transfusion blood
Okochi	1970	Blood transfusion and Au-Ag
Dane	1970	Hepatitis B virus particle
Almeida	1971	HBcAg & HBsAg
Mayumi, Okochi, Nishioka	1971	HBsAg assay method (IAHA)
Obayashi	1971	Familial clustering of HBsAg and cirrhosis
Shikata	1972	HBsAg inclusion body
Ling, Overby	1972	HBaAg assay method (RIA)
Le Bouvier, Bancroft	1972	HBsAg subtypes
Magnius and Murakami	1972	e antigen
WHO report	1973	HCC and HBsAg
Kaplan	1973	DNA polymerase in HBV core
Feinstone, Purcell	1973	HA virus discovered, immune-electronmicrography
Robinson	1974	DNA double chain from Dane particulates
Prince	1974	Existence of Hepatitis C suggested
Juji, Sekine, Mayumi	1975	RPHA of HBsAg assay
Houghton et al.	1988	Hepatitis C antibody

Table 2. Pattens of hepatitis B prevalence[a] [10]

	Low	Intermediate	High
HBsAg	0.2%–0.5%	2–7%	8–20%
Anti-HBs	4–6%	20–55%	70–95%
Childhood infection	infrequent	frequent, neonatal infection frequent	infection highly frequent, neonatal infection highly frequent
Location	Australia, central Europe, North America	Eastern Europe, Japan, Mediterranean, South-west Asia, USSR	Some parts of China, Southern Asia, Tropical Africa

[a] Prevalences up to 50% have been identified in some isolated Pacific islands

of them live in Asia-Pacific region. It is to be noted that the WHO guidance for the vaccination strategy was taken up in the task force meeting held in Nagasaki in 1985 [10] (Table 2). According to these reports, in Africa and the Asia-Pacific region, HBV carriers account for 5%–20% of the whole population. In these regions, the incidence of HCC is also high with the maximum incidence of 150 cases in every 100,000. HBsAg is detected in 50%–80% of these HCC patients, and these are HBV carriers. In contrast, there is only a small number of HBV carriers in North America and Europe: only 0.13%–1.0% of the whole population. Also the incidence of HCC is very low with 1–3 cases in every 100,000. In these areas, 5%–30% of HCC patients are HBV carriers.

From the other investigations of HCC in Africa, Asia, and other parts of the world, one report stated that of the total 2,387 cases studied, there were 1,439 cases (53.6%) in which HBs antigen was detected, while for the 20,251 cases in the control group, there were 823 (4.1%) in which the antigen was detected. The region that showed the highest percentage (71.9%) was the Pacific region (control group 0.3%). In the US and Europe, the main cause of LC is alcoholic liver injury, and both the number of HBV carriers and positivity rate of HBsAg in HCC are small. Except in cases accompanied by alcoholic cir-

Table 3. Recommendations for hepatitis B vaccine prophylaxis to prevalence of HBV [11, 18]

low prevalence		intermediate or high prevalence	
pre-exposure	post-exposure	pre-exposure[a]	post-exposure
high risk groups (health care personnel, dialysis patients, institutionalized patients, drug addicts, male homosexuals, military recruits)	accidental percutaneous exposure, infants of HBsAg positive mothers, sexual contacts of acute cases, and carriers	all infants or selected	infant of HBsAg-positive mothers

[a] on the basis of *"selected"* in Japan

rhosis, the positivity rate of HBsAg in HCC is still high, namely it is the same with the region where there are many HCC patients.

It can be said that in regions with many HBV carriers, a large number of HCC cases are reported and the ratio of HBV carriers relative to HCC patients is high in number. Therefore, it is almost certain that there is an etiological relationship between HBV sustained infection and HCC. In Japan, an investigation was conducted by the Liver Cancer Study Group of Japan [11] for a two-year period of 1980–1981 covering 405 facilities throughout the country. Results showed that of 1,645 cases of HCC, HBs Ag was detected in 517 cases (31.4%). According to the clinical tracking report, the most dangerous infection occurred in the neonatal period which most probably induces HBV carriers.

4 HCC associated with hepatitis C virus (HCV)

In Japan HCC is one of the most prevalent cancers. However, at most, 25% of HCC patients are positive for HBsAg. If so, there must be another virus which is involved in the carcinogenesis of the liver. To investigate a potential role for HCV in the development of HCC, the following study was done through the HCV antibody assay Chiron devised in 1988.

Sera from 105 HBsAg-negative HCC patients were collected and assayed for antibody to HCV antigen (HCVAb). Most of these patients (76.2%) were found to be positive for HCVAb, even though the prevalence in sera from blood donors is 1.1%. A history of blood transfusion was found in 39.6% of the cases positive for HCVAb, which was significantly different to the lower rate (4.7%) observed in HCC patients who

were both positive for HBsAg and negative for HCVAb ($P < 0.001$) [12].

Statistics in Japan indicate that the numbers of fatal cases of liver cancer reported to the Ministry of Health and Welfare of Japan have dramatically increased from 1978 to 1985, as compared with those from 1968 to 1977. The number of deaths with liver cancer a year per 10^5 were 9.5 in 1968 to 1977, and 16.0 in 1984 to 1985 [12]. However, the numbers of the HBsAg-positives among the HCC patients have decreased from 1968 to 1985 according to the reports by the Liver Cancer Study Group of Japan: 40.7% (1968–1977), down to 24.6% (1984–1985) [11]. Based on these figures, it is estimated that the mortality rate in association with liver cancer and HBsAg positivity is 3.9 (1968–1977) and 4.0 (1984–1985) per year per 10^5, respectively. In striking contrast, the mortality rate, with respect to HBsAg negative liver cancer per year per 10^5 has increased significantly by 2.14 times from 5.6 (1968–1977) to 12.1 (1984–1985). Therefore, HCV should be noted in the elucidation of the causative agent of HBsAg-negative HCC cases, which are 75% of the HCC cases in recent years.

6 Carcinogenesis of the liver by viruses

No doubt there is a relationship between hepatitis and HBV, and our experience shows that the HCV virus may play an important role. Japan should determine at which point the HBV-DNA integrates in the process leading to chronic hepatitis. The cloning of human viruses triggered a rush of studies on carcinogenic mechanisms at gene level, and we now need close cooperation between the basic research side and the clinical side to track such cases over time. HCV studies should then be carried out with reference to the HCC problem.

The integration of genes of DNA tumor viruses or RNA tumor viruses into cellular chromosomes through the action of reverse-transcriptase is a common phenomenon. Some tumor viruses possess oncogenes (viral oncogene, v-onc), but this is not the case with HBV. Therefore, studies using recombinant HBV are now being conducted into the conditions that allow the existence of HBV-DNA in HBV-infected liver cells, HCC cells, and cultured cells derived from HCC. The main concern is to determine what effect such a virus has on the cellular oncogene (c-onc), e.g. the effect of the HB-X gene [13] on the c-onc.

7 HCC-diagnosis and treatment

Analysis of α-Fetoprotein levels (Abelev, 1963; Tatarinov, 1965) has enabled serum diagnosis of HCC. It is this serum diagnosis that realized Greenstein's thesis II (proposed by Nakahara) in a practical way. It can be said that the protein is the first example of actual genetic reversion. It will not help so much in the early detection of HCC but will be truly helpful with time in follow-up observations. The shortcomings, however, should be accepted to a certain degree as far as peripheral blood is concerned. On the contrary, supersonic tomography, computer tomography, and also angiography are found to be more effective on the strength of their directness of procedure. In treatment of HCC, partial hepatectomy or embolization of the hepatic artery have shown great effects so far. It is to be hoped that the so-called missile therapy will make progress in the near future.

8 Future of HCC study

HCC should be considered as one of the viral-infectious diseases. In recent years, growing attention has been paid to viral genes involved in the carcinogenic process. It is natural that now much effort should be made towards prevention and treatment of the disease. The prevention of HBV mother-to-child transmission is one of the most important efforts to prevent the occurrence of viral hepatitis and also HCC. Another concern is of course the existence of a third hepatitis virus, and it seems likely that this induces hepatitis and

HCC. Researchers around the world are focusing on a much more powerful, worldwide strategy against infection by hepatitis viruses.

Of the hepatitis cases that occur in about 15% of blood transfusion cases, about 10% are hepatitis B and the remaining 90% HCV and others. As many as about half of all chronic liver disorders are caused by HCV. We have most recently obtained a screening method for HCV. It is, however, likely that there will be some difficulty in handling viruses that produce chronic inflammation.

It is very important to know how the host human body reacts to viral attack. As with all bacterial and viral infections, the host reaction is one of the key factors in the progress of infectious diseases, not to mention the character of the attacking viruses. In other words, it is necessary to make clear the mechanisms yielding viral carriers and carcinogenesis. Once this carcinogenic mechanism is clarified, it will surely help very much in the treatment of cancers, including HCC. There have been many developments in the diagnosis and treatment of hepatitis and HCC , and I put my hope in missile therapy and human monoclonal antibodies. Viewing the steady progress of the study of HCC, I pray that efforts will be continued and that our further understanding of the carcinogenic processes will occur and lead to the prevention of cancer.

References

1. Amano S, Yamamoto H (1960) Infectious hepatitis and cirrhosis as its sequela in Japan. Annual Report of the Institute for Virus Research, Kyoto University 3:185–334
2. Sheldon WH, James DF (1948) Cirrhosis following infectious hepatitis. A report of five cases, in two of which there were superimposed primary liver cell carcinoma. Arch Intern Med 81:666–689
3. Walsche JW, Wolffe HH (1952) Primary carcinoma of the liver following viral hepatitis. Report of two cases. Lancet 2:1007–1010
4. WHO report: Viral hepatitis. (1973) WHO Tech Rep Ser No. 512
5. Nishioka K, Hirayama T, Sekine T, Okochi K, Marumi M, Sung J-L, Liu C-H, Lin T-M (1973) Australia antigen and HCC. Gann Monograph Cancer Research 14:167–175
6. Nishioka K, Levin A, Simons MJ (1975) Hepatitis B antigen, antigen subtypes, and hepatitis B antibody in normal subjects and patients with liver disease. Result of collaborative study. Bull. WHO 52:293–300

7. Nishioka K (1978) Hepatocellular carcinoma and hepatitis B virus. In: Oda T (ed) Hepatitis Virus. Tokyo University Press, Tokyo, pp 247–255
8. Obayashi A, Okochi K, Marumi M (1972) Familial clustering of asymptomatic carriers of Australia antigen and patients with chronic liver disease or primary liver cancer. Gastroenterology 62:618–625
9. Shikata T, Uzawa T, Yoshihara N, Akatsuka T, Yamazaki S (1974) Staining methods for Australia antigen in paraffin section. Jap J Exp Med 44: 25–36
10. Assaad F (1985) Global overview of hepatitis B vaccine, WHO-WPR, 3rd Task Force Meeting on Hepatitis B
11. The Liver Cancer Study Group of Japan (1984) Primary liver cancer in Japan. Cancer 54: 1747–1755
12. Nishioka K, Watanabe J, Furuta S, Tanaka E, Iino S, Suzuki H, Tsuji T, Yano M, Kuo G, Choo Q-L, Houghton M, Oda T (1991) A high prevalence of antibody to the hepatitis C virus in patients with HCC in Japan. Cancer 67:429–433
13. Kim C, Koike K, Saito I, Miyamura T, Jay G Nature 351:317–320, 1991 HB-X gene of hepatitis B virus induces hepatic carcinoma in transgenic mouse. Nature

CHAPTER 7

The role of HBV in hepatocellular carcinoma

Satoshi Tanaka and Nobu Hattori[1]

1 Introduction

Hepatocellular carcinoma (HCC) is one of the most common malignancies worldwide. The incidence of HCC is particularly high in Africa [1, 2] and Asia [3–6]. There is apparently strong epidemiological evidence for an important role of hepatitis B virus (HBV) in the pathogenesis of HCC. However, the precise mechanism by which HBV infection might lead to malignant transformation of hepatocytes is still far from clear.

Recently in Japan, the proportion of patients with HCC which is related to chronic HBV infection is approximately 26% of all HCC patients [7]. While the number of HCC patients with chronic HBV infection has not increased, the number of patients who died from HCC which is considered to be related to chronic hepatitis C virus (HCV) infection [8] is clealy increasing.

The risk factor concerning malignant transformation of hepatocytes due to chronic HBV infection is discussed from the clinical aspect.

2 Recent incidence of HCC worldwide

2.1 High risk geographic regions of HCC

HCC is one of the most common malignancies worldwide. Geographically, there are three types of regions: high-risk regions, intermediate-risk regions, and low-risk regions. Third World countries such as South Africa [1, 2] and Far East countries such as China [3, 4], Senegal [5] and The Philippines [6] are included in the high-risk regions. Greece [9] and Japan are intermediate-risk regions, and the United States [10], the United Kingdom [11] and the other developed countries are low-risk regions. The incidence of HCC has been reported to be as high as 150 per 100,000 population per year for China, but a low of 4 for the United States [12].

Among Africans and Chinese, very close association between HCC and chronic HBV infection is reported. The estimate of the fraction of HCC which is due to chronic HBV infection varies from 60–90% in high- risk regions and 1–50% in the low- to intermediate-risk regions. These data suggest that there is a strong epidemiological relationship between chronic HBV infection and HCC. More than 250 million people throughout the world are chronically infected by HBV. Chronic HBV infection may be implicated as an initiator of as much as 80% of HCC worldwide.

2.2 Recent incidence of HCC in Japan [13]

Age-adjusted death rates per 100,000 population for selected malignancy sites compiled every 5 years show that malignancy of the liver is the third most common cause of death among males; the first and second most common are stomach and lung cancer. Among females, malignancy of the liver is the fourth leading cause of death, while the first three causes are stomach, lung and breast cancer.

Table 1 presents the age-adjusted death rates per 100,000 population for malignancy in the liver every 5 years from 1960 to 1988. Little change is observed for females from 5.7 to 4.5, while there is an obvious increase among males from 8.2 to 14.3. HCC constitutes more than 90% of malignancies in the liver in Japan [7, 14, 15].

[1]Tokyo Metropolitan Komagome Hospital, Komagome, Bunkyo-ku Tokyo, 113 Japan

Table 1. HBV carriers with hepatocellular carcinom in Japan (1968–1987)

Year	Percentage of HBV carriers	Number of cases reported[a]	Number of institutions	Number of HBV carriers
1968–77	40.8[b]	2,829	155	1,154[c]
1978–79	34.0[b]	954	246	325[c]
1980–81	28.8	1,546	405	445
1982–83	25.1	1,624	429	407
1984–85	23.4	1,877	507	442
1986–87	21.8	2,472	601	539

[a] Excluding the cases which were not clearly HBV carriers
[b] Percentage of HBsAg positive in serum (no inquiry about HBV carrier)
[c] Cases with HBsAg in serum
From [7, 14, 15]

Table 2. Age-adusted death rates per 100,000 population for selected malignancy sites

Liver	1960	1965	1970	1975	1980	1985	1988
Male	9.6	8.2	8.6	8.5	11.0	13.5	14.3
Female	6.6	5.7	5.0	4.4	4.5	4.5	4.5
Ratio	1.5	1.4	1.7	1.9	2.4	3.0	3.2

Standardized for age based on the 1935 Japanese population
From [4]

2.3 HBV carriers with HCC in Japan (Table 2)

The Liver Cancer Study Group of Japan reported various aspects of primary liver cancer in Japan. According to their report, in 1968–77, HCC patients who were positive for the HBsAg antigen was 40.8% of all HCC reported, and in 1986–87 it was 21.8%, which showed the proportion of HCC which occurred in HBV carriers is declining. As stated before, the number of HCC cases in Japan is increasing, but the HCC in HBV carriers is remaining stable in the number. Therefore, the increased HCC cases are suspected to be related to chronic HCV infection.

3   Characteristics of HCC in HBV carriers

The following characteristics of HCC in HBV carriers were noted in our hospital. Out of 455 cases, 79 (17.4%) which were diagnosed with HCC from 1982 to 1991 were HBV carriers, as determined by HBsAg positive (R-PHA) and/or high titre of HBcAb (EIA) in serum. HCC is determined by pathological findings (biopsy or autopsy).

3.1 Sex

Out of the 79 cases, 67 were male and 12 were female. The ratio of M:F was 5.6:1. Regardless of the presence of cirrhosis, the ratio of M:F was almost the same.

3.2 Age

The age distribution of patients is listed in Table 3. The peak of the age distribution occurs from the age of 50 to 60, both in males and females. In males, 4 cases were under 30 years old: one was 19 years old and one was 22 years old.

3.3 Co-existing liver injury

Cirrhosis co-exists with HCC in 66 of the 79 cases (83.5%). In three of the 4 cases under 30 years old, HCC co-existed with cirrhosis, although cirrhosis did not co-exist with HCC in 6 of the 33 cases over 60 years old.

3.4 Stages of HBV infection in HCC patients with HBsAg and/or high titre of HBcAb in serum

In 68 of the 79 HBV carriers, HBeAg and HBeAb in serum were tested by EIA at the time HCC was discovered. Among these 68 cases, 8 cases were HBeAg positive, 36 cases were HBeAb positive, and the remaining 24 cases were negative for both. Among 12 non-cirrhotic cases, only one was found to be HBeAg positive, although 6 cases were HBeAb positive and 5

Table 3. Age distribution of HBV carriers at time of HCC[a] diagnosis

Age	~19	20~	30~	40~	50~	60~	70~	Total
Male	1 (1)	1	2	9 (2)	25 (2)	22 (3)	7 (3)	67 (11)
Female	0	0	0	1 (1)	7 (1)	2	2	12 (2)
Total	1 (1)	1	2	10 (3)	32 (3)	24 (3)	9 (3)	

Non-cirrhotic cases in parenthesis
[a] Hepatocellular carcinoma

cases were negative for both of them. Among the 56 cirrhotic cases, 7 cases were HBeAg positive and 30 cases were HBeAb positive.

The prevalence of HBeAg was 11.8% in all 68 cases 12.5% in cirrhotic cases, and 8.3% in non-cirrhotic cases.

Most HCC cases were HBeAg negative. Among 6 male cases over 70 years old, 3 cases were without cirrhosis. Among those 3 cases, one was HBeAg positive and the others were HBeAb positive. Both of the 2 female cases over 70 years old were with cirrhosis and HBeAg positive. Even among the aged people, some HCC cases were HBeAg positive and without cirrhosis. On the other hand, the 19 year-old male was HBeAb positive and non-cirrhotic, and the 22 year-old male was HBeAg positive and with cirrhosis. Among young people some HCC cases were HBeAg positive and with cirrhosis.

3.5 Familial clustering of HCC

Families in which HCC was clustered is shown in Fig. 1. Patient no. 7 of the second generation in Fig. 1 was the first patient to be evaluated, and her 19 year-old son was detected to have HCC with chronic hepatitis type B. The present study includes only those two cases. Familial findings (Harada E and Ohbayashi A, manuscript in preparation) revealed that her father died from HCC, and four elder sisters and two elder brothers of hers were diagnosed as having HCC. Another sister was an HBV carrier and had cirrhosis. In this family, 6 out of 7 members of the second generation and 2 out of 17 members of the third generation had HCC. Six of 10 patients with HCC were tested for serum HBsAg and all 6 were both HBsAg positive and HBV carriers. Five of them were female. Agents such as aflatoxin, alcohol, and drugs (oral contraceptives, and so on) have been implicated as common etiological factors of HCC, but they were not associated with these cases.

In the second generation, including patient no. 7, the development of HCC was suspected to have occurred in their 40's, based on the age at which they died.

4 Discussion

4.1 Sex

HCC in the presence of cirrhosis is far more common among males than among females regardless of geographical region. In high-risk regions, male predominance is also present but is less striking when HCC occurs in non-cirrhotic patients. However, in low risk regions, the sex ratio in HCC patients without cirrhosis is about parity. In our hospital, the ratio of M:F among HCC patients who were also HBV carriers was 5.6:1; regardless of the presence of cirrhosis, the ratio of M:F with HCC was almost the same. The Liver Cancer Study Group of Japan also reported similar results in 1990 [7].

4.2 Age

In low-risk regions, the age of patients diagnosed with HCC and cirrhosis is 8–10 year older than that of HCC patient without cirrhosis [11, 16]. The number of HBV carriers with HCC and cirrhosis is bigger than that of those without cirrhosis. However, for HBV carriers in high-risk regions, there is no difference in the age of HCC development, whether they have cirrhosis or not [2, 4]. The report from our hospital shows the same result as the latter.

It has been estimated that it takes 30–50 years between HBV infection and the appearance of HCC [17]. The peak age at which patients are diagnosed with HCC is 50–60 years-old, but there were 4 male patients who were under 30 years old, as stated previously.

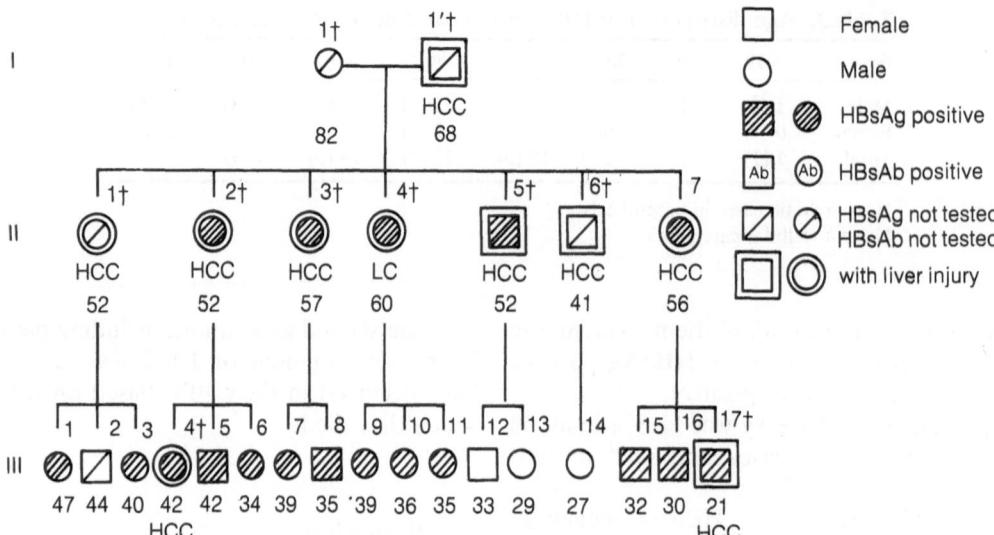

Fig. 1. Familial clustering of hepatocellular carcinoma

4.3 Cirrhosis and chronic HBV infection

In high risk regions, 60–80% of HCC co-exists with cirrhosis; this condition is usually related to chronic HBV infection. Chronic HBV infection is more common in patients with both HCC and cirrhosis than in those with cirrhosis alone. Serum HBsAg in HCC patients with cirrhosis was present 60.5% of the time in Africa, and 88% in China; and in those patients without cirrhosis, serum HBsAg was present in 52.8% and 38.0%, respectively. Therefore, there is a difference between the percentage of HBV carriers with HCC, with and without cirrhosis in China, but not in Africa.

On the other hand, the number of HCC patients with cirrhosis is bigger than that without cirrhosis in the low-risk region. While HBV-related HCC is reported to be rare, in low-risk regions, the incidence of HBV infection is found to be higher than in patients with cirrhosis and HCC than those with cirrhosis alone, e.g., 19.2% and 9.2% of Austrian patients, respectively [18].

In our hospital, there were 13 (16.5%) HBV-related HCC patients without cirrhosis out of 79 and 66 with cirrhosis (83.5%). The latter outnumbers the former by a wide margin.

Being cirrhotic is not a prerequisite for development of HCC in HBV carriers. However, in high-risk regions and in Japan, the majority of HBV-related HCC patients also have cirrhosis. In low-risk regions, most of the patients with HCC also have cirrhosis, regardless of whether they are HBV carriers or not. Therefore, cirrhosis is considered to play an important role in HCC development in HBV carriers.

While 1 out of 4 patients under 30 years old had HCC without cirrhosis, 6 out of 33 patients over 60 years old also had HCC without cirrhosis. HCC developed in patients under 30 years old and over 60 years old, whether or not cirrhosis co-exists.

4.4 Stage of HBV infection

In our hospital, HBeAg in serum was positive in 11.8% of tested 68 cases and HBeAb in serum was positive in 50%. HBeAg was positive in 8.3% of HCC cases with cirrhosis and in 12.5% of those without cirrhosis.

In China among the HCC patients with cirrhosis, 17.0% were HBeAg positive and 48.3% were HBeAb positive; and among those without cirrhosis, the percentages were 10.0% and 63.9%, respectively. It is reported that the correlation between HBeAg and HBeAb positive patients, and cirrhosis is not statistically significant.

The result in our hospital was the same; i.e., a lot of HCC development was observed when HBeAg was negative. In other words, HCC occurred when the replication of complete HBV decreased. However, the following two example of HCC development were reported in our hospital; one was a young patient with cirrhosis and HBeAg positive and the other was without cirrhosis and HBeAb positive.

4.5 Familial clustering of HCC

The presence of familial clustering of HBV carriers was not rare in Japan with HBV being transmitted from mother to baby in most cases. However, familial clustering of HCC is rare.

In this family (Fig. 1), most HCC patients were females and contributory factors such as oral contraceptives or alcohol were denied. The factors of virus and a host should be investigated further to find out if clustering occurs. It is estimated that a genetic factor of a host may predispose an individual to hepatocarcinogenesis.

4.6 Mechanism of hepatocarcinogenesis

DNA molecules from HCC tissue was analyzed, and it was found that the viral DNA sequences were integrated into the chromosomes of the tumor cells [19]. Recently, the altered gene expression in tumor cells has been studied intensively [20–24]. The variety of alterations of cellular genes such as mutations, chromosomal translocation, and rearrangement were reported, and these alterations were discussed in terms of whether or not they are precursors to malignant transformation of hepatocytes. Integrated HBV DNA sequences, which are often extensively rearranged, may be involved in hepatocarcinogenesis.

Although the integration of HBV DNA was mainly observed in tumor cells, it was also found in non-tumor cells from HCC patients [25]. Integrated HBV DNA was occasionally detected in the liver of HBV carriers without HCC [26]. These observations indicate that HBV DNA integration may occur either before or at a very early stage of hepatocarcinogenesis.

While analysis of tumor cells and cell lines have shown that HBV can insert its DNA at many different sites in human hepatocyte chromosomes, it is conceivable that a single gene which was altered by integration of HBV DNA may initiate a cascade of events that inexorably progresses to malignant transformation.

Other possibilities for hepatocarcinogenesis are also considered. The unregulated expression of the HBV X gene product which displays transcriptional trans-activating properties [27] or the HBV DNA polymerase which displays reverse transcriptase activity [28] may contribute to the malignant transformation of the infected hepatocyte. These mechanisms are not completely understood as yet. Chisari et al. [29] has developed a transgenic mouse system in which each of the individual HBV genes can be expressed in the liver, and reports that this way may one can determine the extent to which any given HBV gene product is directly hepatotoxic and the role which it plays in the immune response in the development of liver cell injury and HCC.

The mechanism responsible for hepatocarcinogenesis by chronic HBV infection is poorly defined. HBV might directly trigger hepatocarcinogenesis, or HCC may arise indirectly because of the chronic inflammation, cirrhosis and cell regeneration which take place in the HBV infected hepatocytes.

4.7 Summary

HBV belongs to the hepadnavirus family, which is a retro virus-like agent [30]. The ability of an oncogenic virus to damage DNA through integration or by causing mutations of cellular genes through cell regeneration are probably important factors in the HBV mediated multistep mechanism in the development of HCC.

HBV replication may directly or indirectly cause hepatocarcinogenesis. HCC usually develops several decades after the original infection, but HCC develops in only a minority of patients with chronic HBV infection.

In order to probe the mechanism of hepatocarcinogenesis, the clinical aspects given below and the results of the basic studies should be reconciled:

1. The presence of geographic differences (Racial differences).
2. Sex differences, i.e., the relatively higher rate of HCC development among males than among females. The presence of familial clustering should be considered.
3. HCC often co-exists with cirrhosis. However, the characteristics of HBV-related HCC in Japan are that HCC is just as likely to occur without cirrhosis and that patients could be either young or aged.
4. HCC sometimes occurs in HBcAg positive patients.

1 and 2 above show that the condition of a host, especially regarding a genetic predisposition, may be associated with HCC development.

HBV integration undoubtedly plays an important role, and may play an initiating role, for the development of HCC.

The majority of HBV-related HCC co-exists with cirrhosis, although the role of cirrhosis in carcinogenesis is not clear yet, but HCC occurs among the young who are both without cirrhosis and HBeAg positive.

These facts imply that there may be other mechanisms of carcinogenesis than integration.

References

1. Vogel CL, Anthony PP, Mody N, Barker LF 1970) Hepatitis-associated antigen in Ugandan patients with hepatocellular carcinoma. Lancet 2:621–624
2. Kew MC, Geddes EW, Macnab GM, Bersohn I (1974) Hepatitis-B antigen and cirrhosis in Bantu patients with primary liver cancer. Cancer 34: 539–541
3. Beasley RP (1982) Hepatitis B virus as the etiologic agent in hepatocellular carcinoma—Epidemiologic considerations. Hepatology 2:21s–26s
4. Gibson JB, Wu PC, Ho JCI, Lauder JJ (1980) HBsAg hepatocellular carcinoma and cirrhosis in Hong Kong. A necropsy study. Br J Cancer 42: 370–377
5. Prince AM, Szmuness W, Michon J, Desmaille J, Diebolt G, Linhard J, Quenum C, Sankale M (1975) A case-control study of the association between primary liver cancer and hepatitis B infection in Senegal. Int J Cancer 16:376–383
6. Ligao AL, Domingo EO, Nishioka T (1981) Hepatitis B profile of hepatocellular carcinoma in the Philippines. Cancer 48:1590–1595
7. The Liver Cancer Study Group of Japan (1990) Primary liver cancer in Japan: Clinicopathologic features and results of surgial treatment. Ann Surgery 211:277–287
8. Kuo G, Choo QL, Alter HJ, Gitnick GL, Redecker AG, Purcell RH, Miyamura T, Dienstag JL, Alter MJ, Stevens CE, Tegtmeier GF, Bonino F, Colombo M, Lee WE, Kuo C, Berger K, Shuster JR, Overby LR, Bradley DW, Houghton M (1989) An assay for circulating antibodies to a major etiologic virus of non-A, non-B hepatitis. Science 244:362–364
9. Trichopoulos D, Day NE, Kaklamani E, Tzonou A, Munoz N, Zavitsanos X, Koumantaki Y, Trichopoulou A (1987) Hepatitis B virus, tobacco smoking and ethanol consumption in the etiology of hepatocellular carcinoma. Int J Cancer 39:45–49
10. Austin H, Delzell E, Grufferman S, Levine R, Morrison AS, Stolly PD, Cole P (1986) A case-control study of hepatocellular carcinoma and the hepatitis B virus, cigarette smoking, and alcohol consumption. Cancer Res 46:962–966
11. Johnson PK, Krasner N, Portmann B, Eddleston ALWF, Williams R (1978) Hepatocellular carcinoma in Great Britain: Influence of age, sex, HBsAg status and etiology of underlying cirrhosis. Gut 19:1022–1026
12. Adrian MD (1988) Hepatocellular carcinoma. Ann Intern Med 108:390–401
13. Health and Welfare Statistics Association (1990) The trend of the national health and welfare in 1990 (in Japanese). J Health Welfare Statistics 37:58–59
14. The Liver Cancer Study Group of Japan (1984) Primary liver cancer in Japan. Cancer 54: 1747–1755
15. The Liver Cancer Study Group of Japan (1987) Primary liver cancer in Japan. Cancer 60: 1400–1411
16. Omata M, Ashcavai M, Liew CT, Peters R (1979) Hepatocellular carcinoma in the USA: Etiologic considerations. Gastroenterology 76:279–287
17. Zur Hausen H (1986) Intracellular surveillance of persisting viral infection. Lancet 2:489–491
18. Ferenci P, Dragosics B, Morosi L, Kiss F (1984) Relative incidence of primary liver cancer in cirrhosis in Austria: Etiological consideration. Liver 4:7–14
19. Brechot C, Pourcel C, Louise A, Rain B, Tiollais P (1980) Presence of integrated hepatitis B virus DNA sequences in cellular DNA of human hepatocellular carcinoma. Nature 286:533–535
20. Rogler CE, Sherman M, Su CY, Shafritz DA, Summers J, Show TB, Henderson H, Kew M (1985) Deletion in chromosome 11p associated with a hepatitis B integration site in hepatocellular carcinoma. Science 230:329–332
21. Hino O, Shows TB, Roger CE (1986) Hepatitis B virus integration site in hepatocellular carcinoma at chromosome 17;18 translocation. Proc Natl Acad Sci USA 83:8338–8342
22. Dejean A, Bougueleret L, Grzeschik KH, Tiollas P (1986) Hepatitis B virus DNA integration in a sequence homologous to v-erb-A and steroid receptor genes in a hepatocellular carcinoma. Nature 322:70–72
23. Yaginuma K, Kobayashi M, Yoshida E, Koike K (1987) Hepatitis B virus integration in hepatocellular carcinoma DNA: Duplication of cellular flanking sequences at the integration site. Proc Natl Acad Sci USA 82:4452–4462
24. Benbrook D, Lernhardt E, Pfahl M (1988) A new retinoic acid receptor identified from a hepatocellular carcinoma. Nature 333:669–672
25. Shafrits DA, Shouval D, Sherman (1981) Integration of hepatitis B DNA into the genome of liver cells in chronic liver disease and hepatocellular carcinoma. N Engl J Med 305:1067–1073
26. Kam W, Rall LB, Smuckler EA, Schmid R, Rutter WJ (1982) Hepatitis B viral DNA in liver and serum of asymptomatic carriers. Proc Natl Acad Sci USA 79:7522–7526
27. Two JS, Schloemer RH (1987) Trans criptiona trans-activating function of hepatitis B virus. J Virol 61:3448–3453

28. Summers J, Manson WS (1982) Replication of the genome of a hepatitis B-like virus by reverse transcription of an RNA intermediate. Cell 29: 403–415

29. Chisari FV, Klopchin K, Moriyama T, Pasquinell C, Dunsford HA, Sell S, Pinkert CA, Brinster RL, Palmiter RD (1989) Molecular pathogenesis of hepatocellular carcinoma in Hepatitis B virus transgenic mice. Cell 59:1145–1158

30. Toh H, Hayashida H, Miyata T (1983) Sequence homology between retroviral transcriptase and putative polymerases of hepatitis B virus and cauliflower mosaic virus. Nature 305:827–829

CHAPTER 8

Hepatitis C virus infection and hepatocellular carcinoma

Toshio Shikata[1]

1 Introduction

For the past two decades, hepatitis B virus (HBV) has been believed to be one of causative factors in hepatocellular carcinoma (HCC) in humans, especially in areas where HBV is endemic [1–3]. There is some evidence to support the close relationship between chronic HBV infection and development of HCC; for instance, areas where there is a high prevalence of HCC correspond to endemic areas of HBV. In Asia and Africa, both the HBV carrier rate and HCC incidence are very high. On the contrary, in areas where HBV infection is uncommon, such as the United States, the incidence of HCC is also low. Furthermore, the percentage of patients testing positive for HBsAg (hepatitis B surface antigen) is high among patients with HCC in those endemic areas, for example, 80% in Taiwan [4] and 72% in Uganda [5]. In addition, HBV DNA has been proved to be integrated into cellular DNA of tumor cells in patients with HBsAg-positive HCC [6–9] and non-tumor hepatocytes [10].

Further evidence to support the role of HBV in hepatocarcinogenesis is the existence other hepadna viruses, such as the woodchuck hepatitis virus and duck hepatitis B virus [11, 12]. In the woodchuck, some are infected by a very similar virus to HBV and the infected animals develop chronic hepatitis and HCC. Liver cirrhosis has not been observed, and HCC usually develops on the basis of mild chronic hepatitis [13], indicating woodchuck hepatitis virus is a stronger carcinogen than HBV.

Recently in Japan, however, the situation has changed a little. The incidence of HCC has

markedly increased in the past 15 years, but the positive rate of HBsAg among patients with HCC has decreased [14–16]. The rate was about 40% 20 years ago, and is now only 20% of HCC cases (Table 1). Increasingly, new cases of HCC have been negative for HBsAg and positive for anti-HCV (hepatitis C virus antibody), which is probably associated with hepatitis C virus (HCV) infection. Now, it is supposed that 80% of the cases with HCC in Japan are associated with persistent infection of HCV.

2 Characterization and molecular cloning of HCV

Recently, the virus causing the majority of cases of post-transfusion non-A, non-B hepatitis has been cloned [17], identified, and named as the hepatitis C virus. HCV was the first example of a virus identified through characterization of the viral genome.

HCV is a single positive strand RNA virus and probably is a togavirus, which is very similar to flavivirus or pestivirus. The virus is 36–72 nm in diameter and has an envelope and spikes [18]. The virus particles are usually found in the concentrated sera of infected chimpanzees and human patients with non-A, non-B hepatitis. Similar virus-like particles have been found in the lysosomes of the hepatocytes of infected chimpanzees. The viral RNA is 9.4 Kb in length and divided from the 5'-terminal into the 5' noncoding region, core (C), envelope (E), nonstructural protein (NS)1, NS2, NS3, NS4, NS5, and the 3' non-coding region.

Many Japanese scientists have now successfully cloned the HCV genome from Japanese patients or carriers [19–23]. My colleagues and I tried to

---

[1] Department of Pathology, Nihon University School of Medicine, Itabashi-ku, Tokyo, 173 Japan

Table 1. Chronological changes of positive rate of HBsAg among patients with HCC (histologically proved clinical cases [14–16])

	1968–1977	1978–1979	1980–1981	1982–1983	1984–1985	1986–1987
No of cases	654	954	1,645	1,779	1,933	2,480
HBsAg +	266	325	517	489	476	556
%	40.7	34.1	31.4	27.5	24.6	22.4

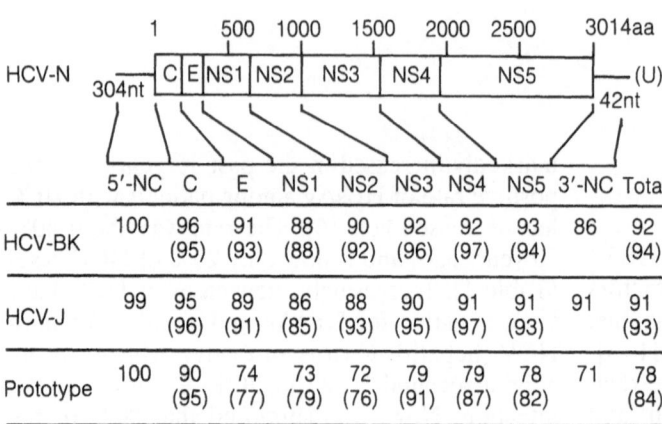

Fig. 1. Homology of HCV genome in Japan and United States. *Upper column* indicates nucleic acid homology and *lower column* (parenthesis) indicates amino acid homology. *HCV-N*, cloned and sequenced in our laboratory; *HCV-BK*, Dr. Okayama's clone [22]; *HCV-J*, Dr. Shimotono's clone [21]; *Prototype*, Dr. Houghton's clone [18]

clone the HCV genome using an immunoscreening method [19]. Houghton [18] used infected chimpanzee serum as the starting material but we used human sera. We pooled HBsAg negative sera with a high transaminase titer from donor blood samples from the Japanese Red Cross. RNA was extracted from the pooled sera and a cDNA library was constructed in the bacteriophage λ gtll. This library was then screened immunologically using infected chimpanzee sera as the antibody. Finally, we obtained one clone from the NS5 region of the virus genome. To determine the entire sequence of the Japanese strain of HCV, we took overlapping clones of almost all the HCV genome from 2 ml of serum from a single carrier of HCV by means of the PCR (polymerase chain reaction) technique. Finally we sequenced the whole genome of the Japanese HCV clone and compared it to that of Chiron obtained by Houghton [18].

We found marked differences between both of the nucleotide sequences (Fig. 1). The homology of the nucleotide sequence between both clones was varied from part to part. The 5'-terminal non-coding region and the core coding region were fairly constant and the homology was estimated as high as 90%. However, in other parts of the genome, homology was very low; at the envelope coding region, homology was as low as 74%. The 3'-terminal non-coding region was variable and

the length was also variable. In other NS regions, homology was 72%–79%. When we compared the amino acid sequence of both clones, homology was about 80% in the variable region. It can be seen that Chiron's clone and the Japanese clone are very different to each other.

We also compared several Chinese and Korean clones to the two previous clones. The Chinese and Korean clones were fairly similar to the Japanese clone and very different to Chiron's clone. Therefore, we have named these clones the American clone and Asian clones. In Japan, we have imported many blood products from the United States over the last 30 years, and therefore we have some patients with chronic hepatitis due to the American stain of HCV.

3 Antibody assay system and RNA assay system

An antibody assay system for HCV infection has been developed and is already widely used in the world [24]. The system uses a recombinant peptide from the NS3 and NS4 regions as antigen. Research has showed that this C-100-3 antibody is found among patients with chronic HCV infection. It has been postulated that the positive rate

Table 2. Chronological changes of the incidences of liver cancer [HCC and cholangiocellular carcinoma (CCC)], stomach cancer, and lung cancer among total autopsy cases in Japan

	1978	1979	1980	1981	1982	1983	1984	1985	1986	1987	1988	Total
Autopsy	30,067	32,859	36,134	39,021	39,050	39,737	39,918	40,250	40,021	39,399	39,333	415,789
Malignant tumor	17,259	18,397	20,382	21,941	23,937	24,803	25,212	23,302	23,433	23,332	23,243	245,241
Liver cancer	1,777	2,098	2,488	2,644	2,933	3,105	3,262	3,408	3,525	3,588	3,596	32,424
% Autopsy	5.9	6.4	6.9	6.8	7.5	7.8	8.2	8.5	8.8	9.1	9.1	7.8
% Malignant tumor	10.3	11.4	12.2	12.1	12.2	12.5	12.9	14.6	15.0	15.4	15.5	13.2
HCC	1,582	1,679	2,024	2,117	2,380	2,555	2,743	2,844	3,013	3,068	3,040	27,045
CCC	273	199	244	192	194	224	180	187	213	202	246	2,460
Stomach cancer	3,046	3,428	3,497	3,815	3,840	3,862	3,816	3,799	3,732	3,616	3,585	40,036
% Malignant tumor	17.6	18.6	17.2	17.4	16.0	15.6	15.1	16.3	15.9	15.5	15.4	15.8
Lung cancer	2,562	2,776	3,176	3,488	3,574	3,755	3,874	3,814	3,902	3,880	4,062	38,863
% Malignant tumor	14.8	15.1	15.6	15.9	14.9	15.1	15.4	16.4	16.7	16.6	17.5	15.8

% Autopsy, percentage among total autopsy cases; % Malignant tumor, percentage among total malignant tumors

of C-100-3 among patients infected with HCV is about 75% and this antibody appears usually 3–6 months after onset of the disease.

In Japan, the positive rate of C-100-3 in various liver diseases was found to be as follows: 70% of post-transfusion non-A, non-B hepatitis showed positive reaction for C-100-3. The positive rate of C-100-3 among patients with community-acquired acute non-A, non-B hepatitis was about 40%. For patients with chronic liver diseases, such as chronic hepatitis, liver cirrhosis, and hepatocellular carcinoma, the positive rate of C-100-3 was about 70% in HBsAg negative cases and 10%–20% in HBsAg positive cases. It seems that there are some cases of double infection of HBV and HCV among the patients with chronic liver diseases [25].

Japanese investigators have also developed other assay systems; four or five groups have developed core antibody assay systems that use recombinant or synthetic core peptide. Our group is using a 120-amino acid of the core region called CP120 (JCC); Dr. Shimotono's group are using a 163-amino acid (Shimotono 1991, personal communication); Dr. Mayumi's group is using rather small peptides called CP9 and CP10 (Mayumi 1991, personal communication); Dr. Miyamura's group has also developed a core assay system called P22 (Miyamura 1991, personal communication). Those core antibodies usually appear at the early stage of HCV infection and these core antibody assay kits can be used for diagnosis of acute hepatitis due to HCV. The positive rate of core antibody among patients

infected with HCV is also in the high range of 90%–95%. Furthermore, almost all researchers agree that if we used a recombinant peptide from the NS3 region, we would get the highest positive rate for HCV carriers. The PCR method is widely used in the many laboratories to detect the HCV genome. If we use the 5′-terminal as the primer, we can detect almost all strains of HCV, but if we use other regions we can only detect either the Japanese or the American clone. If we use PCR with the Chiron-antibody negative cases with chronic non-A, non-B hepatitis, in almost all cases we can detect HCV RNA.

4 HCV infection and HCC

HCC is one of the most common carcinomas in Japan. The number of male patients with stomach cancer, lung cancer, and liver cancer was found to be almost the same in autopsy cases (Table 2). Also, HCC showed a marked male predominance. The male to female ratio of acute hepatitis is 1.3:1, whereas the male to female ratio fo liver cirrhosis is 2 or 3:1. Furthermore, the male to female ratio of HCC is 5 or 6:1 (Table 3).

The incidence of HCC has increased since 1975 in Japan, especially among males, but not so markedly among Japanese females. As mentioned earlier, the rate of HCC patients testing positive for HBsAg in Japan was about 40% in the 1970s. However, this rate is gradually coming

Table 3. Male to female ratio of liver cancer, HCC, and CCC in autopsy cases

	Autopsy	Malignant tumor	Liver cancer	% Autopsy	% Malignant tumor	HCC	% Autopsy	% Malignant tumor	CCC	% Autopsy	% Malignant tumor
Total	415,789	245,241	32,424	7.8	13.2	27,045	6.5	13.2	2,460	0.6	1.0
Male	254,202	155,889	25,265	10.0	16.3	21,894	8.6	14.0	1,377	0.5	0.9
Female	159,061	88,336	6,918	4.3	7.8	5,015	3.1	5.7	971	0.6	1.1

% Autopsy, percentage amomg total autopsy cases; % Malignant tumor: percentage among total malignant tumors

down and recently the rate has been only 20%. Therefore, recent cases of HCC in Japan are almost all HBsAg negative, and if we examine anti-HCV using the C-100-3 kit, the positive rate of C-100-3 is 70% among HBsAg negative cases and 18% among HBsAg positive cases. Furthermore, if we analyze the incidence of HCC with sex and age, we find that, among males in their 50s, a marked increase in HCC incidence was observed from 1975. From 1975 to 1985, the incidence of liver cirrhosis and HCC in this age group almost doubled. In contrast, among females in their 50s, the incidence of liver cirrhosis and HCC decreased by half between 1960 and 1985.

A possible explanation is as follows: after World War II, in Japan, there were many patients with lung tuberculosis, and almost all were around 20 years old. Some of these patients received operations such as lobectomy or thoracoplastic surgery, and in the course of this were infected by HBV or HCV or both via the blood transfusions. If immunologically competent adults are infected by HBV, they usually develop acute hepatitis, and after recovery they clear the virus and rarely develop chronic hepatitis. However, with hepatitis C, 50%–60% of cases develop into chronic hepatitis and 20–30 years later some of them develop liver cirrhosis and HCC. Females infected by HCV become chronic carriers, but they rarely develop liver cirrhosis and HCC. However, they transmit HCV to their husbands and sexual partners and some of these then develop liver cirrhosis and HCC. Of course, patients, with other diseases also received blood transfusions and were infected by HCV at that time in Japan and other countries. However, these patients were usually aged between 50 and 60 years and died before development of liver cirrhosis and HCC, because it takes 20–30 years after infection to develop liver cirrhosis and HCC [26]. In the United States there were fewer cases of lung tuberculosis and in developing countries there were many cases of lung tuberculosis, but those patients did not received operations. In the United States, HCV has spread among drug abusers, and this might be the reason why the HCV carrier rate is almost same as in Japan but the HCC incidence is not as high in the United States.

The mechanisms of hepatocarcinogenesis due to HCV are still obscure. The HCV genome not thought to integrate into cellular DNA like HBV, because HCV is a single strand RNA virus and the existence of a reverse transcription for its replication has not been proved.

5 Conclusion

It has been postulated that chronic HBV infection and the development of HCC in humans is closely related. However, in Japan, chronic HCV infection is probably more important in hepatocarcinogenesis, because the rate of HCC patients testing positive for HBsAg is only 20%, but 80% of cases are associated with HCV infection. A follow-up study of HCV infection indicated that it might take about 20–30 years after infection with HCV for HCC to develop. The mechanism of hepatocarcinogenesis by HCV is still obscure.

References

1. Szmuness W (1978) Hepatocellular carcinoma and the hepatitis B virus: Evidence for a causal association. Prog Med Virol 24:40–69
2. Shikata T (1976) Primary liver carcinoma and liver cirrhosis. In: Okuda K, Peters RL (eds) Hepatocellular Carcinoma. Wiley, New York, pp 53–71
3. Blumberg BS, Larouze B, London WT, Werner B, Hesser JE, Millman I, Saimot G, Payet M (1975) The relation of infection with the hepatitis B agent to primary hepatic carcinoma. Am J Pathol 81: 669–682

4. Tong MJ, Sun SC, Scheffer BT, Chang N, Lo K, Peters RL (1971) Hepatitis-associated antigen and hepatocellular carcinoma in Taiwan. Ann Intern Med 75:687–691

5. Tabor E, Gerty RJ, Vogel CL, Bayley AC, Anthony PP, Chen CH, Barker LF (1977) Hepatitis B virus infection and primary hepato-cellular carcinoma. J Nat Cancer Inst 58: 1197–1200

6. Shafritz D, Kew MC (1981) Identification of inte-grated hepatitis B virus DNA sequences in human hepatocellular carcinoma. Hepatology 1:1–8

7. Brechot C, Pourcel C, Hadchouel M, Scotto J, Fonk M, Potet F, Vyas GN, Tiollais P (1982) State hepatitis B virus DNA in liver disease. Hepatology 2 (Suppl):27–34

8. Hino O, Kitagawa T, Koike K, Kobayashi M, Hara M, Mori W, Nakashima T, Hattori N, Sugano H (1984) Detection of hepatitis B virus DNA in hepatocellular carcinoma in Japan. Hepatology 4:90–95

9. Miller RH, Lee SC, Liaw YF, Robinson WS (1985) Hepatitis B viral DNA in infected human liver and hepatocellular carcinoma. J Inf Dis 151:1081–1092

10. Tanaka Y, Esumi M, Shikata T (1988) Frequent integration of hepatitis B virus DNA in non-cancerous liver tissue from hepatocellular car-cinoma patients. J Med Virol 26:7–14

11. Summers J, Smolec JM, Snyder R (1978) A virus similar to human hepatitis B virus associated with hepatitis and hepatoma in woodchucks. Proc Natl Acad Sci USA 75:4533–4537

12. Abe K, Kurata T, Shikata T (1988) Localization of woodchuck hepatitis virus in the liver. Hepatology 8:88–92

13. Mason WS, Seal G, Summers J (1980) Virus of Peking ducks with structural and biological related-ness to human hepatitis B virus. J Virol 36:829–836

14. Okuda K, The Liver Cancer Study Group of Japan (1980) Primary liver cancer in Japan. Cancer 45:2663–2669

15. The Liver Cancer Study Group of Japan (1984) Primary liver cancer in Japan. Cancer 54: 1747–1755

16. The Liver Cancer Study Group of Japan (1987) Primary liver cancer in Japan. Cancer 60: 1400–1411

17. Choo QL, Kuo G, Weiner AJ, Overby LR, Bradley DW, Houghton M (1989) Isolation of a cDNA clone derived from a blood-borne non-A, non-B viral hepatitis genome. Science 244:359–362

18. Abe K, Kurata T, Shikata T (1989) Non-A, non-B hepatitis: Visualization of virus-like particles from chimpanzee and human sera. Arch Virol 104:351

19. Maeno M, Kaminaka K, Sugimoto H, Esumi M, Hayashi N, Komatu K, Abe K, Sekiguchi S, Yano M, Mizuno K, Shikata T (1990) A clone closely associated with non-A, non-B hepatitis. Nucleic Acids Res 18:2685–2689

20. Okamoto H, Okada S, Sugiyama S, Yotsumoto S, Tanaka T, Yoshizawa H, Tsuda F, Miyakawa Y, Mayumi M (1990) The 5'-terminal sequence of the hepatitis C virus genome. Jap J Exp Med 60: 167–177

21. Kato N, Hijikata M, Ootsuyama Y, Nakagawa M, Ohkoshi S, Sugimura T, Shimotono K (1990) Molecular cloning of the human hepatitis C virus genome from Japanese patients with non-A, non-B hepatitis. Proc Natl Acad Sci USA 87:9524–9528

22. Takamizawa A, Mori C, Fuke S, Manabe S, Murakami S, Fujita J, Onishi E, Andho T, Yoshida I, Okayama H (1991) Structure and organization of the hepatitis C virus genome isolated from human carriers. J Virol 65: 1105–1113

23. Kubo Y, Takeuchi K, Boonmar S, Katayama T, Choo QL, Kuo G, Weiner DW, Bradley DW, Houghton M, Saito I, Miyamura T (1989) A cDNA fragment of hepatitis C virus isolated from an implicated donor of post-transfusion non-A, non-B hepatitis in Japan. Nucleic Acids Res 17: 10367–10372

24. Kuo G, Choo QL, Alter HJ, Gitnick GL, Redeker AG, Purcell RH, Miyamura T, Dienstag JL, Alter MJ, Stevens CE, Tegtmeier GE, Bonono F, Colombo M, Lee WS, Kuo C, Berger K, Shuster JR, Overby LR, Bradley DW, Houghton M (1989) An assay for circulating antibodies to a major etiologic virus of human non-A, non-B hepatitis. Science 244:362–364

25. Nishioka K, Watanabe J, Furuta S, Tanaka E, Suzuki H, Iino S, Tsuji T, Yano M, Kuo G, Choo QL, Houghton M, Oda T (1991) Antibody to the hepatitis C virus in acute hepatitis and chronic liver diseases in Japan. Liver 11:65–70

26. Kiyosawa K, Sodeyama T, Tanaka E, Gibo Y, Yoshizawa K, Nakano Y, Furuta S, Akahane Y, Nishioka K, Purcell RH, Alter HJ (1990) Inter-relationship of blood transfusion, non-A, non-B hepatitis and hepatocellular carcinoma: Analysis by detection of antibody to hepatitis C virus. Hepatology 12:671–675

CHAPTER 9

Molecular biology of hepatitis B virus and hepatocellular carcinoma

Shinako Takada, Katsuyuki Yaginuma, Masayuki Arii, Ikuo Nakamura, Yumiko Shirakata, Midori Kobayashi, and Katsuro Koike[1]

1 Introduction

Hepatitis B virus (HBV) is a causative agent of acute and chronic hepatitis in humans, and its chronic infection is closely related to the development of hepatocellular carcinoma (HCC) [1, 2]. Chronic hepatitis is considered to be a premalignant stage of HCC, since HCC frequently developes via chronic hepatitis; woodchuck carriers experimentally infected by woodchuck hepatitis virus (WHV) developed HCC in all cases [3]. The HBV genome possesses four open reading frames (ORF) for the expression of pregenome RNA, C/e antigen, polymerase, preS/S antigen, and X protein [4], as shown in Fig. 1. Southern blot analyses by us and other investigators [4–7] demonstrated HBV DNA integration in some chronic and acute hepatitis tissues. For clarification of the early stage of tumor development, integrated forms of HBV DNA in chronic hepatitis were extensively studied by molecular cloning to provide an indication of their structural features. HBV DNA integration was found in most chronic hepatitis samples and rearrangement of viral DNA and/or cellular flanking DNA was also apparent [8, 9]. Moreover, some data suggest viral DNA rearrangement possibly occurs prior to integration in the chronically-infected liver [10–12].

The integration of HBV DNA also occurs in HCC tissues at a high frequency [8, 13] and is considered to be important in the initial stage of hepatocarcinogenesis. Structural analyses of integrated HBV DNA were carried out on many HCC samples [7, 14–22], and several characteristics became evident. The cellular site of HBV integration is random and one end of the integrated HBV DNA is close to the 5' end region of the negative or positive viral strand (*DR1* or *DR2*, respectively). Various integrated structures could be seen with or without rearrangement of the viral genome. However, no common structure has been found in HCC at a high frequency so far. Thus, the rearrangement of HBV DNA as well as that of cellular flanking DNA are not specific for HCC cells.

One virus-cell junction is close to the 5' end of the minus-strand DNA and the major part of the *X* ORF (for 154 amino acid residues) and enhancer-promoter sequences are preserved [8]. It should thus be reasonable to consider the expression of cellular gene(s) to be activated in a trans-acting manner through increase in the HBV gene product at the time of chronic infection. Recently, the function of the X-gene product was found by several groups, using the chloramphenicol acetyl transferase (CAT) assay method, to be trans-activation of homologous and heterologous transcriptional enhancers [23, 24].

Using antibodies against synthetic peptides corresponding to *X* ORF, an antigenic polypeptide was detected in an HBV-infected liver [25]. Antibodies that had anit-X reactivity were also found in HBV carriers [26, 27]. We recently used several approaches to clarify the function of the *X* gene. In one case, the expression of the *X* gene in mouse NIH3T3 cells was studied for this purpose. To examine the transforming potential of the X-gene product of HBV, *X* gene was introduced into NIH3T3 cells. Each stably transformed cell line expressed X-coding mRNA to a different degree. A positive correlation was found between the level of X-coding mRNA and cell saturation density. In *X*-gene-transformed cells which bring about a high level of X-coding mRNA and cell saturation density, c-*myc* expression increased [8]. Such growth stimulation is

[1] Department of Gene Research, Cancer Institute JFCR, Kami-Ikebukuro, Toshima-ku, Tokyo, 170 Japan

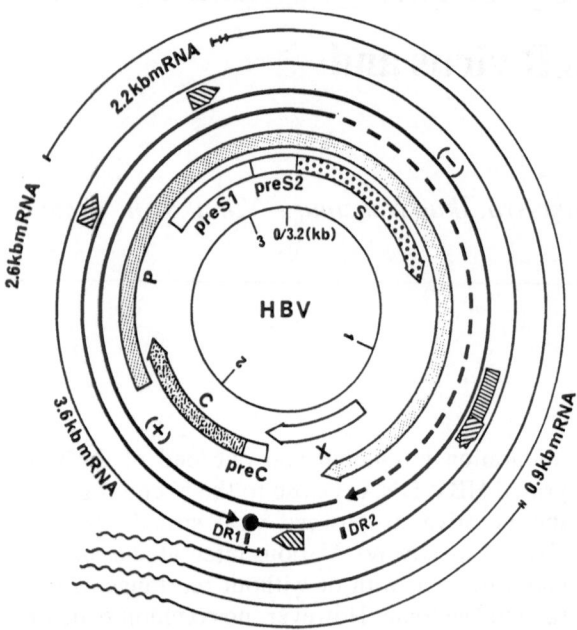

Fig. 1. Genetic organization and transcription map of the HBV genome. The HBV DNA was derived from the virus of adr subtype and its complete nucleotide sequence (3215 base-pairs) has been described. The positions of promotor and enhancer region are indicated by *diagonal and vertical hatching*, respectively. The 4 different transcripts are indicated with a poly(A) tail (*wavy line*). The primer protein (*solid circle*) is attached to the 5' end of the minus strand. *DR1* and *DR2* represent 11 base-pair direct repeats

probably due to activation of a cellular gene(s) by the X-gene product. However, no gross rearrangement in the c-*myc* allele was observed in the *X*-gene-transformed cells. The *X*-gene-transformed cell line exhibited X protein production and tumor formation in nude mice [8, 28]. In another case, determination was made of the trans-acting effect of *X* gene DNA on the expression of CAT gene under the control of SV40 sequences in the NIH3T3 cells by a transient transfection assay. Our findings, therefore, indicate the possibility that the X-gene product activates a cellular oncogene(s) by a trans-acting mechanism.

Although the direct role of the X-gene product for the HBV life cycle has still to be elucidated further, our previous findings indicated that the production of HBV particles as well as viral mRNAs by the transient expression of transfected HBV DNA was not strongly influenced in HuH7 cells but was remarkably inhibited in HepG2 cells following the introduction of a frame-shift mutation into *X* ORF [29]. The X-gene product

probably regulates virus replication as well as transcription by activating a cellular transcription factor. In addition, we described the unique properties of the X-gene product.

As to cellular oncogenes detected in a variety of human tumor cells by the DNA transfection technique using mouse NIH3T3 cells as a recipient [30, 31], the majority of cellular oncogenes so far detected are related to a family of evolutionarily conserved genes, designated as *ras* [32, 33]. Activation of *ras* oncogenes in human tumors is most commonly due to a point mutation at codon 12 or 61 in their coding sequences [34–36].

To search for HCC-specific oncogenes, our laboratory utilized an assay for transforming genes based on the focus induction following cotransfection with a selection marker and DNA from HCC cells. Using this assay, two types of transforming DNAs were obtained from the DNAs of the HCC cell lines and tissues. One transforming DNA corresponded to the activated N-*ras* oncogene [37], but the other was previously named *hcc-1*. The *hcc-1* DNA was obtained from the hepatoma cell line huH2-2, which contained a single copy of 1895 bp integrated HBV DNA [38]. The huH2-2 DNA had a weak focus-inducing activity in NIH3T3 cells, but first and second transformants efficiently grew in nude mice. We cloned 70 kb of human DNA, which was incorporated into the second transformant 2f5. We have recently characterized its structure as a truncated proto-*dbl* oncogene [39].

2 Integration of HBV DNA in chronic hepatitis and hepatocellular carcinoma tissues

Cellular DNAs from chronic hepatitis tissues of 16 patients at different ages were analyzed by Southern blot hybridization using HBV DNA as the probe (Table 1). Of the 16 samples, 15 exhibited hybridization signals in the high molecular weight region, when blot hybridization was conducted without restriction enzyme digestion. When the DNAs were digested with *Hind*III, the hybridization signals became dispersed. Data clearly indicate that most of the chronic hepatitis tissues have HBV DNA integrated to cellular DNA and that heterogeneous cell populations exist with respect to the HBV DNA integration site. Hybridization signals in the low molecular

Table 1. Histological, serological, and hybridization results

Patient	Sex	Age (yrs)	Histological diagnosis	Serological marker(s)	HBV DNA in liver	
					Integrated	Free
N1	M	6	CAH	sAg/cAb/eAg	+	+
N2	M	5	CAH	sAg/cAb/eAg	+	+
NG	F	12	AC	sAg/eAg	+	+
NO	M	15	CAH	eAg	+	+
NS	M	15	CH	sAg/eAb	+	+
T1	M	23	CAH	sAg/eAg	+	+
T2	M	42	CAH	sAg/eAg	+	+
T3	M	39	CAH	sAg/cAb/eAg	?	+
T4	M	44	CH	sAg/cAb/eAg	+	+
T5	M	28	CAH	sAg/eAg	+	+
T6	M	36	CH	sAg/cAb/eAg	+	+
Sa	F	20	CH	sAg/eAg	+	+
Mo	M		CH	cAb/eAg	+	+
Ta	M	27	CAH, LC		+	+
Se	M	41	CH	sAg/eAg	+	+
Ni	M	49	CH	sAg/eAg	+	+

CAH, chronic active hepatitis; AC, asymptomatic carrier; CH, chronic hepatitis; LC, liver cirrhosis; sAg, HBV surface antigen; cAb, antibody to HBV core antigen; eAg, HBV e antigen

weight region showed free viral DNA [9]. As a control experiment, the DNA from a blood sample of a HBV carrier, whose blood contained HBV in high titer, was examined. No hybridization signal was detected in the high molecular weight region. Therefore, signals in the high molecular weight region are attributed to integrated HBV DNA, but not attributed at all to free viral DNA trapped in high molecular weight cellular DNA.

A series of Southern blot experiments were also performed to clarify the state of HBV DNA integration in 48 HCC cases divided into two different groups according to the serological status of HBsAg [8] (Table 2). Among 27 HBsAg positive patients, integration of HBV DNA sequence was observed in 25 HCC DNAs following digestion with *Hind*III or *Eco*RI. The restriction pattern exhibited discrete band(s), but varied from patient to patient. The HBV DNA integration site was found to be random with respect to the cellular DNA. These results may be due to clonal development of the tumor cell population containing integrated HBV DNA. The free viral DNA was infrequently detected in the tumor part.

Of 15 HCC cases from HBsAg-negative patients, but with other HBV markers in their serum, integrated HBV DNA sequences were detected in 6 patients, but 4 of the remaining 9 patients had ambiguous results, in which HBV DNA was detected by dot blot hybridization but not by Southern blot hybridization. Five of the 6

Table 2. Integrated HBV DNA in hepatocellular carcinoma samples from HBsAg positive and negative patients

HBsAg in serum	Ratio of patients	Other HBV marker in serum	Ratio of patients	HBV DNA integration
+	27/48			25/27
−	21/48	+	15/21	6/15
		−	6/21	1/6

patients without any HBV markers showed no hybridization signals. In the HBsAg-negative patients, integrated HBV DNA was found as a weak band in the blot in general, suggesting that only a small part of the HBV genome remained in the cellular DNA or that the tumor cell population without integrated HBV DNA generated in HCC tissues as a result of chromosomal non-disjunction during progression.

3 Structures of integrated HBV DNA in chronic hepatitis and hepatocellular carcinoma tissues

Cellular DNA fragments containing integrated HBV DNA were molecularly cloned from three chronic hepatitis samples and their structures were characterized by restriction enzyme map-

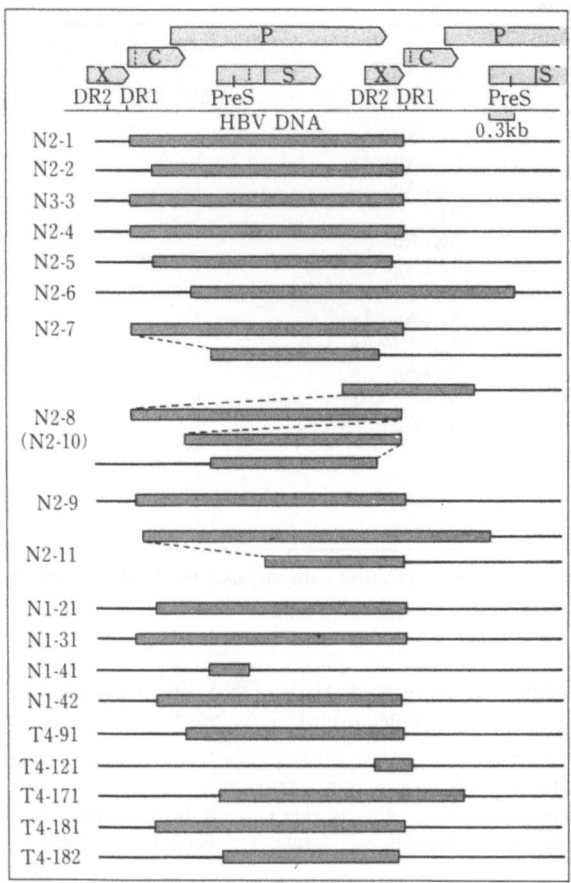

Fig. 2. Restriction map and genetic organization of integrated HBV DNA cloned from chronic hepatitis tissues. *N2-1* to *N2-11* were cloned from chronic active hepatitis tissue N2. *N1-41* was from chronic active hepatitis tissue N1. *T4-91* to *T4-182* were from chronic persistent hepatitis tissue T4. *C, preS, S,* and *X* represent the *C(HBcAg)* gene, *preS* region, *S(HBsAg)* gene, and *X* gene respectively. The *boxes* represent the integrated HBV DNA. *Solid lines* indicate cellular flanking DNAs. The gene organization of the HBV DNA is shown at the top of the figure, where HBV DNA is tandemly arranged at 1.7 genome length. *DR1* and *DR2* indicate the 11bp directly-repeated sequences

ping and hybridization mapping using a gene-specific DNA probe [7, 8]. As shown in Figs. 2 and 3, 12 out of 19 clones included subgenomic HBV DNA spanning from the *DR1* region to the *preS* or *C* gene region through the *X* gene as was often noted in our studies on HCC and chronic hepatitis samples [7, 18, 21]. Two clones, N2-6 and T4-171, had colinear HBV DNA, but both ends of the viral DNA were in the *preS* or its upstream region, possibly the second hot spot of recombination with cellular DNA or within viral

DNA [9, 18, 22]. In these 2 clones, the region corresponding to 0.9 kb X mRNA was conserved. We obtained 3 clones with gross rearrangement of HBV DNA and inverted duplication (N2-7, -8, and -11). This is the first direct evidence for the rearrangement of integrated HBV DNA from chronic hepatitis tissues. Virus-virus junction was most frequently seen in the 5′ end region of the negative viral strand and also in the virus-cell junction. Two clones, N1-41 and T4-121, each containing a very small fragment of HBV DNA were also obtained. To characterize these small viral DNA fragments, chromosome assignment was made of cellular flanking DNAs from clone N1-41 using a human-mouse hybrid panel having 12 hybrid clones. It became clear that translocation occurred between cellular flanking DNAs. It appears evident that rearrangement of HBV DNA as well as cellular flanking DNA is not specific for HCC cells.

Structural analyses of integrated HBV DNAs were carried out with many HCC samples and the following integrated structures were seen: a colinear structure of HBV DNA having the 5′ end region of the negative or positive viral strand as one end, with or without cellular DNA rearrangement; an inversely duplicated structure of HBV DNA accompanied by the cellular flanking DNA; and a highly rearranged structure of HBV DNA without rearrangement of cellular flanking DNAs (HCY-23 is an example in Fig. 3). No common structure became evident in HCC in high frequency. Thus possibly, rearrangement at the site of HBV DNA integration is not responsible for hepatocarcinogenesis. Rather, rearrangement appears due to the individual characteristics and conditions of the host or viral replication, since its frequency was totally independent of whether the sample was from HCC or chronic hepatitis [7, 9, 18].

4 HBV DNA rearrangement with or without cellular DNA

To examine details of virus-cell junctions of clone N2-7, cellular counterpart DNA from the gene library of human thymus DNA was cloned using cellular flanking DNA as the probe. Restriction enzyme mapping and sequence analysis of the cellular counterpart DNA demonstrated no gross change in cellular DNA except a small deletion of 30 bp at the integration site of inversely

Fig. 3. Structure of the cellular DNA before and after HBV DNA integration. Cellular counterpart DNAs of N2-7 and HCY-23 were molecularly cloned and structures were analysed by DNA sequencing (upper restriction maps in each figure). In both cases, no change except a small deletion at the junction site was found in cellular DNA. Restriction endonuclease sites are: *H*, *Hind*III; *P*, *Pvu*II; *F*, *Hin*fI; *Bg*, *Bgl*II; *E*, *Eco*RI

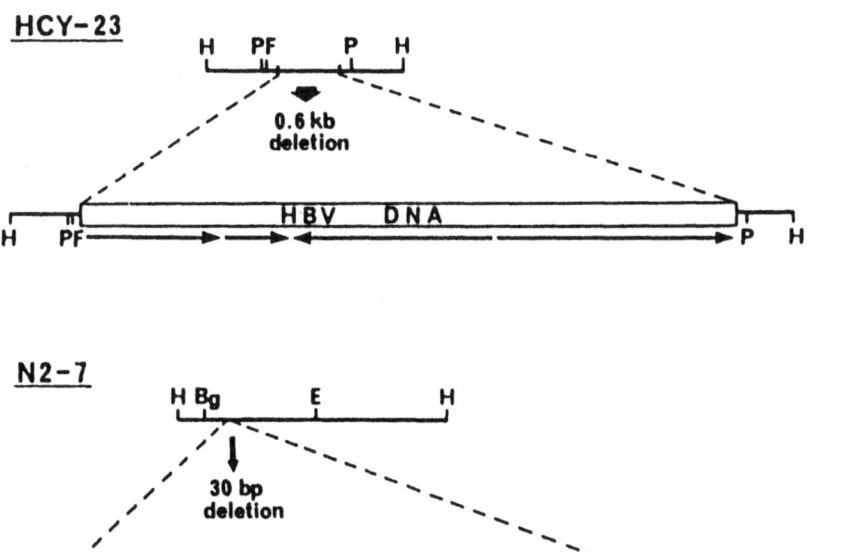

duplicated HBV DNA (Fig. 3). Essentially the same was found from analysis of the clone HCY-23 from the HCC sample (HCY-23), in which a single copy of highly rearranged HBV DNA was integrated (Fig. 3). A similar structure was also reported by Hsu et al. [40], in which highly rearranged WHV DNA was inserted 600 bp upstream of c-*myc* exon 1 with only a 3 bp cellular DNA deletion. Therefore, inverted duplication possibly occurs prior to integration. That is, previously rearranged HBV DNA integrates into cellular DNA at least in some cases, simply because N2-7 and HCY-23 are not likely to be produced by recombination between two distantly integrated HBV DNAs nor by inverted duplication of one original integrant.

To clarify the mechanism of HBV DNA rearrangement and also that of integration into cellular DNA, analysis of these junction sequences was made. At most virus-virus junctions, there is 1–3 nucleotide homology between the two viral DNA strands [9]. In such cases, on one side of the junction, two viral sequences were found to be weakly homologous to each other (a patchy homology box). It is possible that HBV DNA rearrangement may occur by an illegitimate recombination mechanism, which brings about template switching or jumping of polymerase and the 3′ end of the nascent DNA strand to either the complemental strand or to within the same template. As for the virus-cell junctions, 1–5 nucleotide homology between HBV and cellular DNAs was observed in all cases analyzed. From

the data obtained, integration may occur basically by a similar mechanism to that of HBV DNA rearrangement.

The so called novel form of circular viral DNA of more than two genome equivalents with extensive rearrangements is assumed to exist as in the WHV and ground squirrel hepatitis virus (GSHV) systems [10, 11, 12]. Though the mechanism for this is not fully clarified, it appears a reasonable assumption that a novel form of HBV DNA integrates into the cellular DNA through illegitimate recombination between viral and cellular DNAs using patchy homology. This recombination would occur most frequently in the 5′ end region of the negative viral strand and secondly in the *preS* or its upstream region. These regions have been noted as a recombination hot spot [18, 22].

Data from analyses of integrated HBV DNAs performed on chronic hepatitis and HCC samples indicated the following functional characteristics. Since one virus-cell junction was close to the 5′ end of the *DR1*, the major part of the *X* ORF and enhancer sequence were retained [8]. It should thus be reasonable to consider the expression of cellular genes to be activated in trans through an increase in the HBV X-gene product at the time of chronic infection. Meanwhile, the function of the X-gene product was found to be transactivation of homologous and heterologous transcriptional enhancers or promoters [23, 24, 41]. Therefore, the function of the HBV *X* gene should be examined in this regard.

S. Takada et al.

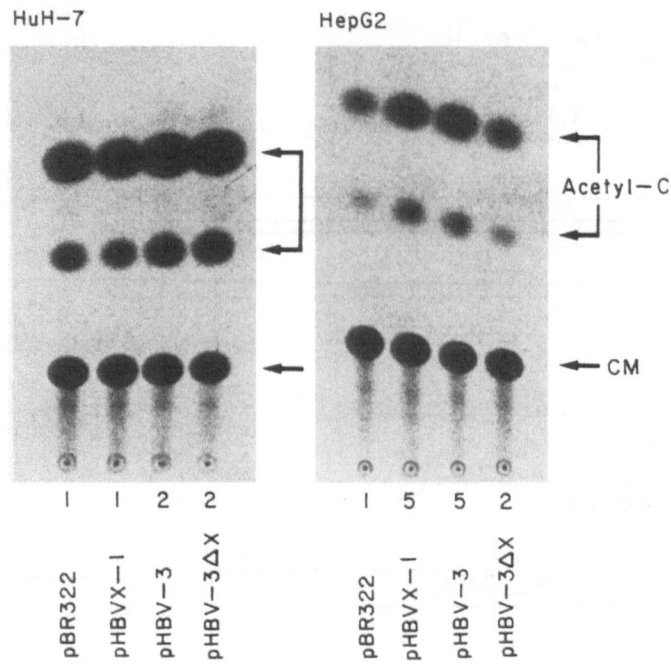

HuH-7   HepG2

Acetyl—CM

CM

1	1	2	2	1	5	5	2
pBR322	pHBVX-1	pHBV-3	pHBV-3ΔX	pBR322	pHBVX-1	pHBV-3	pHBV-3ΔX

Fig. 4. Trans-activation of pSV2CAT by the template plasmids pHBV-3 and pHBV-3ΔX. Human hepatoma cells HuH-7 or HepG2 were transfected with 5 µg of pSV2CAT. CAT activities after cotransfection with 15 µg of one of the plasmids are shown in the indicated lanes. Control activity is shown as 1 under the lane of pBR322. Relative CAT activity is indicated under each lane

5 Effect of X gene on viral transcription in hepatoma cells

We previously established a transient expression system, whose hepatoma cells, HuH-7 or HepG2 cells were capable of producing HBV particles by transfection of HBV DNA [29]. In the transfected cells, four classes of mRNAs were identified during HBV replication. The 3.6 kb mRNA is involved in the expression of the C/e antigen and polymerase. It also functions as a pregenome for virus replication. The 2.2 kb mRNA is involved in the production of preS2/S proteins. 2.6 kb mRNA produces the preS1 protein and 0.9 kb mRNA is related to the X gene expression (Fig. 1).

An attempt was made to clarify the function of the X gene by examination of the transient expression of the viral transcripts by transfected pHBV-3 or pHBV-3ΔX into HuH-7 or HepG2 cells. In the template plasmid pHBV-3, the intact X gene was situated at the one end. In the plasmid pHBV-3ΔX, the linker was inserted into the DraI site on the X ORF. The mutant pHBV-3ΔX DNA produced a defective product in the carboxyl-terminal region of the X protein. Interestingly, almost no reduction in any of the 4 different mRNAs was observed in the HuH-7 cells by pHBV-3ΔX, while in HepG2 cells they were reduced remarkably. Thus, the trans-acting function of the X-gene product was differently exhibited in two different hepatoma cells.

6 Trans-acting function of X gene expressed in HBV replication in human hepatoma cells

To assess the significance of X mutations in the trans-acting function of the X gene, plasmids pHBV-3, pHBV-3ΔX and pHBVX-1 were used in the CAT assay, where the CAT gene is under the control of SV40 promoter/enhancer sequences. Consistent with the above findings, cotransfection of plasmid pHBV-3 into HepG2 cells increased the CAT activity of pSV2-CAT by about five times that in the case of the pBR322 vector (Fig. 4). The X mutant exhibited no such stimulation in CAT expression. Plasmid pHBVX-1 increased CAT activity to about the same degree as did pHBV-3. It is thus quite clear that the X-gene product is able to trans-activate the SV40 promoter/enhancer sequences in HepG2 cells. However, on transfecting the same plasmid pHBV-3 DNA to HuH-7 cells, no such enhancement of CAT activity was observed although high production of X mRNA was observed. Similar results were obtained in the case of pHBVX-1. Virtually no enhancement of CAT activity occurred by pHBVX-1 DNA in HuH-7 cells, but it increased by almost five times as much in HepG2 cells. Thus, there may be a difference in ability to respond to X-gene product in the two types of cells. It would thus be of interest to determine whether there is a cellular transcription factor which interacts with the X-gene product at a transcriptional regulatory sequence, most likely a promoter/enhancer, and whether the amount of this factor differs in the two hepatoma cell lines. The detection and characterization of such a transcription factor in the cells will be important for determining the oncogenic potential and pathogenecity of the hepatitis B virus.

7 Activation of c-*myc* expression by introduction of the *X* gene into mouse NIH3T3 cells

In the previous study, a positive correlation was noted between the level of X-coding mRNA and the saturation density of *X*-gene-introduced mouse NIH3T3 cells [28, 41]. To examine the production of X protein in *X*-gene-introduced cell lines, cell lysates were assayed for the presence of X protein using antisera generated in rabbits for synthetic X peptides [25]. Immunoblots showed 17 kDa protein reacted with antisera to synthetic X peptides [28]. If increases in this cell saturation density is mediated by cellular gene activation due to the trans-acting effect of the X-gene product, a significant change in the growth-related gene, i.e., c-*myc*, should be detectable. The expression of mouse c-*myc* gene was thus examined. Total RNAs were isolated from *X*-gene-introduced NIH3T3 cells at the confluent stage and analysed by Northern blot hybridization using the human c-*myc* gene probe under stringent conditions. As expected, a hybridization signal of mouse c-*myc* mRNA was weak because of their homology but increased greatly in these *X*-high-expression cell lines (lanes 1–3) in contrast to the low expression cell lines (lanes 4 and 5) and NIH3T3 cells (Fig. 5). A great difference in mouse c-*myc* expression between *X*-gene-introduced and control cells became evident at the confluent stage consistent with the previous observations [41]. It thus appears quite likely that growth stimulation arises from c-*myc* activation triggered by expression of the *X* gene. The size of c-*myc* mRNA was found to be 2.4 kb and this

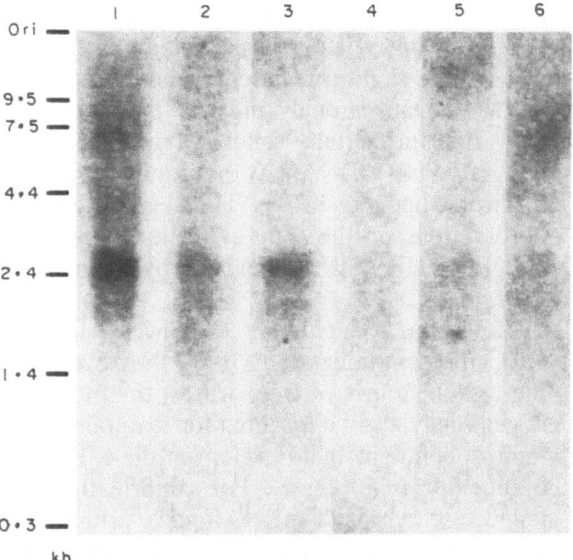

Fig. 5. c-*myc* expression of HBx-transformed NIH3T3 cells. Total RNA of 10 μg from the HBx-transformed cells at the confluent stage was analyzed. For the ^{32}P-labeled probe of the human c-*myc* gene, the ClaI-EcoRI fragment containing exon 3 was used. *Lane 1*, NHBx-1; *lane 2*, NHBx-21; *lane 3*, NHBx-32; *lane 4*, NHBx-22; *lane 5*, NHBx-33; *lane 6*, NIH3T3

indicates possibly that no gross structural change occurs in mouse c-*myc* exons.

The *X* gene is located at the 3′ end of the pregenome RNA of HBV, as in the case of retroviral oncogene(s) [42]. The codon usage of *X* ORF for 154 amino acids is probably similar to that of the genes of eukaryotic cells, whereas, other HBV genes are similar to viral genes in origin [43]. Previous analyses demonstrated the major part of *X* ORF and its upstream sequence to be frequently retained in many integrated HBV DNAs examined to date [8]. Tumorigenicity in nude mice was observed in these transformed NIH3T3 cell lines by introducing the *X* gene with many copies [28].

8 Trans-activation function of integrated HBV DNA

Products of a series of integrated HBV DNAs were examined for the presence of this trans-activation function [44]. The integrated HBV DNA obtained from chronic hepatitis tissues was co-transfected into HepG2 cells with pSV2CAT and subjected to the CAT assay. As shown in Fig. 6, many clones had trans-activation activity in spite of the slight truncation at the 3' end of the X ORF. Data strongly indicate that the trans-activation of certain cellular target genes by integrated HBV DNA may occur quite frequently in chronic hepatitis tissues. This is consistent with observations on the trans-activation function of integrated HBV DNA from HCC by Wollersheim et al. [45].

Based on accumulating evidence that many HCCs possess integrated HBV DNA even after the disappearance of free viruses, the integrated X gene may also be essential for maintaining the tumor phenotype that develops at the early stage of hepatocarcinogenesis. For confirmation, detailed research on X mRNA and X protein produced from integrated HBV DNA in chronic hepatitis and hepatoma tissues should be done. The cDNA structure of X mRNA from integrated HBV DNA indicated that X-cell fusion mRNA and also truncated X protein can be produced and many 3'-truncated X-gene products retain the trans-activation function. Truncation at the carboxyl-terminal end is sufficiently small so that this function is maintained. The results of 5 amino

acid residue truncation support this possibility. In GSHV, X protein has the trans-activation function [44], in spite of missing the carboxyl-terminal region corresponding to the last 12 amino acid residues of HBV X protein. On the other hand, the deletion of the last 22 amino acid residues caused the complete loss of the trans-activation function, indicating that the 7 subtracted amino acid residues (L-G-G-C-R-H-K) are important for this trans-activation function.

9 X protein possesses a serine protease inhibitor domain-like structure

As the 7 amino acid residue sequence (L-G-G-C-R-H-K) in the carboxyl-terminal region of X protein is an essential region for trans-activation (Fig. 7), a search was made to determine the manner in which the protein brings about transcriptional trans-activation of various genes [46]. When the amino acid sequence of X protein was subjected to computer analysis, the amino

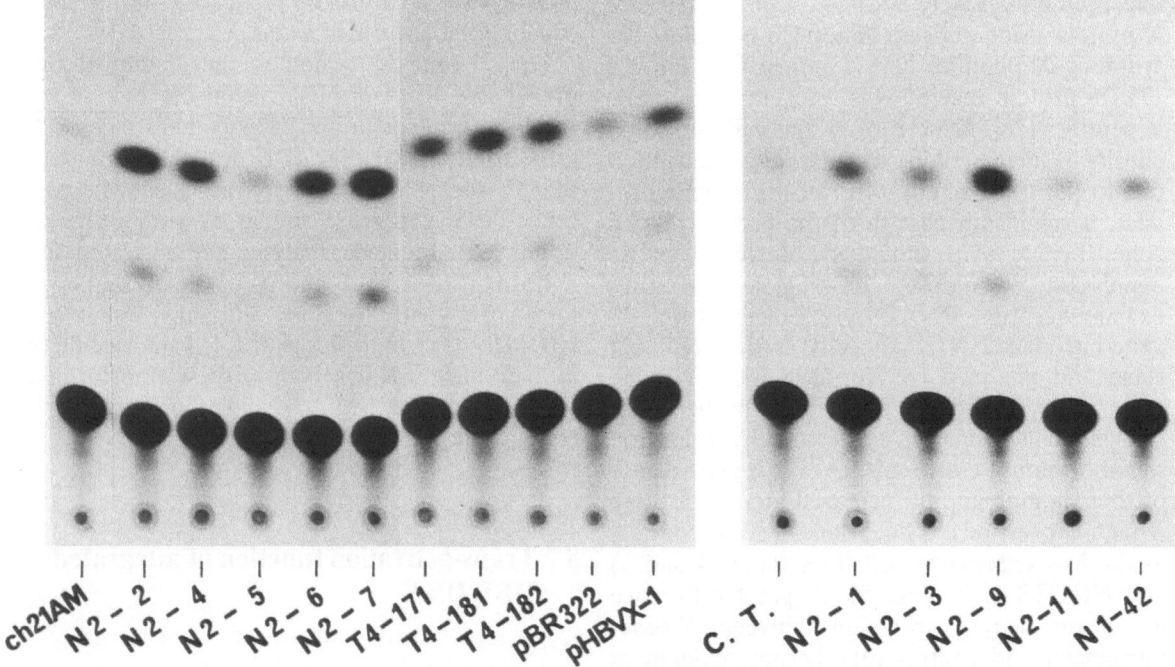

Fig. 6. CAT assay for the trans-activation function of various integrated HBV DNAs. HepG2 cells were cotransfected with 30–40 µg of integrated HBV DNA cloned in the phage ch21AM vector and 5 µg of pSV2CAT DNA as the reporter plasmid, ch21AM, C.T. (calf thymus DNA), and pBR322 DNAs were used as controls. Plasmid pHBVX-1 was used for X mRNA expression

Fig. 7. Amino acid sequences of hepadna virus X proteins. Amino acid sequences of hepadna virus X proteins from human (*HBV*), woodchuck (*WHV*), ground squirrel (*GSHV*) are aligned and represented by single-letter amino acid codes. Common amino acid sequences among hepadna viruses are enclosed by hatched boxes. *P stop* indicates the position of polymerase gene stops and *DR 2* shows the location of 11bp directly-repeated sequences

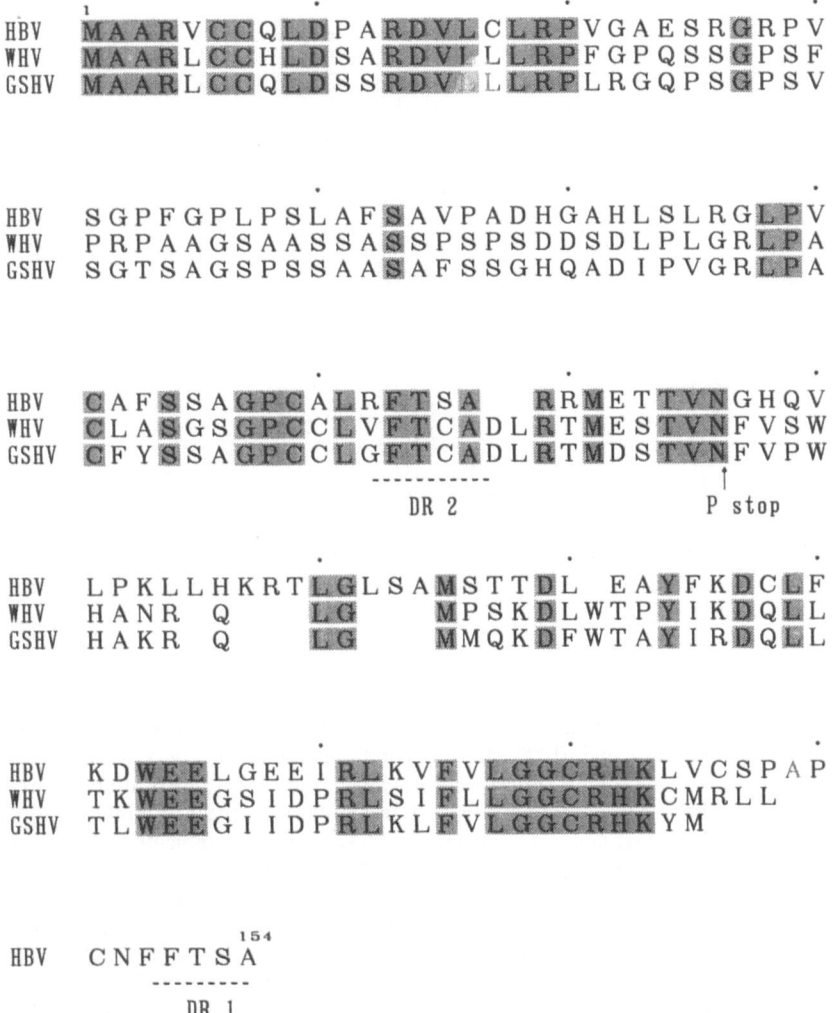

acid residues at position 132-140 in the carboxyl-terminal region, which is conserved among hepadna viruses, was found to be highly homologous to the consensus amino acid sequence (F-V/I-X-G-G-C-R/K) within the serine protease inhibitor domain (Kunitz domain) essential for Kunitz-type serine protease inhibitor [47–49] and incidentally to p18 protein in the *abl* gene of Abelson murine leukemia virus (A-MuLV), whose function is unknown (Fig. 8). Serine protease inhibitors are intracellular polypeptides present in many tissues and inhibit one of the various serine proteases, such as trypsin, kallikrein, chymotrypsin, and plasmin, by virture of their binding to the active center of the protease.

Serine protease inhibitors also possess the consensus amino acid sequence (G-P-C) within their protease inhibitor domain, in which the reaction site (R or K) is next to the (G-P-C) sequence [47–49]. This reaction site is situated close to the former consensus sequence (F-V/I-X-G-G-C-R/K) by means of an intramolecular disulfide bond. The X proteins of hepadna viruses and p18 of A-MuLV also possess this (G-P-C) sequence, though the distance to the (F-V/I-X-G-G-C-R/K) sequence is different from that of known protease inhibitors with respect to the primary structure (Fig. 1). The C residue 6 or 7 amino acid residues upstream from the (G-P-C) sequence is conserved in X protein. The R residue (position 15) corresponding to the cleavage site of bovine basic protease inhibitor precursor (BBPI) on releasing the inhibitor molecule is also conserved (Fig. 8). Thus, X protein possesses all the conserved amino acid residues within the protease inhibitor domain of Kunitz-type serine protease inhibitor except for the Y (at position 49 of BBPI) and the

84

S. Takada et al.

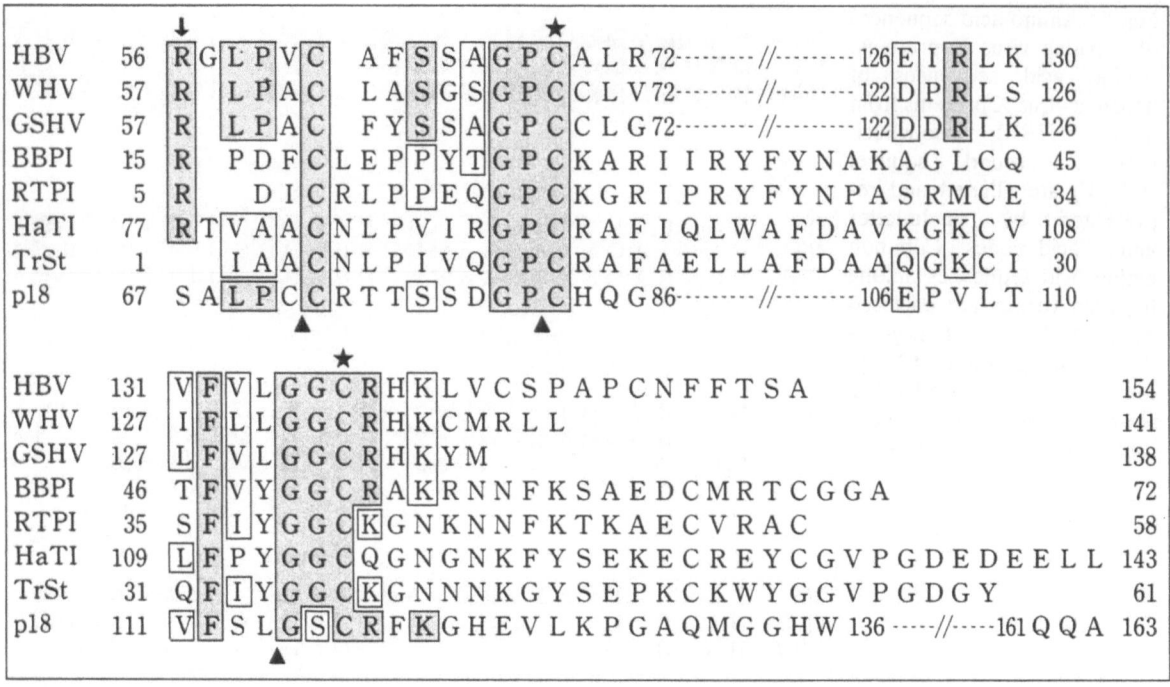

Fig. 8. Comparison of amino acid sequences of proteins from hepadna viruses, the Kunitz domains of serine protease inhibitors and p18[abl], showing common amino acids between any one of serine protease inhibitors and hepadna virus X proteins (*boxed with shadows*), conserved substitutions (*boxed without shadows*), and common amino acids of p18[abl] compared with those of serine protease inhibitor and X protein (*boxed*). Amino acid numbers of the first and last residues in each sequence are indicated on both sides. *HBV*, hepatitis B virus [57]; *WHV*, woodchuck hepatitis virus [58]; *GSHV*, ground squirrel hepatitis virus [58]; *BBPI*, bovine basic protease inhibitor precursor [59]. *RTPI*, rea sea turtle basic protease inhibitor [60]; *HαTI*, human inter-α-trypsin inhibitor [61]; *TrSt*, trypstatin from rat mast cells [61]. *Stars* denote two C residues possibly linked together by a disulfide bond in X protein. The *arrow* indicates position 15 R residue of BBPI, the cleavage site for releasing an inhibitor molecule. Disulfide bonds in BBPI are as follows: C(19)-C(69), C(28)-C(52), C(44)-C(65). The carboxylterminal 30-amino-acid sequence (positions 125–154) of HBV X protein was subjected to local homology search using the NBRF protein database with program SEQFP in IDEAS (Integrated Database and Extended Analysis System for nucleic acids and proteins)

three C residues (positions 44, 65, and 69 of BBPI) (Fig. 8) [47–49].

If, in fact, X protein resembles serine protease inhibitors or related proteins, the mutation of the possible protease inhibitor domain would have a deleterious effect on its function. Deletion of the last 22 amino acids of HBV X protein was found to result in the complete abolition of trans-activation, and the conserved amino acid sequence (L-G-G-C-R-H-K) to be essential for the trans-activation function of X protein. Another mutant X gene was subsequently made and compared with a wild type X gene. Amino acid residues at positions 67, 68, 69 of protein G-P-C were converted to R-C. This mutant X completely lost its capacity to bring about trans-activation. The (G-P-C) sequence was thus essential for X protein to exert its trans-activation

function. However, as shown in Fig. 8, owing to the absence of the K or R residue next to the (G-P-C) sequence possessing affinity for the serine residue in the reactive center of known proteases [47], X protein may be incapable of inactivating the target protease. Even if this should be the case, the X protein might nevertheless contribute to the formation of the tertiary structure about the reaction site. The duck hepatitis virus (DHBV) genome lacks these two sequences in the X + C region [50] and has no trans-activation activity [51]. This supports the view that trans-activation by the X gene occurs by way of a protease inhibitor-like structure.

Chisari et al. recently found the accumulation of toxic quantities of HBsAg within hepatocytes results in severe, prolonged hepatocellular injury which in turn leads to neoplasia, and that regardless of etiology, chronic cell injury and associated inflammatory and regenerative responses constitute a preneoplastic condition which inevitably proceeds toward malignancy [52]. Imbalance of protease and protease inhibitor action may also cause the accumulation of abnormal protein. Some protease inhibitors have been shown to be identical to growth stimulatory factors [53, 54] or cell division cycle genes [55]. Although the mechanism for growth stimulation is unclear, these properties are similar to those of HBV X protein, which exhibits some growth-stimulatory effect [28, 56]. Thus, X protein may contribute to hepatocarcinogenesis in multiple modes as a protein containing a serine protease inhibitor-like structure, that is, through trans-activation of certain genes, growth stimulation, and the promotion of liver cell injury. Thus, hepadna virus X proteins may comprise a new oncogene family, giving rise to multiple changes in the cellular transcription and replication.

References

1. Szmuness W (1978) Hepatocellular carcinoma and the hepatitis B virus: Evidence for causal association. Prog Med Virol 24:40–69
2. Beasley RP, Hwang LY, Lin CC, Chien CS (1981) Hepatocellular carcinoma and hepatitis B virus. Lancet 11:1129–1133
3. Popper H, Roth L, Purcell RH, Tennant BC, Gerin JL (1987) Hepatocarcinogenicity of the woodchuck hepatitis virus. Proc Natl Acad Sci USA 84:866–870
4. Brechot C, Hadchonuel M, Scotto J, Degos F, Charnay P, Trepo C, Tiollais P (1981) Detection of hepatitis B virus DNA in liver and serum: A direct appraisal of the chronic carrier state. Lancet II: 765–767
5. Brechot C, Hadchouel M, Scotto J, Fonck M, Potet F, Vyas GN, Tiollais P (1981) State of hepatitis virus DNA in hepatocyte of patients with hepatitis B surface antigen-positive and -negative liver diseases. Proc Natl Acad Sci USA 78:3906–3910
6. Shafritz DA, Shouval D, Shermann HI, Hadziyannis SJ, Kew MC (1981) Integration of hepatitis B virus DNA into the genome of liver cells in chronic liver disease and hepatocellular carcinoma. N Engl J Med 305:1067–1073
7. Yaginuma K, Kobayashi H, Kobayashi M, Morishima T, Matsuyama K, Koike K (1987) Multiple integration site of hepatitis B virus DNA in hepatocellular carcinoma and chronic active hepatitis from children. J Virol 61:1808–1813
8. Koike K, Kobayashi M, Yaginuma K, Shirakata Y (1987) Structure and function of integrated HBV DNA. In: Robinson WS, Koike K, Will H (eds) Hepadna Viruses Alan R Liss, New York, pp 267–286
9. Takada S, Gotoh Y, Hayashi S, Yoshida M, Koike K (1990) Structural rearrangement of integrated hepatitis B virus DNA as well as cellular flanking DNA is present in chronically infected hepatic tissues. J Virol 64:822–828
10. Marion P, Robinson WS, Rogler CE, Summers J (1982) High molecular weight GSHV-specific DNA in chronically-infected ground squirrel liver. J Cell Biochem Suppl 6:203
11. Rogler CE, Summers J (1982) Novel form of woodchuck hepatitis virus DNA isolated from chronically infected woodchuck liver nuclei. J Virol 44:852–863
12. Rogler CE, Summers J (1984) Cloning and structural analysis of integrated woodchuck hepatitis virus sequences from a chronically infected liver. J Virol 50:832–837
13. Tiollais P, Pourcell C, Dejean A (1985) The hepatitis B virus. Nature 317:489–495
14. Dejian A, Sonigo P, Wain-Hobson S, Tiollais P (1984) Specific hepatitis B virus integration in hepatocellular carcinoma DNA through a viral 11-base-pair direct repeat. Proc Natl Acad Sci USA 81:5350–5354
15. Koch S, Freytag von Loringhoven A, Kahmann R, Hofschneider PH, Koshy R (1984) The genetic organization of integrated hepatitis B virus DNA in the human hepatoma cell line PLC/PRF/5. Nucleic Acids Res 11:5391–5402
16. Koshy R, Koch S, Freytag von Loringhoven A, Kahmann R, Murray K, Hofschneider PH (1983) Integration of hepatitis B virus DNA: Evidence for integration in the single-stranded gap. Cell 34:215–223
17. Mizusawa H, Taira M, Yaginuma K, Kobayashi M, Yoshida E, Koike K (1985) Inversely repeating integrated hepatitis B virus DNA and cellular flanking sequences in the human hepatoma-derived cell line huSP. Proc Natl Acad Sci USA 82:208–212
18. Nagaya T, Nakamura T, Tokino T, Tsurimoto T, Imai M, Mayumi T, Kamino K, Yamamura K, Matsubara K (1987) The mode of hepatitis virus DNA integration in chromosome of human hepatocellular carcinoma. Genes Dev 1:773–782
19. Rogler CE, Shermann M, Su CY, Shalfitz DA, Summers J, Show TB, Henderson A, Kew M (1985) Deletion in chromosome 11p associated with a hepatitis B integration site in hepatocellular carcinoma. Science 230:319–322
20. Tokino T, Fukushige S, Nakamura T, Nagaya T, Murotsu T, Shiga K, Aoki N, Matsubara K (1987) Chromosomal translocation and inverted

duplication associated with integrated hepatitis B virus in hepatocellular carcinomas. J Virol 61:1808–1813

21. Yaginuma K, Kobayashi M, Yoshida E, Koike K (1985) Hepatitis virus integration in hepatocellular carcinoma DNA: Duplication of cellular flanking sequences at the integration site. Proc Natl Acad Sci USA 82:4458–4462

22. Ziemer M, Garcia P, Shaul Y, Rutter WJ (1985) Sequence of hepatitis B virus DNA incorporated into the genome of a human hepatoma cell line. J Virol 53:885–892

23. Spandau DF, Lee CH, (1988) Trans-activation of viral enhancers by the hepatitis B virus X protein. J Virol 62:427–434

24. Seto E, Benedict Yen TS, Matija Perterlin B, Ou J-H (1988) Trans-activation of the human immunodeficiency virus long terminal repeat by the hepatitis B virus X protein. Proc Natl Acad Sci USA 85:8286–8290

25. Moriarty AM, Alexander H, Lerner RA, Thornton GB (1985) Antibodies to peptides detect with new-hepatitis B antigens: Serological correlation with hepatocellular carcinoma. Science 227:429–433

26. Kay A, Madart E, Trepo C, Galibert F (1985) The HBV HBx gene expressed in E.coli is recognised by sera from hepatitis patients. EMBO J 4:1287–1292

27. Meyers ML, Trepo LV, Nath N, Sninsky JJ (1986) Hepatitis B polypeptide X: Expression of Escherichia coli and identification of specific antibodies in sera from hepatitis B virus-infected humans. J Virol 57:101–109

28. Shirakata Y, Kawada M, Fujiki Y, Sano H, Oda M, Yaginuma K, Kobayashi M, Koike K (1989) The X gene of hepatitis B virus induced growth stimulation and tumorigenic transformation of mouse NIH3T3 cells. Jpn J Cancer Res 80:617–621

29. Yaginuma K, Shirakata Y, Kobayashi M, Koike K (1987) Hepatitis B virus (HBV) particles are produced in a cell culture system by transient expression of transfected HBV DNA. Proc Natl Acad Sci USA 84:2678–2682

30. Cooper GM (1982) Science 218:801–806

31. Land H, Parada LF, Weinberg RA (1983) Science 222:771–778

32. Chang EH, Gonda MA, Ellis RW, Scolnick EM, Lowy DR (1982) Human genome contains four genes homologous to transforming genes of Harvey and Kirsten murine sarcoma viruses. Proc. Natl. Acad. Sci. USA 79:4848–4852

33. Shimizu K, Goldfarb M, Suard Y, Perucho M, Li Y, Kamata T, Feramisco J, Stavnezer E, Fogh J, Wigler M (1983) Three human transforming genes are related to the viral ras oncogenes. Proc. Natl. Acad. Sci. USA 80:2112–2116

34. Tabin CJ, Bradley SM, Bargmann CI, Weinberg RA, Papageorge AG, Scolnick EM, Dhar R, Lowy DR, Chang EH (1982) Mechanism of activation of a human oncogene. Nature 300:143–149

35. Yuasa Y, Srivastava SK, Dunn CY, Rhim JS, Reddy EP, Aaronson SA (1983) Acquisition of transforming properties by alternative point mutations within c-bas/has human proto-oncogene. Nature 303:775–779

36. Yuasa Y, Gol RA, Chang A, Chiu I-M, Reddy EP, Tronick SR, Aaronson SA (1984) Mechanism of activation of an N-ras oncogene of SW-1271 human lung carcinoma cells. Proc. Natl. Acad. Sci. USA 81:3670–3674

37. Takada S, Koike K (1989) Activated N-ras gene was found in human hepatoma tissue but only in a small fraction of tumor cells. Oncogene 4:189–193

38. Koike K, Takada S, Iwami M, Yaginuma K, Kobayashi M (1986) Characterization of a transforming gene in human hepatoma cells containing integrated hepatitis B virus DNA. In: Oda T, Okuda K (eds.) New trends in hepatology. Medical Tosho, Tokyo, pp 150–164

39. Takada S, Iwami M, Kobayashi M, Koike K (1991) An oncogene obtained from human hepatocellular carcinoma was identified as the dbl Oncogene (Abstract). In: 2nd Meeting on The Molecular Basis of Human Cancer, Frederic, Md, USA, p 26

40. Hsu TY, Morony T, Etiemble J, Jouise A, Trepo C, Tiollais P, Buendia MA (1988) Activation of c-myc by woodchuck hepatitis virus insertion in hepatocellular carcinoma. Cell 55:627–635

41. Koike K, Shirakata Y, Yaginuma K, Arii M, Takada S, Nakamura I, Hayashi Y, Kawada M, Kobayashi M (1989) Oncogenic potential of hepatitis B virus. Mol Biol Med 6:151–160

42. Molnar-Kimber KL, Summers JW, Mason WS (1984) Mapping of a cohesive overlap of duck hepatitis B virus DNA and of the site of initiation of reverse transcription. J Virol 51:181–191

43. Miller RH, Robinson WS (1986) Common evolutionary origin of hepatitis B virus and retroviruses. Proc Natl Acad Sci USA 83:2531–2535

44. Takada S, Koike K (1990) Trans-activation function of a 3'-truncated gene-cell fusion product from integrated hepatitis B virus DNA in chronic hepatitis tissues. Proc Natl Acad Sci USA 87:5628–5632

45. Wollsersheim M, Debelka U, Hofschneider PH, (1988) A trans-activating function encoded in the hepatitis B virus X gene is conserved in the integrated state. Oncogene 3:545–552

46. Takada S, Koike K (1990) X protein of hepatitis B virus resembles a serine protease inhibitor. Jpn J Cancer Res 81:1191–1194

47. Laskowski M Jr, Kato I (1980) Protein inhibitors of proteinases. A Rev Biochem 49:593–626

48. Wunderer G, Machleidt W, Frotz H (1981) The broad-specificity proteinase inhibitor 5 II from the sea anemone Anemonia sulcata. Methods Enzymol 80:816–820

49. Strydom DJ, Joubert FJ (1981) Amino-acid sequence of a weak trypsin inhibitor-B from *Dendroaspis-polylepisé* (Black-mamba) Hoppe-Seyler's Z Physiol Chem 362:1377–1384

50. Mandart E, Kay A, Galibert F (1984) Nucleotide sequence of a cloned duck hepatitis B virus genome: Comparison with woodchuck and human hepatitis B virus sequences. J Virol 49:782–792

51. Colgrove R, Simon G, Ganem D (1989) Transcriptional activation of homologous and heterologous genes by the hepatitis B virus X gene product in cells permissive for viral replication. J Virol 63:4019–4020

52. Chisari FV, Klopchin K, Moriyama T, Pasquinelli C, Dunsford HA, Sell S, Pinkert CA, Brinster RL, Palmiter RD (1989) Molecular pathogenesis of hepatocellular carcinoma in hepatitis B virus transgenic mice. Cell 59:1145–1156

53. Mckeehan WL, Sakagami Y, Hoshi H, Mckeehan KA, (1986) Two apparent human endothelial cell growth factors from human hepatoma cells are tumor-associated proteinase inhibitors. J Biol Chem 261:5378–5383

54. Gasson JC, Golde DW, Kaufman SE, Westbrook CA, Hewick RM, Kaufman RJ, Wong GG, Temple PA, Leary AC, Brown EL, Orr EC, Clark SC (1985) Molecular characterization and expression of the gene encoding human erythroid-potentiating activity. Nature 315:768–771

55. Edwards DR, Waterhouse P, Holman ML, Denhardt DT (1986) A growth-responsive gene (16C8) in normal mouse fibroblasts homologous to a human collagenase inhibitor with erythroid-potentiating activity: Evidence for inducible and constitutive transcripts. Nucleic Acid Res 14:8863–8878

56. Höhne M, Schaefer S, Seifer M, Feitelson MA, Paul D, Gerlich WH (1990) Malignant transformation of immortalized transgenic hepatocytes after transfection with hepatitis B virus DNA. EMBO J 9:1137–1145

57. Kobayashi M, Koike K (1984) Complete nucleotide sequence of hepatitis B virus DNA of subtype *adr* and its conserved gene organization. Gene 30:227–232

58. Kodama K, Ogasawara N, Yoshikawa H, Murakami S (1985) Nucleotide sequence of a cloned woodchuck hepatitis virus genome. J Virol 56:978–986

59. Anderson S, Kingston IB (1983) Isolation of a genomic clone for bovine pancreatic trypsin inhibitor by using a unique-sequence synthetic DNA probe. Proc Natl Acad Sci USA 80:6838–6842

60. Kato I, Tominaga N (1979) Trypsin-subtilisin inhibitor from red sea turtle eggwhite consists of two tandem domains—one Kunitz—one of a new family. Fed Proc 38:832

61. Kido H, Yokogoshi Y, Katunuma N (1988) Kunitz-type protease inhibitor found in rat mast cells. J Biol Chem 263:18104–18107

Part 4 Diagnosis

Section 1 Clinical Features and Diagnosis

CHAPTER 10

Clinical features and diagnosis of primary liver cancer

Yutaka Inagaki, Masashi Unoura, and Kenichi Kobayashi[1]

1 Introduction

Primary liver cancer is one of the most common causes of cancer death in Japan, and approximately 23,000 patients died of this cancer in 1989 [1]. Moreover, the number of deaths due to primary liver cancer is increasing markedly every year. Hepatocellular carcinoma (HCC) accounts for 90% of primary liver cancer in Japan, and 80 to 90% of HCC is associated with liver cirrhosis [2, 3]. Poor hepatic functional reserve due to underlying cirrhosis is the major factor which limits extended surgical resection in many cases. Obviously it is important to detect HCC at an early stage for curative treatment.

HCC is usually insidious in onset and during its early stages. Therefore, it is difficult to diagnose small HCCs before they have reached an advanced stage. However, recent advances in diagnostic methods, especially ultrasonography [4, 5] and computed tomography (CT) [6, 7], have made it possible to detect early stages of HCC [8]. Indeed, small HCCs less than 2 cm in diameter are now frequently found in Japan, and some smaller than 1 cm are found. The Liver Cancer Study Group of Japan defines small liver cancer as a solitary liver neoplasm smaller than 2 cm in diameter confirmed by surgical resection or necropsy [9], and such small HCCs now account for approximately 10% of the total cases and 15% of the surgically resected cases in Japan [10]. On the other hand, it is still true that there are also many patients with advanced stages of HCC for which we cannot offer any effective therapy.

In this chapter, we describe the clinical features and diagnosis of HCC, with special emphasis on the risk factors for development of HCC and the screening methods for early detection of HCC.

2 Symptoms

No specific symptom is helpful to indicate the presence of a small HCC. In advanced stages of HCC, patients exhibit many symptoms, but most of them are not specific for the cancer. Table 1 indicates the frequency of the first presenting symptoms in patients with HCC, as summarized by the Liver Cancer Study Group of Japan [10, 11]. Periods I and II indicate observation periods from 1980 to 1981, and from 1986 to 1987, respectively. Some patients complained of two or more symptoms simultaneously. It is clearly shown that the frequency of presenting symptom(s) at the initial diagnosis of HCC is decreasing in period II. This decrease reflects an increase in diagnosis of HCC at earlier stages.

General malaise is the most common symptom in patients with HCC. Anorexia, abdominal pain, and sensation of abdominal fullness are also found frequently. However, none of these are specific for the presence of HCC; they reflect hepatomegaly and retention of ascites due to both HCC and underlying cirrhosis. A tumor may be palpable in the abdomen in advanced stages of HCC.

Fever is one of the most important clinical signs which we should keep in mind. It can be derived not only from infection and endotoxemia associated with cirrhosis but also from several important HCC-related conditions such as rupture into the peritoneal cavity, obstruction of the biliary tract followed by infection, and the tumor itself (tumor fever).

Tumor rupture into the peritoneal cavity usually occurs suddenly. It is characterized by

[1] First Department of Internal Medicine, School of Medicine, Kanazawa University, Kanazawa, Ishikawa, 920 Japan

Table 1. Frequency of the first presenting symptoms in patients with hepatocellular carcinoma

Period	I (1980–1981)	II (1986–1987)
Any symptom	78.4%	47.7%
General malaise	65.0%	59.4%
Anorexia	56.0	43.8
Abdominal pain	55.6	45.3
Abdominal fullness	52.1	43.4
Weight loss	42.2	25.7
Mass in abdomen	38.8	21.7
Ascites	28.7	22.7
Fever	23.0	14.7
Jaundice	20.7	14.7
Nausea/Vomiting	18.3	15.4
Edema	16.9	14.3
Hematemesis/Melena	7.1	5.4

shock and progressive anemia, and patients complain of severe abdominal pain and a sensation of abdominal fullness. Tumor rupture is usually observed in patients with advanced HCC, but it sometimes occurs in those with a smaller tumor. Some HCC nodules have a tendency toward extrahepatic growth [12]. This, combined with the fact that most HCC nodules are hypervascular [13], can result in rupture into the peritoneal cavity even at an early stage. Abdominal ultrasonography and paracentesis are necessary for diagnosis.

Jaundice may appear at a relatively late stage of HCC. It is due to hepatic failure and/or obstruction of the biliary tract by the tumor [14]. We observed a patient with HCC who presented with hemobilia due to rupture of lymph node metastasis into the common hepatic duct [15]. Again, abdominal ultrasonography is recommended for the differential diagnosis of jaundice, and magnetic resonance imaging (MRI) as well as endoscopic observation of the papilla of Vater is especially useful for the diagnosis of hemobilia.

Vessel invasion is the most characteristic feature of HCC. Portal vein thrombosis is frequently found in HCC, and more than 60% of autopsy cases present tumor emboli in the portal vein or its branches. Moreover, even in surgically resected HCC, portal vein thrombosis is found in 15% of the cases [10]. In patients with liver cirrhosis and accompanying esophageal varices, growth of HCC into the portal vein results in a marked change in hemodynamics in the portal system. Rapid worsening of portal system function and subsequent rupture of an esophageal varix sometimes follow tumor thrombus in the

portal vein. Bleeding from gastric ulcer and hemorrhagic gastritis are also common causes of hematemesis and melena in patients with liver cirrhosis with or without HCC. Emergency endoscopy should be performed to determine the origin and etiology of gastrointestinal bleeding.

Hepatic vein thrombosis is less common than portal vein thrombosis, but one fourth of HCC autopsy cases have associated tumor emboli in the hepatic veins [10]. Growth of the tumor into the hepatic portion of the inferior vena cava results in Budd-Chiari syndrome, which is characterized by the appearance of ascites, edema of the lower limbs, and dilated ascending veins on the back and anterior abdominal wall, as well as hepatosplenomegaly. Because most of these physical findings are common features of patients with liver cirrhosis who are in a decompensated state, the diagnosis of Budd-Chiari syndrome due to tumor invasion is sometimes difficult without imaging studies.

Invasion into the right atrium is occasionally found in patients with advanced HCC. We observed five HCC cases with right atrial invasion, and two of them presented with the ball valve thrombus syndrome [16]. In such cases, the tumor thrombus covers the orifice of the tricuspid valve, resulting in a sudden onset of dyspnea and weakness or absence of pulse. Recent advances in cardiac ultrasonography and angiography have made it easier to detect tumor growth into the inferior vena cava and right atrium, even at the asymptomatic stage.

HCC has been considered to have a relatively low incidence of distant metastasis [17, 18]. However, some patients with HCC complain of symptoms due to metastasis as the first clinical manifestation. Bone metastases may cause severe pain, pathologic fracture and paralysis. Transverse spinal cord interruption and Brown-Sequard's syndrome sometimes occur in patients with HCC with metastasis to vertebrae. Lung metastasis is usually asymptomatic at an early stage, but it can cause respiratory symptoms as it progresses. Lymph node metastasis and peritoneal dissemination are also restricted to a small proportion of patients with HCC [10]. The left supraclavicular lymph node is rarely palpable in patients with HCC, and cytology for malignant cells in the peritoneal fluid is negative except for the patients with tumor rupture into the peritoneal cavity.

Hypoglycemic attacks related to paraneoplastic syndrome are usually observed in advanced stages of HCC.

Table 2. Liver function tests in patients with early and advanced stages of hepatocellular carcinoma

Stage[a]	Early (I, II)	Advanced (III, IV)
Bilirubin (mg/dl)	1.2 ± 0.5	3.3 ± 7.3
Albumin (g/dl)	3.7 ± 0.5	3.8 ± 0.6
γ-Globulin (g/dl)	1.9 ± 0.3	1.8 ± 0.6
ZTT (KU)	21.1 ± 3.9	18.6 ± 7.8
TTT (KU)	14.0 ± 5.2	13.2 ± 9.3
ALP (IU/l)*	268 ± 65	382 ± 172
γ-GTP (IU/l)	114 ± 143	211 ± 261
GOT (IU/l)	93 ± 71	80 ± 46
GPT (IU/l)**	75 ± 48	51 ± 29
LDH (IU/l)	346 ± 87	395 ± 118
HPT (%)	71 ± 20	72 ± 23
ICGR$_{15}$ (%)	24 ± 9	29 ± 15

*$P < 0.01$ **$P < 0.05$

ZTT, Zinc turbidity test; TTT, thymol turbidity test; ALP, alkaline phosphatase; γ-GTP, γ-glutamyl transpeptidase; GOT, glutamic oxaloacetic transaminase; GPT, glutamate-pyruvate transaminase; LDH, lactate dehydrogenase; HPT, hepaplastin test; ICGR$_{15}$, indocyanine green retention rate at 15 minutes

[a] according to the general rules for the clinical and pathological study of primary liver cancer in Japan

3 Laboratory data

Liver function tests in patients with HCC can detect underlying cirrhosis but will not reveal the presence of HCC. Table 2 shows a comparison of the results of liver function tests in patients with early stages of HCC and those with advanced stages of HCC who were admitted to our department. The stage of each tumor was determined according to the general rules for the clinical and pathological study of primary liver cancer in Japan [9]. Although the differences in serum ALP and GPT levels in the two groups are significant

statistically, both values vary widely in each case. Serum levels of total bilirubin seem to increase in many patients with advanced stages of HCC, but the difference is not significant statistically.

Regarding liver function tests in patients with cirrhosis, we should keep in mind the presence of clinically latent cirrhosis [19]. Table 3 shows the findings in eight patients with latent cirrhosis who were admitted to our department. In all of these cases, liver function tests including the indocyanine green (ICG) retention rate were within normal limits [20]. The diagnosis of liver cirrhosis was based on the findings of peritoneoscopy and/or liver biopsy in each case. Serum HBsAg was positive in seven of eight cases, and anti-HBs antibody was positive in the remaining case. It seems that there are some reasons why latent cirrhosis is frequently found in HBV carriers. First, HBsAg is measured routinely in Japan on blood donation and on admission to hospitals, even because of non-liver diseases. HBV carriers are diagnosed unexpectedly in such cases, and some of them suffer from latent cirrhosis. Second, most HBV carriers undergo seroconversion from HBeAg to anti-HBe antibody. The disease activity usually decreases after seroconversion [21], and liver function tests return to within normal ranges in some patients with early stages of liver cirrhosis. Clinical use of the recently developed assay for anti-HCV antibody [22, 23] will reveal whether latent type C cirrhosis is present as well. It should be noted that two of the eight cases were associated with HCC. Ultrasonography was the first diagnostic method used to detect HCC in both cases. As described later, good hepatic functional reserve in patients with liver cirrhosis is the most significant risk factor for development of HCC. It is there-

Table 3. Liver function tests in patients with latent cirrhosis

Patient No. (Age/Sex)	Bilirubin (mg/dl)	Albumin (%)	γ-Globulin (%)	ZTT (KU)	γ-GTP (IU/l)	GOT (IU/l)	GPT (IU/l)	PT (sec)	ICGR$_{15}$ (%)
1. 50/Male[a]	0.45	63.9	18.4	11.6	34	31	32	13.4	4.0
2. 54/Male[a]	1.12	66.9	14.1	8.3	15	27	16	13.9	9.0
3. 51/Female	0.78	63.2	17.0	11.7	24	25	21	13.1	10.0
4. 30/Male	1.30	66.1	14.6	9.7	29	40	42	13.0	5.5
5. 34/Male	1.16	62.6	15.9	7.3	16	18	6	12.2	6.0
6. 53/Male	0.30	65.4	16.0	8.5	43	22	26	10.9	9.5
7. 40/Male	0.30	66.0	13.3	7.8	38	12	14	12.2	8.5
8. 67/Male	0.75	60.8	18.1	11.8	28	25	34	12.5	10.0
Normal range in our hospital	0.36~ 1.30	60.3~ 73.7	7.2~ 18.4	3.2~ 13.1	4~ 43	10~ 40	3~ 47	11.9~ 13.9	~10.0

[a] cases with associated hepatocellular carcinoma
PT, prothrombin time

fore important to perform ultrasonography as the first screening method for the detection of HCC in older patients with HBV and possibly in HCV carriers, even if their liver function tests are within normal range.

Several tumor markers are useful for the detection of HCC. Alpha-fetoprotein (AFP) has been most widely used for the diagnosis and monitoring of HCC [24, 25]. Recently, protein induced by vitamin K absence or antagonist-II (PIVKA-II) has been found to be a useful marker of HCC [26]. The clinical use and diagnostic value of tumor markers of HCC is described in another chapter.

Patients with HCC often present with the paraneoplastic syndrome. It is usually found in patients with advanced stages of HCC. According to the summary by the Liver Cancer Study Group of Japan, hypercholesterolemia is the most common paraneoplastic manifestation in patients with HCC, and hypercalcemia, erythrocytosis and hypoglycemia are found occasionally [10]. Leukocytosis, thrombocytosis and an increase in plasma fibrinogen and thyroxin binding globulin (TBG) levels are also reported. Table 4 is a summary of the laboratory findings in fourteen patients in our department who presented with paraneoplastic syndrome. Some patients presented with two or more paraneoplastic symptoms simultaneously. We have reported that paraneoplastic syndrome is frequently found in juvenile patients with HCC who are younger than forty [27]. Production of erythropoietin and

parathyroid hormone or related substances by the tumor is demonstrated in some cases [28, 29], but it does not account for all cases with paraneoplastic syndrome. Production of insulin-like substance(s) by the tumor is now thought to be unlikely as a causal mechanism of hypoglycemia. Consumption of a large amount of glucose and/or abnormality in the metabolic pathway of glucose in the tumor is speculated to be the cause.

4 Risk factors for HCC development

As already described, no specific symptoms or laboratory data, except for tumor markers, are available to detect HCC. Even measurement of tumor markers such as AFP and PIVKA-II is insufficient for an early recognition of small HCC [30, 31]. Much clinical concern should be focused how we can detect HCC at an early stage and treat it curatively. Although it is unknown whether or not a cirrhotic liver is a true precancerous lesion, patients with liver cirrhosis are a high risk group for the association of HCC. In Japan, more than 90% of HCC accompanies cirrhotic or precirrhotic chronic liver disease, and HCC seldom occurs in normal liver [2, 3]. It will be of great clinical value if we can predict an association of HCC in patients with liver cirrhosis and detect HCC at an early stage. It is also significant from the viewpoint of cost and efficacy

Table 4. Laboratory data in patients with hepatocellular carcinoma presenting with paraneoplastic syndrome

Patient No. (Age/Sex)	Cholesterol (mg/dl)	Minimum BS (mg/dl)	RBC ($\times 10^4$)	WBC ($\times 10^3$)	Platelet ($\times 10^4$)	Calcium (mEq/l)	Fibrinogen (mg/dl)	Association of cirrhosis
1. 38/Male	267	48	375	6.4	25.3	4.7	283	(−)
2. 63/Male	214	102	455	6.7	36.4	5.2	644	(−)
3. 23/Male	438	32	575	8.2	82.2	4.9	255	(−)
4. 61/Male	182	73	606	7.5	15.8	4.8	214	(+)
5. 53/Female	249	85	407	10.1	58.7	4.9	578	(−)
6. 60/Male	254	80	556	29.7	35.3	5.0	312	(+)
7. 52/Male	142	43	454	11.9	29.1	4.7	287	(+)
8. 54/Male	451	82	426	13.3	57.6	4.7	308	(+)
9. 38/Female	498	71	487	5.9	50.0	4.6	205	(−)
10. 59/Male	130	88	297	10.6	17.0	6.9	245	(+)
11. 68/Male	333	109	393	8.0	12.9	4.5	160	(+)
12. 55/Male	205	24	304	11.2	22.0	4.5	295	(−)
13. 66/Male	117	92	410	10.0	13.0	4.5	440	(+)
14. 58/Male	169	45	268	11.3	26.7	4.5	75	(+)
Normal range in our hospital	132~220	70~110	400~520	5.4~8.0	13.0~35.0	4.3~5.2	170~410	

Abnormal data are indicated by shading
BS, blood sugar; RBC, red blood cells; WBC, white blood cells

Table 5. Risk factors for development of hepatocellular carcinoma in patients with liver cirrhosis

Factors	Relative risk	Chi-squared test
1. Good hepatic reserve (group A in Child's classification)	5.9	$P < 0.0001$
2. Familial clustering of liver diseases	4.3	$P < 0.01$
3. Age (older than fifty)	3.8	$P < 0.001$
4. History of blood transfusion more than 10 years ago	1.5	NS
5. Positive HBsAg	1.3	NS
6. History of alcohol drinking[a]	1.1	NS
7. Sex (male)	0.7	NS

[a] more than 80 g of ethanol per day for more than 5 years
NS, not significant

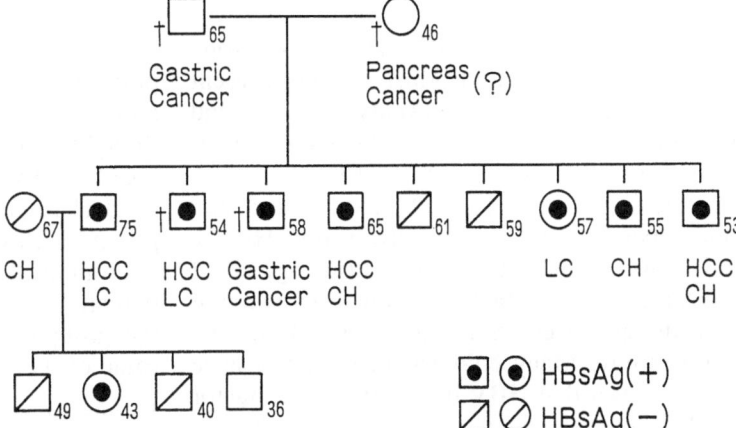

Fig. 1. A representative family showing a clustering of HBV infection and hepatocellular carcinoma. Other kinds of neoplasms were also found in the family members. *HCC*, hepatocellular carcinoma; *LC*, liver cirrhosis; *CH*, chronic hepatitis

to distinguish patients with liver cirrhosis who are in a "super" high risk group for development of HCC.

We investigated the risk factors for the association of HCC in patients with liver cirrhosis. A multivariate analysis using a multiple logistic model was performed in 125 patients with cirrhosis who developed HCC, and in 140 patients who did not developed HCC during the observation period. Of the several factors indicated in Table 5, good hepatic functional reserve (group A according to Child's classification), familial clustering of liver diseases and age of patients (older than fifty) were found to be independent risk factors for development of HCC. As to the contribution of each of these risk factors, good hepatic functional reserve has the largest relative risk (RR = 5.9) and familial clustering of liver diseases is second in importance (RR = 4.3).

Patients with liver cirrhosis in group A of Child's classification have no jaundice, ascites or encephalopathy. They are in a good nutritional state, and the serum albumin levels exceed 3.5 g/dl. They seldom die of hepatic failure, and even

if esophageal varices develop in such cases, esophageal trans-section and endoscopic infusion sclerotherapy are useful to stop the bleeding or prevent rupture of the varices. Consequently, they have a higher incidence of the association of HCC. Moreover, HCC development might be suppressed in the patients who are in a decompensated state of liver cirrhosis, in which regeneration of normal hepatocytes is also disturbed.

Familial clustering of liver diseases indicates not only the vertical and horizontal transmission of HBV but also some genetic factor(s) in the hosts leading to advanced liver disease and HCC development. Although most healthy HBV carriers are asymptomatic and have no specific histological findings in the liver, we have observed several families with a clustering of HBV infection and HCC. A representative family is shown in Fig. 1.

HCC is frequently found in patients with liver cirrhosis who are more than fifty years old, and this is true for most other neoplasms. However, a large proportion of HBV infections occur by vertical transmission from mother to infant in

Table 6. Comparison of the clinical features and prognosis of hepatocellular carcinoma found in regularly followed-up and non-regularly followed-up patients with liver cirrhosis

Group	Regularly followed-up	Non-regularly followed-up	
No. of cases	44	68	*P* value
Solitary tumor	25 (57%)	9 (13%)	*P* < 0.01
Tumor smaller than 3 cm	31 (70%)	9 (13%)	*P* < 0.01
Portal vein invasion	4 (9%)	18 (27%)	*P* < 0.05
Good hepatic reserve[a]	18 (41%)	20 (29%)	NS
Operated cases	19 (43%)	7 (10%)	*P* < 0.01
50% survival period	32 months	12 months	*P* < 0.001

[a] Expressed as the number and proportion of patients in clinical stage I according to the general rules for the clinical and pathological study of primary liver cancer in Japan

Japan, resulting in the HBV carrier state during the perinatal period [32]. Most of them present with hepatitis when around twenty years old, and it is unknown why at least a 30-year period is needed for the development of HCC.

Interestingly, a history of blood transfusion more than 10 years ago, positive serum HBsAg and a history of heavy alcohol drinking, all of which are important factors for the progression of liver disease, were not significant risk factors in this study. Many epidemiologic studies have clearly shown that HBV infection is a risk factor for HCC development [33, 34]. It is not significant, however, at least in the step from cirrhosis to HCC. Moreover, as described in another chapter, the relative frequency of serum HBsAg positivity among all HCC cases has been steadily decreasing every year [10]. In contrast, the incidence of a history of blood transfusion is increasing markedly in patients with HCC [35], and HCV infection is now found to be responsible for most of these cases [36]. Anti-HCV antibody is also found frequently in patients with HCC who have no history of blood transfusion and in those who have a history of heavy drinking [37, 38]. HCC seldom develops in Japan in patients with "pure" alcoholic cirrhosis who are seronegative for both HBV and HCV infection. These recent findings as to the etiology of HCC suggest that all patients with posthepatitic cirrhosis, regardless of HBV serology, have a high risk for HCC development.

Another great clinical problem in the treatment of HCC seems to be its recurrence after surgical resection. As described in another chapter, HCC has a much higher incidence of recurrence when compared to other neoplasms [39]. The recurrence rate of HCC after curative resection in our hospital was 20% within 1 year, 50% after 2 years, and 60% after 3 years. A high incidence of portal vein invasion, even at an early stage [40], and the multifocal origin of HCC [41, 42], are thought to be major reasons for the recurrence of HCC. In any event, patients who have undergone surgical resection of HCC are again a high risk group for further HCC development.

From all these findings, we propose that some patients with liver cirrhosis are a "super" high risk group for the association of HCC if they have some of the following risk factors:

1. surgical resection of HCC
2. group A of Child's classification
3. familial clustering of liver diseases
4. older than fifty
5. seropositive for hepatitis B or C virus

Screening methods for early detection of HCC should be performed especially in these patients, and will contribute to improvement in the survival of patients with HCC.

5   Screening methods for early detection of HCC

Since 1983, abdominal ultrasonography and AFP measurement have been performed systematically in patients with liver cirrhosis in our department [43]. Until now, a total of 112 patients with cirrhosis were diagnosed as having associated HCC. Table 6 indicates the clinical features and prognosis of HCC found in 44 regularly followed-up patients and 68 non-regularly followed-up patients. The incidence of solitary tumors and that of tumors smaller than 3 cm in diameter were significantly higher in the regularly followed-up

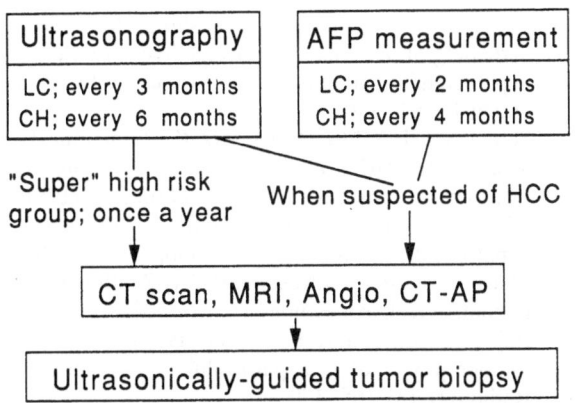

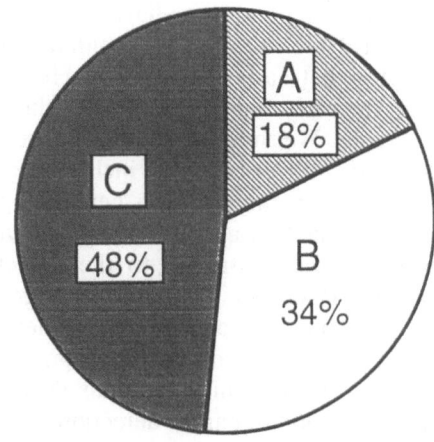

A : Appearance of multiple HCC nodules

B : Without regular examinations

C : Simultaneous diagnosis of HCC
     and liver cirrhosis

Fig. 2. Screening methods for early detection of hepatocellular carcinoma among patients with liver cirrhosis or chronic hepatitis. *AFP*, alpha-fetoprotein; *CT*, computed tomography; *MRI*, magnetic resonance imaging; *Angio*, hepatic arteriography; *CT-AP*, computed tomography during arterial portography; *LC*, liver cirrhosis; *CH*, chronic hepatitis

Fig. 3. The reasons that earlier diagnosis was not possible in 61 patients with advanced stages of HCC

group, and the incidence of portal vein invasion was significantly lower in this group compared to the non-regularly followed-up group. Although there was no significant difference in the hepatic functional reserve between the two groups, the 50% survival period of regularly followed-up patients (32 months) was significantly longer than that of non-regularly followed-up patients (12 months), indicating the clinical value of regular examinations in groups at high risk for HCC.

We propose the systemic screening methods shown in Fig. 2 for early detection of HCC. Patients with liver cirrhosis should undergo abdominal ultrasonography every three months and serum AFP measurement every two months. For patients with chronic hepatitis, ultrasonography should be performed every six months and serum AFP values should be measured every four months. When ultrasonography and/or elevation of serum AFP values is suggestive of HCC, various imaging studies such as CT scan, MRI, hepatic arteriography [13] and CT scan during arterial portography (CT-AP) [44] are recommended for further evaluation. In the case of the "super" high risk group, these imaging studies should be performed routinely once a year, even if HCC is not suspected as a result of ultrasonography and AFP measurement. It should be noted that a small HCC, especially smaller than 1 cm in diameter, is well-differentiated and does not necessarily present typical imaging patterns [8]. Nor is the measurement of serum AFP and PIVKA-II levels useful for the detection of

small HCC [30, 31]. Ultrasonically-guided tumor biopsy using a fine needle is recommended for the final diagnosis of HCC in such cases [45].

6 Current problems and future perspectives

As already discussed, recent advances in various imaging studies and regular examinations in the high risk group have contributed to the detection of HCC at an early stage. It is still true, however, that there are also many patients with advanced stages of HCC, for which we can offer no effective therapy. We analyzed the reasons why an earlier diagnosis was not made in 61 patients with advanced stages of HCC who were admitted to our department in a recent period of eight years. The patients were divided into three different categories. As shown in Fig. 3, 18% of the patients received regular examinations as described above, but multiple HCC nodules were detected simultaneously. Although 34% of the patients had been diagnosed as having liver cirrhosis, they did not receive regular examinations in the outpatient clinic. Finally, 48% of the patients were not aware that they were suffering from liver disease, and the diagnosis of liver cirrhosis and HCC was made simultaneously. This indicates that early detection of HCC still depends on the early diagnosis of liver cirrhosis in half of the cases. We should take much more care in the diagnosis of liver cirrhosis, including latent cirrhosis. Mass screening of the general population by combined assay of HBsAg and anti-HCV antibody will contribute to the detection of asymptomatic carriers, and ultrasonography should be performed to determine the underlying liver disease in such carriers. Once diagnosed as liver cirrhosis, the screening methods described above can contribute to earlier detection of HCC which can be treated curatively.

Another problem in the diagnosis of HCC is the management of adenomatous hyperplasia (AH) [46] and similar hyperplastic lesions. This is also discussed in another chapter. Various imaging techniques can detect small lesions in the liver, and sometimes the diagnosis of AH is made by ultrasonically-guided tumor biopsy. There has been increasing evidence that AH is a precancerous lesion and has a tendency toward malignant transformation [47, 48]. Moreover, there is a borderline lesion, "atypical" AH, which can be hardly distinguished from extremely well-differentiated HCC. Common diagnostic criteria are needed to clarify the nature and prognosis of ordinary and atypical AH and to determine whether or not we should treat these equivocal lesions.

Acknowledgments. We are grateful to Drs. K. Notsumata and K. Nishimura in our department for their clinical analyses of patients with HCC, and to Drs. T. Takashima and O. Matsui in the Department of Radiology, Kanazawa University, for their kind cooperation throughout the work.

References

1. Ministry of Health and Welfare (1990) Annual report of demographic statistics in Japan, 1989. Health and Welfare Statistics Association, Tokyo
2. Miyaji T (1976) Association of hepatocellular carcinoma with cirrhosis among autopsy cases in Japan during 14 years from 1958 to 1971. Gann Monogr Cancer Res 18:129–149
3. The Liver Cancer Study Group of Japan (1990) Primary liver cancer in Japan. Clinicopathologic features and results of surgical treatment. Ann Surg 211:277–287
4. Okazaki N, Yoshida T, Yoshino M (1984) Screening of patients with chronic liver disease for hepatocellular carcinoma by ultrasonography. Clin Oncol 10:241–246
5. Shinagawa T, Ohto M, Kimura K, Tsunetomi S, Morita M, Saisho H, Tsuchiya Y, Saotome N, Karasawa E, Miki M, Ueno T, Okuda K (1984) Diagnosis and clinical features of small hepatocellular carcinoma with emphasis on the utility of real-time ultrasonography. A study in 51 patients. Gastroenterology 86:495–502
6. Itai Y, Nishikawa J, Tasaka A (1979) Computed tomography of hepatocellular carcinoma. Radiology 131:165–170
7. Kunstinger F, Federle MP, Moss AA, Marks W. (1980) Computed tomography of hepatocellular carcinoma. Am J Roentgenol 134:431–437
8. Okuda K (1986) Early recognition of hepatocellular carcinoma. Hepatology 6:729–738
9. The Liver Cancer Study Group of Japan (1987) The general rules for the clinical and pathological study of primary liver cancer, 2nd edn. Kanehara, Tokyo
10. The Liver Cancer Study Group of Japan (1990) Follow-up investigation of primary liver cancer. 9th report. Shinko Press, Kyoto
11. The Liver Cancer Study Group of Japan (1984) Follow-up investigation of primary liver cancer. 6th report. Shinko Press, Kyoto
12. Horie Y, Katoh S, Yoshida H, Imaoka T, Suou T, Hirayama C (1983) Pedunculated hepatocellular carcinoma. Report of three cases and review of literature. Cancer 51:746–751
13. Takashima T, Matsui O (1980) Infusion hepatic angiography in the detection of small hepatocellular carcinoma. Radiology 136:321–325
14. Nakashima T, Okada K, Kojiro M, Jimi A, Yamaguchi R, Sakamoto K, Ikari T (1983) Pathology of hepatocellular carcinoma in Japan. 232 consecutive cases autopsied in ten years. Cancer 51:863–877
15. Hayakawa Y, Urabe T, Yoneshima M, Terada M, Mizuno Y, Matsushita E, Inagaki Y, Unoura M, Kobayashi K, Hattori N (1989) A case of hepatocellular carcinoma associated with hemobilia in which endoscopic nasobiliary drainage and urokinase infusion was useful for improving jaundice. Gastroenterol Endoscopy 31:2472–2477
16. Kato Y, Tanaka N, Kobayashi K, Ikeda T, Hattori N, Nonomura A (1983) Growth of hepatocellular carcinoma into the right atrium: report of five cases. Ann Intern Med 99:472–474
17. Edmondson HA, Steiner PE (1954) Primary carcinoma of the liver. A study of 100 cases among 48,900 necropsies. Cancer 7:462–503
18. Anthony PP (1973) Primary carcinoma of the liver: a study of 282 cases in Ugandan Africans. J Pathol Bacteriol 110:37–49
19. Sherlock S (1985) Clinically latent cirrhosis. In: Sherlock S (ed) Diseases of the liver and biliary

system, 7th edn. Blackwell Scientific Publications, London, p 340

20. Kobayashi K, Inagaki Y, Unoura M, Tanaka N, Kato Y, Hattori N (1991) Studies of clinically latent cirrhosis. Hepatogastroenterology 37:77–80, 1991

21. Hoofnagle JH, Seeff LB (1982) Natural history of chronic type B hepatitis. In: Popper H, Schaffner F (eds) Progress in liver diseases, vol VII. Grune and Stratton, New York, p 469

22. Choo QL, Kuo G, Weiner AJ, Overby LR, Bradley DW, Houghton M (1989) Isolation of a cDNA clone derived from a blood-born non-A, non-B viral hepatitis genome. Science 244:359–362

23. Kuo G, Choo QL, Alter HJ, Gitnick GL, Redeker AG, Purcell RH, Miyamura T, Dienstag JL, Alter MJ, Stevens CE, Tegtmeier GE, Bonino F, Colombo M, Lee WS, Kuo C, Berger K, Shuster JR, Overby LR, Bradley DW, Houghton M (1989) An assay for circulating antibodies to a major etiologic virus of human non-A, non-B hepatitis. Science 244:362–364

24. Kew MC (1975) Alpha-fetoprotein. In: Read AE (ed) Modern trends in gastroenterology, vol 5. Butterworths, London, p 91

25. Alpert E (1976) Human alpha-1 fetoprotein. In: Okuda K, Peters RL (eds) Hepatocellular carcinoma. John Wiley and Sons, New York, p 353

26. Liebman HA, Furie BC, Tong MJ, Blanchard RA, Lo KJ, Coleman MS, Furie B (1984) Des-r-carboxy (abnormal) prothrombin as a serum marker of primary hepato-cellular carcinoma. N Engl J Med 310:1427–1431

27. Furusawa A, Unoura M, Notsumata K, Morioka T, Hayakawa K, Matsushita E, Kobayashi K, Hattori N, Makino H, Fukuoka K, Tanaka N, Nakagawa H, Nishimura K, Kanai M, Sugimoto T (1989) Clinico-pathological study of juvenile hepatocellular carcinoma. Jpn J Gastroenterol 86:2765–2772

28. Kew MC, Fisher JW (1986) Serum erythropoietin concentration in patients with hepatocellular carcinoma. Cancer 58:2485–2488

29. Knill-Jones RP, Buckle RM, Parsons V, Calne RY, Williams R (1970) Hypercalcemia and increased parathyroid-hormone activity in a primary hepatoma. N Engl J Med 282:704–708

30. Kubo Y, Okuda K, Musha H, Nakashima T (1978) Detection of hepatocellular carcinoma during a clinical follow-up of chronic liver disease. Observations in 31 patients. Gastroenterology 74:578–582

31. Hattori N, Ohmizo R, Unoura M, Tanaka N, Kobayashi K (1988) Abnormal prothrombin measurements in hepatocellular carcinoma. J Tumor Marker Oncol 3:207–216

32. Okada K, Kamiyama I, Inomata M, Imai M, Miyakawa Y, Mayumi M (1976) e Antigen and anti-e in the serum of asymptomatic carrier mothers as indicators of positive and negative transmission of hepatitis B virus to their infants. N Engl J Med 294:746–749

33. Popper H, Gerber MA, Thung SN (1982) The relation of hepatocellular carcinoma to infection with hepatitis B and related viruses in man and animals. Hepatology 2:1S-9S

34. Beasley RP, Lin CC, Hwang LY, Chien CS (1981) Hepatocellular carcinoma and hepatitis B virus: A prospective study of 22,707 men in Taiwan. Lancet II:1129–1132

35. Ohbayashi A, Tanaka S, Ohtake H, Harada H, Komachiya K, Kodama T, Okada Y, Takahashi K, Tanaka N, Yamada H, Sakamoto H, Shimizu M (1983) Clinico-pathological observations on relationship of blood transfusion to liver cirrhosis and hepatocellular carcinoma. Acta Hepatol Jpn 24:521–525

36. Kiyosawa K, Sodeyama T, Tanaka E, Gibo Y, Yoshizawa K, Nakano Y, Furuta S, Akahane Y, Nishioka K, Purcell RH, Alter HJ (1990) Interrelationship of blood transfusion, non-A, non-B hepatitis and hepatocellular carcinoma: analysis by detection of antibody to hepatitis C virus. Hepatology 12:671–675

37. Saito I, Miyamura T, Ohbayashi A, Harada H, Katayama T, Watanabe Y, Koi S, Onji M, Ohta Y, Choo QL, Houghton M, Kuo G (1990) Hepatitis C virus infection is associated with the development of hepatocellular carcinoma. Proc Natl Acad Sci USA 87:6547–6549

38. Shimizu S, Kiyosawa K, Sodeyama T, Tanaka E, Yosizawa K, Nakano Y, Usuda S, Furuta S (1990) Prevalence of antibody to hepatitis C virus in heavy drinkers with liver disease. Acta Hepatol Jpn 31:589–590

39. Nagao T, Inoue S, Yoshimi F, Sodeyama M, Omori Y, Mizuta T, Kawano N, Morioda Y (1990) Postoperative recurrence of hepatocellular carcinoma. Ann Surg 211:28–33

40. Kanai T, Hirohashi S, Upton MP, Noguchi M, Kishi K, Makuuchi M, Yamasaki S, Hasegawa H, Takayasu K, Moriyama N, Shimosato Y (1987) Pathology of small hepatocellular carcinoma. A proposal for a new gross classification. Cancer 60:810–819

41. Esumi M, Aritaka T, Arii M, Suzuki K, Tanikawa K, Mizuo H, Mima T, Shikata T (1986) Clonal origin of human hepatoma determined by integration of hepatitis B virus DNA. Cancer Res 46:5767–5771

42. Blum HE, Offensperger WB, Walter E, Offensperger S, Wahl A, Zeschnigk C, Gerok W (1987) Hepatocellular carcinoma and hepatitis B virus infection: molecular evidence for monoclonal origin and expansion of malignantly transformed hepatocytes. J Cancer Res Clin Oncol 113:466–472

43. Kobayashi K, Sugimoto T, Makino H, Kumagai M, Unoura M, Tanaka N, Kato Y, Hattori N (1985) Screening methods for early detection of hepatocellular carcinoma. Hepatology 6:1100–1105

44. Matsui O, Kadoya M, Suzuki M (1983) Work in progress: dynamic sequential computed tomography during arterial portography in the detection of hepatic neoplasms. Radiology 146:721–727
45. Majima Y, Fujimoto T, Iwai I, Tanaka M, Sakai T, Abe M, Abe H, Tanikawa K (1988) Histological diagnosis of hepatocellular carcinoma by a new technique of ultrasound-guided fine needle biopsy. Acta Hepatol Jpn 29:628–636
46. Edmondson HA (1976) Benign epithelial tumors and tumor-like lesions of the liver. In: Okuda K, Peters RL (eds) Hepatocellular carcinoma. John Wiley and Sons, New York, p 309
47. Arakawa M, Sugihara S, Kenmochi K, et al. (1986) Small mass lesions in cirrhosis: transition from benign adenomatous hyperplasia to hepatocellular carcinoma. J Gastroenterol Hepatol 1:3–14
48. Takayama T, Makuuchi M, Hirohashi S, Sakamoto M, Okazaki N, Takayasu K, Kosuge T, Motoo Y, Yamazaki S, Hasegawa H (1990) Malignant transformation of adenomatous hyperplasia to hepatocellular carcinoma. Lancet 336:1150–1153

Section 2   Diagnostic Imaging

An overview of diagnostic imaging techniques for detecting hepatocellular carcinoma

Choichiro Kido[1]

1 Introduction

The frequency of hepatocellular carcinoma (HCC) is increasing in Japan where it is now the third leading cause of death among males. HCC is relatively uncommon in the West but it is more common in Africa, Southeast Asia and Japan; and it is also known to have a high incidence in areas where the HBs antigen is prevalent.

Recent advances in imaging techniques have made significant contributions to the detection and elucidation of pathological changes in the liver. Based on clinical experience, it is relatively simple to define the population at the risk of developing HCC, and it is becoming inceasingly simple to survey such populations and detect relatively small lesions. Through these diagnostic techniques it has become possible to establish interventional radiology (IVR) and to obtain unequivocal results. This chapter concentrates on the characterisitics, effectiveness and limitations of the various imaging techniques for HCC, and also discusses IVR.

2 Ultrasonography

The main features of Ultrasonography (US) are that it is a noninvasive method that permits imaging from all angles. In addition, US can be used as a monitoring method under which needle cytology can be performed or anhydrous alcohol can be instilled, and is effective for IVR. As such, US is an extremely important imaging method that should be the first method of choice. With recently developed US equipment, it has become possible to detect HCC covered with a fibrotic capsule, which is common in Japan, and HCC lesions smaller than 2 cm in diameter. The Doppler method can demonstrate changes in the rate of blood flow accompanying the development of HCC or impedance of blood flow as a result of tumor-related thrombi in the protal vein. However, areas immediately below the diaphragm, such as S_7, S_8 and S_3 can be blind spots. With liver cirrhosis, the blind spot resulting from contraction of the anterior segment of the right lobe can be large. In addition, distinguishing between regenerative nodules and small HCC lesions can be difficult with this method.

The following list includes some of the characteristic US findings of HCC:

1. As the HCC increases in size, the appearance tends more towards a mosaic pattern with fibrosis and necrosis developing within the lesions as well as lobulation
2. In non-tumorous areas of hepatitis or cirrhosis, there is no decrease in the US waves and the image appears as a posterior echo because the tumor is soft
3. The lateral echo and halo deriving from the fibrotic pseudocapsule are characteristic findings in many of the HCC cases detected in Japan
4. In embolism of the portal vein, which frequently occurs in HCC, US shows an extremely well-filled portal vein. Incidentally, the rate of detection of HCC lesions measuring 2–3 cm in diameter is 98% [1], and it is 100% for larger lesions

Recently, the US color Doppler system has been employed to measure hemodynamics for the diagnosis of HCC [2]. In HCC tumors less than 2 cm in size, a signal is detected in 85% of the cases, while there is no signal detected from

[1] Aichi Cancer Center, Chigusa-ku, Nagoya, Aichi, 464 Japan

non-tumorous areas or intrahepatic regenerative nodules.

The diagnostic accuracy of needle biopsy using a 21G needle inserted under US supervision is 86–97%, but the accuracy varies according to the size of the lesion [1]. It is only natural that the results of cytology are not as satisfactory as those of histologic diagnosis, but the method of cytologic harvesting under US monitoring deserves attention as it is safe and simple, and the degree of invasiveness is relatively low.

In the case of HCC, the presence of daughter lesions or thrombi can significantly affect the prognosis. It is, therefore, extremely important to recognize such conditions intraoperatively and to take appropriate counteractive measures. The ability to recognize such conditions macroscopically or by palpation is understandably limited. Therefore, examination by 5 MHz or 7.5 MHz US probes during the operation can help in determining the appropriate extent of resection. Since structures that cause blind spots on extracorporeal examination can be circumvented. While US examination does involve some blind spots, it is non-invasive and, unlike CT, it is easy to perform the examination from a variety of angles, giving a relatively three-dimensional understanding of the blood vessels and the intrahepatic bile duct.

There are also limitations regarding spatial analysis which makes it difficult to detect HCC lesions less than 15 mm in size. Apart from HCC lesions possessing pseudocapsules and their distinctive lateral shadow and halo, other HCC lesions are difficult to distinguish from blood vessels or regenerative nodules. However, US is considered to be the diagnostic imaging modality of choice in the group of subjects at high risk for HCC.

3 Computed tomography

Computed tomography (CT) is becoming widely employed as a routine radiographic technique. In addition to plain CT, there are now various types of enhanced CT techniques which can permit not only the detection of lesions but also yield qualitative information concerning the internal structure of the lesion. Various methods can contribute to qualitative diagnostic CT imaging, such as drip infusion CT, bolus injection CT, dynamic

CT, CT angiography, and dynamic sequential CT with table incrementation during arterial portography [3]. In addition, 3-dimensional computerized imaging and helical CT are being highly evaluated. CT is effective in imaging splenomegaly, atrophy of the right hepatic lobe, hypertrophy of the left hepatic lobe, esophageal varices, ascites, and space occupying lesions with low absorption, accompanying hepatic cirrhosis. Contrast medium can also yield further information concerning the histological characteristics of these internal structural changes. Furthermore, conventional CT images involve slices of fixed thickness so that sometimes only part of a small lesion can be seen in cross-section. Changes in absorption might occur or a lesion might not be detected because of the partial volume phenomenon. These problems can be overcome by the use of thin slice CT or helical CT.

While the ability of CT to detect encapsulated HCC is lower than that of US (87% vs. 94%) [4], CT has no blind spots and it is also unaffected by the relative experience of the examiner. Furthermore, by the planned use of contrast medium, the lesion can be revealed dynamically, and differential diagnosis with this method has a high level of reliability. Infusion of Lipiodol into the hepatic artery has been shown to embolize the tumor [5]. Since Lipiodol remains in extremely small HCC lesions or metastatic liver lesions, it can be employed for diagnostic imaging, but it must be remembered that it does not necessarily penetrate all small lesions.

HCC lesions 2 cm in diameter or less are referred to as extremely small lesions and their prognosis is good. They generally appear on CT as round lesions with low or homogenous absorption, and they can be detected by reducing the window level of the plain CT and by either increasing the contrast or by employing a contrast medium. Unlike tumors larger than 2 cm, extremely small lesions do not possess characteristic findings such as internal changes or necrosis. Many of the HCC lesions detected in Japan that are 1–2 cm in size have a capsule, but in most cases the capsule is thin and difficult to detect.

Tumor embolism of the portal vein is easily detected by both US and CT. For tumors less than 3 cm in size, the detection rate of CT (79%) is slightly less than that of US (82%) [6].

The accuracy of CT in nodular or massive type-lesions is high. However, in diffuse-type cases in which the liver tissue is replaced by numerous small nodules surrounded by connective tissue, diagnosis by CT is difficult, just as it is in cancer of the intrahepatic bile duct.

In summary, CT, like US, provides cross-sectional images from a variety of planes and its accuracy can be increased by enhancement with a contrast medium. HCC is accompanied by hepatic cirrhosis in approximately 80% of cases, but in cases unaccompanied by this condition it is important to make a differential diagnosis taking into account other conditions resembling HCC such as focal nodular hyperplasia, adenoma, liver cell adenoma and hemangioma.

4 Angiography

Selective arteriography used to be performed for the diagnosis of liver parenchymal diseases, but due to the recent progress in noninvasive methods such as US, CT and MRI, this technique is now largely restricted to interventional radiology, which will be described later. The vascular findings of HCC show a distinct pattern including irregular dilatation, proliferation of meandering vessels, tumor stain, A-V shunt, A-P shunt, avascular areas within the tumor, venous threads and streaks, and pooling of the contrast medium.

There are also cases of HCC which do not show tumor stain even after administration of contrast medium or which do not show the classical vascular findings associated with HCC. These are seen in cases with a high level of fibrous components, such as those accompanied by cirrhotic changes, necrosis or marked metamorphosis, highly differentiated Edmondson's type I cases, and those with sarcomatous changes. Such cases are difficult to distinguish from hemangiomas. As a result of the improvement of angiography catheters, it has become easier to perform super-selective angiography and digital subtraction angiography (DSA) which enables a diagnosis to be made with an extremely small amount of contrast medium.

At present, angiography is more commonly employed in IVR rather than for the detection or differential diagnosis of HCC. TAE (Trans-arterial embolization) is performed using a metal coil, a mixture of Lipiodol, and a chemo-therapeutic agent. Other methods are avaliable for the preoperative elucidation of vascular distribution, determination of the site of the lesions, and detection of the presence of intrahepatic metastasis or portal vein tumor thrombus. The significance of arteriography is extremely important in the detection of very small lesions.

5 Magnetic resonance imaging

Magnetic resonance imaging (MRI) is a relatively new technique that can naturally be applied to HCC [7, 8]. It has the advantages of not involving radiation, and allowing a free selection of the cross-section plane. It is not influenced by bone or the presence of intracolonic gas, it permits observation of the portal and venous systems without using a contrast medium, and the contrast between areas of tumor and normal areas is high.

However, with presently available equipment, the time required for the examination is considerable so it cannot be performed in cases which cannot undergo examination for an extended period of time or who have magnetic implants. However since this method provides much valuable information future progress with this method is anticipated including reducing the time required for the examination.

HCC lesions generally appear as a low signal on T1-weighted images and as a high signal on the T2-weighted images. The images also reveal many morphological characteristics. Capsules appear as a ring-like low signal region and mosaic patterns reflecting septal walls within the tumor appear strongly on the T1-weighted image. This type of imaging potential is said to be the same as that of CT. However, as mechanical improvements continue to overcome various obstacles and problems, reports of MRI being more effective in the diagnosis of HCC are beginning to appear. For HCC lesions 2 cm or less, the detection rate by CT is 72%, whereas by MRI it is 93%. In lesions larger than that, detection by MRI is 100% [9].

Since HCC generally yields a high signal on T2-weighted images, detection is generally simple. On the T1-weighted images, the signal is either homogenous, low or high. Tumorous lesions of the liver that yield a high signal include HCC, hemorrhagic hepatic cyst, and liver cell adenoma. Because other entities generally yield a low signal, it is important to examine the correlation between T1- and T2-weighted images to make a differential diagnosis. To improve the quality of the diagnostic imaging, dynamic MRI involving bolus arterial injection of G-DTPA and short-term imaging will no doubt be developed [10].

6 Interventional radiology

Interventional radiology has been widely promoted by Margulis, Wallace and others and is now commonly employed not only in vascular but also in non-vascular areas. IVR techniques applied in HCC include TAE (arterial injection of Lipiodol and a chemotherapeutic drug), continuous infusion of a high concentration of chemotherapy drugs by a reserver, and selective hepatic arteriography. There is also the PEIT method involving injection of anhydrous alcohol directly into the HCC lesion, and accurate puncture of the lesion under US monitoring. All of these procedures can provide important information to preoperatively determine the stage of the disease.

7 Diagnosis of small hepatocellular carcinomas

The HCC high risk group consists primarily of hepatic cirrhosis, which accounts for 80% of HCC cases, as well as B type or A type chronic hepatitis plus rarer conditions such as those with a history of Thorotrast or vinyl chloride, or oral contraceptives. In high risk cases, it is important to follow changes in HCC tumor markers such as AFP (alpha-fetoprotein) and PIVK-II (protein-induced vitamin K absence or antagonist-II) in combination with regular diagnostic imaging of the liver in order to detect small lesions at a treatable stage.

As has previously been noted, US is the first examination of choice. In cases in which a typical US image cannot be obtained or differential diagnosis from hepatic hemangioma cannot be obtained, then the next examination method of choice is MRI [11]. However, if MRI is not available, the findings can be clarified by enhanced CT (dynamic CT is the most effective). Once HCC has been confirmed, angiography can be performed for the purposes of IVR or preoperative work-up. In such cases, instillation of Lipiodol can be performed to elucidate small lesions that had previously not been noted on

diagnostic imaging followed by repeat evaluation by CT. When resection is performed, intraoperative US should be performed. Biopsy under US guidance can be performed at the stage of localization.

8 Conclusion

Progress in diagnostic imaging has caused a revolution in the diagnosis of HCC. Less invasive yet more accurate methods have been developed and, when combined logically, they permit the selection of the optimal therapeutic strategy which in turn holds hope for extension of survival and improvement of the quality of life for HCC patients. Each type of procedure has its own distinct features, and it should be the aim of the radiologist not to perform as many different procedures as possible and compare the respective accuracy but rather, knowing the limits of each type of procedure, to decide on the most appropriate method. Also, when the indications are present, effective IVR must be performed. Be that as it may, it must be remembered not to merely perform examinations for the sake of examinations, but rather to permit the patient to be treated with time-saving and cost-saving methods.

References

1. Ebara M, Nihira T, Yashiro K, Ohto M (1990) Ultrasonography of the small hepatocellular carcinoma (in Japanese). J Med Imag 8:1274–1281
2. Taylor KJW, Ramos I, Morse SS (1987) Focal Liver masses: Differential diagnosis with pulsed Doppler US. Radiology 164:643–647
3. Matsui O, Kadoya M, Suzuki M, Takashima T (1983) Dynamic sequential computed tomography during arterial portography in the direction of hepatic neoplasms. Radiology 146:721–727
4. Kuroda T, Marukawa T, Hosoki T, Masuike M, Tokunaga K, Kozuka T (1988) CT diagnosis of hepatoma (in Japanese). J Med Imag 8:1283–1288
5. Ohishi H, Uchida H, Yoshimura H, Ohue S, Ueda J, Katsuragi M, Matsuo N, Hosogi Y (1985) Hepatocellular carcinoma detected by iodized oil. Radiology 154:25–29
6. Matsui O, Takashima T, Kadoya M, Kitagawa K, Kamimura R, Itoh H, Suzuki M, Ida M (1984) Segmental staining on hepatic arteriography as a

sign of intrahepatic portal vein obstruction. Radiology 152:601–606

7. Ebara M, Ohto M, Watanabe Y, Kimura K, Saisho H, Tsuchiya Y, Okuda K, Arimizu N, Kondo F, Ikehira H, Fukuda N, Tateno Y (1986) Diagnosis of small hepatocellular carcinoma: Correlation of MR imaging and tumor histologic studies. Radiology 159:371–377

8. Itai Y, Kokubo K, Makita T, Okuda Y, Yashiro N (1986) MR imaging of hepatocellular carcinoma. J Comput Assist Tomogr 10:963–968

9. Itoh K, Nishimura K, Togashi K, Fujisawa I, Noma S, Minami S, Sagoh T, Nakano Y, Itoh K, Mori K, Ogawa K, Torizuka K (1987) Hepatocellular carcinoma: MR imaging. Radiology 164:21–25

10. Hirai K, Ono N, Tanikawa K (1990) MRI in Hepatocellular carcinoma—correlation with US, CT Angiography. J Med Imag 10:1299–1304

11. Itoh K, Shibata T, Konishi J (1990) MRI of Hepatocellular Carcinoma—On the basis of pathology (in Japanese) J Med Imag 10:1292–1298

CHAPTER 12

Ultrasonographic diagnosis of hepatocellular carcinoma

Seigo Sakaguchi, Keiji Tohara, and Yoshihiko Oka[1]

1 Introduction

The liver is the largest soft tissue organ in the body and, acoustically, it consists of roughly homogeneous parenchyma. Its position in the body allows negligible interference caused by gas in the digestive canal. Therefore, the liver is an excellent organ to evaluate by means of ultrasonography, especially for the detection of hepatocellular carcinoma (HCC). Normal hepatic parenchyma is seen as a homogeneous and fine echogenic pattern, and focal disorders in the liver cause focal alteration in acoustic impedance which are easily recognizable as abnormally and irregularly localized hypoechoic, isoechoic, hperechoic, or anechoic areas either alone or in combination.

The value of hepatic ultrasonography has not been completely elucidated. Radionuclide study, computed tomography (CT), magnetic resonance imaging (MRI), and angiography of the liver are alternative examinations that have been proven to be valuable in detecting hepatic lesions. These methods are often used in combination to correctly diagnose or treat many cases of HCC.

In this chapter the ultrasonic diagnosis and its differential diagnosis of HCC in Japan are presented and discussed.

2 General remarks for diagnosis of HCC

2.1 Ultrasonographic techniques

Abdominal scanning for hepatic diseases using ultrasound (US) ordinarily starts laterally on the right near the spleen and left kidney or left

---

[1] First Department of Internal Medicine, School of Medicine, Fukuoka University, Fukuoka, 814-01 Japan

adrenal gland. Next, with the patient supine, both lobes of the liver, the hepatic vein and inferior vena cava, portal system, biliary system and pancreas, and lymph nodes are examined. Longitudinal, transverse, oblique and intercostal scanning are suitable for these observations. Then, with the patient in a left lateral position, the hepatic right lobe, common bile duct, right adrenal gland, and right kidney are examined.

To prevent interruption by gas in a lung or the digestive canal, or the shadowing of a rib, hepatic movement by deep inspiration and expiration, either sitting or standing, are recommended to obtain the best results.

2.2 Variables in the diagnosis of HCC

Variables which must be determined to properly diagnose HCC are as follows:

2.2.1 Form of the liver
In a normal subject, the hepatic edge is sharp and its surface is smooth [1]. Rounded edge, uneven surface, and an enlarged caudate lobe are often encountered in chronic diseases of the liver [1]. The hump sign suggests the existence of a tumor near the hepatic surface. An enlarged right lobe suggests the complication of chronic hepatitis, and an atrophic liver suggests hepatic cirrhosis [1].

2.2.2 Parenchymal echogenicity of the liver
Homogeneous echogenic parenchyma of the liver is observed in normal or non-focal disorders. Increased echogenicity of hepatic parenchyma is encountered in patients with fatty metamorphosis or fibrosis in the liver [2–4]. Decreasing echogenicity is observed in cellular infiltration such as with acute hepatitis [4].

Abnormally localized and heterogeneous hyperechoic, isoechoic, hypoechoic, or anechoic areas are important findings for the detection of focal disorders such as HCC.

2.2.3 Size of the spleen:
The anterior-posterior size of the spleen in right lateral position is estimated to be less than 8 cm in normal Japanese subjects [5].

Splenomegaly may suggest the presence of chronic disease of the liver such as chronic hepatitis, hepatic cirrhosis, or HCC.

2.2.4 Portal system, hepatic vein, inferior vena cava and biliary system
A normal splenic vein near the pancreas, the main trunk of the portal vein, and its umbilical portion are 0.7–0.8 cm, 1.1 cm and 0.9 cm, respectively [6]. Dilated or tortuous portal vein, varices and collateral circulation of the portal system such as spleno-renal shunt suggests the presence of portal hypertension.

2.2.5 Other abnormalities
Normally, the adrenal gland, lymph nodes and ascites are not detected. When these are detected, some abnormal situations are suggested such as metastasis or decompensation of hepatic function.

Minimal ascites can be identified as collections of fluid, especially between the right hepatic lobe and the right kidney, around a root of the mesentery, and adjacent to the urinary bladder.

2.3 Indications of ultrasonography for HCC

The indications of ultrasonography for HCC are as follows:

2.3.1 Detection of masses in the liver
Malignant tumors in the liver such as cholangio-cellular carcinoma or metastatic carcinoma; benign tumors such as cavernous hemangioma; and tumor-like lesions such as focal nodular hyperplasia, regenerative nodule, regional fatty infiltration, or a focal area with relatively less fat than the rest of the liver are easily detected with US.

2.3.2 Differentiation of HCC from other malignant tumors and benign focal disorders in the liver
These indications for the differential diagnosis of HCC using US are somewhat limited at the present time. However, expectations for US due to its non-invasiveness in diagnosis of HCC are increasing as equipment is improved newer systems such as the ultrasonic Doppler

method and ultrasonic contrast enhancement.

2.3.3 Locating the mass
Using ultrasonographic scanning, one can observe the portal vein, hepatic vein, and a part of the intrahepatic bile duct simultaneously. Thus, hepatic segments [7, 8] are easily recognizable. It is important to grasp the segmentation of the liver and hepatic vessels to the tumor for surgical treatment or for transcatheter arterial embolization.

2.3.4 Evaluation of hepatic complications in HCC
Evaluation of underlying hepatic changes associated with HCC such as hepatic cirrhosis and portal hypertension; and emboli in the portal veins, hepatic veins, and inferior vena cava are essential for the differential diagnosis of HCC from metastatic carcinoma. These findings are also essential to determine the proper modality of treatment. Other abnormal findings may include enlarged lymph nodes or ascites.

2.3.5 Ultrasonically-guided insertion of a needle into the liver
Ultrasonically-guided insertion of a needle for percutaneous transhepatic portography, measurement of the portal pressure, needle biopsy for the histological diagnosis, or percutaneous transhepatic ethanol injection are newly developed techniques that employ ultrasonography. The details concerning these techniques will appear in Chap. 11.

3 Special treatise for diagnosis of HCC

3.1 Ultrasonography of hepatic focal disorders

3.1.1 Diagnostic criteria for detection of masses by ultrasonography
The diagnostic criteria for ultrasonography for the definitive existence of masses in the liver proposed by the Japan Society of Ultrasonic Medicine and Biology are given below [9].

Echo levels of the hepatic tissue surrounding a mass can be hypoechoic, isoechoic, hyperechoic, or anechoic. They reveal homogeneous or heterogeneously combined, mosaic or mixed type, or the formation of septa. Demonstration of a mass on two different scanning planes at right angles to each other, such as right subcostal and intercostal scans, indicates the presence of

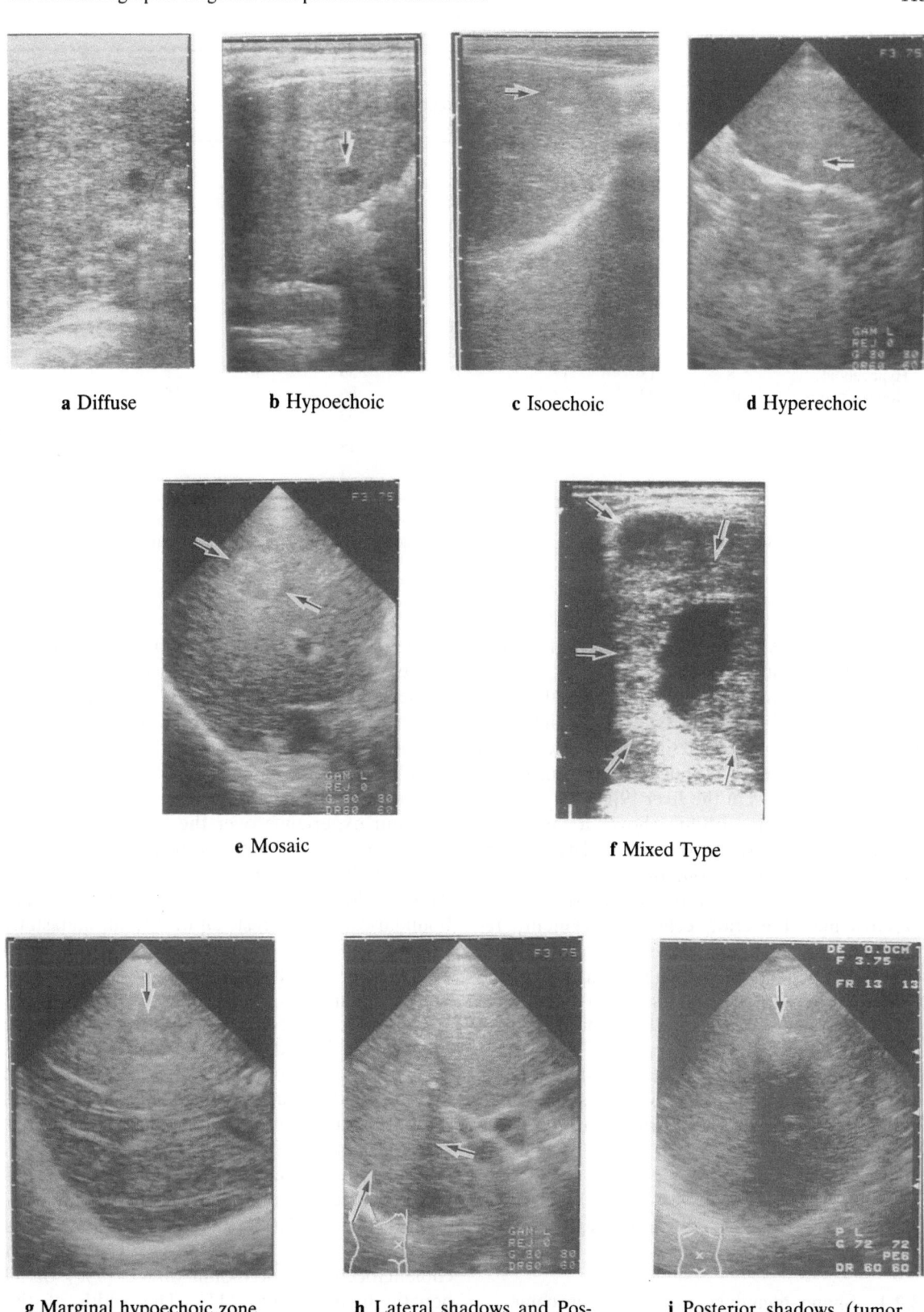

a Diffuse   **b** Hypoechoic   **c** Isoechoic   **d** Hyperechoic

e Mosaic   **f** Mixed Type

g Marginal hypoechoic zone   **h** Lateral shadows and Posterior echo-enhancement   **i** Posterior shadows (tumor with hyperechoic ring)

Fig. 1. Ultrasonographic findings of hepatocellular carcinoma

Table 1. Ultrasonic findings of small hepatic masses 3 cm or less in diameter

	HCC					Meta	CHA	AH	RN
	≦1.0	≦1.5	≦2.0	≦3.0 (cm)	Total				
No. of lesions	10	22	33	33	98	4	15	4	14
Boundary									
Sharp	9	19	28	25	81	4	15	4	14
Blurred	1	3	5	8	17				
Smooth	8	16	27	21	72	4	9	4	11
Irregular	1	3	1	12	17		6		3
MHZ positive	1	6	6	16	29		1		
Internal echoes									
Hyperchoic	2	7	16	8	33	1	14	1	8
Isoechoic		2		13	15				
Hypoechoic	8	13	17	12	50	3	1	3	6
Homogeneous	10	20	28	8	66	4	15	4	14
Mosaic		2	5	25	32				
PEE positive		1		17	18				
LS positive				4	4				

HCC, hepatocellular carcinoma; Meta, metastatic carcinoma; CHA, cavernous hemangioma; AH, adenomatous hyperplasia; RN, regenerative nodule of cirrhosis; MHZ, marginal hypoechoic zone; PEE, posterior echo enhancement; LS, lateral shadows

a mass. If this is impossible, however, narrower angles are also acceptable.

A compression, interruption, or irregularity of the wall of the blood vessels, a hump sign on a hepatic surface, or an edge sign on hepatic margin are important indirect findings to estimate the presence of masses in the liver [9].

Focal disorders often show a marginal hypoechoic zone around the lesion. The acoustic shadows are formed from the lateral edges of a lesion extending towards the interior of the parenchyma. Posterior echo-enhancement, reinforcement, posterior acoustic shadow, or a comet sign beneath the lesion is detected in some patients. These findings may serve to detect focal lesions in the liver, especially in patients with isoechoic lesions.

A dilated hepatic bile duct suggests the existence of a mass in or near the biliary system, and in a few cases, intraductal infiltration of HCC into the bile duct [10].

3.2 Characterization of ultrasonographic findings of HCC

3.2.1 Shape, boundary, marginal hypoechoic zone, internal echoes, posterior echo and lateral shadows

There are two types of HCC: the diffuse type (Fig. 1a) and the tumor-forming type (Fig. 1b–f).

The shape of the tumor-forming type is round, and its boundary is sharp and smooth. A marginal hypoechoic zone is present, although thin. Internal echoes show a mosaic pattern and the anechoic area appears starry. Posterior echo is enhanced and lateral shadows are present occasionally [9].

In our experience over the last 6 years, HCC 3 cm or less in diameter were round or oval in shape in all 98 of our cases. Seventeen (17%) of 98 were blurred and 17 (19%) in 89 had irregular boundaries. In contrast, all of 4 small metastatic carcinomas and 15 hemangiomas showed sharp boundaries, and 40% of the latter revealed irregular boundaries (Table 1).

Marginal hypoechoic zones (Fig. 1g) were observed in 29 (30%) of the 98 HCCs. In contrast, only 7% of small hemangiomas were accompanied by such zones (Table 1). Similarly, in another analysis including larger masses, this zone was detected in 76 (29%) of 265 HCCs [11]. However, it was also detected in 13 (81%) of 16 metastatic carcinomas of the liver, more frequently than in HCC. In other tumors, it was detected in only 1 (10%) of 10 cases with cholangiocellular carcinoma and 2 (7%) of 30 hepatic hemangiomas [11]. The width of the marginal hypoechoic zone (Mean ±SD) around the tumor in these cases are 3 ± 3 mm in 76 of HCC, 7 mm in 1 cholangiocellular carcinoma, 3 ± 3 mm in 13 metastatic carcinomas of the liver and

Table 2. Detectability of small HCC by US, RI, CT and angiography

(%)

Diameter Total No. of Lesions		≦ 1.0 cm 14	≦ 2.0 cm 32	≦ 3.0 cm 29	Total 75
US	detectable	11 (79)	29 (91)	27 (93)	67 (89)
	detectable after TAE	1 (7)	2 (6)	2 (7)	5 (7)
	undetectable	2	1	0	3
RI	detectable	0 (0)	4 (31)	4 (27)	8 (24)
	undetectable	5	9	11	25
	not tested	9	19	14	42
CT	detectable	9 (64)	17 (53)	24 (83)	50 (67)
	undetectable	5	15	5	25
AG	detectable	9 (64)	23 (77)	19 (95)	51 (80)
	undetectable	5	7	1	13
	not tested	0	2	1	3

US, ultrasonic examination; RI, radionuclide hepatic scan; CT, computed tomography; AG, hepatic angiography; TAE, Transcatheter arterial embolization

3 mm in 2 hepatic hemangiomas [11]. Furthermore, the width of the marginal hypoechoic zone compared to the radius of the tumor was 21 ± 13%, 39%, 22 ± 10% and 24% and 44%, for HCC, cholangiocellular carcinoma, metastatic carcinoma, and hepatic hemangiomas, respectively [11]. Therefore, it is impossible to differentiate HCC from other tumors by the width of the marginal hypoechoic zones.

Marginal hypoechoic zones are detected around tumors which have capsules more than 1 mm in width and the zone represents the capsule itself [12–14]. Its formation is not affected by the existence of cirrhosis [13].

Additionally, some cases of HCC have a hyperechoic rim around the tumor which represents fatty degeneration [15].

Posterior echo-enhancement and lateral shadows (Fig. 1h,i) were detected in 18 (18%) and 4 (4%) of the 98 HCCs 3 cm or less in diameter, however, these findings were usually not detected in small metastatic carcinoma or hemangioma (Table 1). Posterior echo-enhancement represents decreasing attenuation in the tumor compared to the surrounding parenchyma [14, 16].

3.2.2 Internal echoes

There are three types of the internal echogenicity in HCC: hypoechoic (Fig. 1b), isoechoic (Fig. 1c), and hyperechoic (Fig. 1d). Mostly they are homogeneous but some HCC are found to be heterogeneous and consist of a mosaic (Fig. 1e) or mixed type (Fig. 1f).

In our 10 cases of small HCC 1 cm or less in diameter, 8 (80%) were hypoechoic, and 2 (20%) were hyperechoic. In the 55 cases that were 2 cm or less, 30 (55%) were hypoechoic, 2 (4%) were isoechoic, and 23 (42%) were hyperechoic. In 33 cases that were 3 cm or less, the values were 12 (36%), 13 (39%) and 8 (24%), respectively (Table 1). It can be concluded that hyperechoic lesions were more frequent in smaller HCC, and these findings make it difficult to differentiate HCC from hemangiomas.

Hyperechoic lesions in small HCC are indicative of fatty degeneration, clear cell changes or pseudoglandular arrangement of the cancer cells, peliotic changes of the vascular space in the tumor or sclerotic changes in the tumor [17]. However, there is a report that fatty degeneration occurs focally in the tumor when it is over 3 cm [18]. If there is no necrosis, the tumor is seen as either hypoechoic or isoechoic [12]. Necrosis and coagulation necrosis [19] in the tumor causes it to appear more hyperechoic [12].

Internal echoes of those 98 small HCCs in Table 1 were homogeneous in 66 (67%) and mosaic in 32 (33%), but all of the small metastatic carcinomas and hemangiomas were homogeneous.

When both necrotic and non-necrotic areas, are present, the internal echoes show a mosaic pattern [12], and it is consistent with the lobulation of the tumor histologically [16]. Anechoic areas in HCC appear starry [9]. Twenty-seven percent of the HCC revealed combined echogenic and transonic areas, and this combined type is considered to be the manifestation of necrosis in the tumor [20]. However, only one of our cases had an anechoic area in the tumor and it resembled an abscess (Fig. 1f). In this case, brown fluid was obtained after puncture. Nonetheless, there is a report of a multilocular cystic HCC [21].

3.3 Detectability of HCC

In patients with small HCC, 2 cm or less in diameter, the surgical prognosis is better than that of larger lesions. Their survival rates at 5 years are 60.5% for 2 cm or less, 39.3% for 2–5 cm and 26.8% for more than 5 cm [22]. These days, the percutaneous transhepatic ethanol injection is widely accepted in Japan as a viable therapy for small HCC less than 3 cm in diameter [23]. Therefore, early detection of HCC is essential.

In our clinic, 11 (79%) of 14 cases of HCC 1 cm or less in diameter, 29 (91%) of 32 of 2 cm or less and 27 (93%) of 29 of 3 cm or less were detected by ultrasonography (Table 2). These detection rates are better than those of radionuclide scintigraphy, CT, and angiography in small HCC [24]. Similar results have also been obtained in other reports [25, 26], however, satellite nodules of HCC are rarely detected [26].

Most HCC are the nodular type, conglomerate type of some nodules or the massive type. However, 6–19% of HCC including relatively larger masses are the diffuse type [12, 19, 27]. In this type of HCC, almost all of the hepatic parenchyma are replaced by the cancer, and parenchymal echoes do not make focal nodular changes, but show diffusely spread abnormal but homogeneous echoes (Fig. 1a). This diffuse type of HCC is hard to recognize in some cases. Usually, careful observation, makes it possible to diagnose the abnormal intensity and distribution of the hepatic parenchymal echoes.

Analyzing 62 patients with small HCC 3 cm or less in diameter, 14 (23%) of undetectable masses were later found to be located in hepatic segments S2 (2/5), S8 (4/16), S6 (4/16), S5 (2/8), S4 (1/5), and S7 (1/10), but none in S3 (0/2) [24].

3.4 Hepatic tumors mimicking HCC

3.4.1 Malignant tumors of the liver

Cholangiocellular carcinoma (CCC) (Fig. 2a). The shape is potato- or cauliflower-like and the boundary is coarsely irregular. There is a thick marginal hypoechoic zone and its internal side is blurred. The internal echoes have a target-like distribution, and an anechoic area is observed at the center that is convex to the outside. Posterior echoes are attenuated or even, and lateral shadows are absent [9].

Dilated bile ducts in the liver are one of the characteristic signs of biliary obstruction by the CCC. Partially dilated bile ducts with irregular walls and partial occlusion are important findings of cholangiocellular carcinoma.

Squamous cell carcinoma. The mass has a blurred boundary and its internal echoes are irregular (heterogeneous) [28]. The irregularity of internal echoes is caused by the partial calcification in the mass.

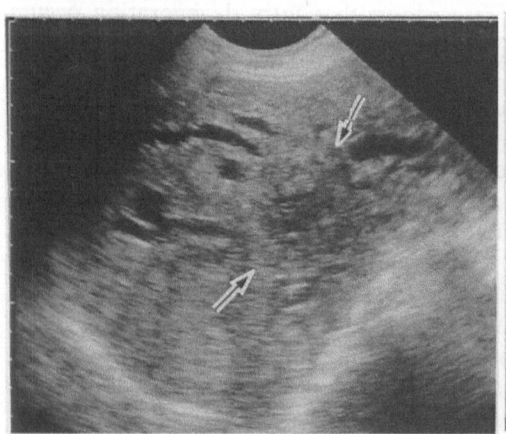 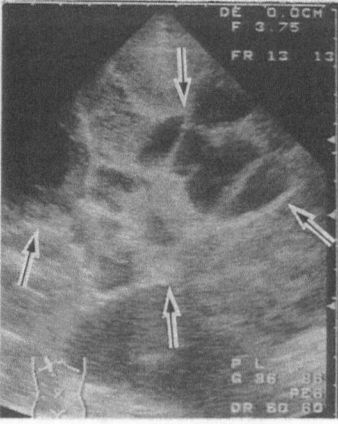 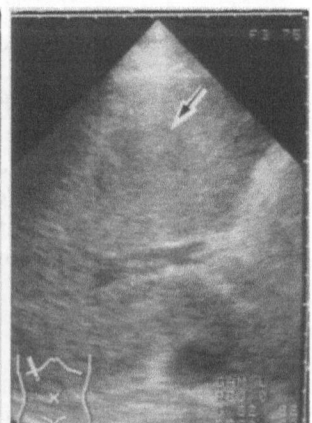

a Cholangiocellular carcinoma   b Cystadeno-carcinoma   c Epithelioid hemangio-endothelioma

Fig. 2. Tumors in the liver

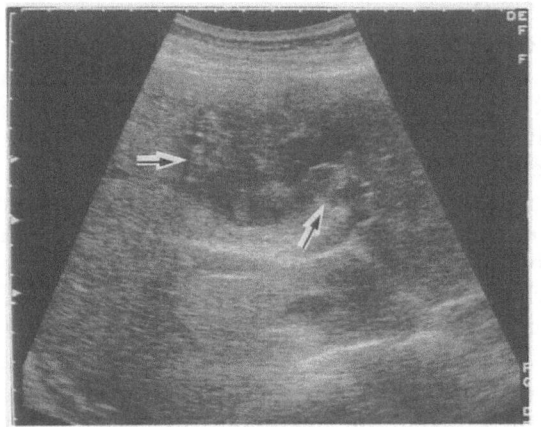

d Leiomyosarcoma with portal emboli

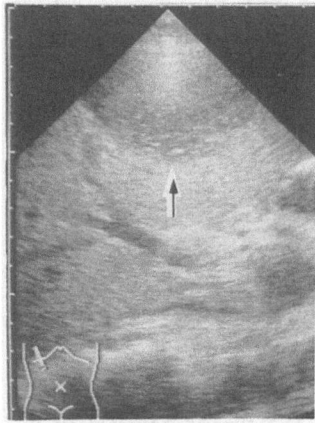

e Malignant lymphoma

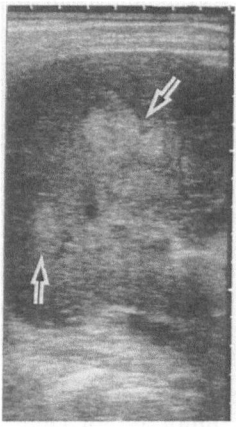

f Multiple myeloma

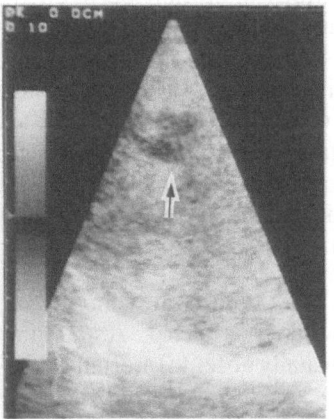

(i) Lung cancer

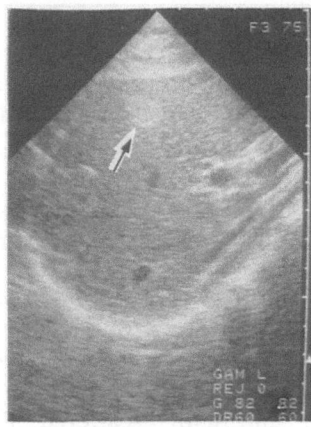

(ii) Gastric cancer

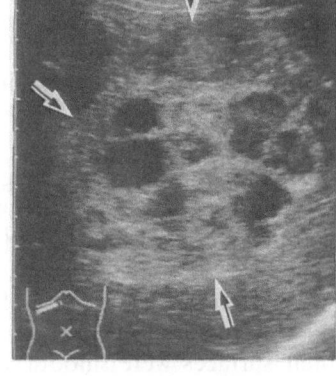

(iii) Gastrinoma

g Metastatic carcinoma

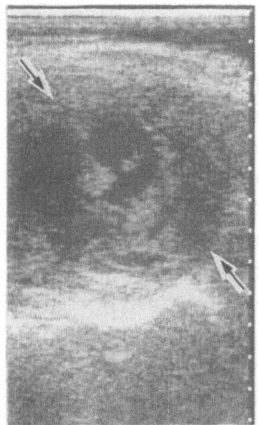

h Hepatocellular adenoma

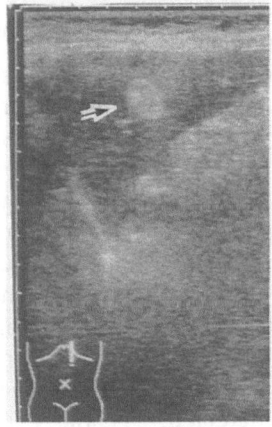

i Angiomyolipoma

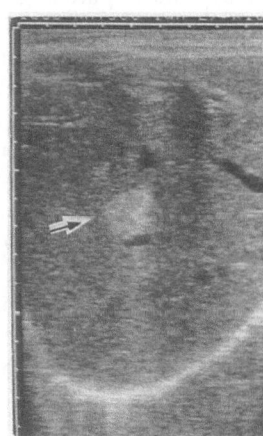

j Cavernous hemangioma

Fig. 2. (*Continued*)

Cystadenocarcinoma (Fig. 2b). Ultrasonographic tomogram shows some anechoic, transonic lesions resembling benign cysts in some cases. However, some parts of the cystic wall are irregular and show an abnormal tumorous area. This abnormal echogenic area suggests cystadenocarcinoma.

Malignant epithelioid hemangioendothelioma of the liver. In the patients with this disease shown in Fig. 2c, there are hypoechoic and isoechoic areas 3 cm in diameter and a few acoustic shadows are detected without a clear tumorous border.

Hepatic leiomyosarcoma. The boundary of this tumor is not clear and the tumor consists of a hypoechoic mass, usually with a mosaic pattern [29]. However, in the patient in Fig. 2d, the boundary is clear, internal echoes are mosaic, and emboli were detected in a portal vein.

Hematological malignancies of the liver. Malignant lymphoma, show well demarcated, round or oval hypoechoic tumors (Fig. 2e). In Fig. 2f, one case with multiple myeloma in the liver is shown. In this ultrasonogram, there are 4 hyperechoic lesions.

Ultrasonographic scanning of the liver was undergone in 73 patients with malignant lymphoma over 5 years [30]. According to the analysis of these patients, space occupying lesions were detected in 5 (7%) of them. They were relatively homogeneous and hypoechoic, and their surfaces were smooth and clear, and there was no marginal hypoechoic zone, lateral shadows or posterior echo-enhancement. Enlargement of intraperitoneal lymph nodes (41%), splenomegaly (29%), a space occupying lesion in the spleen (4%), and hepatomegaly (11%) were additional findings associated with this disease [30]. With leukemia, including adult T-cell leukemia, a hypoechoic area was detected in a few cases with either a clear boundary [31], a blurred boundary [32], or with a target sign [33] near the portal vein [34].

Metastatic carcinoma of the liver (Fig. 2g). In patients with metastatic carcinomas of the liver, the findings of chronic disease of the liver, especially cirrhosis, are absent. Internal echoes of the tumor are mostly hyperechoic (62%) [11]. In a few cases of metastatic carcinoma, mostly from a colon, an anechoic area is detected. Marginal hypoechoic zones are frequently detected (81%) in metastasis, but only 29% in HCC [11]. Seventy-nine percent of HCC are based on cirrhotic liver or chronic hepatitis in Japan

[35]. On the other hand, it is well-known that metastasis of the carcinoma to a cirrhotic liver is relatively rare [36]. Therefore, the detection of a tumor in the liver with cirrhotic changes on ultrasonic tomogram is a remarkable difference between HCC and metastatic carcinoma.

The metastasis of malignant tumors to the liver has a variety of presentations. The so-called "bulls-eye" lesion presents as slightly more echogenic than normal hepatic parenchyma, and it is surrounded by an anechoic rim [37]. Lesions more echogenic than normal hepatic parenchyma are frequently seen in a metastatic carcinoma from a colon. In metastatic carcinoma, either severe necrosis comprises more than 20% of the malignant area, or fatty degeneration forms. A hyperechoic tumor and marginal hypoechoic zone are made by edematous alteration between the tumor and the surrounding parenchyma [38]. Another common variety of metastasis is a relatively anechoic lesion. Multiple small sonolucent lesions result in the so-called diffuse pattern of metastasis [37]. Calcification, for example, in a metastatic malignancy of the liver causes acoustic shadows, and air in the tumor may reveal a comet sign.

Metastatic sarcoma. The tumors are smooth and round, and the boundary is sharp. A marginal hypoechoic zone is usually absent. Internal echoes are uniform and the anechoic area is round and scattered. Posterior echo is even or enhanced, and lateral shadows are rarely present [9].

Carcinoid. The findings of this tumor are similar to those of metastatic sarcoma [9]. The dense lesion is a metastatic carcinoid [9].

3.4.2 Benign tumors

Hepatocellular adenoma (Fig. 2h). This is considerably more frequent in women, promoted by the estroprogestational hormones, and is associated with the risk of hemorrhage. Ultrasonography allows recognition of the tumor, but has no histological specificity. The mass may appear round or oval, and its ultrasonographic structure may be variable. Often, it is hypoechoic, and sometimes hyperechoic. The center of a mass may appear heterogeneous because of the frequency of necrosis and bleeding causing a hypoechoic, even anechoic, area [39, 40].

In Fig. 2h, a case of hepatocellular adenoma is presented. The tumor shows a combined type with hyperechoic, hypoechoic and anechoic areas and its boundary is blurred. The anechoic area

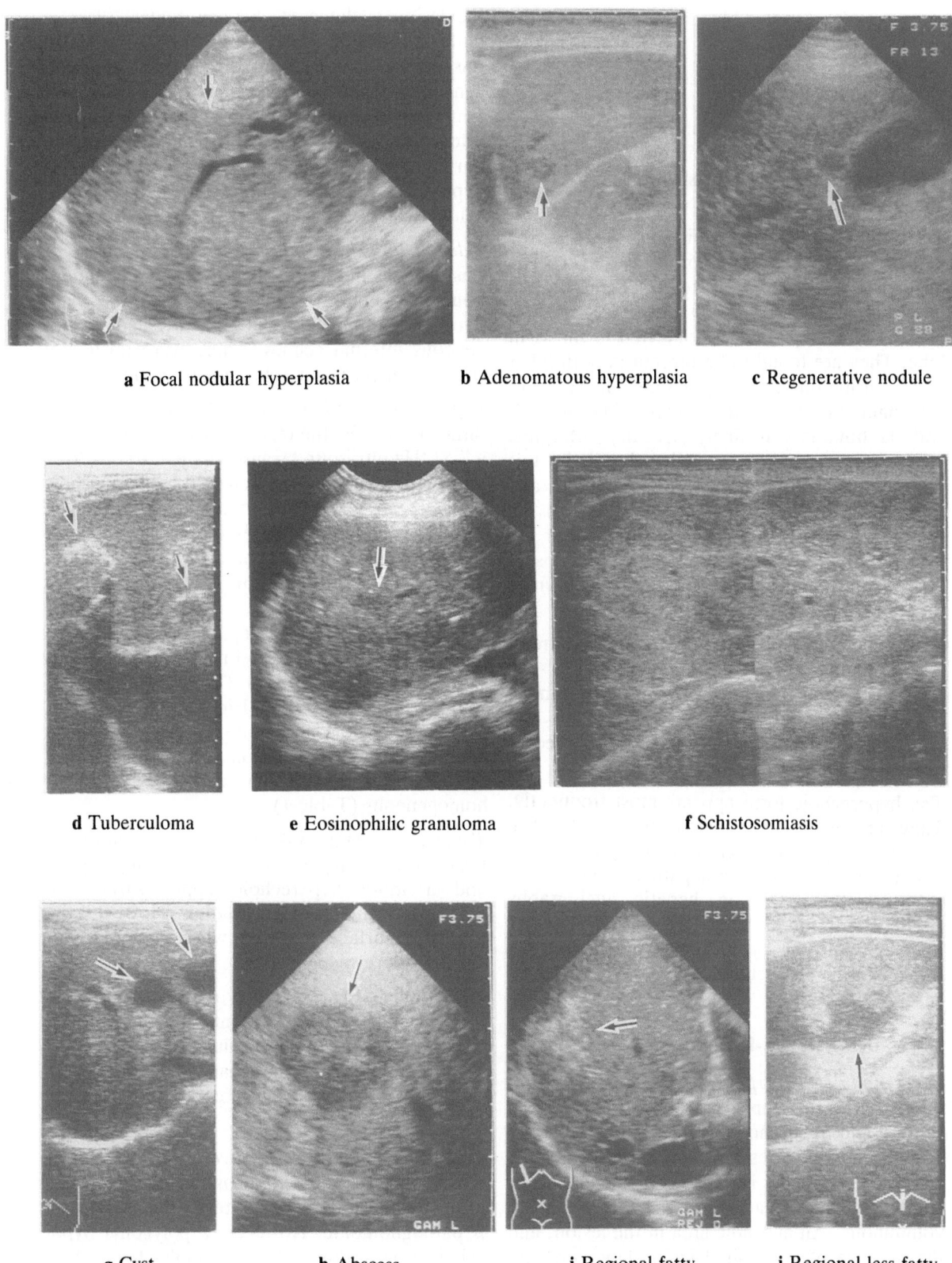

a Focal nodular hyperplasia   **b** Adenomatous hyperplasia   **c** Regenerative nodule

d Tuberculoma   **e** Eosinophilic granuloma   **f** Schistosomiasis

g Cyst   **h** Abscess   **i** Regional fatty   **j** Regional less fatty

Fig. 3. Tumor-like lesions in the liver

was ascertained to be a bleeding hematoma in the tumor by the operation.

Angiomyolipoma. In Fig. 2i, a case of angiomyolipoma is demonstrated. The tumor has a clear boundary, and its internal echoes are more hyperechoic than cavernous hemangioma. Some of these tumors show slight posterior echo-enhancement [41].

Cavernous hemangioma (Fig. 2j). This is the most common benign tumor of the liver. The incidence has been evaluated as being 2% in one autopsy series of 2,400 cases [42]. In 50% of cases, hemangiomas are detected in the right lobe. They are found to be present in both lobes in 25% using ultrasonography [43]. The shape of a hemangioma is round or shaped like an "8", and its boundary is finely irregular. Marginal hypoechoic zones are usually absent in this disease. Internal echoes are echogenic and shaped like an "8", and anechoic areas in the tumor are usually round. Posterior echoes are even or enhanced, and lateral shadows are absent [9]. From the ultrasonographic point of view, three variants are described [44]:

1. A hyperechoic image whose outline is more or less regular.
2. A hypoechoic image with a central septum.
3. The association of a hypoechoic image and internal echoes in it with posterior echo-enhancement, suggesting a fluid content.

The hyperechoic form appears most frequently. They are generally isolated and small. The location is quite characteristic in apposition to either a hepatic vein or a hepatic capsule.

Strong "pooling" on hepatic angiography is detected more frequently in hypoechoic hemangioma than hyperechoic, and the former has posterior echo-enhancement in 62% of the cases [45].

3.3.3 Benign tumor-like disorders

Focal nodular hyperplasia. This condition produces lesions that appear as rounded, mostly as a solitary and hypoechoic or hyperechoic area [39, 46–48], and the sizes are 2–10 cm. Again, they can sometimes be isoechoic, hyperechoic, or combined and can lead to a mass effect if they are voluminous. An anechoic area in the lesion, and the absence of a marginal hypoechoic zone are typical findings with this disease. These findings are due to bleeding in the necrotic lesion [39]. There is no capsule formation around the lesion. In some cases, a stellate hyperechoic structure in the lesion is detected showing central scarring [46]. In Fig. 3a, one of the ultrasonogram of this disease is shown. In this patient, a homogeneous hypoechoic lesion with a blurred boundary is detected, and branches of a hepatic artery are recognized in it. In another case in our clinic, internal echoes were heterogeneously hyperechoic, and there was no stellate hypoechoic structure.

Adenomatous hyperplasia (Fig. 3b). In 4 cases of this disease, the lesions had a sharp and smooth boundary. One was hyperechoic, and 3 were hypoechoic and all of them revealed homogeneous internal echoes. There were no lateral shadows or posterior echo-enhancement.

Regenerative nodules (Fig. 3c). Usually, it is difficult to detect the regenerative nodule without a 7.5 MHz ultrasound transducer in cirrhotic liver [49]. However, if it is detected, a hypoechoic mass is more frequent than hyperechoic. The former is difficult to differentiate from HCC [50], and the latter from hemangioma. The latter suggests fatty degeneration in the hyperechoic area [51].

In 14 patients with the diagnosis of regenerative nodules by needle biopsy in our clinic, all had sharp boundaries, and 11 (79%) of them had smooth boundaries [52]. Eight (57%) of them were hyperechoic and some of them had fatty degeneration in the lesions. Six (43%) were hypoechoic, and all of their internal echoes were homogeneous (Table 1).

Tuberculoma (Fig. 3d). The tuberculoma of the liver reveals a hyperechoic area in a upper part, and a more hyperechoic upper surface of the lesion with an acoustic shadow. However, the posterior surface and the whole boundary of the lesion are recognizable.

Granuloma (Fig. 3e). The eosinophilic granuloma in the liver represents a homogeneous hypoechoic area with a blurred margin. The findings of these lesions changed in the course of follow-up studies, and some lesions actually disappeared.

Parasitic diseases of the liver. In the case of schistosomiasis, the hepatic parenchyma forms an echogenic tortoise-shell pattern (Fig. 3f) which is pathognomonic. However, a polygonal hypoechoic area in this pattern resembles hypoechoic HCC or conceals tumors like hemangioma, therefore, some cases are recommended for needle biopsy for differential diagnosis. Some fascioliasis show tumorous echoes [53, 54].

Hydatid cysts. This disease is exclusively found in the northern part of Japan. Ultrasonographic findings are described in many papers [55–60], however, the differential diagnosis from HCC is difficult in some cases [58, 59].

The solitary or multiple hydatid cysts are characterized by a well-demarcated, rounded anechoic zone of a fluid nature. Its wall is echogenic, and is sometimes duplicated internally by a fine dense line corresponding to the germinal membrane. The existence of germinal vesicles is indicated by presence of fine echoes located in the lower part of the cyst. When fissuration occurs, this feature disappears, resulting in a completely modified, very heterogeneous appearance. The sonograms obtained of biliary cysts, in contrast, are quite characteristic and shows single or multiple well-demarcated, rounded or oval formations that are anechoic, and have smooth and regular borders with posterior echo-enhancement (Fig. 3g). It is hard to recognize the wall. Usually, hydatid cysts are easily differentiated from HCC.

Hepatic abscesses (Fig. 3h). An abscess appears as an echo-free area that presents some echogenic structure corresponding to septa and necrotic remnants of variable sizes. The outlines of these zones are irregular and roughly circular. The wall of an abscess is not recognized and some irregular echogenic areas are detected around the hypoechoic area. Posterior echo-enhancement is not always found. Here, ultrasonography is useful for precise localization of certain deep-seated abscesses, to exclude the presence of further lesions, and to ensure the correct arrangement of a drainage system inserted. With necrotic metastasis, mostly from a colon, the hyperechoic wall around the anechoic area is recognized and this is one of the most important findings for the differential diagnosis of these two anechoic areas. Their sizes vary from a few millimeters to several centimeters.

Regional fatty degeneration in a less fatty area or a regional less fatty area in more fatty area in a liver. Regional fatty degeneration in a less fatty area in the liver makes a hyperechoic lesion (Fig. 3i), and a regional less fatty area in a more fatty area makes a hypoechoic area (Fig. 3j). The shape is irregular, not round, and sometimes a regional less fatty area makes a hypoechoic area and is showed by hepatic vessels.

Other diseases. Some patients with Wilson's disease, which have a tumor-like appearance [61, 62] of scale-like echo-texture [63]. Again, some do not represent tumorous area, but rather cirrhotic parenchyma [64].

3.4 Differential diagnosis of HCC

The criteria for the differential diagnosis of hepatic tumors are proposed by the Japan Society of Ultrasonic Medicine and Biology [9]. However, the differential diagnosis of the HCC is not easy. Especially with small HCC, the detectability of characteristic findings of the tumor is decreased [52, 65].

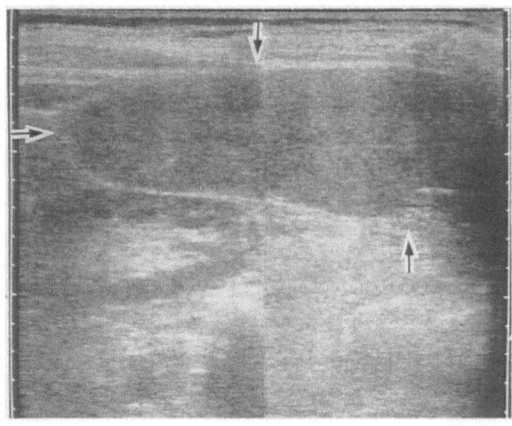 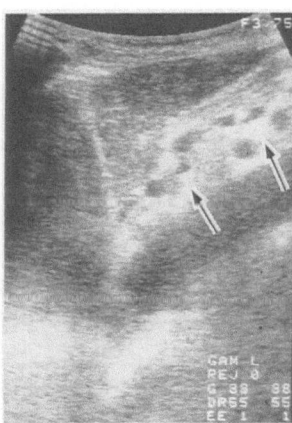 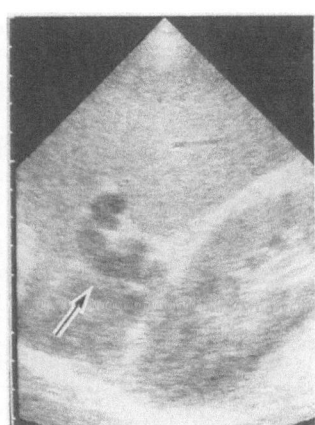

a Splenomegaly   b Esophago-cardial varices   c Spleno-renal shunt

Fig. 4. Complications of hepatocellular carcinoma

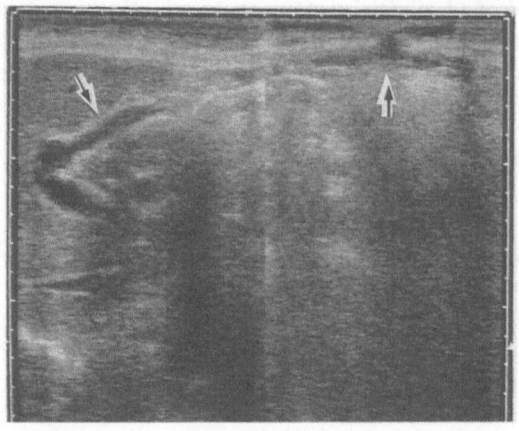

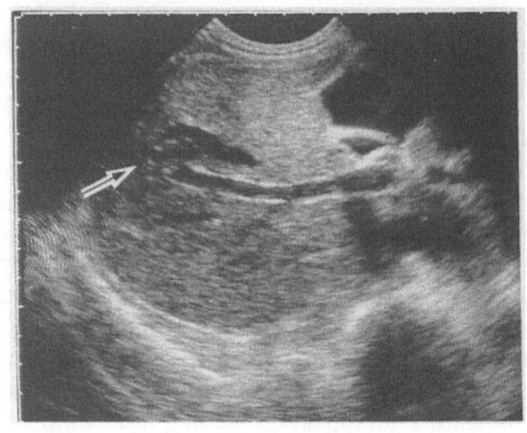

d Recanalization of ligament teres hepatis with caput medusae

e Porto-hepatic shunt

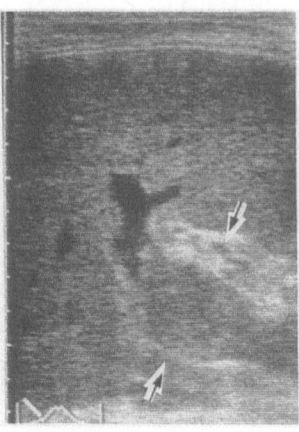

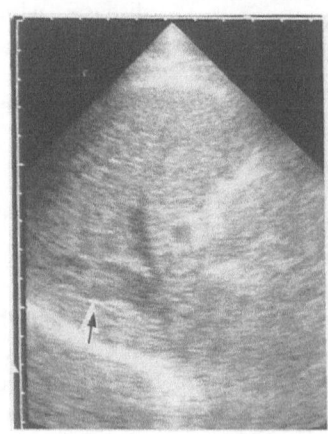

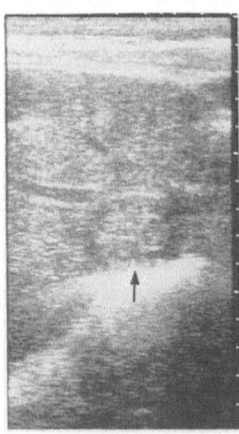

f Tumor emboli in portal vein with cavernous transformation

g Tumor emboli in hepatic vein

h Tumor emboli in vena cava

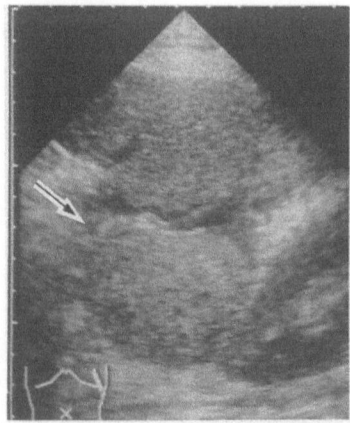

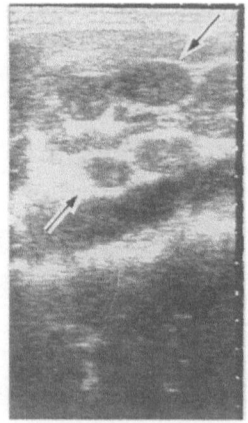

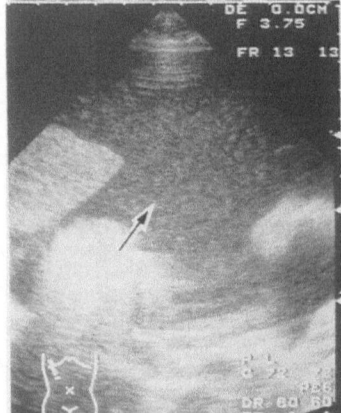

i Adrenal metastasis

j Lymph nodes metastasis

k Carcinomatous peritonitis

Fig. 4. (*Continued*)

For differential diagnosis, the smooth boundary [66, 67], marginal hypoechoic zone, posterior echo-enhancement [66], internal echoes [66–68], lateral shadows [66] are noteworthy. The internal echoes are hypoechoic and make a mosaic pattern in HCC [66, 67] and are hyperechoic in metastasis [67, 68]. Because of the difference of echogenicity of the surrounding non-tumorous parenchyma of the liver, fluid-filled lesions are clearly and easily defined as a transonic area. These lesions such as dissolved or liquefied necrosis in metastatic carcinomas of the liver, abscess or cyst in the liver, are diagnostically detected and differentiated by ultrasonic examination.

Evaluation of underlying hepatic changes in HCC (Fig. 4), especially hepatic cirrhosis and portal hypertension (Fig. 4a–e), or emboli in the portal veins (Fig. 4f), hepatic veins (Fig. 4g), inferior vena cava (Fig. 4h) are essential for the differential diagnosis of HCC from a metastatic carcinoma of the liver.

Ultrasonic Doppler adds useful information for the differential diagnosis of HCC from other diseases mimicking HCC [69, 70].

3.5 Complications of HCC

In contrast to metastatic carcinoma, HCC was complicated with hepatic cirrhosis in 85.5% of autopsy cases in one study in Japan [22]. Metastatic carcinoma of the liver is rarely complicated by emboli in the portal vein, whereas HCC sometimes is. In HCC patients, the formation of thrombi in the portal vein were detected in a few cases after endoscopic injection sclerotherapy for esophageal varices. Also, emboli are occasionally detected in the portal vein, hepatic vein [71], or the inferior vena cava. Emboli in the portal vein are easily detected by ultrasonography [72].

Debris-like echoes in the gallbladder are commonly detected after transcatheter arterial embolization for the treatment of HCC or in hemobilia following a needle biopsy of the liver.

The metastasis of HCC to the right adrenal gland is occurs in 15.0% of the autopsy cases in one study [22]. The boundary of the tumor is clear and smooth (Fig. 4i), and internal echoes are mostly hypoechoic [73].

Enlarged lymph nodes may be suggestive of a metastasis of a malignant disease to these lymph nodes. When metastasis of HCC occurs in the intraperitoneal lymph nodes, either round or oval, mostly hypoechoic masses are detected near the liver (Fig. 4j).

Ascites with small fine echoes are usually observed in ruptured HCC or carcinomatous peritonitis (Fig. 4k).

4 New technique for diagnosis of HCC

4.1 Ultrasonic color Doppler

Recently, the newly developed ultrasonic color Doppler was adopted for clinical use. It allows easy detection of vessels, and the direction, speed, volume, and wave form of the blood stream, whether pulsating or continuous, can be determined.

In tumors or tumor-like lesions, there are three or four kinds of color Doppler signals (Fig. 5). One of them is a feeding signal with a pulsating or continuous wave which goes into the lesion from the outside. The second is a signal with a pulsating or continuous wave which is detected in a lesion as spotty or short linear signals. The third is a drainage signal with a continuous wave which goes from the inside to the outside of the lesion. The last one is a penetrating signal with a pulsating or continuous wave which penetrates all the way through the lesion [74].

For differential diagnosis of a tumor or tumorous lesion from HCC, these 4 types of color Doppler signals are useful. They were detected in HCC most frequently (69%), but also in 41% of metastatic carcinoma in a liver, and in 20% of cavernous hemangiomas. Furthermore, the feeding signals and drainage signals were detected in HCC but not in metastasis or hemangioma. The penetrating signals were detected in metastasis but not in HCC or hemangioma (Table 3).

This new Doppler system gives an excellent information for the differential diagnosis of HCC.

4.2 Ultrasonic contrast enhancement

For the detection as well as differential diagnosis of HCC, a new ultrasonographic technique has been developed recently [75, 76]. When the mixture of carbon dioxide and autologous blood is injected into a hepatic artery, changes of the echogenicity in the tumor are observed. These changes are used for the differential diagnosis of the tumors in certain cases.

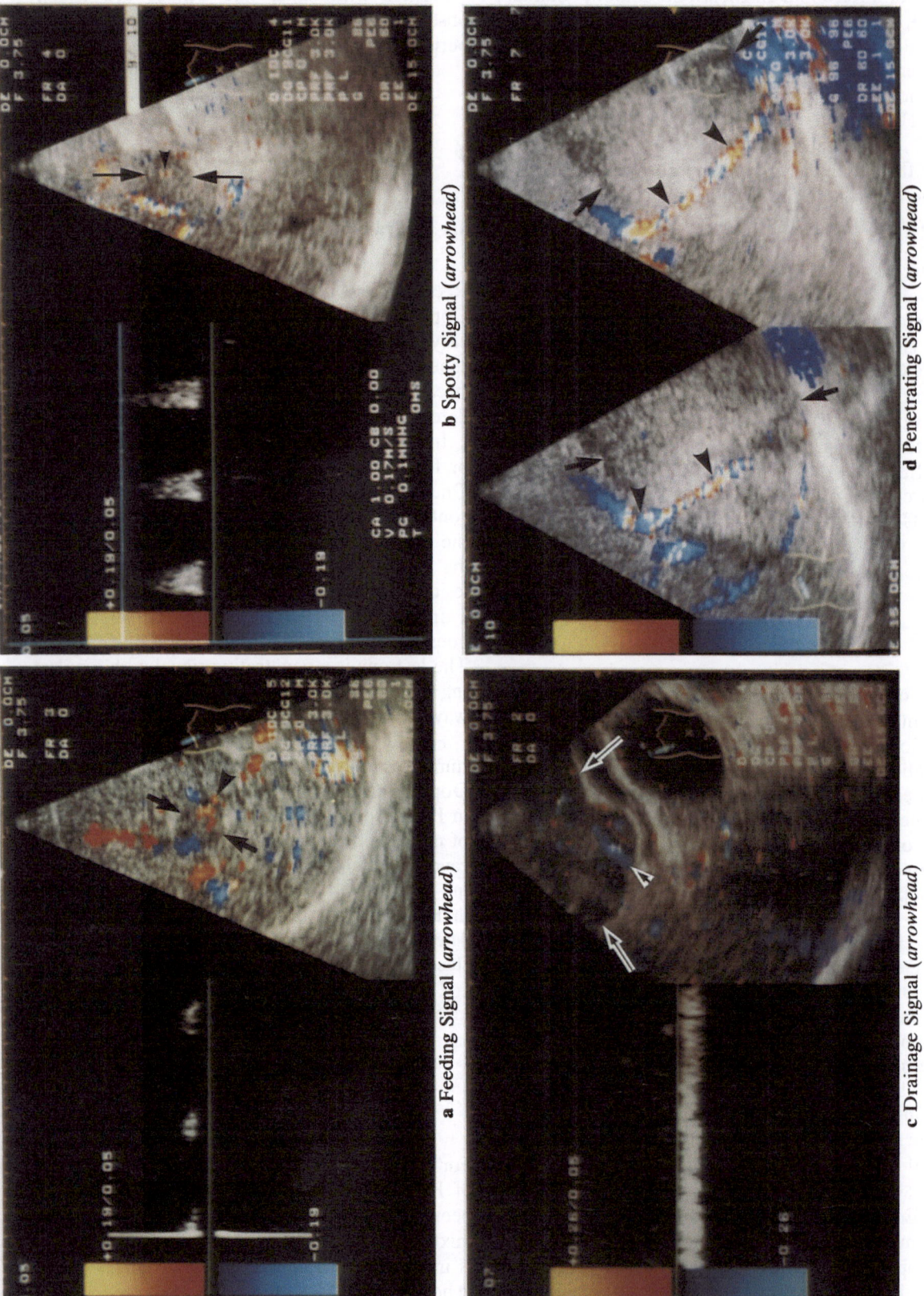

a Feeding Signal (*arrowhead*)

b Spotty Signal (*arrowhead*)

c Drainage Signal (*arrowhead*)

d Penetrating Signal (*arrowhead*)

Fig. 5. Doppler color flow mapping of hepatic masses

Table 3. Color doppler signals of liver masses

	No. of Lesions	Signals (+)	FS	SS	DS	PS
Hepatocellular carcinoma ≦ 2 cm	35	25	14	17		
> 2 cm	54	42	29	36	16	
Total	89	67	43	53	16	
Metastatic liver cancer	20	6		1		5
Leiomyosarcoma	1	1	1		1	
Epithelioid hemangioendothelioma	1	0				
Cavernous hemangioma	14	2		2		
Focal nodular hyperplasia	2	2	2		1	
Hyperplastic nodule	4	0				

FS, feeding signal; SS, spotty signal; DS, drainage signal; PS, penetrating signal

5 Conclusion

For the detection of HCC, several kinds of diagnostic imaging techniques such as ultrasonography, radionuclide hepatic scan, CT, MRI, and angiography are available.

Ultrasonographic indications, techniques and variables for the diagnosis of HCC were discussed, as were the ultrasonograms of several kinds of tumors or tumor-like lesions and their differential diagnosis.

Masses can be detected ultrasonographically in patients with HCC before complications such as hepatic cirrhosis occur by mass screening [77]. However, the differential diagnosis of HCC from other tumors or tumor-like lesions is difficult in some patients. Therefore, the combining various imaging techniques or needle biopsy of the tumor, in some cases, are required for differentiation.

References

1. Sakaguchi S, Tohara K (1990) Ultrasonic diagnosis of chronic hepatitis (in Japanese). Modern Physician 10:1176–1182
2. Rettenmaier G (1974) Quantitative criteria of intrahepatic echo patterns correlated with structural alterations. In: Vlieger M, White DN, McCready VR (eds) Ultrasonics in medicine. Excerpta Medica, Amsterdam
3. Wells PNT, McCarthy CF, Ross FGM, Read AEA (1969) Comparison of A-scan and compound B-scan ultrasonography in the diagnosis of liver disease. Br J Radiol 42:818–823
4. Watanuki S, Kubota H, Fukushima M, Hirakata M (1967) Diagnosis of the hepatic disease by ultrasonic attenuation. Second Report (English abstract). Proceedings of JSUM 11:109–110
5. Ishii K, Doi T, Kurokawa M, Sakaguchi S, Okumura M (1986) Sizes of liver, spleen and portal vein in normal subjects (English abstract). Proceedings of JSUM 48:689–690
6. Doi T, Sakaguchi S (1986) Measurement of the size of the liver, spleen and portal vein in chronic liver diseases (English abstract). Jpn J Med Ultrasonics 13:335–340
7. Cuinaud C (1954) Distribution de l'artère hèpatique dans le foie (in French). Acta anat 22:49–81
8. Takayasu K, Moriyama N, Muramatsu Y, Shima Y, Ishikawa T, Goto H, Ushio K, Matsue H, Sasagawa M, Yamada T (1984) Clinico-radiological anatomy of the intrahepatic portal vein branches studied by percutaneous transhepatic portography. Proposal of a new nomenclature for the branching order and third order (subsegmental) branches (English abstract). Jap J Gastroent 81:56–65
9. The Japan Society of Ultrasonics in Medicine (1989) A Public Announcement of the Diagnostic Criteria for Liver Tumors. Jpn J Med Ultrasonics 16:108–111
10. Kumagaya Y (1979) A histological study of hepatocellular carcinoma—obstruction of the common bile duct by intraductal growth (English abstract). Acta Hep Jap 20:157–163
11. Hatono N, Tohara K, Sakaguchi S, Oka Y, Okumura M (1990) The evaluation of marginal hypoechoic zone of hepatic tumors (English abstract). Proceedings of JSUM 57:67–68
12. Inayoshi A (1983) Clinical studies on ultrasonic diagnosis of carcinoma of the liver: Comparative study between ultrasonograms and pathological findings (in Japanese). Nippon Shokaki Gekka 16:2088–2097
13. Okabe M (1979) Patho morphological studies on hepatocellular carcinoma: A study on a mechanism of capsule formation and septum formation of tumor nodule (English abstract). Acta Hepatol Jpn 20:144–156
14. Akimoto S, Saitoh A, Watayoh T, Isobe Y, Takasaki T (1984) Diagnostic capability and

limitation of ultrasonography in small hepatocellular carcinoma (in Japanese). Fukubu Gazoushindan 4:209–216

15. Majima Y, Fujimoto T, Iwai I, Tanaka M, Sakai T, Miura C, Abe M, Tanikawa K (1988) Pathological background of the characteristic "bright loop" pattern in ultrasonography of small hepatocellular carcinoma (HCC) (English abstract). Proceedings of JUSM 52:17–18

16. Makuuchi M, Hasegawa H, Yamasaki S, Bandai Y, Watanabe G, Ito T (1981) The characteristic features of small hepatocellular carcinoma smaller than 5 cm in diameter (in Japanese). Acta Hep Jap 22:1740

17. Edamitsu O, Kiyomatsu K, Nakashima O, Sugihara S, Kojiro M, Saitsu H, Nakayama T, Majima Y, Tanikawa K (1991) Pathomorphologic study on hepatocellular carcinoma showing hyperechoic pattern (English abstract). Acta Hepatol Jpn 33:618–624

18. Kiyomatsu K (1989) Pathomorphologic study on hepatocellular carcinoma (HCC)—A study of fatty changes in HCC (English abstract). Acta Hepatol Jpn 30:974–979

19. Shinagawa T, Ohto M, Kimura K, Matsutani S, Kimura M, Unosawa T, Ukaji H, Tsunetomi S, Nakano T, Morita M, Saisho H, Tsuchiya Y, Ono T, Okuda K (1981) Real-time ultrasonographic diagnosis of hepatocellular carcinoma: Correlation of echograms and histopathological finding (English abstract). Jap J Gastroent 78:2402–2411

20. Boultbee JE (1979) Grey scale ultrasound appearances in hepatocellular carcinoma. Clin Radiol 30:547–552

21. Mizuno Y, Notsumata K, Furusawa A, Motoo Y, Hirai N, Matsui O, Izumi R, Noda Y, Unoura M, Tanaka N, Kobayashi K, Hattori N, Nakamura Y (1989) A case of multilocular cystic hepatocellular carcinoma without underlying cirrhosis (English abstract). Acta Hepatol Jpn 30:75–81

22. Liver Cancer Study Group of Japan (1990) Follow-up study of the primary liver cancer in Japan. 9th report. (in Japanese). Japanese Liver Cancer Study Group, Kyoto

23. Sugiura N, Kora K, Ohto M, Kunio O, Hirooka N (1983) Treatment of small hepatocellular carcinoma by percutaneous transhepatic ethanol injection under ultrasonographic imaging (in Japanese). Acta Hepatol Jpn 24:920, 1983

24. Sakaguchi S (1987) Diagnosis of liver cancer (in Japanese). Imag Diag. Medicina 24:1592–1597

25. Osada Y (1981) Clinicopathological studies of ultrasonogram in small hepatocellular carcinoma (English abstract). Jpn J Gastroent 78:685–692

26. Hirai T, Ohishi H, Yoshimura K, Honda N, Kitamura I, Ohue S, Nishimine K, Ide K, Suzuki R, Uchida I, Satou N, Uchida H (1989) Ultrasonic detectability of multiple small hepatic nodules (English abstract). Rinsho Hosyasen 34:857–863

27. Kawasaki H, Sakaguchi S, Irisa T, Hirayama C (1978) Value of B-scan ultrasonography in the diagnosis of liver cancer. Am J Gastroent 69:436–442

28. Imai H, Horiguchi Y, Ohsuki M, Kitano T, Takagawa H, Nakano H, Nakajima S, Itoh M, Miyagawa S (1987) A case of squamous cell carcinoma of the liver (English abstract). Jpn J Med Ultrasonics 14:148–152

29. Ishihara A, Kitagawa N, Tsuji Y, Syundo J, Ito S, Kishi S, Mori H, Shimamura Y, Hasegawa H (1989) A Case of Leiomyosarcoma of the Liver (English abstract). Jpn J Med 16:492–498

30. Kurokawa M, Sakaguchi S, Kamachi T, Morioka E, Okumura M (1988) Ultrasonographic study of abdominal lesions in malignant lymphoma (ML)—especially on ultrasonographic findings of hepatic and splenic tumor-forming ML (English abstract). Proceedings of JSUM 52:521–522

31. Teshima T, Morioka E, Ishibashi H, Ikeda K, Ohtsuka T, Niho Y (1987) A Case of Adult T-cell leukemia/lymphoma with nodular lesions ultrasonographically detected in both liver and spleen (English abstract). Jpn J Med Ultrasonics 14:610–613

32. Tanaka K, Egami K, Nakamura E, Natori K, Nakagoshi T, Naito K, Akashi A, Uto K, Nagata O, Natori H, Kaji M, Nakamura S, Yoshida T, Ohtake S, Matsuda T (1987) A Case of ATL Presenting a huge intrahepatic tumor, abated with etoposide (NK-171) therapy alone (English abstract). Rinsyou Ketsueki 28:392–397

33. Koike G, Morioka E, Ishibashi H, Otsuka T, Niho Y (1989) A target appearance of hepatic invasion in adult T-cell leukemia (ATL) (English abstract). Jpn J Med Ultrasonics 16:76–80

34. Karube T, Yano S, Ijima H, Muchi H, Kamoshita S, Itoh K (1985) Ultrasonogram of the liver and brain in a patient with congenital leukemia (English abstract). Jpn J Med Ultrasonics 12:537–542

35. Ishii K, Kurokawa M, Doi T, Simizu M, Sakaguchi S, Okumura M (1987) Twelve Year Observation of Patients with Liver Disease in Fukuoka University Hospital (English abstract). Med Bull Fukuoka Univ 14:47–55

36. Hamaya K, Hashimoto H, Maeda Y (1975) Metastatic carcinoma in cirrhotic liver: Statistical survey autopsies in Japan. Acta Pathol Jpn 25:153–159

37. Raymond HW (1979) Fundamentals of abdominal sonography: A teaching approach. Grune & Stratton, New York

38. Gondoh M, Kasumi F, Yanagisawa A (1987) Correlation between ultrasonographic and histological findings of metastatic liver cancer (English abstract). Jpn J Med Ultrasonics 14:181–188

39. Sandler MA, Petrocelli RD, Marks DS, Lopez R (1980) Ultrasonic features and radionuclide

correlation in liver cell adenoma and focal nodular hyperplasia. Radiology 135:393–397

40. Nakashima T, Ohta G, Okudaira M, Arakawa M (eds) (1984) Hepatic diseases mimicking HCC (in Japanese). Chugai Igakusya, Tokyo

41. Iwai I, Majima Y, Fujimoto T, Tanaka M, Aoki Y, Hirai K, Abe M, Abe H, Tanikawa K, Sugihara S, Fujiyoshi Y (1986) Lipomatous tumors of the liver: Report of two cases (English abstract). Jpn J Med Ultrasonics 13:473–479

42. Ochsner JL, Halpert B (1958) Cavernous hemangioma of the liver. Surgery 43:577–582

43. Tohara K, Sakaguchi S, Hirano M, Okumura M (1987) Comparison of ultrasonographic findings between hyperechoic lesions in the liver (English abstract). Proceedings of JSUM 51:273–274

44. Deixonne B, Makuuchi M, Pissas JM (1988) Ultrasonography of the liver. In: Deizonne B, Lopez FM (eds) Operative ultrasonography. Springer-Verlag, Berlin

45. Tanaka M, Suto T, Kunikane M, Moriyama Y, Kondoh H, Soejima Y, Sasaki D, Yoshida Y (1988) Angiographic pooling findings in cases with hypoechoic hemangiomas of the liver (English abstract). Jpn J Ultrasonics 15:221–230

46. Takehara Y, Nomura M, Matsukawa S, Yasuda T, Yamashita K, Tanaka I, Matsuzawa K, Kojima M, Ohno Y, Matsuda M (1987) Diagnosis of the ultrasonogram: Focal nodular hyperplasia (FNH) (in Japanese). Rinsyou Syoukaki Naika 2:1325–1330

47. Oda T, Sakaguchi S, Okumura M (1990) A case of focal nodular hyperplasia of the liver: Study on diagnostic imaging (English abstract). Fukubu Gazou Shindan 10:81–87

48. Morita S, Okajima K, Tamio T, Kubokawa M, Matsui A, Nakata E, Nakajima T, Ishiga N (1987) A case of focal nodular hyperplasia of the liver and the review of previously reported 44 cases in Japan (in Japanese). Jpn J Gastroent 84:302–306

49. Freeman MP, Vick CW, Taylor KJW, Carithers RL, Brewer WH (1986) Regenerating nodules in cirrhosis: Appearance with anatomic correlation. AJR 146:533–536

50. Ida M, Kitagawa K, Kawamura I, Matsui O, Takashima T, Shinmura K, Kinami Y, Shinozaki K (1984) A case report of regenerative nodule in liver cirrhosis: Ultrasonographically mimicking hepatocellular carcinoma (English abstract). Acta Hepatol Jpn 25:400–404

51. Lee S, Fujita N, Yano A, Kobayashi G, Chonan A, Mochizuki F (1988) A case of hyperechoic regenerating nodules mimicking hemangioma of the liver (English abstract). Jpn J Med Ultrasonics 15:72–78

52. Oka Y, Sakaguchi S, Tohara K, Hatono N, Ueki T, Okumura M (1991) Ultrasonographic findings of small hepatic tumors (less than 2 cm in diameter) (English abstract). Proceedings of JSUM 58:177–178

53. Nambu S, Ichida T, Kojima T, Aoyama K, Matsui S, Yasuyama T, Konda T, Higuchi K, Inoue K, Sasaki H, Yoshimura H, Kasukawa M (1984) A case study of fascioliasis with special reference to immunoserological tests and diagnostic imagings (English abstract). Acta Hepatol Jpn 25:1489–1497

54. Yoon S, Nakata K, Kawara A, Saeki S, Oimomi M, Baba S, Tsuji M (1986) Ultrasonic findings in two patients with human fascioliasis (English abstract). Jpn J Med Ultrasonics 13:375–383

55. Gharbi HA, Hassine W, Brauner MW, Dupuch K (1981) Ultrasound examination of the hydatic liver. Radiology 139:459–463

56. Hadidi A (1982) Sonography of hepatic echinococcal cysts. Gastrointest Radiol 7:349–354

57. Beggs I (1983) The Radiological Appearance of Hydatid Disease of the Liver. Clin Radiol 34:555–563

58. Didier D, Weiler S, Rohmer P, Lassegue A, Deschamps JP, Vuitton D, Miguet JP, Weil F (1985) Hepatic alveolar echinococcosis: Correlative US and CT study. Radiology 154:179–186

59. Chen M, Dong B, Li J, Wan B, Zhang J, Gan L, Ye X, Xu M (1986) Ultrasonographic appearance of echinococcal hydatid cyst (English abstract). Jpn J Med Ultrasonics 13:42–48

60. Amoh K, Arakawa K (1986) Ultrasonographic evaluation of the hepatic alveolar echinococcosis: Experimental and clinical study (English abstract). Jpn J Med Ultrasonics 13:264–271

61. Wakabayashi Y, Suzuki T, Kanesaka N, Kotake F, Kakizaki D, Ike K, Abe K, Amino S (1986) A case of Wilson's Disease with nodular lesion in liver (English abstract). Rinsyo Housyasen 31:425–427

62. Ishibashi H, Tsuchiya Y, Dohmen K, Shimamura R, Kondo H, Hirata Y, Kudo J (1991) The ultrasonographic appearance of the liver in two patients with Wilson's Disease presented as fulminant hepatitis. Jpn J Med Ultrasonics 18:104–110

63. Ohyama Y, Ishida H, Yagisawa H, Morikawa P, Naganuma S, Ishioka T, Masamune O (1990) Two cases of Wilson's Disease (English abstract). Jpn J Med Ultrasonics 17:90–95

64. Sakaguchi S (1988) Storage disease of the liver (in Japanese). Kan Tan Sui 17:67–74

65. Kurioka N, Kanno T, Kim K, Toda S, SO K, Nakajima S, Oka H, Asai H, Kuroki T, Harihara S, Yamamoto S, Monna T (1985) Ultrasonic reevaluation of small hepatocellular carcinoma: On the diagnostic problems and the limits of detectability (English abstract). Jpn J Gastroent 82:247–254

66. Gibo Y, Furuta K, Uemura K, Imai Y, Kiyosawa K, Furuta S, Yokoyama K, Kusano M, Mochizuki A (1990) Examination of the usefullness of ultrasonic diagnostic criteria for hepatocellular carcinoma (HCC) and metastatic liver cancer

(Meta) (English abstract). Jpn J Med Ultrasonics 17:160–167

67. Hui Z, Nakamura M, Itou K (1990) Ultrasonographic study on 502 cases of malignant tumor in the Liver (English abstract). Jpn J Med Ultrasonics 17:250–259

68. Okuno T, Yamato M, Hisa N, Fujikura Y, Izutsu M, Kaneda S, Sato M, Imai Y, Nishioka K (1983) Real-time ultrasonographic manifestation of hepatocellular carcinoma and metastatic liver tumor: Tumor in Tumor Appearance and Lobulation (English abstract). Gazouigakushi 2:112–120

69. Ohnishi K, Nomura F (1989) Ultrasonic Doppler studies of hepatocellular carcinoma and comparison with other hepatic focal lesions. Gastroenterology 97:1489–1497

70. Itoh Y, Kawauchi A, Fukunari N, Naitoh S, Shiga S, Nakayama K, Matsui W, Kamiya K, Koike T, Ishii M, Yoneyama K, Takahashi S, Onuki M, Hatta Y (1990) 2-D Doppler echographical evaluation for the differential diagnosis of liver tumors (English abstract). Jpn J Med Ultrasonics 17:260–266

71. Kuratomi S (1976) A histopathological study of hepatocellular carcinoma: Pathology of advanced hepatocellular carcinoma and intravascular tumor thrombosis in relation to vascular structure and alterations (English abstract). Acta Hepatol Jpn 17:517–527

72. Sugiura N, Ohto M, Kimura K, Okuda K, Kondo F, Hirooka N (1986) Diagnosis and clinical features of portal vein tumor thrombosis in hepatocellular carcinoma (English abstract). Jpn J Gastroent 83:2151–2160

73. Oda T, Sakaguchi S, Tohara K, Hirano M, Kamachi T, Okumura M (1989) Ultrasonic findings of metastatic adrenal tumor in primary liver cancer (English abstract). Proceedings of JSUM 55:735–736

74. Tohara K (to be published) Evaluation of the hemodynamics of liver masses by ultrasonic Doppler method: Usefullness in differential diagnosis of tumor (English abstract). Acta Hepatol Jpn

75. Matsuda Y, Yabuuchi I (1986) Hepatic tumors: US contrast enhancement with CO_2 microbubbles. Radiology 161:701–705

76. Kudo M, Tomita S, Tochio H, Kashida H, Hirasa M, Todo A (1991) Hepatic focal nodular hyperplasia: Specific findings at dynamic contrast-enhanced US with carbon dioxide microbubbles. Radiology 179:377–382

77. Mihara S (1990) Evaluation of ultrasonic mass screening for hepatocellular carcinoma (English abstract). Jpn J Med Ultrasonics 17:639–647

CHAPTER 13

Diagnosis of primary liver cancer by computed tomography

Osamu Matsui[1] and Yuji Itai[2]

1 General considerations

For the early detection of hepatocellular carcinoma (HCC), the effectiveness of ultrasonography (US) has been widely accepted in Japan. However, US examination of the entire liver is occasionally impossible because of intervening bones, air in the gut or lung, or dense fatty tissue, especially in patients with a small cirrhotic liver. In such patients, computed tomography (CT) has begun to play an increasingly important role in detecting HCC as a complementary imaging method for US. CT is also very useful in differentiating various space-occupying lesions of the liver [1, 2], evaluating the location and extension of these lesions, and determining the viability of neoplasms treated by transcatheter arterial embolization (TAE), percutaneous ethanol injection therapy, or chemotherapy. Another advantage of CT is its objectiveness in visualizing the relation between the lesions and the surrounding tissues. For these reasons and because of widespread availability of CT machines in Japan, CT is now performed in almost all patients with HCC and is making a major contribution to the treatment of HCC.

2 CT techniques

For the diagnosis of HCC, both pre- and postcontrast CT are usually performed. Postcontrast CT is done immediately after intravenous injection of 50–150 ml contrast medium. Postcontrast CT demonstrates the distribution of contrast medium in all tissues including arterial, portal and venous spaces, capillary beds and interstitial spaces. Evaluation of the arterial blood supply is very useful in detecting hypervascular lesions and in the differential diagnosis of hepatic tumors. To this end, 30–50 ml of contrast medium is administered intravenously as a single bolus, and sequential CT scans are obtained at the same level. With current instruments, it is possible to scan several to 30 slices in sequence, even in a single breath-holding period (single level dynamic study). Using sequential CT, early scans (10–20 seconds following injection) show dense opacification of the abdominal aorta and its branches while later scans demonstrate the portal and venous systems clearly. However, considering the time required for injection and the long circulation pathway, terms such as "arterial-dominant" and "portal-dominant" phases have come into use [3]. Following the portal-dominant phase, contrast medium distributes over the whole body as in postcontrast CT, and is called the "equilibrium" phase (Fig. 1). The injected contrast agent gradually disappears from the surrounding blood spaces and the contrast medium remaining in the tissues will be visualized as hyperdense areas in the later equilibrium phase (delayed CT scan) [4]. This phenomenon is called "delayed enhancement" (Fig. 2).

The combined use of CT and arteriography is the most precise imaging method for the diagnosis of hepatic tumors. However, it is an invasive method and its indications should be considered the same as those of hepatic angiography. There are three combinations of CT and arteriography: CT during the infusion of contrast medium into the hepatic artery (CT arteriography: CTA) (Fig. 3) [5], CT during arterial portography (CTAP) (Fig. 4) [6] and CT performed after intra-arterial

[1] Associate Professor of Radiology, Kanazawa University School of Medicine, Kanazawa, Ishikawa, 920 Japan
[2] Professor and Chairman, Department of Radiology, Institute of Clinical Medicine, Tsukuba University, Ibaraki, 305 Japan

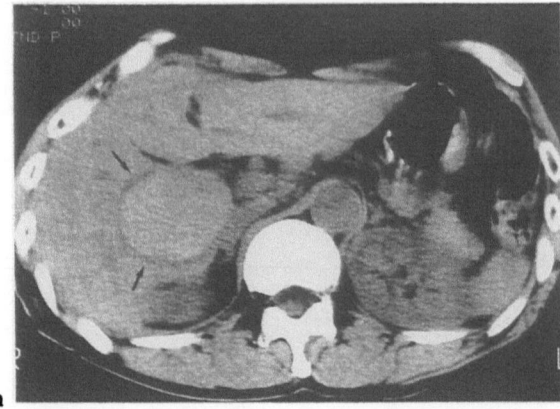 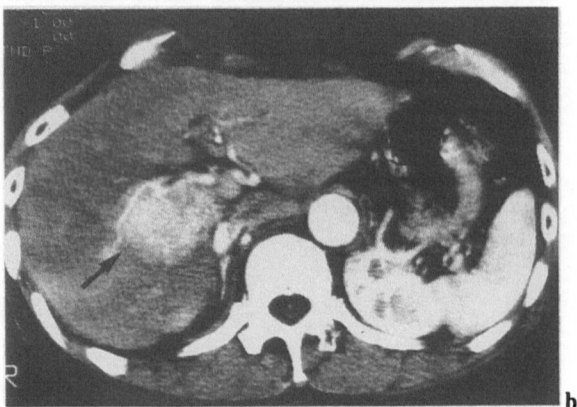

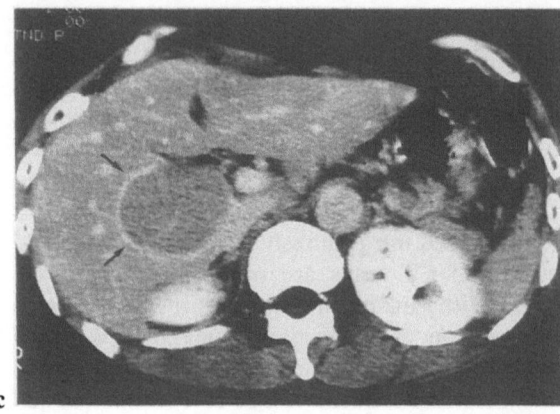

Fig. 1a–c. Hepatocellular carcinoma. a Precontrast CT shows the fibrous capsule as a thin circular hypodense band (*arrows*). b The arterial-dominant phase of dynamic CT shows the clearly opacified tumor (*arrow*) with internal mosaic architecture. The hepatic arteries are also well-visualized. c Postcontrast CT shows the fibrous capsule (*arrows*) and internal septum as a hyperdense band and the hypodense tumor

injection of iodized poppyseed oil (Lipiodol: Andre-Gelbe Laboratories, France) (Lipiodol CT) (Fig. 5) [7]. In CTA, 10–15 ml of contrast medium is infused into the hepatic artery during the scanning of each slice of the liver. For CTAP, 70 ml of contrast medium is injected via a catheter in the superior mesenteric artery at an estimated rate of 0.5–0.8 ml/sec during sequential scanning of the liver with incremental changes in the position of the table. In Lipiodol CT, CT is performed 2–3 weeks following injection of 2–5 ml of Lipiodol into the proper hepatic artery.

3 CT detection of primary liver cancer

Table 1 shows the detectability of 209 surgically confirmed HCC nodules in 148 patients using various imaging methods. CT is inferior to US in the detection of small HCCs less than 2 cm in diameter. However, these methods complement each other and both CT and US are carried out periodically in patients at high risk for HCC. For initial HCC screening, US is performed every three months, and CT every six months to one year. When HCC is suspected by US or elevated serological tumor markers, CT is immediately carried out to help arrive at a qualitative diagnosis of the lesion. As shown in Table 1, CTAP and Lipiodol CT are the most sensitive imaging methods to detect small HCC nodules (Figs. 4, 5). CTAP is more sensitive than Lipiodol CT in the detection of hypovascular tumors [8], while Lipiodol CT is more accurate for hypervascular lesions. HCCs of Edmondson and Steiner grade II or above are usually hypervascular, and therefore, Lipiodol CT is the most reliable in detecting them and their intrahepatic metastases. However, injected Lipiodol occasionally disappears from small viable HCC nodules within 1–2 weeks. Therefore, care should be taken not to attach too much importance to Lipiodol CT when TAE is not performed following Lipiodol injection [9]. On the other hand, well-differentiated HCCs are hypovascular or avascular in nature [10] and CTAP is the most sensitive in visualizing them (Fig. 4) [11]. However, since both CTAP and Lipiodol CT are invasive, they are usually performed as preoperative evaluation methods.

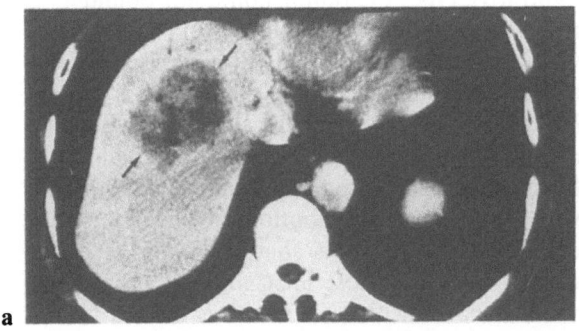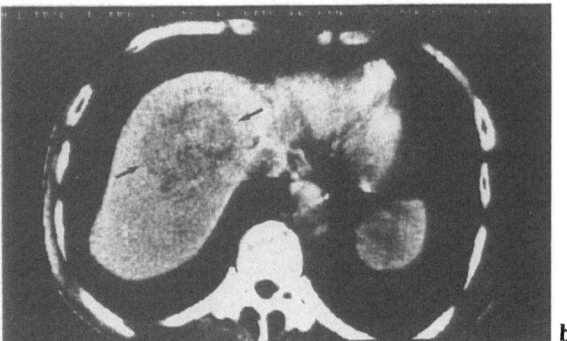

Fig. 2a,b. Scirrhous type of hepatocellular carcinoma. **a** Postcontrast CT shows hypodense nodule with irregular margin (*arrows*). **b** Delayed CT shows delayed enhancement in the tumor (*arrows*)

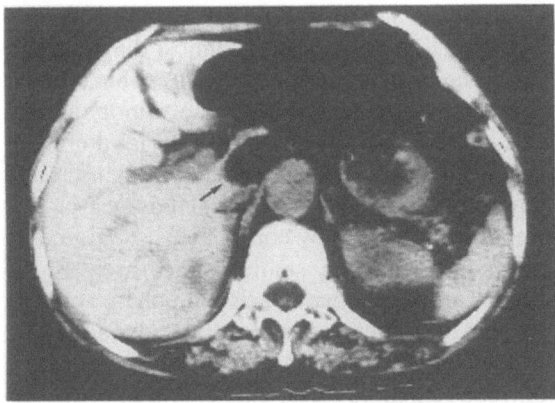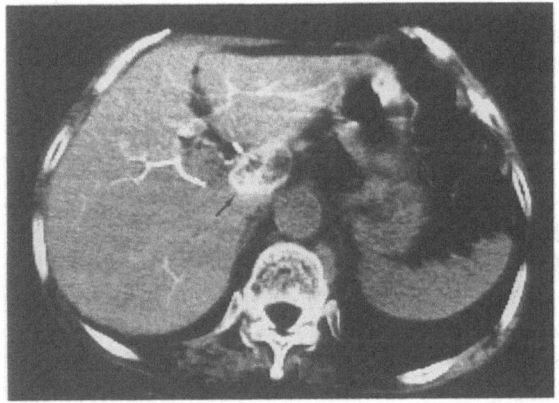

Fig. 3a,b. Hepatocellular carcinoma with marked fatty metamorphosis. **a** Precontrast CT shows an extremely hypodense nodule an attenuation value of −30 HU in the caudate lobe of the liver (*arrow*). **b** CT arteriography shows the mosaic architecture clearly (*arrow*)

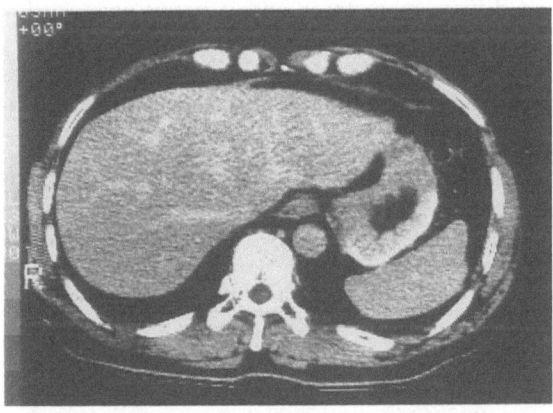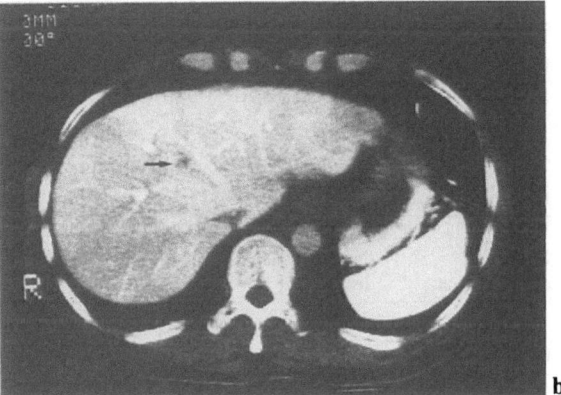

Fig. 4a,b. Well-differentiated hepatocellular carcinoma. **a** Postcontrast CT did not demonstrate the tumor. **b** CT during arterial portography clearly shows it as a hypodense nodule (*arrow*)

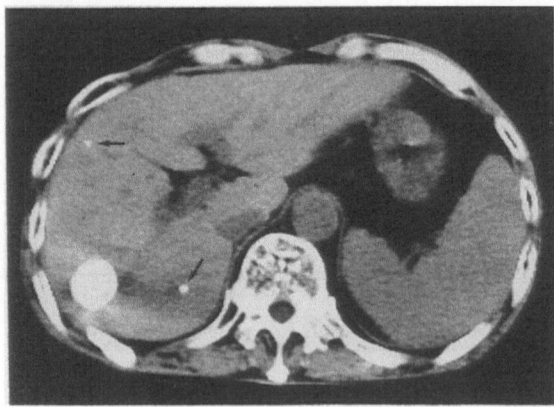

Fig. 5. Hepatocellular carcinoma with intrahepatic metastases. Precontrast CT one month following the injection of Lipiodol and Gelfoam particles into the right hepatic artery shows extremely hyperdense nodules. Minute intrahepatic metastases less than 5 mm in diameter are also definitely demonstrated (*arrows*)

When elevated serological tumor markers strongly suggest the existence of HCC, and US, CT, and hepatic arteriography are all negative, CTAP or Lipiodol CT is of value as a screening modality.

Cholangiocellular carcinomas are usually found at an advanced stage and can usually be demonstrated by all imaging methods. CTAP is very sensitive in demonstrating intrahepatic metastases resulting from these tumors.

4   CT findings of primary liver cancers and their differential diagnosis

The gross pathology of HCCs is divided into five types: infiltrative, expansive, mixed infiltrative and expansive, diffuse, and specific [12]. In the infiltrative type, the tumor-nontumor boundary is irregular and indistinct, and neoplastic foci of varying sizes are fused to form larger foci distributed segmentally. This type of HCC is demonstrated as a mainly segmental uneven hypodense area with unclear margins that is indistinguishable from other wide-spreading malignant neoplasms with segmental distribution. Conversley, the expansive type mass is sharply demarcated and usually nodular. Most HCCs of this type which are associated with liver cirrhosis have a fibrous capsule and internal mosaic architecture (Fig. 1). Since HCCs are being increasingly detected at an early stage, the frequency of expansive HCC has risen sharply, and recently, in our institution, this type of lesion accounts for approximately 90% of all HCCs. These macroscopic features of the expansive (or nodular) type are very specific and their detection by imaging is almost diagnostic of HCC. The fibrous capsule is seen as a thin circular hypodense band surrounding the tumor on precontrast CT and during the arterial-dominant phase of dynamic CT, and as a hyperdense band on postcontrast CT. The internal mosaic architecture is characterized by components separated by thin bands with the same CT features as the fibrous capsule and with each component showing different densities on precontrast, dynamic and postcontrast CT (Fig. 1). The diffuse type shows numerous small nodules, 0.5–1.0 cm in diameter, scattered throughout the liver which do not fuse with each other and are always associated with liver cirrhosis. Diffuse nodules are visualized as diffusely distributed small hypodense nodules on both pre- and postcontrast CT. This CT finding is very similar to that of macroregenerative nodules and diffuse metastases and it is not easy to differentiate these lesions without dynamic CT.

In addition to the morphological features described above, the hypervascular nature is rela-

Table 1. Comparison of the detectability of hepatocellular carcinomas in various imaging modalities (209 lesions in 148 patients)

Largest diameter (cm)	No. of lesions	US	CT	Angiography		Lipiodol CT
				Arteriography	CTAP	
~ < 0.5	14	0/14 (0%)	0/14 (0%)	4/14 (29%)	1/14 (7%)	0/4 (0%)
0.5 ≦ ~ ≦ 1.0	31	4/31 (13%)	3/31 (10%)	12/27 (44%)	26/31 (84%)	5/6 (83%)
1.0 < ~ ≦ 1.5	34	23/34 (68%)	17/34 (50%)	13/19 (68%)	33/34 (97%)	4/6 (67%)
1.5 < ~ ≦ 2.0	30	24/30 (80%)	19/30 (63%)	9/13 (69%)	29/30 (97%)	2/2 (100%)
2.0 < ~ ≦ 3.0	33	27/33 (82%)	26/33 (79%)	26/28 (93%)	33/33 (100%)	9/10 (90%)
3.0 < ~ ≦ 4.0	20	20/20 (100%)	18/20 (90%)	19/20 (95%)	20/20 (100%)	4/4 (100%)
4.0 < ~	47	47/47 (100%)	47/47 (100%)	47/47 (100%)	47/47 (100%)	8/8 (100%)

No. of detected HCC/No. of imaging tests performed (detectability %)
CTAP, CT during arterial portography

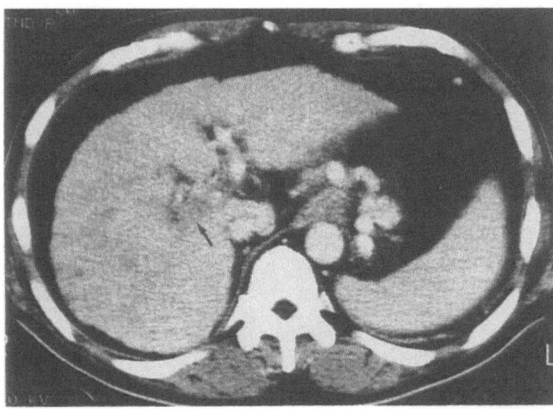

Fig. 6. Hepatocellular carcinoma with tumor thrombus in right branch of intrahepatic portal vein. Postcontrast CT shows hypodense solid mass in the right branch of the intrahepatic portal vein (*arrow*)

tively specific for HCCs. Dynamic CT with bolus injection of contrast medium is one of the best noninvasive methods to evaluate the vascularity of liver tumors (Fig. 1) [13]. Typical HCCs appear hyperdense in the arterial-dominant phase and become hypodense in the portal-dominant or equilibrium phases (Fig. 1). Another peculiar characteristic of HCCs is their tendency to grow into the portal and/or hepatic veins, eliciting tumor thrombi. Tumor thrombi are shown as solid mass lesions in the blood vessels with a marked hypervascularity often seen on dynamic CT due to arteriovenous shunting through them (Fig. 6) [14, 15]. The hepatic segment in which the feeding portal vein is obstructed demonstrates segmental staining [16, 17] in the arterial-dominant phase of dynamic CT probably due to arterial compensation for the decreased portal blood flow. When ischemia is severe, it is visualized as a segmental hypodensity on precontrast CT and hyperdensity on postcontrast CT, probably due to fibrotic changes. The imaging information revealed by dynamic CT is demonstrated in greater detail by CT arteriography (Fig. 3).

CT findings indicating a fibrous capsule are almost diagnostic for HCC, although a fibrous capsule is also seen in hepatic adenomas and, very rarely, in metastatic liver cancers. Mosaic architecture separated by fibrous septa is pathognomonic for HCC, but care should be taken not to misdiagnose uneven CT densities in the tumors due to degeneration, necrosis or bleeding as a true mosaic pattern. Hypervascularity is also seen in some metastatic liver tumors, hepatic adenomas, focal nodular hyperplasias, and

cavernous hemangiomas. Metastatic tumors tend to have a central necrotic area, which results in a "doughnut-shaped" appearance on CT. However, hypervascular metastases from renal carcinomas, medullary carcinomas, endocrine tumors and some non-epithelial tumors rarely demonstrate this doughnut pattern and are indistinguishable from HCCs even by dynamic CT. Hepatic adenomas and focal nodular hyperplasias are also difficult to differentiate from HCCs [18]. In focal nodular hyperplasias, a stellate scar in the center of the lesion is a characteristic histological marker. If the stellate scar is large enough to be visualized on CT, it appears hypodense on precontrast CT and hyperdense on postcontrast CT. Cavernous hemangioma is the most common benign liver tumor and should be differentiated from HCC. Cavernous hemangiomas are composed of vascular channels of various sizes separated by thin fibrous tissue and are usually discrete and well-demarcated. Therefore, they show almost the same density as that of the blood with a clear margin on precontrast CT and dense accumulation of contrast material in or near the periphery which spreads in all directions with time. The hyperdensity of the mass usually persists for more than three minutes with prolonged enhancement [19]. Although this dynamic CT pattern is diagnostic, a conclusive diagnosis is not always possible for small lesions less than 1.5 cm in diameter in which case magnetic resonance imaging or arteriography should be performed.

The histopathology of HCCs varies depending on the combinations of the following features: the structural pattern (trabecular, sclerosing, etc.), differences in the degree of cell differentiation, cytological variants (fatty change, clear cells, etc.), degeneration, and so on. These histological features each modify the imaging findings. For example, it is well-known that HCC shows various degrees of fatty metamorphosis histologically, especially in small HCCs less than 2 cm in diameter (small liver cancer: SLC). Fatty change is usually diffuse in small HCCs (Fig. 3) and focal in larger tumors, and the degree of fat deposition varies among components in mosaic architecture [20]. When fatty deposition is extreme, CT detection is possible because it causes a hypodense area with an attenuation value of less than -1 Hounsfield units (H) on CT (Fig. 3). In these cases, it is important to differentiate between lipoma, liposarcoma and angiomyolipoma. However, HCC with fatty metamorphosis is far more common than these lipomatous tumors in patients

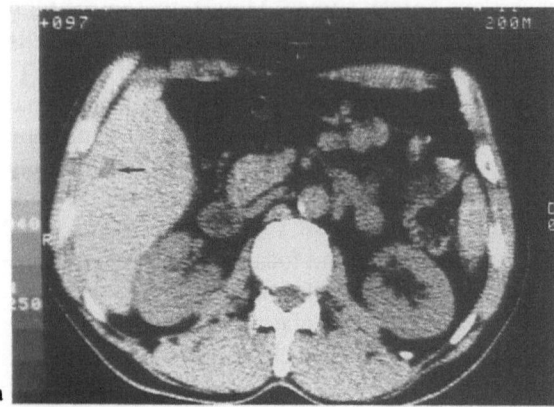

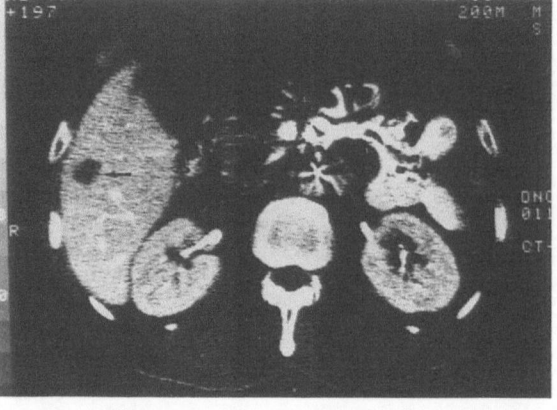

Fig. 7a,b. Hepatocellular carcinoma with moderate fatty deposition. **a** Precontrast CT shows a small hypodense nodule (*arrow*) but recognition of the fat is impossible. **b** CT during arterial portography shows the entire tumor as a definitely hypodense nodule (*arrow*)

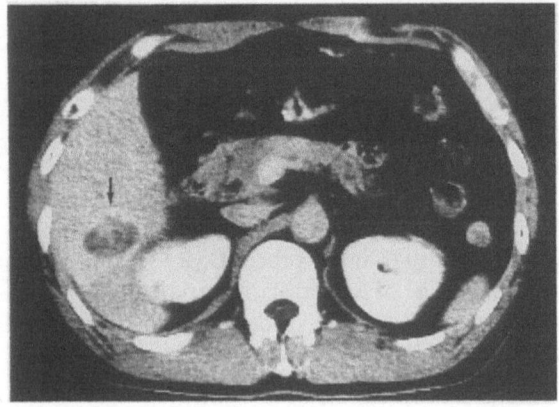

Fig. 8. Hepatocellular carcinoma with massive necrosis. Postcontrast CT shows a cystic mass lesion with irregularly enhanced capsule (*arrow*)

at high risk for HCC. When fatty deposition is moderate, it shows as a definite hypodensity but is more than 0 H on CT, and recognition by CT is impossible (Fig. 7). In these cases, various types of hypodensity mass lesions including focal fatty change should be ruled out. Focal fatty change is usually differentiated from true mass lesions by its segmental configuration and internal portal tracts. However, when it is small, its differentiation from fatty HCC is difficult. Contrary to HCCs, focal fatty changes are not clearly visualized on CTAP because of the existence of internal portal flow [21]. Massive necrosis in small HCCs with a fibrous capsule is occasionally seen, and is shown as a non-enhanced mass with enhanced capsule on post-contrast CT (Fig. 8). This CT finding is very similar to that of organized abcess or hematoma, other necrotic tumors, ciliated hepatic foregut cyst [22], complicated cyst and some biliary cystadenomas or cystadenocarcinomas. HCCs with abundant fibrous stroma separating cords of tumor cells are called the scirrhous type (WHO classification). This type shows hypovascularity on dynamic CT and delayed enhancement on delayed CT. These CT findings are common among hepatic mass lesions with abundant fibrous tissue such as postinflammatory fibrosis (organized granuloma), cholangiocellular carcinoma (Fig. 2), and metastatic liver cancers including gastrointestinal adenocarcinomas [23]. Differentiation among them is occasionally impossible when only CT is performed. The coexistence of sarcomatousappearing cells has been reported as a rare histological feature of HCC. In our experience, HCC with sarcomatous change shows marked hypodensity on pre- and postcontrast CT and hypo- or avascularity on dynamic CT resembling cholangiocellular carcinoma and metastatic adenocarcinoma. Calcification in HCCs is very rare and was seen in less than 0.2% of our cases. Histological examination revealed non-specific dystrophic calcification in a necrotic area in one of the calcified HCCs (Fig. 9). Deposition of copper and copper-binding protein in some HCCs has been recognized, and our recent study revealed that the dense accumulation of these substances is responsible for the hyperdensity on precontrast CT (55–65 H).

In SLCs, fibrous capsule and internal mosaic architecture are underdeveloped and the frequency of their visualization on imaging diagnosis

Table 2. Visualization of the fibrous capsule of hepatocellular carcinomas

Largest diameter of lesions (cm)	No. of lesions	Histologically positive	US	CT
~ < 2.0	26	14	2 (14%)	0 (0%)
2.0 ≦ ~ < 3.0	16	15	5 (33%)	4 (27%)
3.0 ≦ ~	30	27	21 (78%)	23 (85%)
Total	72	56	28 (50%)	27 (48%)

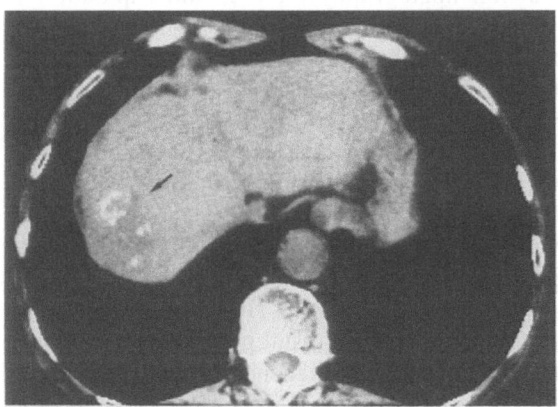

Fig. 9. Hepatocellular carcinoma with calcification. Precontrast CT shows a hypodense nodule with amorphous calcifications (*arrow*)

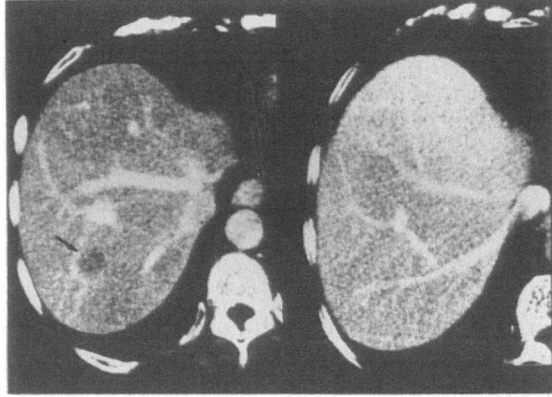

Fig. 10. Adenomatous hyperplasia (AH). Postcontrast CT (*left*) shows a hypodense nodule (*arrow*). It is indistinguishable from a small hepatocellular carcinoma. CT during arterial portography (*right*) did not demonstrate AH because of internal portal blood flow

is decreased (Fig. 7). Table 2 shows the correlation between the size of HCCs and the visualization of fibrous capsule histologically on US and CT. As shown in Table 2, the frequency of fibrous capsule in SLCs less than 1.5 cm is very low, even histologically, and almost zero on US or CT. It is well known that SLCs are more frequently well-differentiated than large HCCs and that Edmondson and Steiner's grade I HCC cells are not uncommon in SLCs. As reported by Takayasu et al. [10], well-differentiated HCCs are hypovascular on arteriography, and SLCs are occasionally not opacified on dynamic CT. Therefore, the imaging findings of SLCs, especially when they are less than 1.5 cm in diameter, are usually non-specific. Among the mass lesions which should be differentiated from SLCs, hepatocytic nodular lesions associated with liver cirrhosis are the most important and the most frequent clinically. Recent advances in imaging modalities have facilitated the detection of small nodular lesions in cirrhotic livers. Some of these lesions are overt HCCs, and others may represent adenomatous hyperplasia (AH) [24]. The CT findings of AHs are nearly indistinguishable from those of well-differentiated small HCCs (Fig. 10). One useful method to differentiate the two lesions is to evaluate the intranodular blood supply using imaging diagnosis. We reported the usefulness of in vivo analysis of intranodular blood supply in estimating the grade of malignancy of hepatocytic nodular lesions associated with liver cirrhosis (Table 3) [25]. The portal blood supply was evaluated by CTAP, with the arterial blood supply evaluated by hepatic arteriography, CTA, and Lipiodol CT, or US following intra-arterial injection of CO_2 microbubbles. A portal blood supply was seen in 96% of AHs and only 6% of HCCs on CTAP (Figs. 4, 7, 10). In contrast, a greater arterial supply relative to that of the surrounding liver was verified in 94% of the HCCs and only 4% of the AHs. The blood supply of AHs with atypical hepatocytes (atypical AH) and well-differentiated HCCs (Edmondson and Steiner's grade I) tended to be intermediate between AHs without atypia (ordinary AH) and HCCs with Edmondson and Steiner's grade II or above. Evaluation of the blood supply of the nodular lesions associated with liver

Table 3. Intranodular portal blood supply evaluated by CT during arterial portography

		Portal supply		
		(−)	(±)	(+)
Hepatocellular carcinoma	(n = 84)	79	4[a]	1[b]
Adenomatous hyperplasia	(n = 25)	1	7	17
Ordinal AH	(n = 10)	0	2	8
Atypical AH	(n = 12)	1	4	7
AH with malignant foci	(n = 3)	0	1	2[b]

AH, adenomatous hyperplasia
Portal supply (−), Visualized as lower density than that of the intrahepatic inferior vena cava on CT during arterial portography; (+), Not visualized on CT during arterial portography; (±), Visualized as intermediate density between (−) and (+) on CT during arterial portography
[a] Three out of five were Edmondson and Steiner's grade I of cancer cell anaplasia
[b] A malignant focus about 0.7 cm in diameter showed portal supply (−) in one of them

cirrhosis using CT is useful clinically in the differential diagnosis and treatment of early stage HCCs.

5 Evaluation of the extension and of primary liver cancer

Before the determination of the best treatment method for HCCs can be made, their precise location must be known, and the presence of intrahepatic metastases or other lesions (multicentricity) and tumor thrombi must be confirmed or ruled out. CT diagnosis of the segment in which the tumor exists is done in relation to hepatic and intrahepatic portal veins. Therefore,

the portal-dominant phase of dynamic CT, high dose contrast enhancement CT, and CTAP in which intrahepatic veins are well-opacified are valuable. Of these three modalities, CTAP visualizes both the entire tumor and veins most distinctly and is the most accurate in determining the segmental location of the tumor (Fig. 11) [26, 27]. Intrahepatic metastases are usually hypervascular in nature and well-visualized by dynamic CT, arteriography (especially using digital subtraction angiography), CTA, and Lipiodol CT. When the lesions are extremely hypervascular, nodules less than 0.5 cm in diameter can be detected by these methods, particularly by Lipiodol CT (Fig. 5). When HCC nodules are hypovascular, they are detected most accurately by CTAP which can visualize nodules measuring 0.5 cm in diameter or more regardless of their vascularity [8, 11]. Tumor thrombi in the major portal branches are easily diagnosed by US, CT (Fig. 6) or arteriography. However, the detection of tumor thrombi in distal portal branches (distal to the third order branches of the intrahepatic portal vein) is usually difficult by these imaging modalities. For the detection of such peripheral tumor thrombi, CTAP is most valuable [27]. CTAP visualizes the portal perfusion defect caused by portal tumor thrombi as a wedge-shaped hypodense area including the tumor (Figs. 11, 12). When a portal perfusion defect is shown as a fan-shaped hypodense area on CTAP, only compression by the tumor of peripheral portal branches is usually verified histologically. However, our previous study showed that the frequency of microscopic tumor thrombi is very high in fan-shaped portal perfusion defects. [27] For these reasons, we perform CTAP for precise evaluation of tumor extension, especially for preoperative examinations.

Type I Fan-shaped   Type II Wedge-shaped

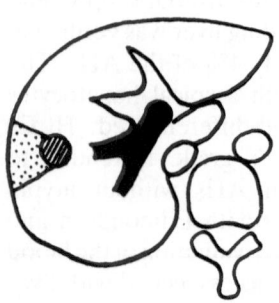 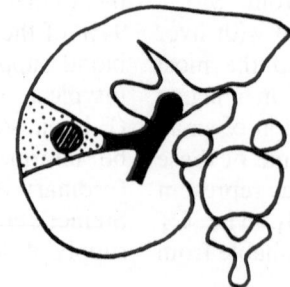

Fig. 11. Two types of portal perfusion defects seen on CT during arterial portography. *Hatched area*, hepatocellular carcinoma; *dotted area*, portal perfusion defect

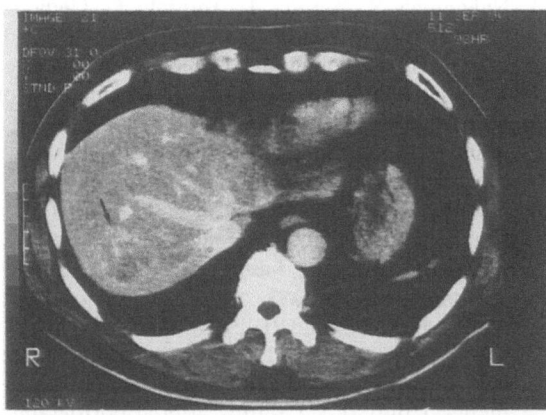

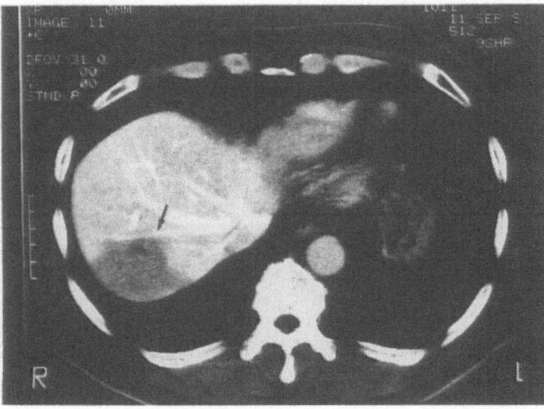

Fig. 12a,b. Hepatocellular carcinoma with tumor thrombus in the peripheral portal vein. **a** Postcontrast CT shows a hypodense nodule with the enhanced capsule and internal mosaic architecture (*arrow*). **b** CT during arterial portography shows a wedge-shaped portal perfusion defect surrounding the tumor (*arrow*)

References

1. Itai Y, Nishikawa J, Tasaka A (1979) Computed tomography in the evaluation of hepatocellular carcinoma. Radiology 131:165–170
2. Itai Y, Araki T, Furui S, Tasaka A (1981) Differential diagnosis of hepatic masses on computed tomography, with particular reference to hepatocellular carcinoma. J Comput Assist Tomogr 5:834–842
3. Itai Y (1987) Imaging diagnosis with computed tomography. In: Okuda K, Ishak KG (eds) Neoplasms of the Liver. Springer-Verlag, Tokyo, pp 289–300
4. Itai Y, Ohtomo K, Yamauchi T, Minami M, Yashiro N, Araki T (1986) CT of hepatic masses: Significance of prolonged enhancement and delayed enhancement. AJR 146:792–733
5. Prando A, Wallace S, Bernardino ME, Lindell MM Jr (1979) Computed tomographic arteriography of the liver. Radiology 130:697–701
6. Matsui O, Kadoya M, Suzuki M, Inoue K, Itoh H, Ida M, Takashima T (1983) Dynamic sequential computed tomography during arterial portography in the detection of hepatic neoplasms. Radiology 146:721–727
7. Ohishi H, Uchida H, Yoshimura H, Ohue S, Ueda J, Katsuragi M, Matsuo N, Hosogi Y (1985) Hepatocellular carcinoma detected by iodized oil: Use of anticancer agents. Radiology 154:25–30
8. Matsui O, Takashima T, Kadoya M, Suzuki M, Hirose J, Kameyama T, Choto S, Konishi H, Ida M, Yamaguchi A, Izumi R (1987) Liver metastases from colorectal cancers: Detection with CT during arterial portography. Radiology 165:65–69
9. Matsui O, Takashima T, Kadoya M, Kitagawa K, Hirose J, Kameyama T, Choto S, Miyata S (1987) Mechanism of Lipiodol accumulation and retention in hepatic tumors: Analysis in cases with simple Lipiodol injection. Nippon Acta Radiol. 47: 1395–1404 [Japanese]
10. Takayasu K, Shima Y, Muramatu Y, Goto H, Moriyama N, Yamada T, Makuuchi M, Yamasaki S, Hasegawa H, Okazaki N, Hirohashi S, Kishi K (1986) Angiography of small hepatocellular carcinoma: analysis of 105 resected tumors. AJR 147:525–529
11. Matsui O, Takashima T, Kadoya M, Ida M, Suzuki M, Kitagawa K, Kamimura R, Inoue K, Konishi H, Itoh H (1985) Dynamic computed tomography during arterial portography: the most sensitive examination for small hepatocellular carcinomas. J Comput Assist Tomogr 9:19–24
12. Kojiro M, Nakashima T (1987) Pathology of hepatocellular carcinoma. In: Okuda K, Ishak KG (eds) Neoplasms of the Liver. Springer-Verlag, Tokyo pp 81–104
13. Araki T, Itai Y, Furui S, Tasaka A (1980) Dynamic CT densitometry of hepatic tumors. AJR 135: 1037–1043
14. Suzuki M, Itoh H, Konishi H, Ida M, Matsui O, Takashima T (1982) Hepatocellular carcinoma involving the portal vein. J Comput Assist Tomogr 6:831–832
15. Itai Y, Furui S, Ohtomo K, Kokubo T, Yamauchi T, Minami M, Yashiro N (1986) Dynamic CT features of arterioportal shunt in hepatocellular carcinoma. AJR 146:723–727
16. Matsui O, Takashima T, Kadoya M, Kitagawa K, Kamimura R, Itoh H, Suzuki M, Ida M (1984) Segmental staining on hepatic arteriography as a sign of intrahepatic portal vein obstruction. Radiology 152:601–606
17. Itai Y, Moss AA, Goldberg HI (1982) Transient hepatic attenuation difference of lobar or segmental distribution detected by dynamic computed tomography. Radiology 144:835–839
18. Kerlin P, Davis GL, McGill DB, Weiland LH, Adson MA, Sheedy PF (1983) Hepatic adenoma and focal nodular hyperplasia: Clinical, pathological and radiologic features. Gastroenterology 84:994–1002

19. Itai Y, Furui S, Araki T, Yashiro N, Tasaka A (1980) Computed tomography of cavernous hemangioma of the liver. Radiology 137:149–155
20. Yoshikawa J, Matsui O, Takashima T, Ida M, Takanaka T, Kawamura I, Kakuda K, Miyata S (1988) Fatty metamorphosis in hepatocellular carcinoma: Radiologic features in 10 cases. AJR 151:717–720
21. Yoshikawa J, Matsui O, Takashima T, Sugiura H, Katayama K, Nishida Y, Tsuji M (1987) Focal fatty change of the liver adjacent to the falciform ligament: CT and sonographic findings in five surgically confirmed cases. AJR 149:491–494
22. Kadoya M, Matsui O, Nakanuma Y, Yoshikawa J, Arai K, Takashima T, Amano M, Kimura M (1990) Ciliated hepatic foregut cyst: Radiologic features. Radiology 175:475–477
23. Muramatsu Y, Takayasu K, Moriyama N, Shima Y, Goto H, Ushio K, Yamada T, Hasegawa H, Koyama Y, Hirohashi S (1986) Peripheral low-density area of hepatic tumors: CT-pathologic correlation. Radiology 160:49–52
24. Nakanuma Y, Terada T, Terasaki S, Ueda K, Nonomura A, Kawahara E, Matsui O (1990) "Atypical adenomatous hyperplasia" in liver cirrhosis: Low-grade hepatocellular carcinoma or borderline lesion? Histopathology 17:27–35
25. Matsui O, Kadoya M, Kameyama T, Yoshikawa J, Takashima T, Nakanuma Y, Unoura M, Kobayashi K, Izumi R, Ida M, Kitagawa K (1991) Benign and malignant nodules in the cirrhotic livers: Distinction based on blood supply. Radiology 178:493–497
26. Nelson RC, Chezmar JL, Sugarbaker PH, Murray DR, Bernardino ME (1990) Preoperative localization of focal liver lesions to specific liver segments: Utility of CT during arterial portography. Radiology 176:89–94
27. Matsui O (1986) Basic and clinical studies of dynamic sequential computed tomography during arterial portography in the diagnosis of hepatic cancers (in Japanese). Nippon Acta Radiol. 46:335–359

CHAPTER 14

Diagnosis of primary liver cancer using magnetic resonance imaging

Yuji Itai,[1] Kuni Ohtomo,[2] and Osamu Matsui[3]

Introduction

Magnetic resonance imaging (MRI) appeared for use in diagnostic radiology in the early 1980s. This method of diagnostic imaging is characterized by excellent contrast resolution and free direction as well as no exposure to radiation. The intensities of organs and tumors reflect multiple factors, such as proton density, longitudinal relaxation time (T1), and transverse relaxation time (T2). The weights of these factors are changed by pulse sequences and their timing parameters, whereas X-CT and radionuclide imaging are determined by only one factor. In addition, there are many pulse sequences that can be used in MRI, such as a set of radiofrequency pulses, gradient pulses and time intervals between pulses. However, the standard technique used is spin echo imaging because of the high signal to noise ratio.

The disadvantages of MRI are the long acquisition time, expensive instrumentation, high running costs, degradation of image quality due to movement and magnetic substances, and, in some rare cases, claustrophobia. When used to image the liver, motion artifacts due to respiration, pulsation, and bowel movement may be critical. However, fairly good images can be obtained in most of patients with conventional spin echo imaging as long as the patients breathe regularly and/or the number of excitations for imaging are suitably increased. There are a large number of papers reporting the usefulness of MRI with the liver [1–4]. Many techniques, such as presatura-

tion, flow compensation, respiratory gating, and fat suppression, have been successfully developed to reduce motion artifacts.

On the other hand, fast acquisition techniques have been also investigated. Gradient echo imaging (3–5 s), turbo FLASH (1 s), and echo planar imaging (100 ms) are now available as commercial or investigative instruments, and this makes it possible to obtain images free from respiratory movement or even pulsation. The fast acquisition method is useful not only for liver imaging in general, but also in dynamic studies of liver tumors using contrast agents. There are still major developments to be made in MRI in the fields of software and hardware as well as contrast agents.

Our experience in primary liver cancer using conventional spin echo and/or gradient echo magnetic resonance images will be presented in this paper.

1 Detection

The detectability of hepatocellular carcinoma (HCC) using MRI is represented in Table 1. To discuss the detection rate with MRI, it is necessary to clarify the conditions of acquisition (kinds of pulse sequence, TR, TE, TI (IR), flip angle (gradient echo), number of excitations, slice thickness, slice interval, with or without contrast agent) as well as the instrument and magnetic field used. For example, Kurume University reported better results using short time-interval inversion recovery (STIR) in addition to short TR and long TR spin echo images working at 0.5 tesla [5].

The best pulse sequence per given time unit has been investigated in the detection of metastatic

[1] University of Tsukuba, 1-1-1 Tennodai, Tsukuba, Ibaraki, 305 Japan
[2] Yamanashi Medical College, 1110 Shimokawahigashi, Tamaho, Yamanashi, 409-38 Japan
[3] University of Kanazawa, 13-1 Takaramachi, Kanazawa, Ishikawa, 920 Japan

Table 1. Detectability of HCC on both long TR, TEs and short TR, TE images

Size (cm)	Positive	Equivocal	Negative	Total
~1	3 (75%)	1	0	4
~2	16 (73%)	3	3	22
~3	15 (88%)	0	2	17
~4	17 (100%)	0	0	17
~5	8 (100%)	0	0	8
5~	19 (86%)	3[a]	0	22
Total	78 (86.7%)	7 (7.8%)	5 (5.6%)	90

[a] unclear extent with thrombosis in the portal vein (1.5T, 1986–1988, University of Tokyo)

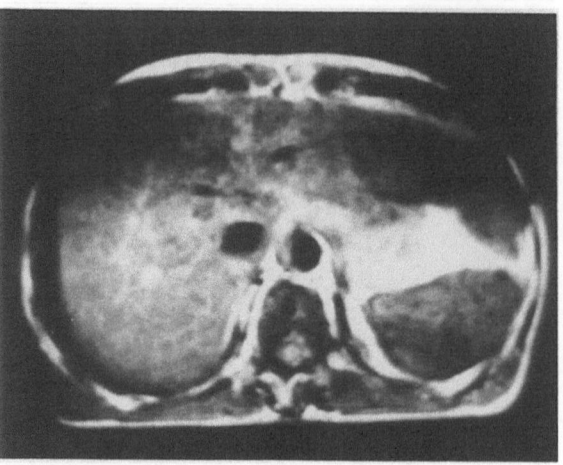

Fig. 1. Proton density image of small HCC. A small high intensity nodule is clearly demonstrated

liver tumors [6]. The results vary according to the field strengths of the instruments as well as the institution where the results were obtained. However, there are no similar studies for primary liver cancer. In many institutions, MRI is as good as or superior to conventional CT in the detection of primary liver cancer.

The minimum tumor size which can be detected is a little less than 10 mm in diameter (Fig. 1) [5]. However, smaller lesions can be detected in the liver with decreased intensity due to the presence of iron (hemosiderin or ferritin). This means iron-containing contrast material can be effective for the detection of liver tumors (Fig. 2).

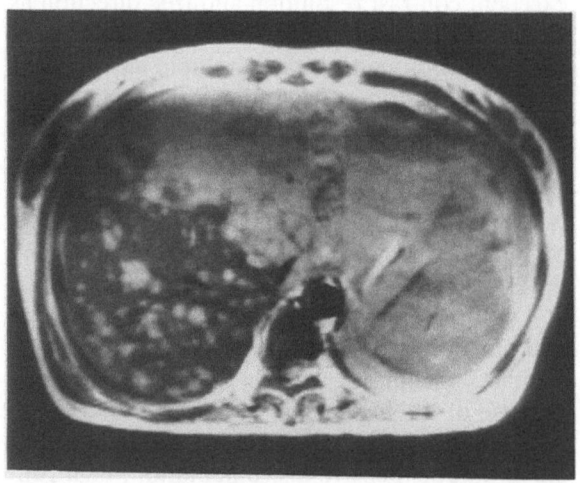

Fig. 2. T2WI (T2-weighted image) of a large tumor and tiny daughter lesions. A large tumor occupies the whole left lobe while a large number of small hyperintense nodules are noted in the right lobe of the liver. The intensity of the right lobe is unusually low

2   Characterization

There are several pathomorphological features important for the characterization of HCC in Japan: capsule, septa, mosaic pattern (nodule in nodule appearance) [3–5] and tumor thrombus in veins [7]. These features can be well depicted by ordinary imaging techniques, but MRI can provide some additional useful findings, such as the T2 value and high intensity on T1-weighted imaging in differential diagnosis of liver tumors.

2.1   Capsule and septa

Encapsulated HCC is the most frequently encountered in Japan and is characterized by a pseudocapsule surrounding the nodular HCC. This capsule appears as a low-intensity ring on

any pulse sequence though it is best seen on T1-weighted imaging (Fig. 3) [3]. It occasionally looks like a double ring consisting of an internal low-intensity ring and an external high-intensity ring [4]. Histopathologically, the internal part consists of fibrous tissue lacking water, while the external part is composed of compressed hepatic parenchyma associated with abundant vessels. Septa also appear as a low-intensity band on any pulse sequence since they consist of fibrous tissue lacking water (Fig. 4).

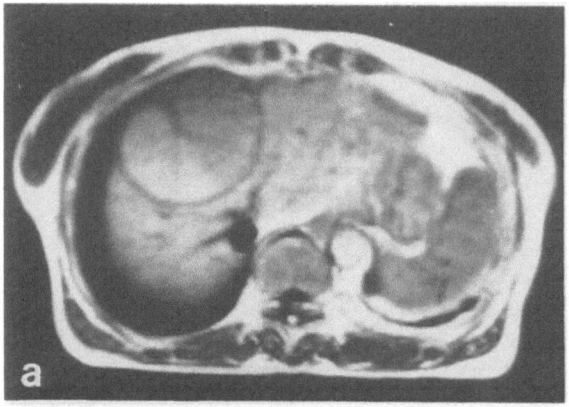

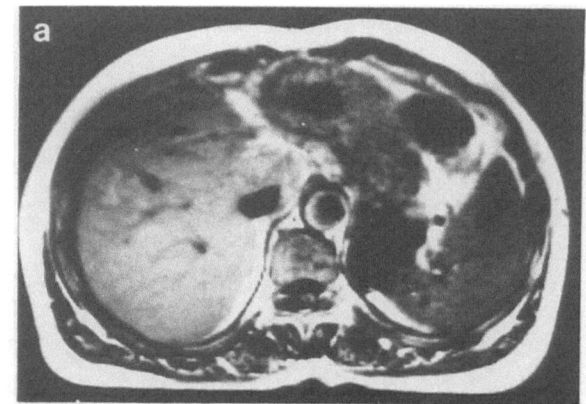

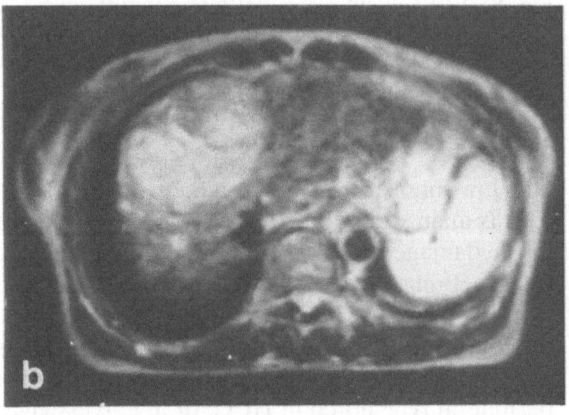

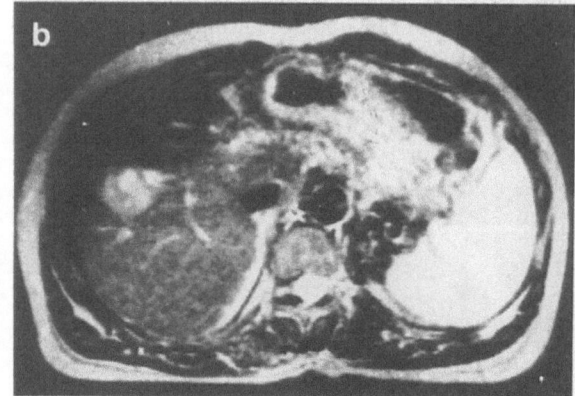

Fig. 3a,b. Capsule, **a** T1WI showing a large isointense or hyperintense mass surrounded by a hypointense rim. **b** T2WI showing a large hyperintense mass surrounded by an internal hypointense and external hyperintense rim

Fig. 5a,b. Mosaic pattern seen on T1WI (**a**) and T2WI. (**b**). On the T2WI, a high-intensity mass is divided by low-intensity septa into three compartments, one of which is hyperintense on the T1WI

2.2 Mosaic pattern

Encapsulated HCC can be seen to have many nodular compartments separated by septa on the cut surface of gross specimens. The HCC may appear as a mass of multiple compartments of different intensities on MRI (Figs. 4, 5) [5]. Detection of a mosaic pattern on MRI spin echo imaging is not necessarily higher than with ultrasound, partly because of the partial volume phenomenon due to the long acquisition time.

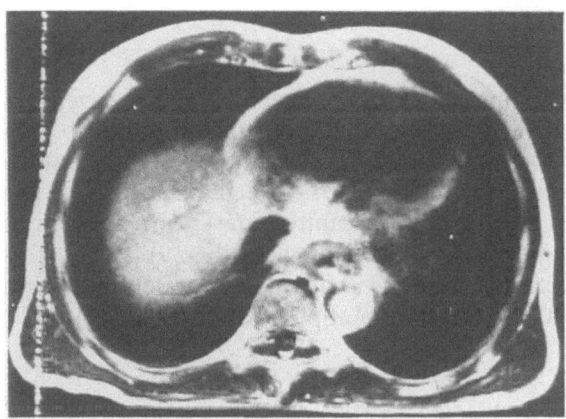

Fig. 4. T1WI of the septa. A hyperintense mass is separated by the hypointense septa. Intensities of individual compartments are fairly different

2.3 Tumor thrombus

On MRI, vessels generally appear as markedly hypointense due to flow void. Flow void on any pulse sequence means blood flow in the vessel. MRI is therefore a good modality in demonstrating the vessels themselves and tumor thrombi

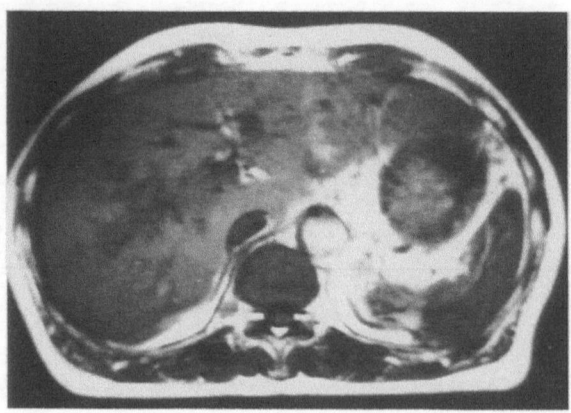

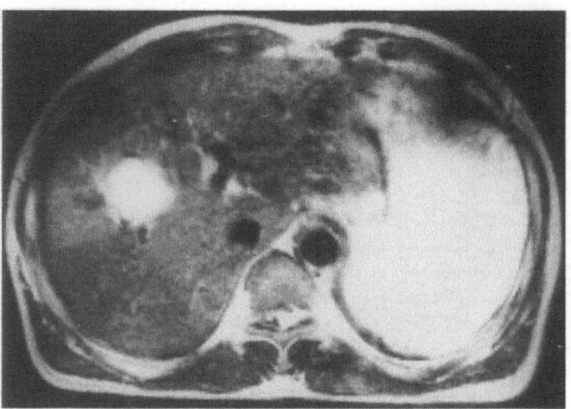

Fig. 6. T1WI of massive tumor thrombi in the portal vein. The arborizing tree-like low-intensity zones in the right lobe of the liver correspond to massive tumor thrombi in the portal vein

Fig. 8. T2WI of subsegmental intensity difference. A high-intensity mass is associated with wedge-shaped zone of slight high-intensity in its periphery. (Reproduced with permission from [8])

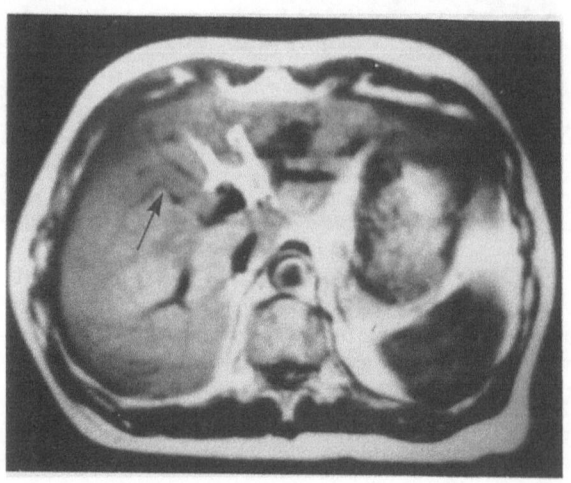

Fig. 7. T1WI of tumor thrombus. A slightly hypointense shadow (*arrow*) is noted in the anterior branch of the right portal vein

therein without any aid of contrast material. Tumor thrombi are high-intensity zones in the areas of veins often abnormally dilated (Figs. 6, 7). However, it should be kept in mind that abnormal signals of various shape and intensity can occur in the vessel due to paradoxical enhancement of slow flow and the use of multislice, multi-echo, flow compensation, or gradient echo imaging.

When venous flow, especially in the portal vein, is blocked, secondary parenchymal changes can be detected as an area of abnormal intensity in the anatomical distribution on MRI (high-intensity on T2-weighted imaging and occasion-

ally low-intensity on T1-weighted imaging) [8]. This is mainly due to an increase in water content in the damaged area. Portal flow stoppage caused by something other than tumor thrombus can also cause a similar phenomenon (Fig. 8). Stoppage by compression of the portal vein by any kinds of tumors, by arterioportal shunt of trunkal or peripheral type noted in HCC, or in abscess gives rise to a wedge- or fan-shaped area of abnormal intensity. This phenomenon is also noted less sensitively on plain CT and most sensitively on CT during arterial portography.

2.4 T2 value

We measured T2 values of HCC and cavernous hemangioma since the contrast of tumor to hepatic parenchyma is usually different between these two tumors on T2-weighted images [9]. The T2 value is significantly different irrespective of tumor size or magnetic field (Fig. 9) [9, 10]. This phenomenon is visually demonstrated on images with the use of multiple and longer TEs [11].

2.5 Signal intensity

About half of all HCCs actually show high-intensity on T1-weighted images, while almost all HCCs appear as hyperintense on T2-weighted imaging [5]. This is an exception to the general rule whereby hypointensity is generally seen on T1-weighted images and hyperintensity on T2-

Fig. 9. Correlation between tumor diameter and T2 value. *Solid circles*, HCC; *open circle*, cavernous hemangioma. (Reproduced with permission from [10])

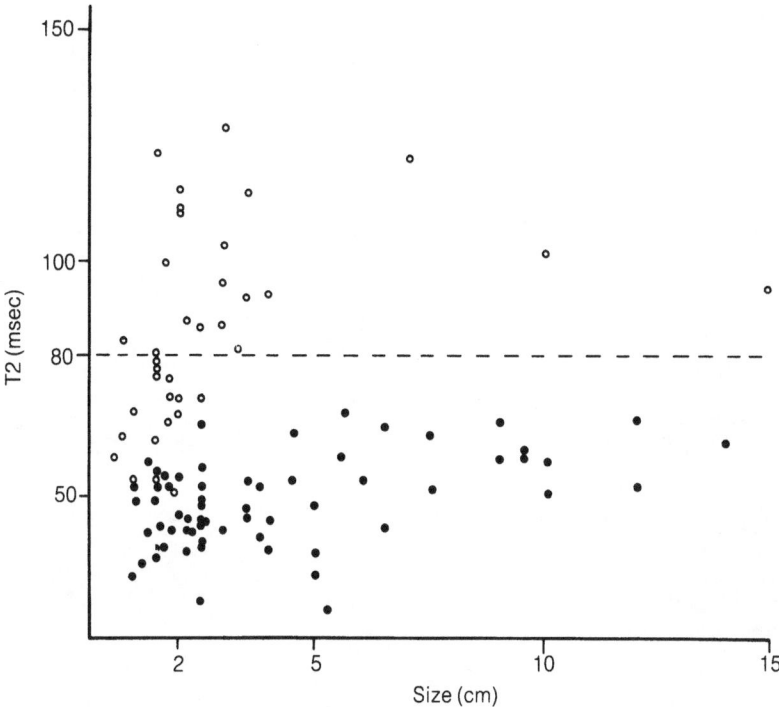

weighted images because of prolonged T1 and T2 in liver tumors, and is of use in characterization of hepatic tumors (Figs. 4, 5). This phenomenon is explained partly by the presence of fat, especially in small, well-differentiated HCC, and partly by prolonged T1, and/or the deposits of iron in cirrhotic liver associated with 80%–90% of all HCC in Japan. However, this phenomenon requires another explanation in many cases since MRI is less sensitive in detecting fat than CT (hyperintense HCC is less frequently markedly hypodense on plain CT) and prolongation of liver T1 is far milder compared with that of HCC. Recently, the presence of copper has been suggested by biopsy work as a possible cause [12].

3 Contrast enhancement

Gd-DTPA (gadopentetate dimeglumine) is the only contrast material permitted for use in human imaging so far. The agent mainly shortens T1, and it has pharmacokinetic properties almost the same as those of water-soluble iodine contrast materials for X-ray examination. For T1-weighted images, changes in signal intensity are interpreted in a similar way to CT; higher intensity means the presence of a relatively large dose of contrast material.

There are two types of contrast enhancement used in liver tumors. One is dynamic MRI (sequential examination of same slice level(s) after bolus injection of 0.05–0.2 mmol/kg of contrast agent) [13] and the other is multisection scans of the whole liver after administration of contrast material [14].

The time-intervals of dynamic MRI depend on the function of instruments, and it ranges from 2 s to 1 min [13, 15–17], as has been the case with dynamic CT for the last 10 years. HCC usually shows similar patterns noted in dynamic CT: transient (peak enhancement in early phase), diffuse, or mosaic enhancement in nodular tumors, and delayed and prolonged enhancement in capsule and septa (Figs. 10, 11) [16]. Additionally, hyperintensity of tumors tends to be prolonged for a longer time than does hyperdensity on dynamic CT (which usually becomes isodense or hypodense within a minute). Dynamic MRI images of HCC are in striking contrast to the spreading and prolonged enhancement with final fill-in in cavernous hemangioma (Fig. 12) [14, 16] and irregular ring enhancement in nonhypervascular metastatic liver tumors. The advantages of dynamic MRI over dynamic CT include less patient discomfort, safety (absence of fatal shock), and rapid injection of small volume and reduced viscocity.

Enhanced, multisection MRI is taken immediately or several minutes after administration

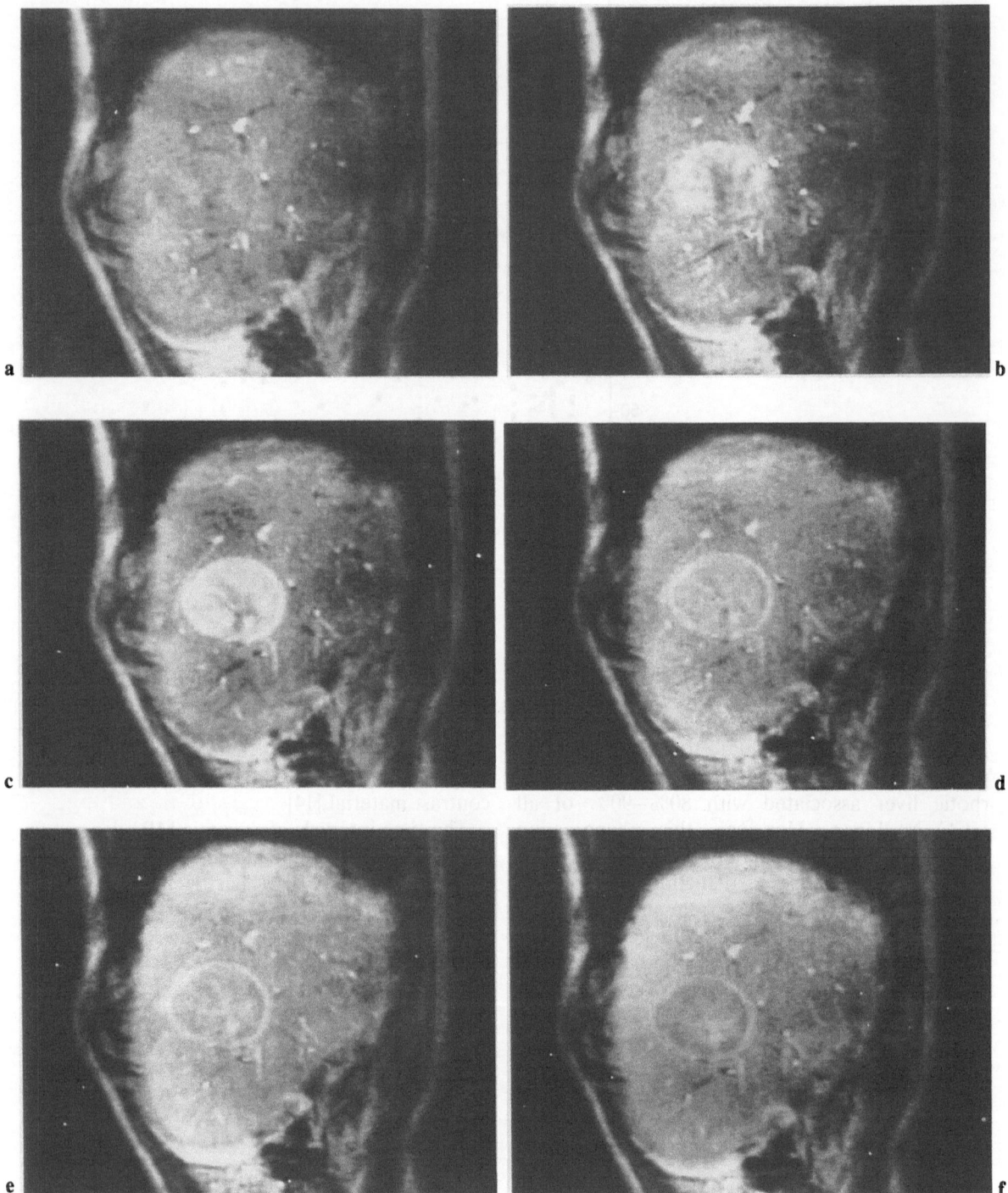

Fig. 10a–f. Dynamic MRI of HCC. **a** Before bolus injection of 0.05 mmol/kg Gd-DTPA, FLASH 19/12, 90°, 2 excitations. A hypointense ring is partially visible on plain MRI. **b** After 10 s. Diffuse enhancement sparing central asteroid region is noted. After 40 s (**c**) and 70 s. (**d**) There is dense ring-enhancement which is prolonged after mass lesion become isointense. **e** After 2 min. **f** After 3 min central low-intensity area becomes hyperintense

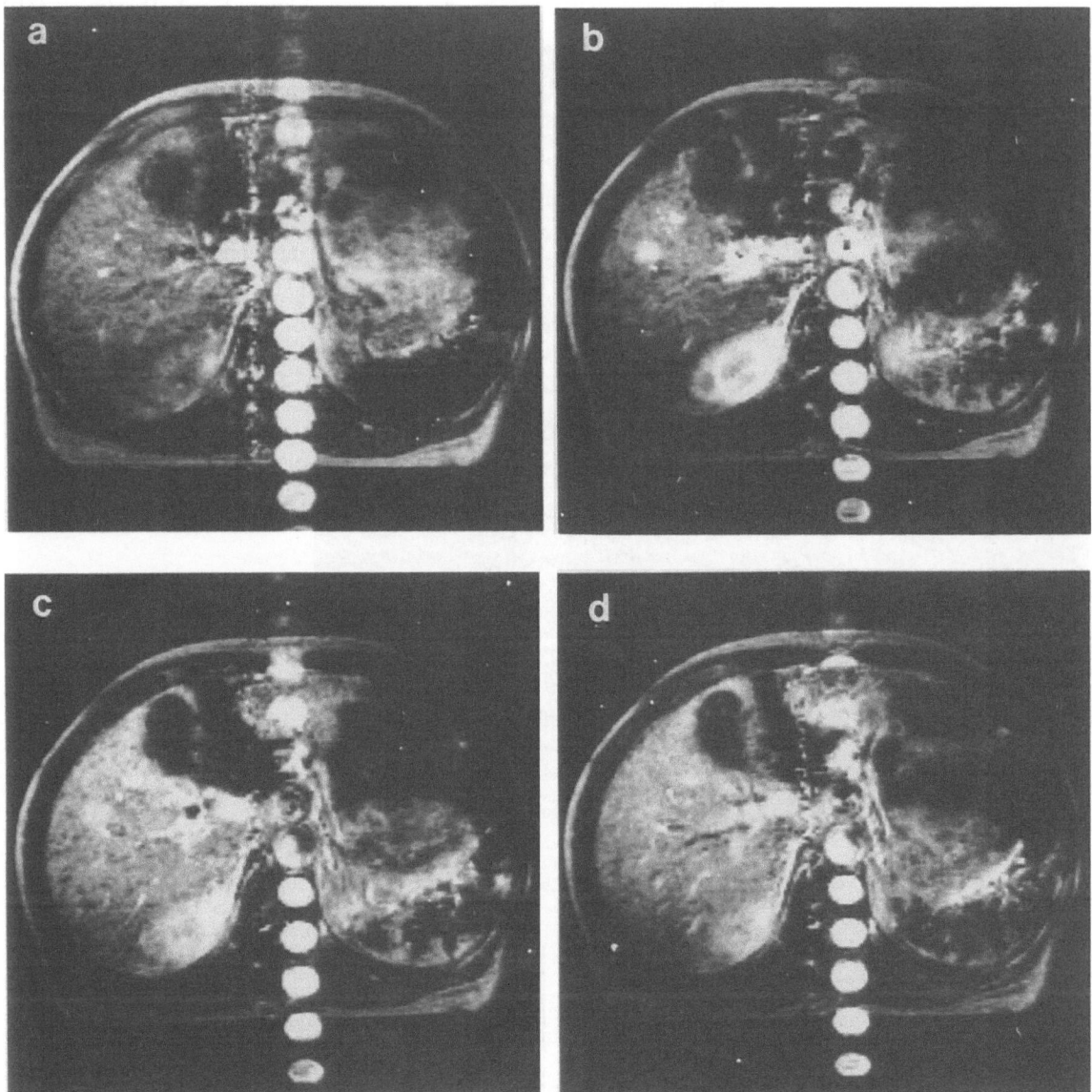

Fig. 11a–d. Dynamic MRI of small HCC. **a** Before bolus injection of Gd-DTPA (same conditions as Fig. 10). **b** After 10 s. An isointense mass shows prominent enhancement of the entire region. This enhancement rapidly decreases in degree but is still fairly noticable in the late scan after 40 s (**c**) and 70 s (**d**)

to the contrast agent. Lately, dynamic MRIs have produced much more enhanced images than CTs since a large dose of contrast material can be safely administered. Thus, cavernous hemangioma changes from a hypo- and/or iso-intense mass to a hyperintense mass, and fibrotic portions such as the central zone of metastatic adenocarcinoma and capsule and septa of HCC, also show prolonged enhancement (Fig. 10) [14].

One of the fascinating points of enhanced MRI is multisection dynamic MRI which combines the advantages of both types mentioned above [18]. Possible drawbacks of dynamic study, especially dynamic CT, are respiratory misregistration in small tumors and incomplete application to multiple tumors. Although a shortening of acquisition time and an increase in the number of slices taken simultaneously are essentially contradictionary, multisection MRI can be taken in the period of respiratory holding (Fig. 13). For example, a series of 11 slices covering the whole liver is taken in 26 s and is repeated once every

Y. Itai et al.

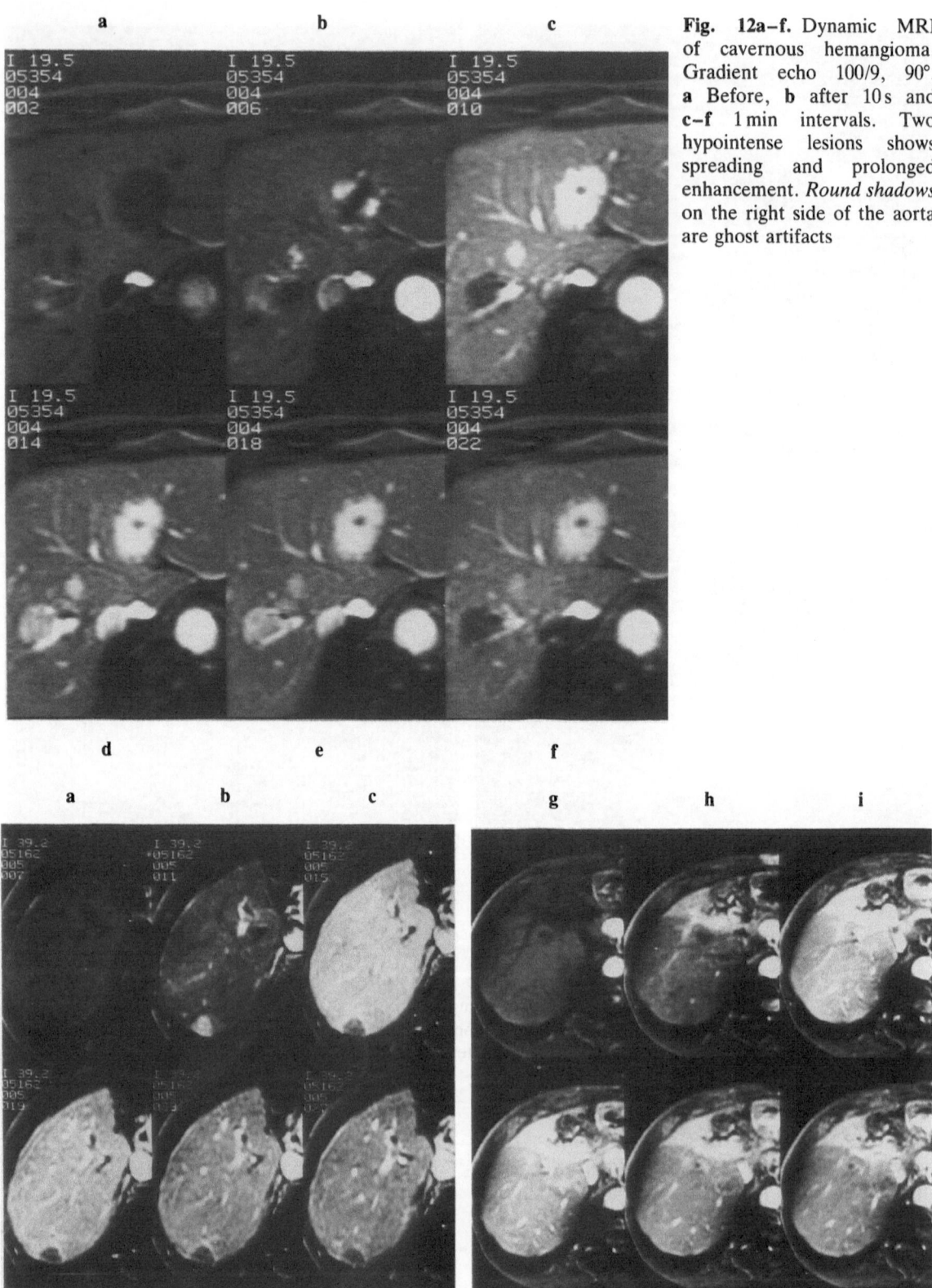

Fig. 12a–f. Dynamic MRI of cavernous hemangioma. Gradient echo 100/9, 90°. **a** Before, **b** after 10 s and **c–f** 1 min intervals. Two hypointense lesions shows spreading and prolonged enhancement. *Round shadows* on the right side of the aorta are ghost artifacts

Fig. 13a–l. Multisection dynamic MRI for HCC (**a–f**) and radiation hepatitis (**g–l**). **a** before, bolus injection of Gd-DTPA, gradient echo 100/9, 90°. **b** After 10 s and **c–f** at 1 minute intervals. A small HCC represents transient, diffuse enhancement. **g–l** as (**a–f**). *Triangle-shaped* radiation hepatitis shows slower and more prolonged, diffuse enhancement

minute [19]. Thus, multiple liver tumors can be detected and more correctly differentiated.

4 Evaluation of tumor extent

For determination of treatment, MRI is useful in detecting tumors in any part of the liver and depicting normal vessels and tumor thrombi. However, angiography or lipiodol CT for hypervascular tumors, and CT during arterial portography or intraoperative ultrasound for hypovascular tumors are mandatory for critical or preoperative cases since MRI frequently fails to pick up daughter lesions less than 7–10 mm under ordinary conditions. Metastatic lesions outside of the liver are less sensitively detected by MRI than by CT.

5 Differential diagnosis

5.1 Metastatic liver tumor

Metastatic liver tumors have less characteristic features in individual masses than do other types of tumors. Wittenberg, et al. reported amorphous appearance, target sign, halo, and changes in morphology on different pulse sequences as rather characteristic of metastatic tumors and claimed one or more of them were noted in 92% of tumors [20]. In our opinion, a non-spherical, three-layer appearance and subcapsular, lentiform mass are almost characteristic of metastatic tumors but are infrequently encountered. Late enhanced MRI shows prolonged, central enhancement changing a hypointense mass on plain MRI to a central hyperintense mass associated with a peripheral low intensity zone [21]. This is the same as reported with CT (Fig. 14) [22, 23]. This finding is noted in metastatic liver tumors (mainly adenocarcinoma) and cholangiocellular carcinoma.

5.2 Cavernous hemangioma

Large cavernous hemangioma shows bizarre shapes with a prominent protrusion and notch, hypointense septa, and hyperintense clefts on T2-weighted imaging [24], and are apt to be peripherally located, contacting with the hepatic

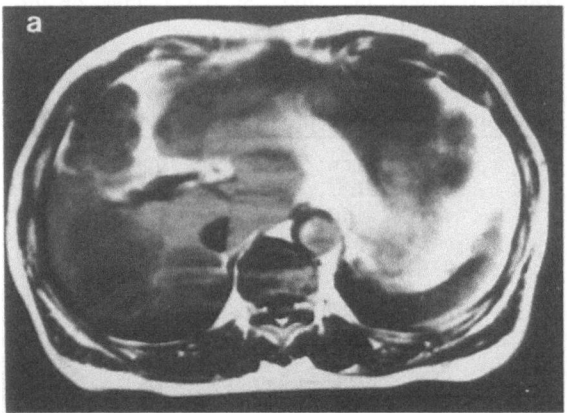
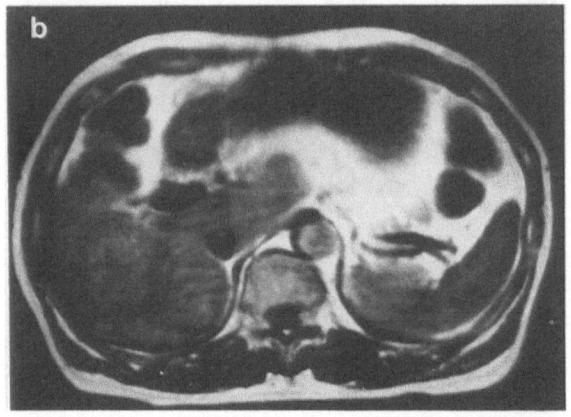

Fig. 14. T1WI of delayed, central enhancement of metastatic liver tumor. **a** Precontrast. **b** Postcontrast. A hypointense mass on plain MRI reveals delayed and prolonged enhancement in the central area

contour for a long distance but rendering no change to this contour. The smaller the size, the less frequently encountered are the characteristic morphological features. Prolonged T2 values and enhancement patterns on dynamic and/or late enhanced MRI are useful even in small lesions (Table 2). Hepatic cysts also have prolonged T2 values and appear very hyperintense on T2-weighted imaging [25]. However, the morphological features and intensity on proton density imaging are quite different from each other: spherical and isointense in cysts, and nonspherical and hyperintense in hemangioma.

5.3 Hepatic adenoma and focal nodular hyperplasia

Adenoma may mimic HCC [26] although there are no large series of adenoma found on MRI.

Table 2. Signal intensities of the lesions on pre/postcontrast T1-weighted images

Signal Intensity of Lesions		Numbers of Lesions	
Precontrast	Postcontrast	Hemangioma	HCC
Low	Low	0	1
	Iso	2	3
	High	47	1
	Mixed	4	1
Iso	Iso	3	3
	High	7	0
High	Iso	0	4
	High	0	6
	Mixed	0	1
Mixed	High	0	1
	Mixed	0	2

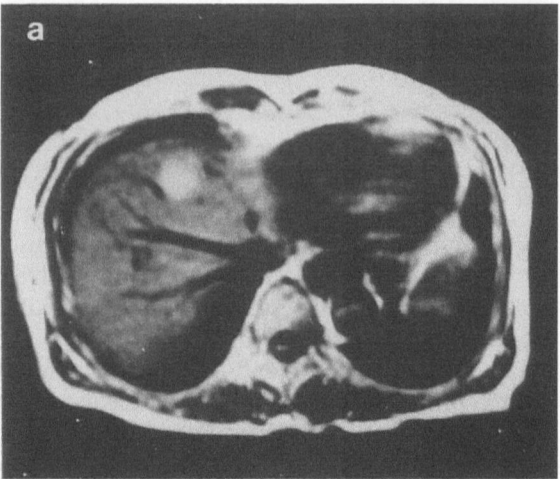

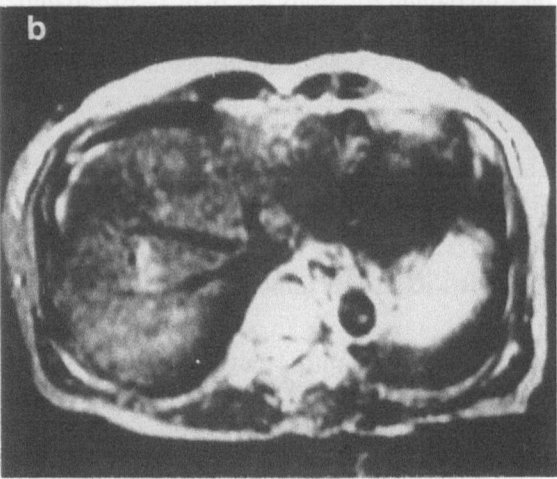

Fig. 16a,b. Adenomatous hyperplasia containing HCC. **a** T1WI. The mass shows hyperintensity. **b** T2WI. The mass shows hypointensity. However, a hyperintense region is noted in the center of the mass and histologically HCC in adenomatous hyperplasia. (Reproduced with permission from [30])

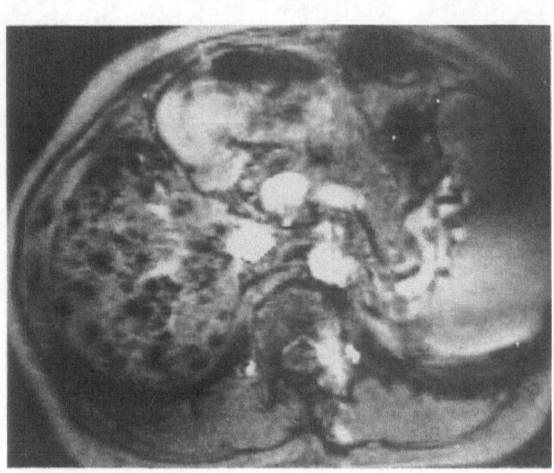

Fig. 15. Regenerating nodules containing iron. Gradient echo (19/12, 90°). Many hypointense nodules of varying size are clearly demonstrated

Focal nodular hyperplasia (FNH) has been well known because of isointensity on both T1- and T2-weighted imaging. However, a large series published recently classified a wide variation of intensities [27]. A central scar (hyperintense on T2-weighted imaging) and homogeneity (except scar and isointensity on either T1- or T2-weighted imaging) are rather characteristic findings of FNH.

5.4 Adenomatous hyperplasia

Adenomatous hyperplasia is a nodular parenchymal lesion found in cirrhotic livers, and is appreciably larger than surrounding regenerative nodules [28]. Its clinical significance as well as subtypes have already been discussed in a previous section. Regenerating nodules of liver cirrhosis are not infrequently demonstrated as a large number of small low-intensity nodules on T2-weighted imaging while rarely on T1-weighted imaging [29]. Regeneraling nodules containing iron are clearly demonstrated using gradient echo techniques (Fig. 15). The MR appearance of adenomatous hyperplasia is quite characteristic: hyperintense on T1-weighted imaging and hypointense on T2-weighted imaging [30]. This is contrary to the general rule of hepatic mass on MRI, and is rarely encountered in HCC with massive necrosis. Focal HCC occasionally noted

Table 3. Correlations between signal intensity on MRI and nodular lesions associated with liver cirrhosis

T2 \ T1	hypo	iso	hyper
hypo	◎		△ △ △ △ ▲ ▲ ▲ ▲ ▲ ▲ ▲ ● ● ◎
iso	○		△ △ ▲ ▲ ▲ ● ● ● ● ● ○ ○
hyper	○○○○○○○ ○○○○○○○ ○○○○○○○ ○○ ◎	● ○○○○○○○ ○	▲ ● ● ● ○○○○○○○ ○○○○○○○ ○○○○○○

Open triangles, ordinary adenomatous hyperplasia; solid triangles, atypical adenomatous hyperplasia; solid circles, well differentiated hepatocellular carcinoma (Edmondson I); open circles, hepatocellular carcinoma (≤Edmondson II); double circles, hepatocellular carcinoma with massive necrosis

within adenomatous hyperplasia appears as a central high-intensity area within a hypointense mass on T2-weighted imaging which corresponds to adenomatous hyperplasia (Fig. 16) [30]. Comparison of signal intensity on T1- and T2-weighted imaging is useful in determing the borderline and whether it is benign or malignant in nodules noted in liver cirrhosis (Table 3) [31].

6   Role of MRI

The role of MRI in diagnostic imaging has not yet been settled. Ignoring poor throughput and tight time scheduling, MRI may be the second most common method of diagnostic imaging next to ultrasound in the evaluation of HCC. MRI is certainly of great use in the differential diagnosis of nodular lesions in cirrhotic livers and in the diagnosis of cavernous hemangioma in patients at high risk for HCC [9, 10, 30].

MRI may also be effective in evaluating treatment for HCC in transcatheter arterial embolization (TAE) or percutaneous ethanol injection [32]. Coagulation necrosis caused by both treatments results in a signal intensity change from high to low on T2-weighted imaging.

New pulse sequences, such as multishot RARE (rapid acquisition relaxation enhanced sequence), gives T1- and T2-weighted multisection imaging higher quality in respiratory holding [33].

7   Future of MRI

In addition to steady progress in hardware and software, development of new contrast agents will undoubtly increase the usefulness of MRI, and throughput will be improved a great deal. Gd-DTPA is a nonspecific contrast agent with intravascular and interstitial space distribution which enhances both tumor and surrounding liver according to their vascularity (in early phase) and interstitial space (in equibrilium phase).

New contrast agents now under development include hepatobiliary agents (e.g., Mn-DPDP, Fe-EHPG, Gd-BOPTA [34]. A reticuloendothelial (particulate) contrast agent such as superparamagnetic iron oxide [35] will soon be available for clinical application. Both agents are accumulated in the normal liver by hepatocyte receptors or by phagocytosis of the reticuloendothelial system, and they increase the contrast between the tumor and the liver. With such contrast agents, tumor detection will be improved. Tumor-targeting contrast agents are ideal but they are not practical compared to radionuclide agents in nuclear medicine from the viewpoint of concentration of the agent.

References

1. Moss AA, Goldberg HI, Stark DD, Davis PL, Margulis AR, Kaufman L, Crooks LE (1984) Heptic tumors: Magnetic resonance and CT appearance. Radiology 150:141–147

2. Itai Y, Ohtomo K, Furui S, Yamauchi T, Minami M, Yashiro N (1985) Noninvasive diagnosis of small cavernous hemangioma of the liver: Advantage of magnetic resonance imaging. AJR 145:1195–1199

3. Ebara M, Ohto M, Watanabe Y, Kimura K, Saisho H, Tsuchiya Y, Okuda K, Arimizu N, Kondo F, Ikehira H, Fukuda N, Tateno Y (1986) Diagnosis of small hepatocellular carcinoma: Correlation of MR imaging and tumor histologic studies. Radiology 159:371–377

4. Itoh K, Nishimura K, Togashi K, Fujisawa I, Noma S, Minami S, Sagoh T, Nakano Y, Itoh H, Mori K, Ozawa K, Torizuka K (1987) Hepatocellular carcinoma: MR imaging. Radiology 164:21–25

5. Inayoshi G, Nishimura H, Tanaka T (1989) MR imaging of hepatocellular carcinoma (in Japanese). Jpn J Magnet Reson in Med 9:216–221

6. Stark DD, Wittenberg J, Edelman RR, Middleton MS, Saini S, Butch RJ, Brady TJ, Ferrucci JTJr (1986) Detection of hepatic metastases: Analysis of pulse sequence performance in MR imaging. Radiology 159:365–370

7. Ohtomo K, Itai Y, Furui S, Yoshikawa K, Yashiro N, Iio M (1985) MR imaging of portal vein thrombus in hepatocellular cacinoma. J Comput Assist Tomogr 9:328–329

8. Itai Y, Ohtomo K, Kokubo T, Okada Y, Yamauchi T, Yoshida T (1988) Segmental intensity difference of the liver on MR imaging: A sign of intrahepatic portal flow stoppage. Radiology 167:17–19

9. Ohtomo K, Itai Y, Furui S, Yashiro N, Yoshikawa K, Iio M (1985) Hepatic tumors: Differentiation by transverse relaxation time (T2) of magnetic resonance imaging. Radiology 155:421–423

10. Ohtomo K, Itai Y, Yoshikawa K, Kokubo T, Iio M (1988) Hepatocellular carcinoma and cavernous hemangioma: Differentiation with MR imaging—efficacy of T2 values at 0.35 and 1.5 T. Radiology 168:621–623

11. Choi BI, Han MC, Kim CW (1990) Small hepatocellular carcinoma versus small cavernous hemangioma: Differentiation with MR imaging at 2.0 T. Radiology 176:103–106

12. Watanabe S, Ebara M, Matsushiro Y, Kita K, Yoshikawa M, Sugiura N, Ohto M, Kondo F (1991) MR imaging of small hepatocellular carcinoma: Characteristic findings with reference to pathology. Jpn J Magn Reson in Med 11 (suppl): 298

13. Ohtomo K, Itai Y, Yoshikawa K, Kokubo T, Yashiro N, Iio M, Furukawa K (1987) Hepatic tumors: Dynamic MR imaging. Radiology 163:27–31

14. Okada Y, Itai Y, Ohtomo K, Kokubo T, Yoshida H, Sasaki Y (1991) MR differentiation of hepatic hemangioma and hepatocellular carcinoma: Value of delayed-phase Gd-DTPA-enhanced images. RöFo 154:621–627

15. Mano I, Yoshida H, Nakabayashi K, Yashiro N, Iio M (1987) Fast spin echo imaging with suspended respiration: Gadolinium-enhanced MR imaging of liver tumors. J Comput Assist Tomogr 11:73–80

16. Yoshida H, Itai Y, Ohtomo K, Kokubo T, Minami M, Yashiro N (1989) Small hepatocellular carcinoma and cavernous hemangioma: Differentiation with dynamic FLASH MRI with Gd-DTPA. Radiology 171:339–342

17. Murakami T, Mitani T, Nishikawa M, Nakanishi K, Marukawa T, Harada K, Tokunaga K, Kuroda C, Kozuka T (1990) Dynamic MRI of liver tumors: Evaluation by inversion recovery snap shot FLASH MR imaging (in Japanese). Nippon Acta Radiol 50:1451–1453

18. Hirohashi S, Tanaka M, Uchida H, Itoh T, Otsuji H, Iwasaki S, Ohishi H (1990) Usefulness of MRI contrast agent in liver diseases (in Japanese). J Medical Imag 10:1330–1338

19. Mirowitz SA, Lee JKT, Gutierrez, E Eilenberg SS, Heiken JP, Perman WH (1990) Dynamic gadolinium-DTPA enhanced rapid acquisition spin echo (RASE) MR imaging of the liver. Radiology 175:131–135

20. Wittenberg J, Stark DD, Forman BH, Hahn PF, Saini V, Weissleder R, Rummeny E, Ferrucci JF (1988) Differentiation of hepatic metastases from hepatic hemangiomas and cysts by using MR imaging. AJR 151:79–84

21. Okada Y, Ohtomo K, Itai Y, Sasaki Y (1990) MR imaging of metastatic liver tumors (in Japanese). J Medical Imag 10:1305–1312

22. Itai Y, Ohtomo K, Kokubo T, Yamauchi T, Minami M, Yashiro N and Araki T (1986) CT of hepatic masses: Significance of prolonged and delayed enhancement. AJR 146:729–733

23. Muramatsu Y, Takayasu K, Moriyama N, Shima Y, Goto H, Ushio K, Yamada T, Hasegawa H, Koyama Y, Hirohashi V (1986) Peripheral low-density area of hepatic tumors: CT-pathologic correlation. Radiology 160:49–52

24. Choi BI, Han MC, Park JH, Kim SH, Han MH, Kim CW (1989) Giant cavernous hemangioma of the liver: CT and MR imaging in 10 cases. AJR 152:1221–1226

25. Stark DD, Felder RC, Wittenberg J, Saini S, Butch RJ, White ME, Edelman R, Mueller PR, Simeone JF, Cohen AM, Brady T, Ferrucci JT (1985) Magnetic resonance imaging of cavernous hemangioma of the liver: Tissue-specific characterization. AJR 145:213–222

26. Rummeny E, Saini S, Wittenberg J, Compton C, Hahn PF, Mueller PR, Simeone JF Stark DD,

Weissleder R, Dousset MG, Ferrucci JF (1989) MR imaging of liver neoplasms. AJR 152:493–499

27. Lee J, Saini S, Hamm B, Taupitz M, Hahn PF, Seneterre E, Ferrucci JT (1991) Focal nodular hyperplasia of the liver: MR findings in 35 proved cases. AJR 156:317–320

28. Nakanuma Y, Terada T, Terasaki S, Ueda K, Nonomura A, Kawahara E, Matsui O (1990) Atypical adenomatous hyperplasia in liver cirrhosis: Low-grade hepatocellular carcinoma or borderline lesion? Histopathology 17:27–35

29. Itai Y, Ohnishi S, Ohtomo K, Kokubo T, Yoshida H, Yoshikawa K, Imawari M (1987) Regenerating nodules of liver cirrhosis: MR imaging. Radiology 165:419–423

30. Matsui O, Kadoya M, Kameyama T, Yoshikawa J, Arai K, Gabata T, Takashima T, Nakanuma Y, Terada T, Ida M (1989) Adenomatous hyperplastic nodules in the cirrhotic liver: Differentiation from hepatocellular carcinoma with MR imaging. Radiology 173:123–126

31. Matsui O, Kadoya M, Yoshikawa J, Arai K, Gabata T, Takashima T, Nakanuma Y, Unoura M, Kobayashi K, Izumi R, Miura M, Mitsui T, Ida M, Kitagawa K (1990) Imaging diagnosis of the grades of malignancy in hepatocytic nodular lesions associated with liver cirrhosis (in Japanese). J Abdominal Imag 10:697–701

32. Sironi S, Livraghi T, DelMaschio A (1991) Small hepatocellular carcinoma treated with percutaneous ethanol injection: MR imaging findings. Radiology 180:333–336

33. Imai Y, Higuchi N (1991) High resolution MR imaging of small hepatocellular carcinoma using the breathhold technique (in Japanese). Jap J Clin Med 49:1832–1836

34. Lim KO, Stark DD, Leese PT, Pfefferbaum, Rocklage SM, Quay SC (1991) Hepatobiliary MR imaging: First human experience with Mn DPDP. Radiology 178:79–82

35. Stark DD, Weissleder R, Elizondo G, Hahn PF, Saini S, Todd LE, Wittenberg J, Ferrucci JT (1988) Superparamagnetic iron oxide: Clinical application as a contrast agent for MR imaging of the liver. Radiology 168:297–301

Hepatic angiography in hepatocellular carcinoma: status among modern imaging modalities and its role as a further examination

Kenichi Takayasu, Yukio Muramatsu, Noriyuki Moriyama, and Fumihiko Wakao[1]

1 Introduction

With the advent of various sectional imaging modalities such as ultrasonography (US), computed tomography (CT) and magnetic resonance imaging (MRI), the role of hepatic angiography, or hepatic arteriography, has changed. Previously, it was merely a way to diagnose liver tumors and to obtain a vascular map for surgery, but it has since become a more precise method of diagnosis which is often combined with CT and other modalities to manage hepatic malignancies [1–4].

In Japan hepatic angiography is commonly combined with CT, angio-CT [5–7] and lipiodol-CT [8–12] to detect small intrahepatic metastases which were not detected by other imaging methods. Using these combined studies, small hepatocellular carcinomas (HCCs) less than 3 cm in diameter are diagnosed easily and frequently and such precise diagnosis has become imperative, especially in surgical candidates [6, 7]. Small hypovascular HCC as small as 3 cm in diameter which could not be diagnosed by arteriography alone, is now demonstrable by angio-CT [13]. Therapeutic oil-chemoembolization following angiography is a most powerful and reliable treatment for inoperable [14–16] and recurrent HCCs [17].

Currently, the diagnosis of adenomatous hyperplasia (AH) and AH containing foci of HCC is one of the major interests in the field of imagings [18]. AH is also of great interest to those studying pathogenesis of HCC [19, 20].

2 Methods and equipment for arteriography

The Seldinger technique is commonly used through the femoral artery in which a 5–7 F size catheter is advanced into the hepatic artery. First, celiac angiography is carried out to obtain general information regarding the liver and coexisting portal hypertension. It is followed by transmesenteric portography and superselective hepatic angiography. Thirty to 40 ml of contrast medium is injected at a speed of 6–8 ml/sec for celiac arteriography, and 50 to 60 ml of contrast medium is injected, following injection of 20 µg of Prostaglandin E1, at a speed of 10–12 ml/sec into the superior mesenteric artery for transmesenteric portography, and 10–20 ml for superselective arteriography.

Recently, new equipment has been developed to facilitate superselective catheterization with a high success rate. This includes the followings: a guide wire coated with a hydrophilic polymer (Terumo, Tokyo) [21] which can be easily inserted into the peripheral hepatic arteries even with severe kinking, a 3 F coaxial parent-baby catheter covered with hydrophilic polymer (Terumo, Tokyo) [22, 23] has made ultrasuperselective catheterization possible, and a 25 cm-long sheath (Cook, Bloomington) that permits the catheter to pass quickly into the hepatic artery even when the aorta winds markedly.

New non-ionized and/or low osmotic pressure contrast agents with lower viscosity have made injection into a coaxial catheter having a narrow inner diameter easier, and has permitted lower doses of contrast medium to be used and thus the incidence of anaphylactic reaction. Digital subtraction angiography (DSA), particularly intra-arterial DSA, is also useful in reducing the amount of contrast medium to one third or one

[1] Department of Diagnostic Radiology, National Cancer Center Hospital, Tsukiji 5-1-1, Chuo-ku, Tokyo, 104 Japan

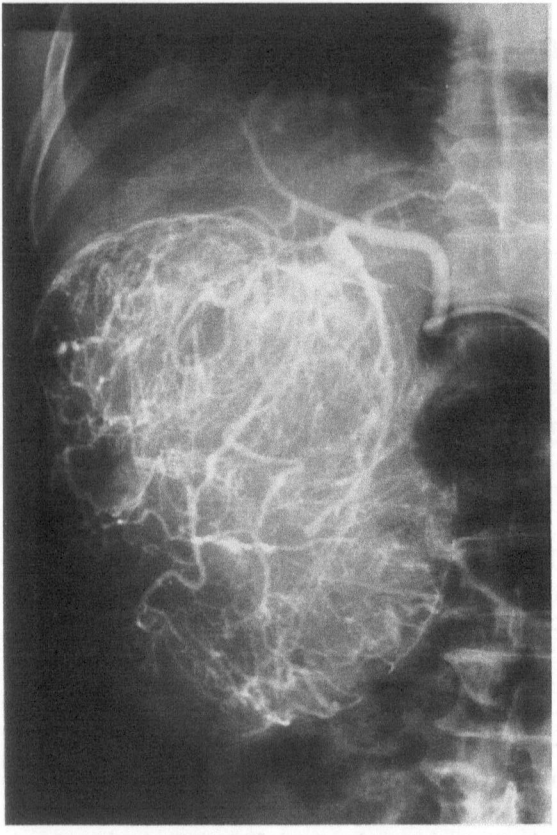

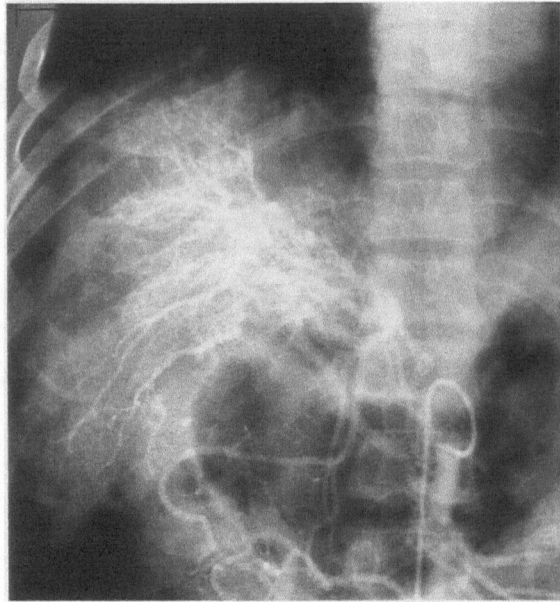

Fig. 2. Tumor thrombus developing in the main portal trunk. Replaced right hepatic arteriography revealing fine network of tumor vessels nourishing tumor thrombus (*thread* and *streaks*)

Fig. 1. A large nodular hepatocellular carcinoma (classical type). Hepatic arteriography in the arterial phase demonstrating a large hypervascular tumor with numerous tumor vessels measuring 12 cm in diameter. These findings are compatible with typical hepatocellular carcinoma. In the late phase, nodular stainings within the mass were clearly disclosed (not shown)

Gelbe Laboratories, France) which is slowly injected into the proper hepatic artery. Follow-up unenhanced CT (lipiodol-CT) is carried out 7 to 10 days later.

3 Classical type hepatocellular carcinoma

The typical angiographic findings of classical (large nodular type) HCC are dilated and markedly tortuous neovasculature seen in the arterial phase, and nodular stainings with a translucent rim around the mass in the venous phase (Fig. 1) [24, 25]. If such HCCs reach an advanced stage, arterio-portal shunts and/or filling defects in large vessels, are frequently recognized which reflect direct tumor invasion. This is especially true in the portal vein. The feeding arteries to a tumor thrombus are visible as the thread and streaks sign (Fig. 2) [26]. If vascular invasion develops in the main portal trunk, multiple intrahepatic metastases are expected, and altered hemodynamics, such as compensatory increase in arterial and portal blood supply through cavernous transformation, make it difficult to diagnose the location and size of the primary lesion. Therefore, the majority of diffuse type HCCs are presumed to be a late stage of another

half of the previous dose. DSA has also made possible the diagnosis of small lesions, especially those whose images are superimposed on the vertebral column.

Especially among surgical candidates, arterial angio-CT and/or portal angio-CT, collectively called angio-CT, is carried out after routine angiography as follows: in arterial angio-CT [5, 7], the catheter tip is placed in the common hepatic artery and 50 ml of 20% contrast medium is injected at a rate of 1 ml/sec and the table incremental CT is begun 1 sec later; in portal angio-CT [5, 7], the catheter tip is placed deeply in the superior mesenteric artery with injection of 100 ml of 20% contrast medium at a rate of 3 ml/sec and the table incremental CT starts 25 sec later. Lipiodol-CT, which is a separate procedure, may follow angio-CT. It is performed with the use of 5 ml of lipiodol (Ethiodol, Andre-

type of HCC rather than the tumor being diffuse from its early stages.

4 Small hepatocellular carcinoma

4.1 Angiographic features
Among a total of 105 small HCCs less than 5 cm in diameter which were resected after angiography, 86 (82%) had been identified and 19 were missed by this modality [13]. Of the 82 small HCCs identified, nodular staining was most frequent (75.6%) and was presumed to reflect the "nodule in nodule" structure of HCC. Hypervascularity was recognized in only 69.8% in this group compared to 95% of advanced HCCs [25]. The incidence of arterio-portal shunt was 9.3%, much less than that found in advanced HCC (52%) [25]. Therefore, the tumor staining in the late phase was the most important finding for detection of small HCCs (Fig. 3).

4.2 Detection rates
The detection rate reported for angiography for small HCC no larger than 3 cm in diameter, was 82% [27] in 22 lesions, and 89% [28] in 17 lesions. Our recent large study on angiography in 100 patients with a total of 135 small HCCs less than 3 cm which were resected and diagnosed histopathologically showed the following detection rates: 81% for all tumors, 87% for tumors between 1 and 3 cm, and 55% for tumors smaller than 1 cm (Table 1) [7]. Compared to US and CT, angiography had a similar detection rate. However, portal angio-CT and lipiodol-CT showed a much higher detection rate (Fig. 3). These results suggest that further study following angiography is necessary in surgical candidates. In the analysis of the detection rate with angiography in relation to tumor size, a significant correlation was found ($P < 0.01$): the smaller the tumor, the lower the detection rate. When the detectability of these lesions was compared with the degree of cancer-cell differentiation according to the Edmondson-Steiner grading system [29], the lesions detected by angiography tended to have more poorly differentiated cancer cells and the undetected ones had better differentiated cells ($P < 0.01$) [13]. Another pitfall in angiography was the detection of two masses superimposed in ventrodorsal direction.

4.3 Anatomical location of small HCCs
When the location of 100 small HCCs less than 5 cm was analyzed on the basis of hepatic segmentation by Healey [30] and Couinaud [31] by angiography as well as CT scanning, 50% of the HCCs resided in the anterior segment of the right lobe (40% in the anterosuperior and 10% in the anteroinferior subsegments), 31% in the posterior segment, 18% in the left lobe, and 1% in the caudate lobe [13]. Kanematsu, et al. [32] also reported similar findings: 60% of 32 solitary HCCs less than 4 cm were located in the anterosuperior area. The reason why HCC frequently emerges in this area is not clear. When diagnosing HCC on imaging, one should pay special attention to this area of the liver.

5 Borderline lesions

5.1 Imaging problems with borderline lesions
A recent interest in hepatology centers around borderline lesions which include AH and AH with small foci of HCC within it. The latter is designated as early HCC (e-HCC) because it may

Table 1. Detection rates with various imaging techniques for small hepatocellular carcinomas (Reference 7)

Size (cm)	No. of lesion	Sonography	CT	Angiography	Arterial angio-CT	Portal angio-CT	Lipiodol-CT	Intraoperative sonography
<1[a]	22	37% (7/19)	42% (8/19)	55% (12/22)	0% (0/1)	67% (2/3)	83% (10/12)	86% (19/22)
1–3[b]	113	92 (101/110)	91 (100/110)	87 (97/112)	88 (14/16)	95 (19/20)	96 (45/47)	98 (111/113)
Total[c]	135	84 (108/129)	84 (108/129)	81 (109/134)	82 (14/17)	91 (21/23)	93 (55/59)	96 (130/135)

[a] $P < 0.05$ for Lipiodol-CT vs sonography and CT and for intraoperative sonography vs CT, angiography, and arterial angio-CT; $P < 0.01$ for intraoperative sonography vs conventional sonography

[b] $P < 0.05$ for intraoperative sonography vs conventional sonography and CT; $P < 0.01$ for intraoperative sonography vs angiography

[c] $P < 0.05$ for angiography vs Lipiodol-CT; $P < 0.01$ for intraoperative sonography vs conventional sonography, CT, angiography, and arterial angio-CT

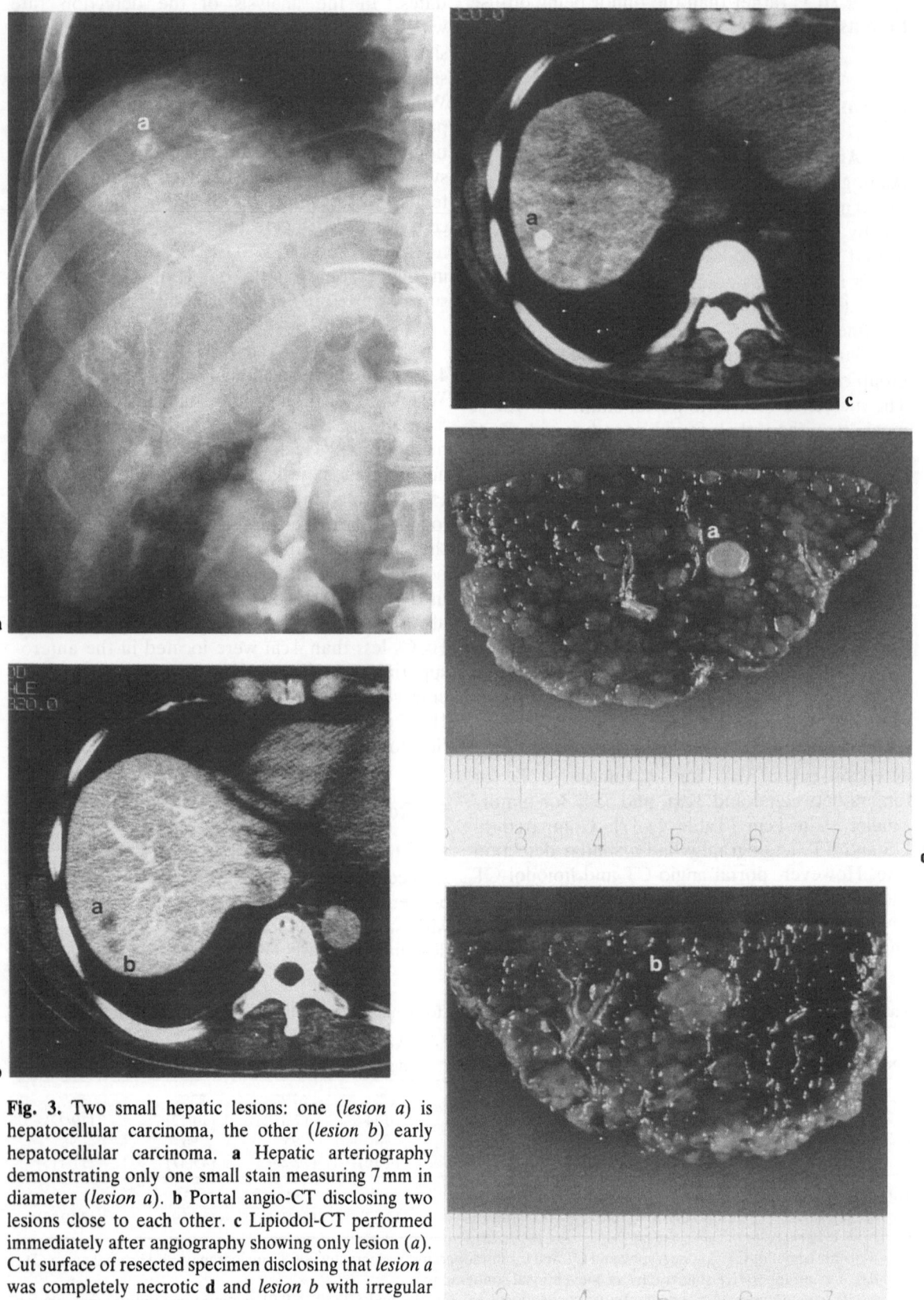

Fig. 3. Two small hepatic lesions: one (*lesion a*) is hepatocellular carcinoma, the other (*lesion b*) early hepatocellular carcinoma. **a** Hepatic arteriography demonstrating only one small stain measuring 7 mm in diameter (*lesion a*). **b** Portal angio-CT disclosing two lesions close to each other. **c** Lipiodol-CT performed immediately after angiography showing only lesion (*a*). Cut surface of resected specimen disclosing that *lesion a* was completely necrotic **d** and *lesion b* with irregular margin was viable **e**. Soft X-ray study showing dense retention of lipiodol not in *lesion b* but in *lesion a* **f**

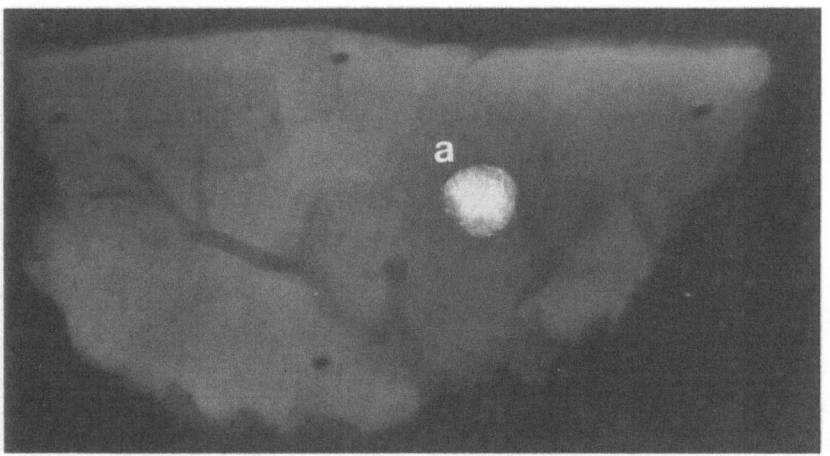

Fig. 3. (*Continued*)   **f**

be an early stage of HCC [16]. The majority of these lesions are small, less than 1.5 cm [14], and frequently found by US as a lesion associated with advanced HCC. However, they are not usually detected by angiography and not enhanced even by arterial angio-CT (Fig. 3). Thus, differential diagnosis of e-HCC from AH and from a large regenerative nodule by imaging is difficult. We are now trying to make differential diagnosis of e-HCC from the others by using arterial angio-CT: if a lesion suspected to be e-HCC is enhanced by arterial angio-CT, it could be clinically diagnosed as e-HCC even though its lesion was neither enhanced by dynamic CT nor detected by angiography (Fig. 4). If non-enhanced e-HCC progresses, only the central portion of the lesion comes to be enhanced by angiography and/or dynamic CT. These temporal changes in enhancement of the tumor (Fig. 4) are presumed to reflect the gradual development of tumor vessels, and they support the concept of multi-step progression of HCC.

5.2   Detection rates for AH and e-HCC

In 41 patients with 54 borderline lesions resected and studied histopathologically, the detectability of these lesions was evaluated. Fifty-four borderline lesions consisted of 14 AH in 9 patients, 28 e-HCC in 22 patients, and 12 atypical AH which fell between AH and e-HCC in 10 patients (Table 2). Most of the 54 lesions was 1.2 ± 0.4 cm in diameter and that of AHs was 0.8 ± 0.3 cm, the latter being significantly smaller than atypical AHs and e-HCCs ($P < 0.01$). Detection rates for all lesions and e-HCCs respectively were: intraoperative US, 70.0%, 87.5%; portal angio-CT, 58.3%, 71.4%; US, 44.4%, 64.3%; and arterial angio-CT, 37.5%, 50.5%. By contrast, detection rates with lipiodol-CT, which showed a high sensitivity in advanced HCC, were only 9.1% for all lesions and 25.0% for e-HCCs. It was presumed that an e-HCC has a poorly developed neovasculature within it because retention of lipiodol in the lesion mainly depends on the vascularity of the tumor [8–12]. In our series, US was the most sensitive for these borderline lesions.

Acknowledgments. This study was supported in part by the Foundation for Promotion of Cancer Research.

References

1. Yamada R, Sato M, Kawabata M, Nakatsuka H, Nakamura K, Takashima S (1983) Hepatic artery embolization in 120 patients with unresectable hepatoma. Radiology 148:397–401
2. Nakamura H, Tanaka T, Hori S, Yoshioka H, Kuroda C, Okamura J, Sakurai M (1983) Transcatheter embolization of hepatocellular carcinoma: Assessment of efficacy in cases of resection following embolization. Radiology 147:401–405
3. Takayasu K, Moriyama N, Muramatsu Y, Suzuki M, Yamada T, Kishi K, Hasegawa H, Okazaki N (1984) Hepatic arterial embolization for hepatocellular carcinoma: Comparison of CT scans and resected specimens. Radiology 150:661–665
4. Ohnishi K, Tsuchiya S, Nakayama T, Hiyama Y, Iwama S, Goto N, Takashi M, Ohtsuki T, Kono K, Nakajima Y, Okuda K (1984) Arterial chemo-embolization of hepatocellular carcinoma with mitomycin C microcapsules. Radiology 152:51–55
5. Moriyama N (1980) Angiographic computed tomography (in Japanese). Gan No Rinsho 26: 1037–1040

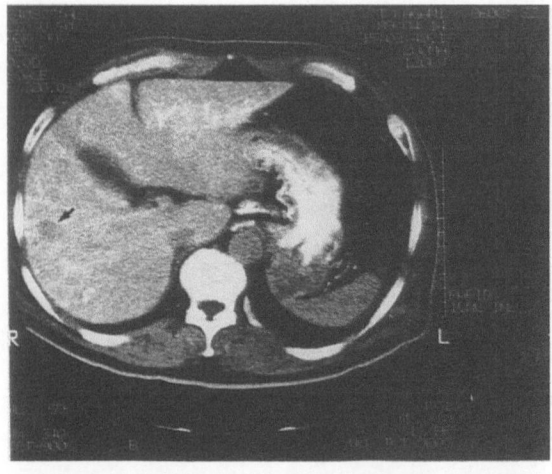
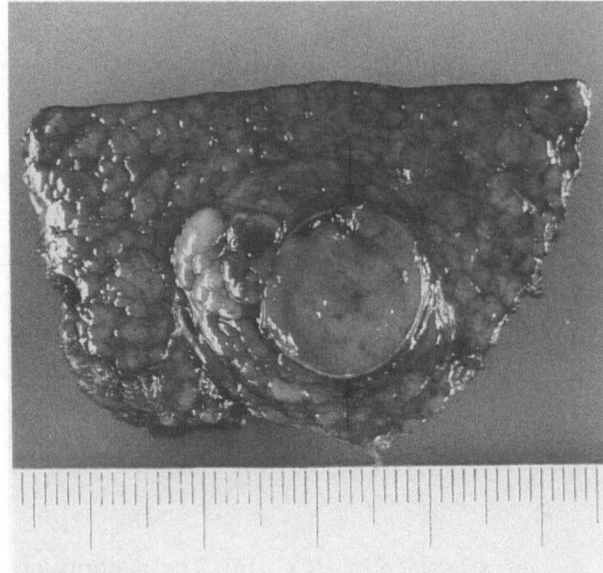
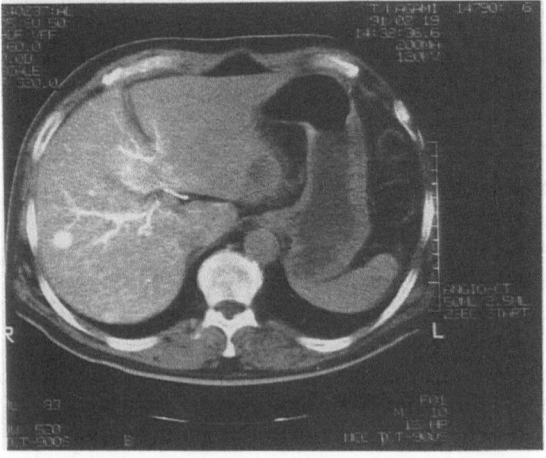

a

b

c

Fig. 4. Temporal change of enhancement of lesion. a A small lesion located in the right lobe demonstrated by arterial angio-CT (*arrow*) was not disclosed by lipiodol-CT nor superselective arteriography. Twenty two months later, the lesion was well enhanced by arterial angio-CT b as well as arteriography. c Cut surface of the resected specimen shows nodule in nodule type HCC. Microscopically, the central portion is composed of moderately differentiated HCC, which was surrounded by well differentiated HCC cells. Interior nodule (arrows) was presumed to make multi-step progression and to be enhanced by contrast medium.

6. Matsui O, Kadoya M, Suzuki M, et al. (1983) Dynamic sequential computed tomography during arterial portography in the detection of hepatic neoplasms. Radiology 146:721–727

7. Takayasu K, Moriyama N, Muramatsu Y, Makuuchi M, Hasegawa H, Okazaki N, Hirohashi S (1990) The diagnosis of small hepatocellular carcinomas: Efficacy of various imaging procedures in 100 patients. AJR 155:49–54

8. Konno T, Maeda H, Iwai K, Tashiro S, Maki S, Morinaga T, Mochinaga M, Hiraoka T, Yokoyama I (1983) Effect of arterial administration of high-molecular-weight anticancer agent SMANCS with lipid lymphographic agent on hepatoma. Eur J Cancer Clin Oncol 19:1053–1065

9. Nakakuma K, Tashiro S, Hiraoka T, Ogata K, Ootsuka K (1985) Hepatocellular carcinoma and metastatic cancer detected by iodized oil. Radiology 154:15–17

10. Yumoto Y, Jinno K, Tokuyama K, Arai Y, Ishimitsu T, Maeda H, Konno T, Iwamoto S, Ohnishi K, Okuda K (1985) Hepatocellular carcinoma detected by iodized oil. Radiology 154: 19–24

11. Ohishi H, Uchida H, Yoshimura H, Ohue S, Ueda J, Katsuragi M, Matsuo N, Hosogi Y (1985) Hepatocellular carcinoma detected by iodized oil: Use of anticancer agents. Radiology 154:25–29

12. Takayasu K, Shima Y, Muramatsu Y, Moriyama N, Yamada T, Makuuchi M, Hasegawa H, Hirohashi S (1987) Hepatocellular carcinoma: Treatment with intraarterial iodized oil with and without chemotherapeutic agents. Radiology 163:345–351

Table 2. Detection rates for adenomatous hyperplasia (AH), atypical adenomatous hyperplasia (AAH) and early hepatocellular carcinomas (e-HCC) by various imaging methods (Reference 18)

Group	No. of lesion	Size (cm)	Sonography	CT	Angiography	Arterial angio-CT	Portal angio-CT	Lipiodo-CT	Intraoperative sonography
AH	14	0.8 ± 0.3^a	0% (0/14)	0% (0/12)	0% (0/10)	0% (0/1)	50% (1/2)	0% (0/10)	35.7% (5/14)
AAH	12	1.2 ± 0.3	50.0 (6/12)	9.1 (1/11)	0 (0/11)	33.3^b (1/3)	33.3 (1/3)	0 (0/4)	75.0 (9/12)
Subtotal	26	1.0 ± 0.4	23.1 (6/26)	4.3 (1/23)	0 (0/21)	25.0^b (1/4)	40.0 (2/5)	0 (0/14)	53.8 (14/26)
e-HCC (I)^c	21	1.3 ± 0.4	61.9 (13/21)	52.6 (10/19)	26.3 (5/19)	50.0^b (2/4)	33.3 (1/3)	16.7 (1/6)	82.4 (14/17)
e-HCC (I > II)^c	7	1.5 ± 0.5	71.4 (5/7)	71.4 (5/7)	42.9 (3/7)	not done	100 (4/4)	50.0 (1/2)	100 (7/7)
Subtotal	28	1.4 ± 0.5	64.3 (18/28)	57.7 (15/26)	30.8 (8/26)	50.0^b (2/4)	71.4 (5/7)	25.0 (2/8)	87.5 (21/24)
Total	54	1.2 ± 0.4	44.4 (24/54)	32.7 (16/49)	17.0 (8/47)	37.5^b (3/8)	58.3 (7/12)	9.1 (2/22)	70.0 (35/50)

^{a} Significant difference ($P < 0.01$) between AH and other groups
^{b} Lesions were demonstrated as low density area
^{c} Cellular atypism according to Edmondson's classification [29]

13. Takayasu K, Shima Y, Muramatsu Y, Goto H, Moriyama N, Yamada T, Makuuchi M, Yamasaki S, Hasegawa H, Okazaki N, Hirohashi S, Kishi K (1986) Angiography of small hepatocellular carcinomas: Analysis of 105 resected tumors. AJR 147:525–529

14. Nakamura H, Hashimoto T, Oi H, Sawada S (1989) Transcatheter oily chemoembolization of hepatocellular carcinoma. Radiology 170:783–786

15. Kasugai H, Kojima J, Tatsuta M, Okuda S, Sasaki Y, Imaoka S, Fujita M, Ishiguro S (1989) Treatment of hepatocellular carcinoma by transcatheter arterial embolization combined with intra-arterial infusion of a mixture of cisplatin and ethiodized oil. Gastroenterology 97:965–971

16. Takayasu K, Suzuki M, Uesaka K, Muramatsu Y, Moriyama N, Yoshida T, Yoshino M, Okazaki N, Hasegawa H (1989) Hepatic artery embolization for inoperable hepatocellular carcinoma: Prognosis and risk factors. Cancer Chemother Pharmacol 23 (Suppl):S123–S125

17. Takayasu K, Muramatsu Y, Moriyama N, Hasegawa H, Makuuchi M, Okazaki N, Hirohashi S, Tsuganc S (1989) Clinical and radiologic assessments of the results of hepatectomy for small hepatocellular carcinoma and therapeutic arterial embolization for postoperative recurrence. Cancer 64:1848–1852

18. Takayasu K, Makuuchi M, Hirohashi S, Okazaki N, Muramatsu Y, Moriyama N, Takayama T, Hasegawa H (1989) Imaging of adenomatous hyperplastic lesions containing and not containing hepatocellular carcinoma in the liver (in Japanese). Nippon Shokakibyo Gakkai Zasshi 86:2404–2412

19. Arakawa M, Kage M, Sugihara S, Nakashima T, Suenaga M, Okuda K (1986) Emergence of malignant lesions within an adenomatous hyperplastic nodule in a cirrhotic liver: Observations in five cases. Gastroenterology 91:198–208

20. Kanai T, Hirohashi S, Upton MP, Noguchi M, Kishi K, Makuuchi M, Yamasaki S, Hasegawa H, Takayasu K, Moriyama N, Shimosato Y (1987) Pathology of small hepatocellular carcinoma: A proposal for a new gross classification. Cancer 60:810–819

21. Takayasu K, Muramatsu Y, Moriyama N, Ohtsu T, Catapia FC (1988) Plastic-coated guide wire for hepatic arteriography. Radiology 166:545–546

22. Hosoki T, Hashimoto T, Masuike M, Marukawa T, Tokunaga K, Kuroda C, Kozuka T (1989) Slippery coaxial catheter system. Radiology 171:858–859

23. Takayasu K, Aoki K, Ichikawa T, Ohmura T, Sekiguchi R, Kasugai H, Terauchi T (1990) New plastic-coated coaxial catheter system for superselective hepatic catheterization. Cardiovasc Intervent Radiol 13:384–386

24. Kido C, Sasaki T, Kaneko M (1971) Angiography of primary liver cancer. AJR 113:70–81

25. Okuda K, Obata H, Jinnouchi S, Kubo Y, Nagasaki Y, Shimokawa Y, Motoike Y, Muto H, Nakajima Y, Musha H, Yamazaki T, Sakamoto K, Kojiro M, Nakashima T (1977) Angiographic assessment of gross anatomy of hepatocellular

carcinoma: Comparison of celiac angiograms and liver pathology in 100 cases. Radiology 123:21–29

26. Okuda K, Musha H, Yoshida T, Kanda Y, Yamazaki T, Jinnouchi S, Moriyama M, Kawaguchi S, Kubo Y, Shimokawa Y, Kojiro M, Kuratomi S, Sakamoto K, Nakashima T (1975) Demonstration of growing casts of hepatocellular carcinoma in the portal vein by celiac angiography: The thread and streaks sign. Radiology 117: 303–309

27. Shinagawa T, Ohto M, Kimura K, Tsunetomi S, Morita M, Saisho H, Tsuchiya Y, Saotome N, Karasawa E, Miki M, Ueno T, Okuda K (1984) Diagnosis and clinical features of small hepatocellular carcinoma with emphasis on the utility of real-time ultrasonography: A study in 51 patients. Gastroenterology 86:495–502

28. Chen DC, Sheu JC, Sung JL, Lai MY, Lee CS, Su CT, Tsang YM, How SW, Wang TH, Yu JY, Yang TH, Wang CY, Hsu CY (1982) Small hepatocellular carcinoma. A clinicopathological study in the thirteen patients. Gastroenterology 83:1109–1119

29. Edmondson HA, Steiner PE (1954) Primary carcinoma of the liver: A study of 100 cases among 48,900 necropsies. Cancer 7:462–503

30. Healey JE Jr, Schroy PC (1953) Anatomy of the biliary ducts within the human liver: Analysis of the prevailing pattern of branchings and the major variations of the biliary ducts. Arch Surg 66: 599–616

31. Couinaud C (1954) Lobes et segments hepatiques: Notes sur l'architecture anatomique et chirurgicale du foie. Presse Med 62:709–712

32. Kanematsu T, Sugimachi K, Inokuchi K (1984) A hepatic unit at high risk for primary hepatocellular carcinoma. IRCS Med Sci 12:721

Section 3   Tumor Markers

Lectin-binding analysis of serum alpha-fetoprotein: Predictive importance of the change of AFP sugar chain in the development of hepatocellular carcinoma

Yasuo Endo[1]

1 Introduction

In Japan, hepatocellular carcinoma (HCC) usually develops on the basis of liver cirrhosis that results from chronic infection by hepatitis virus B (HVB) or C (HVC). One of the most important factors which influences the prognosis of the patient is early detection of the tumor, i.e., detection when it is as small as possible. HCC is diagnosed using a combination of imaging methods, such as ultrasound (US) techniques, computed tomography (CT), angiography, and tumor marker assays. Of the various tumor markers, alpha-fetoprotein (AFP) and protein induced by vitamin K antagonist II (PIVKA-II) are the most reliable, and for an early diagnosis of HCC, it is necessary to regularly check the patient using imaging methods and AFP assays.

Because of recent progress in the development of diagnostic techniques, detection of tumors less than 2 cm in diameter is increasing. In patients with small tumors, 64% do not show elevation of serum AFP levels [1] (Table 1). However, in some patients, regular AFP checks give clues for the early detection of HCC.

In this chapter, I would like to focus on the recent progress in AFP research, especially in relation to the importance of AFP sugar chain analysis in the prediction of HCC development.

2 AFP heterogeneity

AFP is a glycoprotein whose molecular structure consists of about 4% sugar. This glycoprotein is present in the serum during the fetal stage, and during this period is produced mainly by the yolk sac and fetal liver. However, after birth, the synthesis of AFP stops. Serum levels of AFP in the adult are usually under 10 ng/ml. The production of AFP, once stopped, takes place again only under pathological conditions, such as HCC, yolk sac tumor, and some benign liver diseases.

After the reports by Abelev et al. [2] and Tatarinov et al. [3], AFP became one of the most important tumor markers in the clinical field and is now most widely used as a specific marker for HCC. According to Morinaga et al. [4], AFP is composed of 590 amino acid residues. It has one asparagine-linked sugar chain at the 232nd position from the N-terminal of the AFP molecule. The sugar chain of AFP was analyzed by Yoshima et al. [5] and Yamashita et al. [6], and the difference between the sugar chains of HCC AFP and those of yolk sac tumor AFP was demonstrated (Fig. 1). In order to determine the difference between the AFP of HCC and that of other diseases, lectin-binding analysis using concanavalin A (Con A), lens culinaris (LCA), and phytohemagglutinin (PHA-E4) has become a useful tool in the early detection of HCC.

The existence of human AFP heterogeneity was first described by Purves et al. [7]. They used starch gel electrophoresis and found four subfractions in the serum AFP taken from patients with HCC. However, the results from analysis of fetal AFP showed only one subfraction was present. Kortright et al. purified AFPs from cord serum and from ascites fluid [8]. They analyzed the physico-chemical properties of each AFP but could not find any difference between the two AFPs as to the isoelectric point (PI); the PI of cord serum AFP was 4.85 and that of ascites fluid AFP 4.80. Alpert et al. purified AFP originated from patients with HCC and found microheterogeneity in its physico-chemical characteristics [9]. They demonstrated two variants of AFP

[1] Sanraku Hospital, 2-5 Kanda Surugadai, Chiyoda-ku, Tokyo, 101 Japan

Table 1. Tumor size and percentage of patients testing positive for elevated serum AFP levels

Tumor diameter (cm)	Total no. of cases	Positive rate at increasing serum AFP levels (%)			
		<20 ng/ml	21–200	201–1000	1001~
<2.0	359	64.1	23.1	8.4	4.4
2.1–5.0	499	15.6	38.3	26.4	20.0
5.1–10.0	256	33.6	28.5	13.3	24.6
10.1~	101	27.7	24.8	19.8	27.7

From [1]

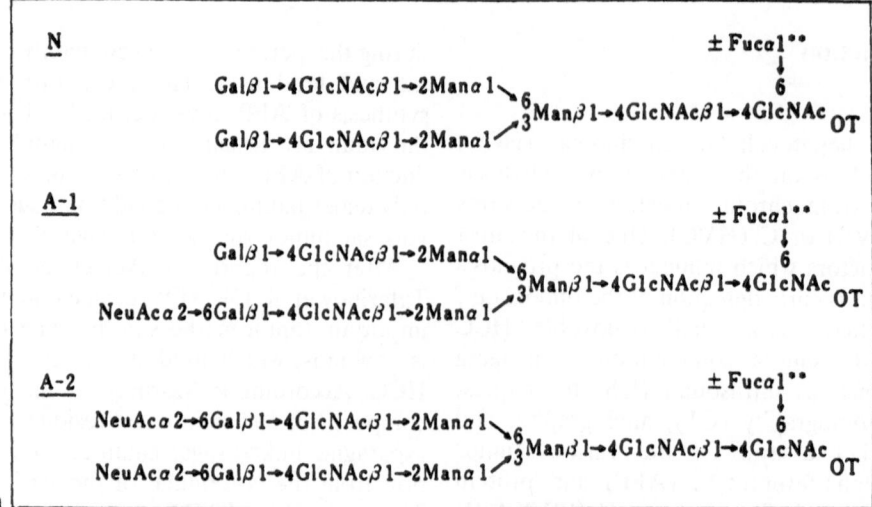

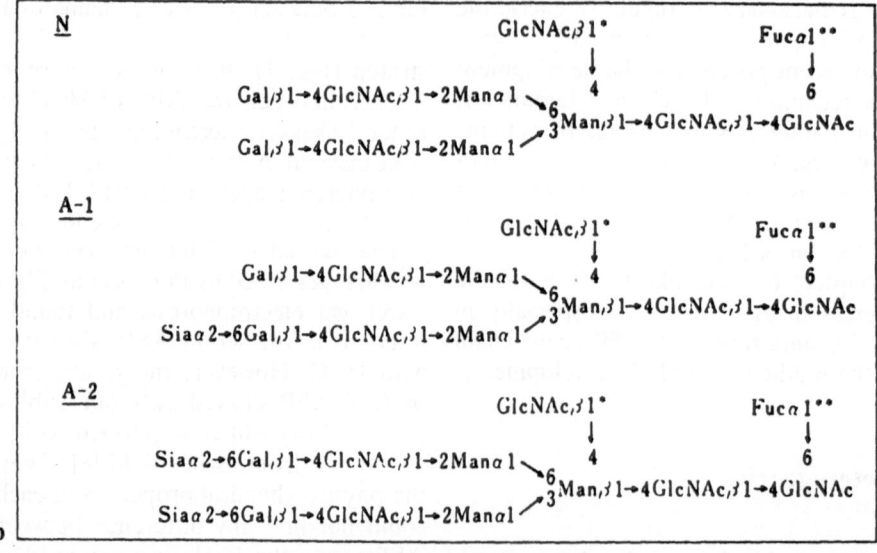

Fig. 1a,b. Molecular structure of AFP. **a** Sugar chain of AFP from ascites fluid of patient with HCC. This AFP was composed mainly of Con A bound fraction. *Fuc*** shows the fucose bound to GlcNAc at the root of sugar chain. From [5] with permission. **b** Sugar chain of AFP purified from yolk sac tumor innoculated into nude mouse. This AFP was composed mainly of Con A nonbound fraction. *GlcNAc** bound to mannose in this figure is called a bisecting GlcNAc and is supposed to interfere with the binding of Con A to this AFP. From [6] with permission

Table 2. Lectins (1)

Group	Lectin	Trivial name	Sugar specificity
1	Ulex europeus I	UEA-I, Ulex-I	α-L-Fuc
	Lotus tetragonolobus	Asparagus pea	α-L-Fuc
2	Arachis hypogaea	PNA	β-Gal
	Bandeiraea simplicifolia I	BS-I	α-Gal > α-GalNAc
	Dolichos biflorus	DBA	α-GalNAc
	Glycine max	Soybean, SBA	α-GalNAc > β-GalNAc
	Phaseolus vulgaris	Red kidney bean, PHA	GalNAc
	Ricinus communis	Castor bean, RCA	β-Gal

From [21]

Table 3. Lectins (2)

Group	Lectins	Trivial name	Sugar specificity
3	Canavalia ensifolmis	Jack bean, Con A	α-Man > α-Glc
	Lens culinaris	Lentil, LCA	α-Man > α-Glc
	Pisum sativum	Pea, PSA	α-Man > α-Glc
	Vicia faba	Faba bean	α-Man > α-Glc
	Bandeiraea simplicifolia-II	BS-II	GlcNAc
	Laburnum alpinum		GlcNAc β1-4GlcNAc
	Triticum vulgaris	Wheat germ, WGA	GlcNAc β1-4GlcNAc
	Ulex europeus II	UEA-II, Ulex II	GlcNAc β1-4GlcNAc

From [21]

existed: AFP with a PI of 4.85 and AFP with a PI of 5.20. Among these variants, some showed changes after neuraminidase treatment and some did not. They concluded that AFP microheterogeneity does not depend only on differences in the sialic acid residues present in the AFP sugar chain.

3 AFP and its lectin-binding properties

Smith et al. [10] reported that there were two subfractions of serum AFP in HCC patients: one was Con A bound and the other Con A nonbound. Ruoslahti et al. [11] analyzed AFPs from amniotic fluids of the first and last trimesters. AFP of the first trimester was about 50% Con-A-bound AFP and about 50% of Con-A-nonbound AFP. In contrast, AFP of the last trimester was mainly Con-A-bound AFP. They supposed that the first trimester AFP was of yolk sac origin and that of the last trimester was of fetal liver origin.

AFP has, as stated above, one asparagine-linked sugar chain. In order to study changes in these sugar chains, several lectins have been used. There are two kinds of lectins: those that bind AFP and those that do not, and the most widely used lectins are listed in Tables 2 and 3. The lectin-binding profiles of AFPs from HCC patients, amniotic fluids, and metastatic liver cancer patients are illustrated in Figs. 2 and 3. Con A, LCA, PHA-E4, Allo A, and RCA 120 are lectins which bind AFP and Fig. 2 shows the peaks of bound and nonbound subfractions determined by crossed immuno-affino electrophoresis. WGA, SBA, UEA-I, UEA-II, and PNA are lectins which do not bind AFP and Fig. 3 shows only one peak as determined by crossed immuno-affino electrophoresis.

The clinical data obtained to date by various authors [12–20] are summarized in the following sections.

3.1 Con-A-binding analysis

According to Con-A-binding analysis, AFP is divided into two subfractions: con A nonbound and bound. During the natal period, serum AFP

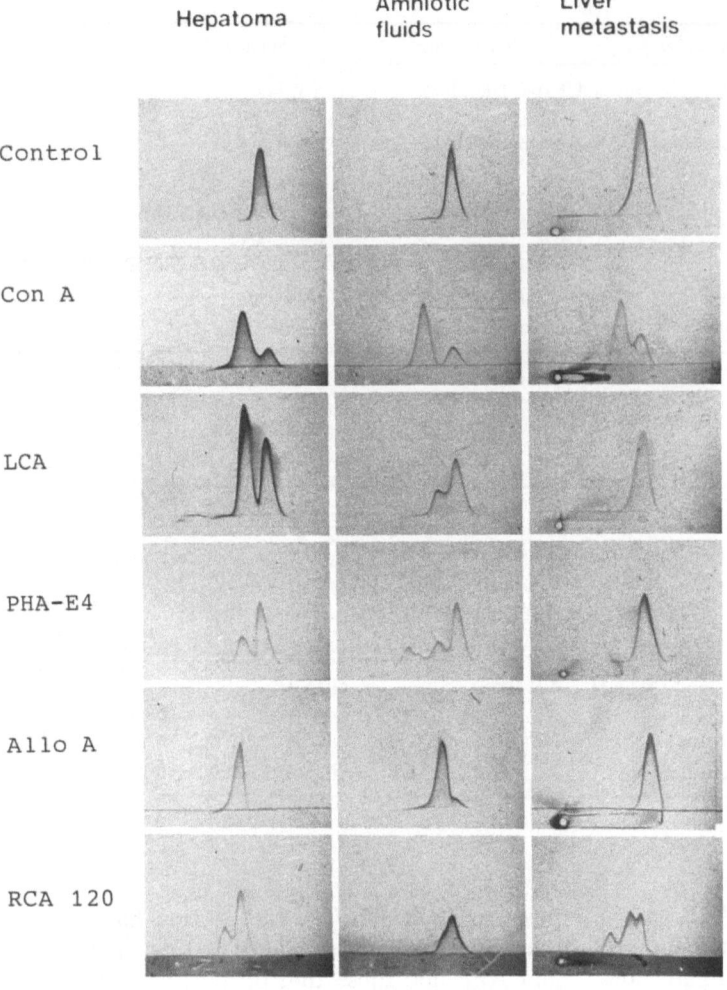

Fig. 2. Lectin-binding profiles of various lectins with AFPs from hepatoma, amniotic fluids and from liver metastasis. Lectin bound and lectin nonbound fractions were subjected to crossed immuno-affino electrophoresis

increases in various diseases; in neonatal hepatitis, congenital biliary atresia, and hepatoblastoma, serum AFP showed a similar lectin-binding profile as that of cord serum AFP. In these diseases, the AFP was composed mainly of the Con-A-bound fraction. In yolk sac tumor, AFP was composed of about 50% Con-A-bound and about 50% Con-A-nonbound fractions, AFP in yolk sac tumor patients was markedly different from that in HCC patients. A similar tendency was observed in adults. AFP from patients with HCC showed very low quantities of the Con-A-nonbound fraction, and AFP from patients with liver cirrhosis showed almost the same profile as in HCC. In metastatic liver cancer (where the origin was the stomach or pancreas), serum AFP showed the same lectin-binding profile as in yolk sac tumor. It is impossible to distinguish liver cirrhosis from HCC by Con A lectin-binding

analysis of AFP. Our data concerning Con A binding are demonstrated in Fig. 4.

3.2 LCA-binding analysis

AFP was divided into three subfractions by LCA-binding analysis: LCA nonbound, weakly bound, and strongly bound. AFP from cord blood and from liver cirrhosis were composed mainly of LCA-nonbound subfractions. AFP from yolk sac tumor and from metastatic liver cancer were composed mainly of LCA-bound subfractions. In HCC, various profiles of AFP-LCA binding were observed.

I compared LCA-binding ratios of AFP in 7 cases of liver cirrhosis and 31 cases of HCC. Results showed that these two diseases could be

Fig. 3. Lectin-binding profiles of various lectins with AFP from hepatoma, amniotic fluids, and from liver metastasis. The lectins do not bind with AFP. They show only one peak in crossed immuno-affino electrophoresis

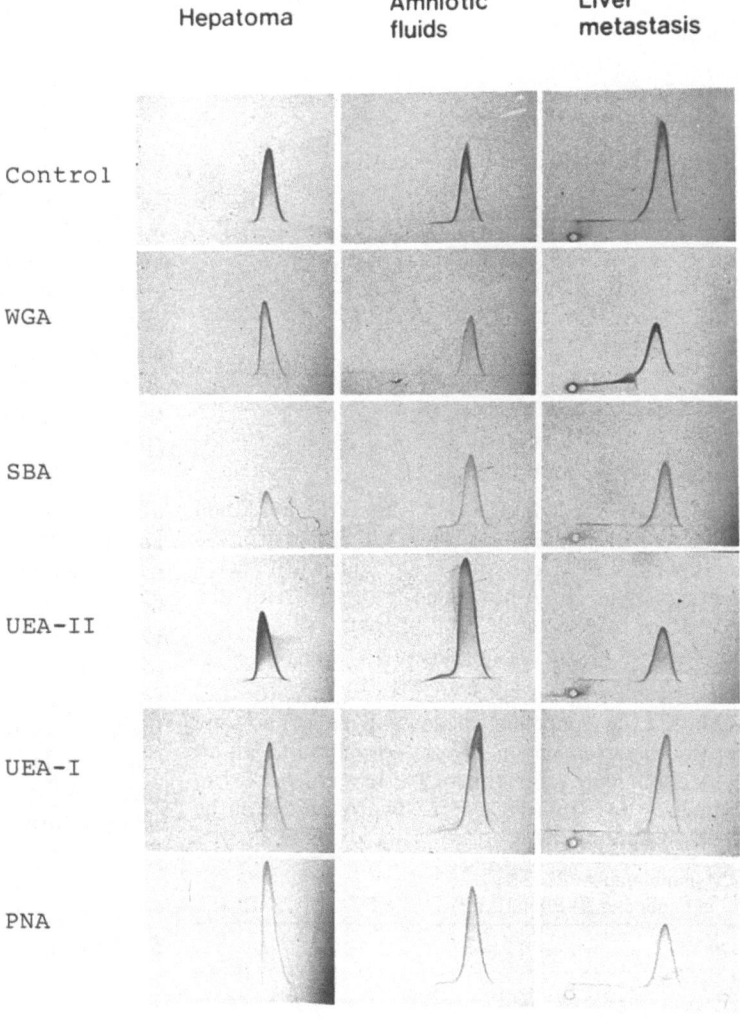

Fig. 4. The rate of Con-A-nonbound AFP (%) in various diseases. AFPs from cord blood, from sera of congenital biliary atresia, neonatal hepatitis, liver cirrhosis, hepatoblastoma, and hepatocellular carcinoma show a low rate (%) of Con-A-nonbound AFP. In cases of metastatic liver cancer and yolk sac tumor, Con-A-nonbound AFP increase to about 50% of total AFP

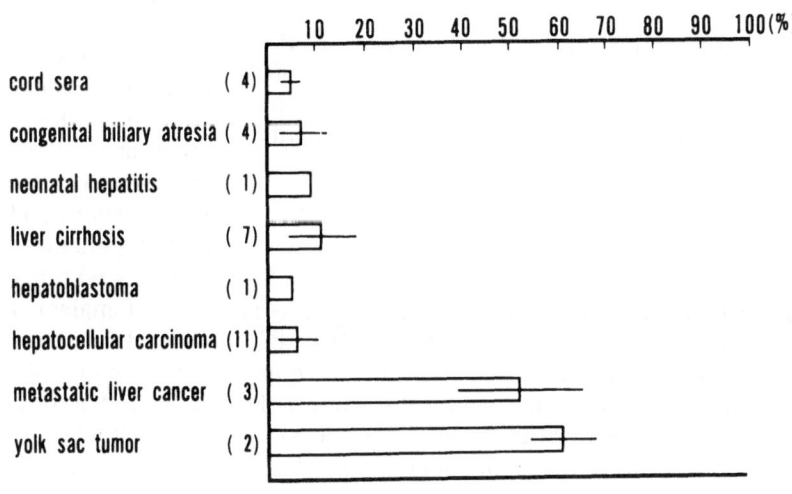

168   Y. Endo

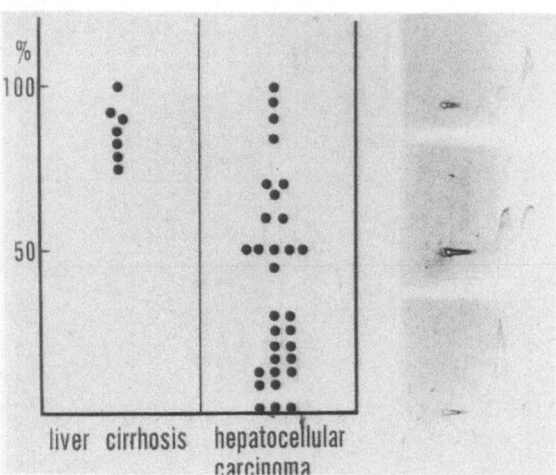

Fig. 5. The percent of LCA-non-bound AFP in LC and HCC. AFP of liver cirrhosis shows a high rate of LCA-non-bound AFP. AFP of hepatocellular carcinoma shows various LCA-nonbound patterns with the increase of LCA-bound AFP (see Table 4)

Table 4. LCA-nonbound fraction in liver cirrhosis and hepatocellular carcinoma. A cut-off value of 70% of LCA-nonbound AFP (mean-2SD) was chosen to distinguish LC from HCC. The two diseases can be clearly differentiated

LCA-nonbound AFP (% of nonbound AFP/total AFP)	LC	HCC
>70	7	4
≦70	0	27 (87%)

Mean ± SD = 87.1 ± 8.2%
Mean − 2SD = 70.7%
Mean − 2SD = 78.9%

differentiated when the cut off value was set at 70% of the LCA-nonbound ratio; in all 7 cases of liver cirrhosis, the LCA-nonbound ratio was over 70%. In contrast, in 87% of the cases of HCC, the LCA-nonbound ratios were under 70% (Fig. 5, Table 4). Increases of the LCA-bound fraction in patients with HCC were also reported.

3.3 PHA-E4-binding analysis

AFP is divided into 5 subfractions by PHA-E4 binding analysis: PHA-E4-nonbound (P1, P2), and bound surfractions (P3, P4, P5). We found that in liver cirrhosis the main subfraction is P2 and P4 is usually low (under 10% of total AFP). P4 appears and increases in patients with HCC.

4 AFP in chronic liver diseases

Serum AFP increases markedly in cases of HCC. AFP, however, also increases in other chronic liver diseases, such as chronic hepatitis, and liver cirrhosis. In my studies, serum AFP increases in about 20% of the cases of chronic hepatitis and in about 50% of the cases of liver cirrhosis. In chronic hepatitis, the increased serum AFP usually remains under 100 ng/ml and in liver cirrhosis, serum AFP usually remains under 400 ng/ml. When serum AFP exceeds 400 ng/ml, this probably indicates the presence of HCC (Fig. 6).

The increases of serum AFP in chronic liver diseases are tentatively classified into three groups: (1) progressive increases, (2) spiky increases, and (3) continuous high levels. The first group usually indicates the development of HCC and the second group is observed in cases of liver cirrhosis after massive destruction and regeneration thereafter. The third group is the most difficult from the view point of differentiating HCC. In order to distinguish between these AFPs the LCA- and PHA-E4-binding analyses are useful.

5 Prediction of HCC development

The most efficient method for the detection of tumor development is regular checks on changes of serum AFP and imaging profiles in patients with a high risk of hepatoma development. High risk patients include middle-aged male patients with liver cirrhosis, with a history of blood transfusion (chronic HVC infection), HBV carriers, heavy drinkers, and so on. I studied retrospectively the serum samples of patients with liver cirrhosis, some of whom had developed HCC and some who had not. The samples had been taken at regular intervals, and kept frozen until analysis, from 35 patients with liver cirrhosis who had developed HCC (24 males and 11 females) and 9 patients with liver cirrhosis or chronic hepatitis who had not developed HCC (5 males and 4 females). Lectin binding was analyzed by using LCA and PHA-E4. Criteria suggesting development of HCC in the near future (the HCC pattern) were set as over 20% of the LCA-bound fraction (L3) and/or over 10% of PHA-E4-bound fraction (P4). In Table 4, the mean

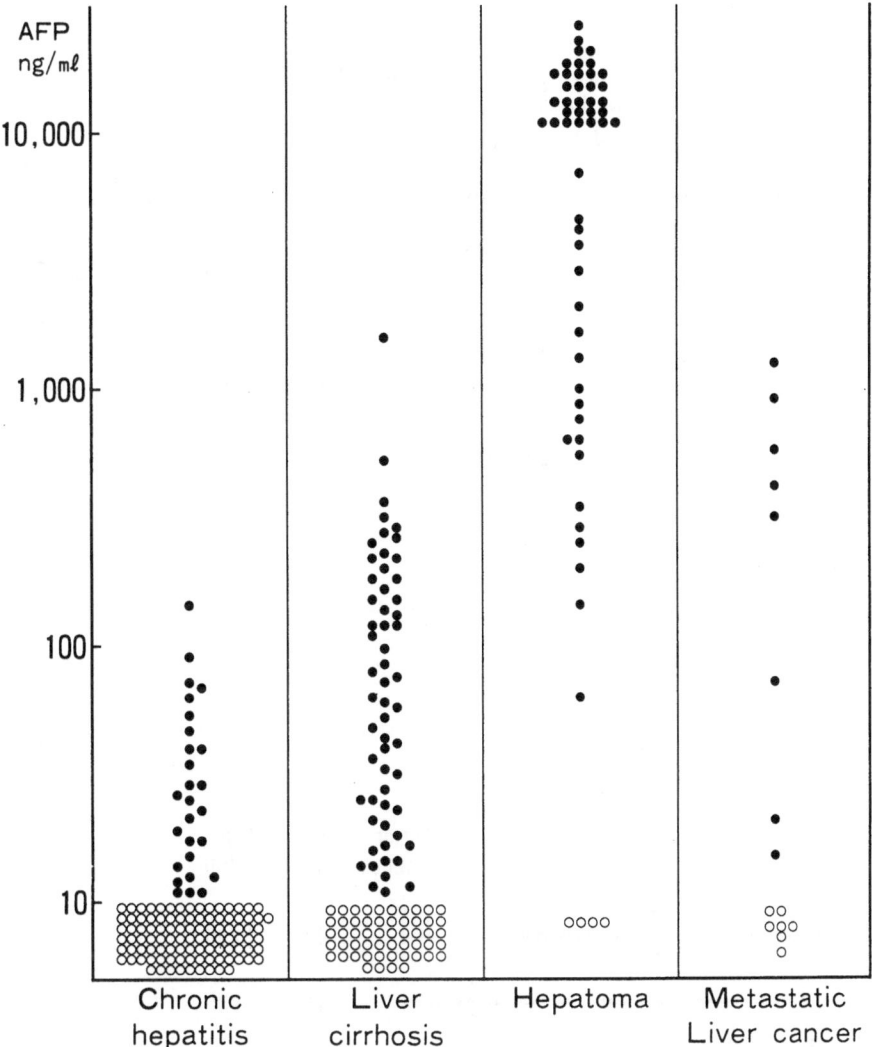

Fig. 6. Serum levels of AFP in chronic hepatitis, liver cirrhosis, hepatoma, and metastatic liver cancer. About 20% of chronic hepatitis and about 50% of liver cirrhosis patients showed elevation of serum AFP. These elevations were usually under 400 ng/ml in liver cirrhosis and usually under 100 ng/ml in cases of chronic hepatitis. Marked elevation was observed in hepatocellular carcinoma. There was some overlapping of the increased serum levels of AFP between HCC and LC

value of nonbound AFP was 87.1% ± 8.2% (mean −SD, 78.9%). We designated the value 20% as the HCC pattern. If these conditions were not met, I termed it the LC pattern (liver cirrhosis pattern).

Figure 7 demonstrates 8 cases of HCC in which L3 and P4 were observed simultaneously at the first analysis. In case S.T., L3 and P4 were observed 1 year and 5 months before tumor detection by imaging techniques. At the time of tumor detection, the tumor size was 1.5 cm in diameter and serum AFP was 2,360 ng/ml.

Figure 8 shows 3 cases of HCC, in which L3 preceeded P4 appearance. In case K.O., L3 was

observed 1 year and 1 month before tumor detection. P4 appeared after L3 appearance.

In Fig. 9, 6 cases of HCC are shown. In these 6 cases P4 appeared first, followed by L3. In case M.S., P4 appeared 2 years and 1 month before tumor detection.

In Fig. 10, 14 cases of HCC were demonstrated. In these cases, only P4 appeared and L3 was not observed. In case Y.M., for example, P4 appeared 4 years and 5 months before tumor detection. In case T.T., P4 first appeared 7 years and 1 month before tumor detection, disappeared once, and then reappeared.

In Fig. 11, 4 cases of HCC, in which L3 and P4

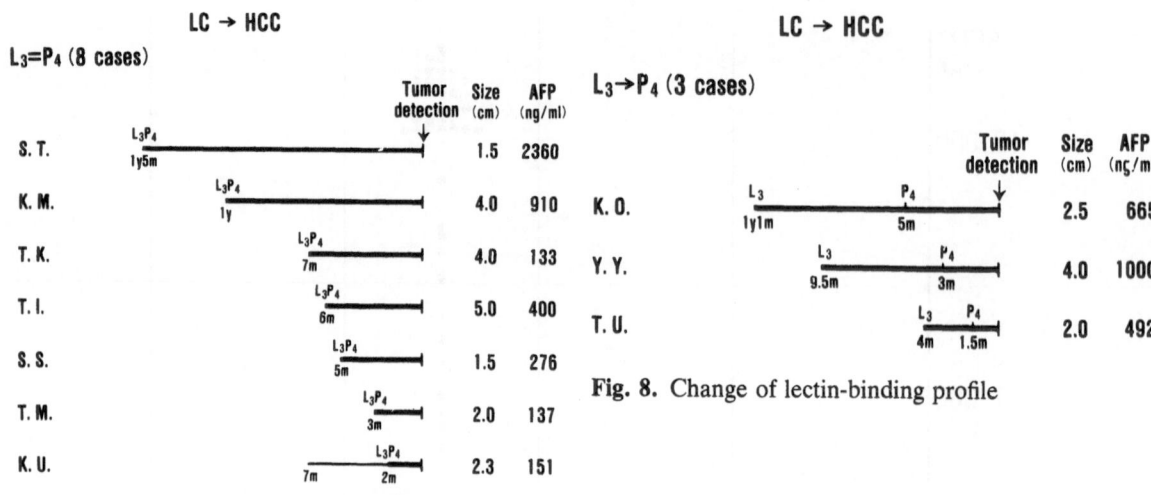

Fig. 7. Change of lectin-binding profile

Fig. 8. Change of lectin-binding profile

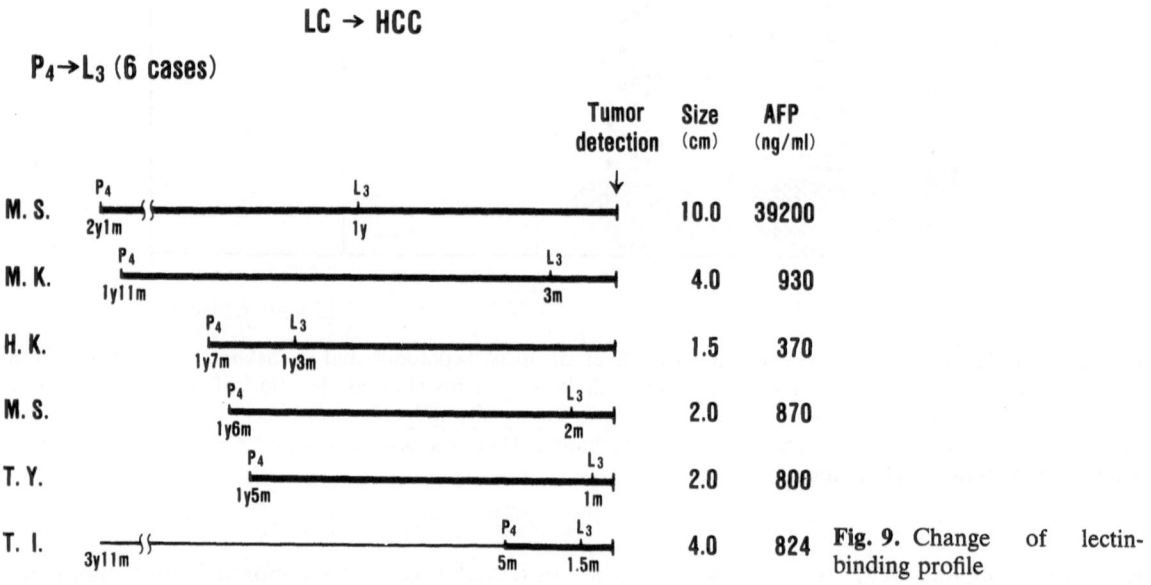

Fig. 9. Change of lectin-binding profile

did not appear, are shown. In Fig. 12, 9 cases of liver cirrhosis and chronic hepatitis are demonstrated. In these cases, no tumors were detected by imaging techniques during 2 years of observation. In these cases, L3 and P4 were not observed.

When the above results are considered, it seems that AFP with an LCA-bound fraction ratio of over 20% (L3) or with PHA-E4-bound fraction ratio of over 10% (P4) in patients with liver cirrhosis strongly suggests HCC development in the very near future. The appearance of P4 is more sensitive than that of L3, and they were both observed between several months and several years before tumor detection by imaging techniques.

The increase of the LCA-bound subfraction (L3) in patients with HCC has been widely

Fig. 10. Change of lectin-binding profile

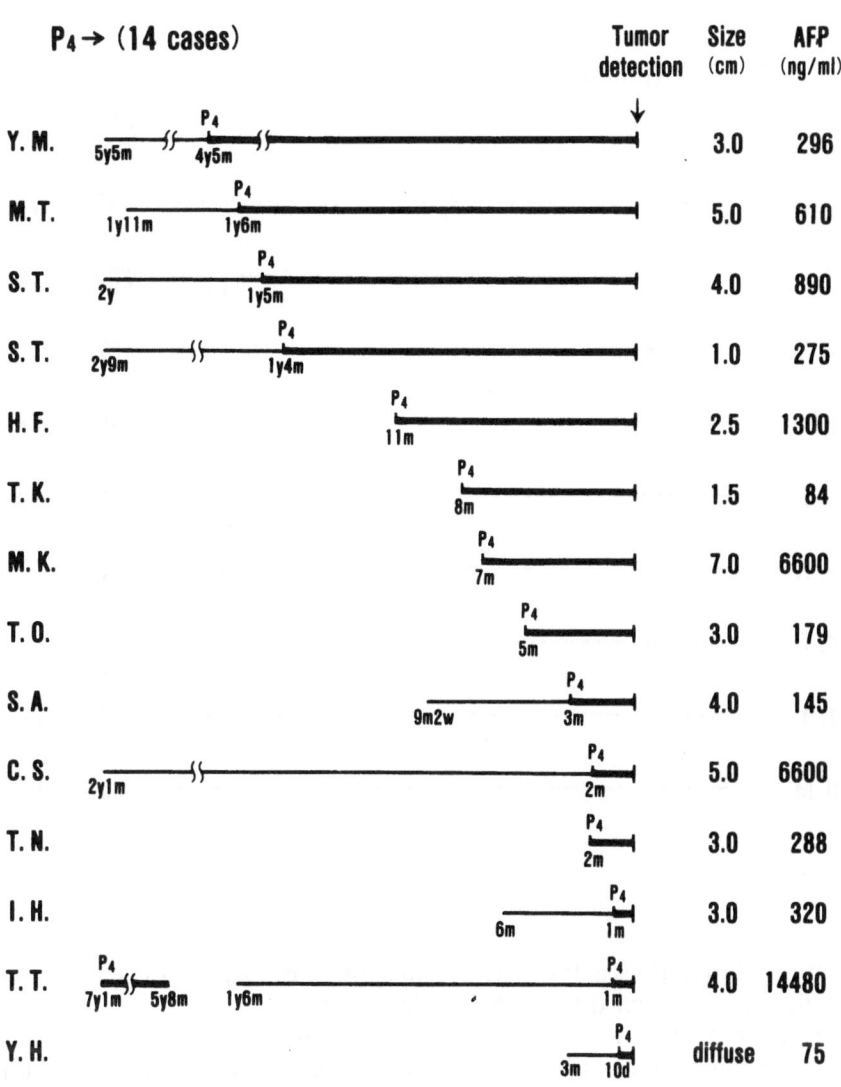

LC → HCC

P₄ → (14 cases)

	Tumor detection	Size (cm)	AFP (ng/ml)
Y. M.		3.0	296
M. T.		5.0	610
S. T.		4.0	890
S. T.		1.0	275
H. F.		2.5	1300
T. K.		1.5	84
M. K.		7.0	6600
T. O.		3.0	179
S. A.		4.0	145
C. S.		5.0	6600
T. N.		3.0	288
I. H.		3.0	320
T. T.		4.0	14480
Y. H.		diffuse	75

LC → HCC

L₃(−), P₄(−) (4 cases)

	Tumor detection	Size (cm)	AFP (ng/ml)
K. E.		1.2	262
M. H.		3.0	62
T. H.		3.0	75
K. T.		8.0	153

Fig. 11. Change of lectin-binding profile

171

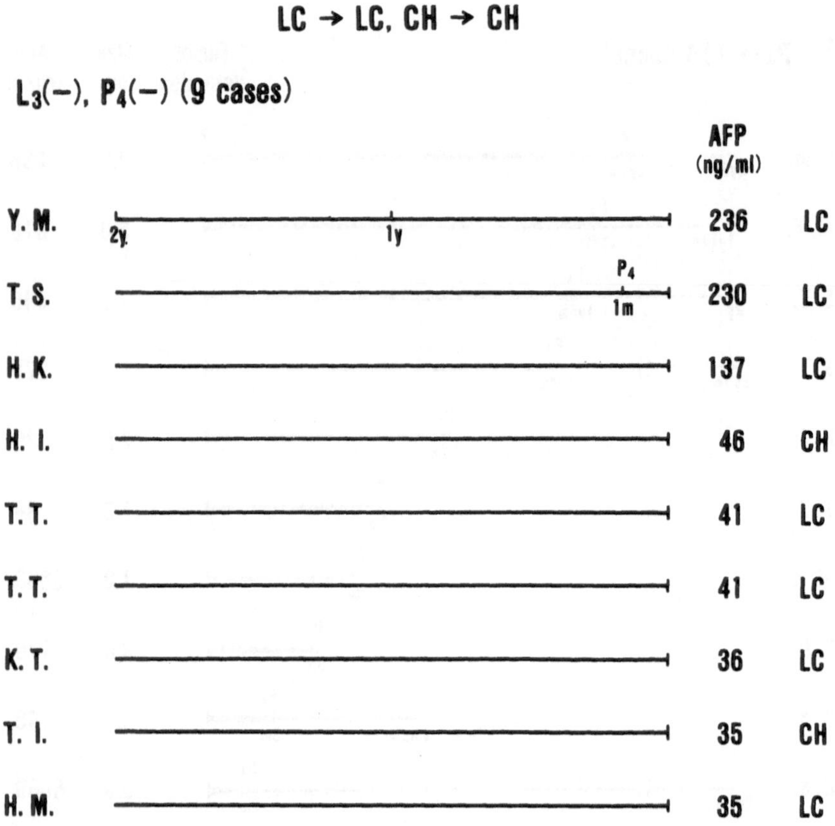

Y. Endo

LC → LC, CH → CH

$L_3(-)$, $P_4(-)$ (9 cases)

Fig. 12. Change of lectin-binding profile

	AFP (ng/ml)	
Y. M.	236	LC
T. S.	230	LC
H. K.	137	LC
H. I.	46	CH
T. T.	41	LC
T. T.	41	LC
K. T.	36	LC
T. I.	35	CH
H. M.	35	LC

observed by various authors. The binding of AFP with LCA is assumed to be due to the presence of fucose at the GlcNAc site of the root of the sugar chain. More AFP binds with LCA when the amount of fucosylated AFP increases. Aoyagi et al. [17] analyzed the purified AFP from patients with HCC and found an increase of fucosylated AFP. They suggested that the activation of fucosyltransferase in the cell because of the development of cancer may play the important role.

The mechanism of the increase of the PHA-E4-bound fraction (P4) in HCC is not clear. The presence of bisecting GlcNAc which binds to the mannose core may play some role, but this has not yet been confirmed. The purification of the P2 and P4 subfractions and analysis of their physico-chemical characteristics may be needed. The sugar chain of AFP synthesized by tumor tissues is thought to be produced by a different metabolic pathway than that used during fetal stage.

References

1. Liver Cancer Study Group of Japan (1990) Primary liver cancer in Japan: Clinicopathologic features and results of surgical treatment. Ann Surg 211:277
2. Abelev GI, et al. (1963) Production of embryonal alpha-globulin by transplantable mouse hepatoma. Transplantation 1:174–180
3. Tatarinov YS (1964) Presence of embryonal alpha-globulin in the serum of patient with primary hepatocellular carcinoma (in Russian). Vopr Med Khim 10:90–91
4. Morinaga T, et al. (1983) Primary structures of human alpha-fetoprotein and its mRNA. Proc Natl Acad Sci USA 80:4604–4608
5. Yoshima H, et al. (1980) Structures of the asparagine-linked sugar chains of alpha-fetoprotein purified from human ascites fluid. Cancer Res 40:4279–4281
6. Yamashita K, et al. (1983) Sugar chain of alpha-fetoprotein produced in human yolk sac tumor. Cancer Res 43:4691–4695
7. Purves LR, et al. (1970) Variants of alpha-fetoprotein. Lancet II:464–465

8. Kortright KH, et al. (1978) Purification and physical characterization of human alpha-fetoprotein from cord blood and from ascites fluid of individuals with hepatocellular carcinoma. Scand J Immunol 8 (suppl 8):347–360

9. Alpert E, et al. (1972) Human alpha-fetoprotein. Isolation, characterization, and demonstration of microheterogeneity. J Biol Chem 247:3792–3798

10. Smith CJ, et al. (1973) Alpha-Fetoprotein: separation of two molecular variants by affinity chromatography with concanavalin A-agarose. Biochem Biophys Acta 317:231–235

11. Ruoslahti E, et al. (1978) Developmental changes in carbohydrate moiety of human alpha-fetoprotein. Int J Cancer 22:515–520

12. Miyazaki J, et al. (1981) Lectin affinities of alpha-fetoprotein in liver cirrhosis, hepatocellular carcinoma, and metastatic liver tumor (in Japanese). Acta Hepatol Jpn 22:1559–1568

13. Breborowicz J, et al. (1981) Microheterogeneity of alpha-fetoprotein in patient serum as demonstrated by lectin affino-electrophoresis. Scand J Immunol 14:15–20

14. Buamah PK, et al. (1986) Lentil-lectin-reactive alpha-fetoprotein in the differential diagnosis of benign and malignant liver disease. Clin Chem 32:2083–2084

15. Taketa K, et al. (1985) Increased asialo-alpha-fetoprotein in patients with alpha-fetoprotein-producing tumors: Demonstration by affinity electrophoresis with erythroagglutinating phytohemagglutinin of *Phaseolus vulgaris* lectin. Tumor Biology 6:533–544

16. Taketa K, et al. (1985) Antibody-affinity blotting, a sensitive technique for the detection of alpha-fetoprotein separated by lectin affinity electrophoresis in agarose gels. Electrophoresis 6:492–497

17. Aoyagi Y, et al. (1988) The fucosylation index of alpha-fetoprotein and its usefulness in the early diagnosis of hepatocellular carcinoma. Cancer 61:769–774

18. Endo Y, et al. (1984) Lectin-affinity analysis of alpha-fetoprotein in liver diseases and in infantile diseases (in Japanese). Seibutsu butsuri kagaku 28:355–360

19. Taketa K, et al. (1990) Lectin-reactive profiles of alpha-fetoprotein characterizing hepatocellular carcinoma and related conditions. Gastroenterology 99:508–518

20. Endo Y, et al. (1991) Analysis of patients with high risk of hepatocellular carcinoma by lectin binding technique of AFP (in Japanese). Seibutsu butsuri kagaku 35:205–208

21. Tsuji T, Osawa T (1983) Lectins and their sugar binding specificity (in Japanese) Tanpakushitsu Kakusa Koso 28:118–131

Part 5   Hepatic Function

CHAPTER 17

Evaluation of hepatic function

Fukashi Imai, Kyoichiro Toshima, Mikio Uematsu, Hiromi Kamoshita, Kazuhito Kuga, and Haruo Kameda[1]

1 Introduction

In the natural course of liver cirrhosis, a very strong correlation with hepatocellular carcinoma (HCC) has been observed regardless of its etiology. Although cirrhosis can be controlled very well, HCC may still occur in the later stages, and it appears that the overall incidence of HCC is increasing. It is clinically interesting to note at which stage in cirrhosis HCC occurs, and moreover, how liver function correlates to the various stages of cirrhosis and HCC [1]. To this end, the incidence of HCC in association with cirrhosis cases treated by this department during the past 14 years was studied. The liver function test results of fatal cases were compared with liver cirrhosis cases with HCC and without HCC at one month, one year, and two years prior to death.

2 Changes in the incidence of cirrhosis and associated HCC

It is widely believed that there exists a difference in the progress of cirrhosis during the last decade before death and the previous decade to this. Major causes of cirrhosis associated deaths are esophageal varices including gastrointestinal bleeding, HCC, hepatic coma, hepatic failure, and renal failure. On one hand, dietary control such as a high-protein, high-calorie diet, development of excellent diuresis, adrenal cortical hormone therapy, administration of blood albumin, lacturose, and branched-chain amino acids (BCAA), and better treatment of esophageal varices, contribute greatly to life prolongation of patients with cirrhosis. On the other hand, cirrhosis complicated by HCC and gastrointestinal bleeding caused by a relapse of esophageal varices have recently emerged as the major causes of death in patients with cirrhotic livers. Therefore, when discussing the progress of cirrhosis, it is necessary to mention the circumstances surrounding the occurrence of HCC, and the details associated with the development of esophageal varices.

Figures 1 and 2 show the changes in cirrhosis observed in this department. One can see that the percentage of HCC is increasing both in admissions and autopsy cases. Although the percentage of HCC was only 12%–30% among the fatal cases of cirrhosis from the 1960s to the early 1970s, it increased to over 50% by the end of the 1970s, and has continued to increase to over 70% of cases diagnosed with HCC from the end of the 1970s to the 1980s. Currently, over 80% of fatal cases of cirrhosis are also diagnosed as having HCC. The same also applies for hospitalized patients in the 1970s when the percentage of HCC was below 30%. By the 1980s it increased to over 30%, and by 1988 had reached 64% [2].

3 HCC incidence in long term observation cases of cirrhosis

Table 1 summarizes the cause and progress of 20 long-term observation cases treated during 1988 who were diagnosed with cirrhosis of the liver through a combination of clinical findings, test results, 15-minute indocyanine green retention (ICGR$_{15}$), laparoscopy, and liver biopsy.

---

[1] The First Department of Internal Medicine, Jikei University School of Medicine, Minato-ku, Tokyo, 105 Japan

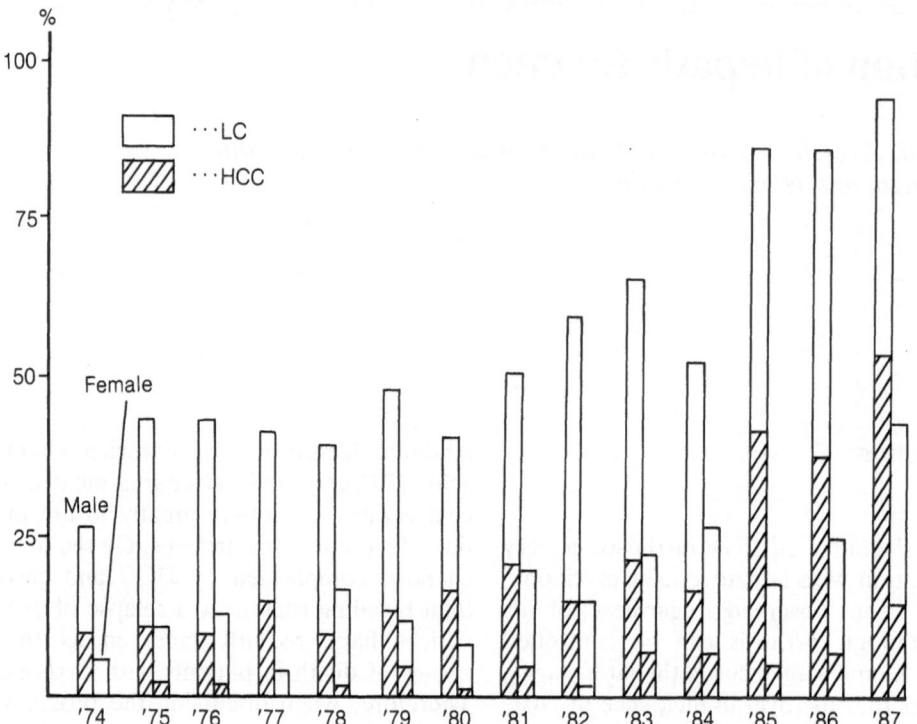

Fig. 1. Hepatocellular carcinoma (HCC) incidence among liver cirrhosis inpatients (1974–1987)

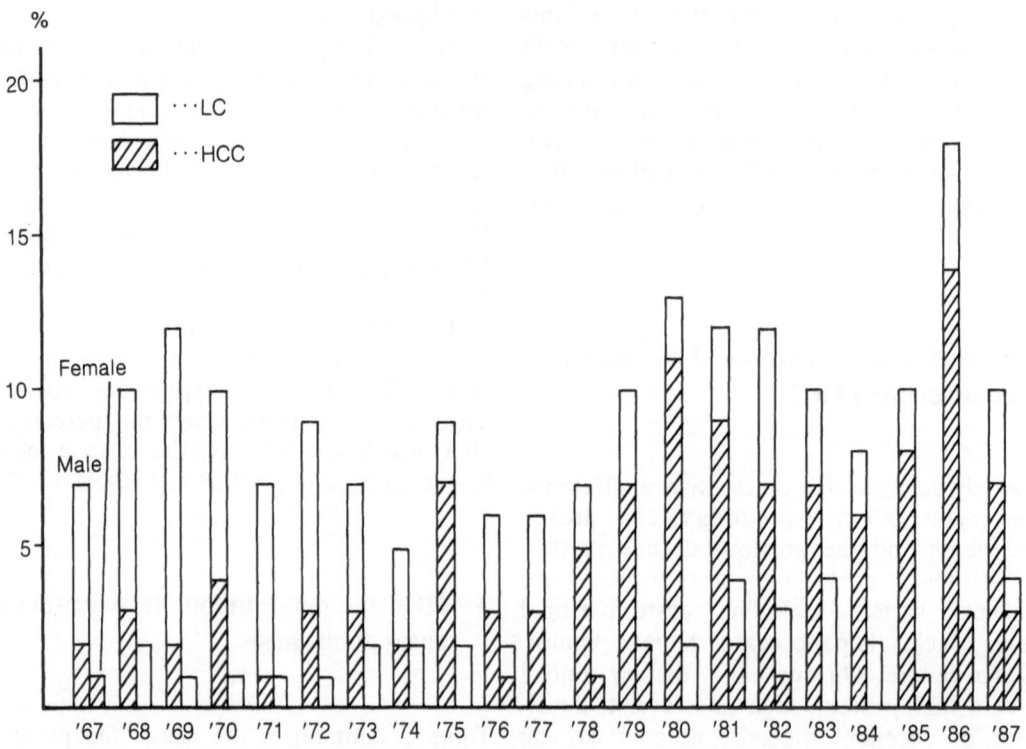

Fig. 2. Number of HCC-diagnosed cases among liver cirrhosis cases (autopsy) (1967–1987)

Table 1. Cases and findings

Case No.	Age	Sex	Years of cirrhosis or severe hepatopathy	Years since blood transfusion	Alcohol-induced cirrhosis	HBs Ag	HBs Ab	ICG (%) 3–5 years ago	ICG (%) now or at death	Hepaplastin test (%) 3–5 years ago	Hepaplastin test (%) now or at death	Maximum albumin value (g/dl)	Minimum albumin value	Esophageal varices	HCC	Ascites	Encephalopathy In progress	Encephalopathy now or at death	Jaundice in progress	Diabetes	Cause or outcome
1	50	M	6	–	+	+	–	41	56	54	38	4.1	3.0	+	+	+	+	+	–	+	HBV carrier, dead
2	69	F	8	+36	–	–	–	26	32	70	82	4.4	3.8	–	+	–	–	–	–	+	Non-A non-B type hepatitis
3	52	F	8	–	+	–	–	38	40	62	58	3.6	2.8	+	–	+	+	–	–	+	Alcohol
4	55	M	13	–	+	–	–	42	46	58	45	4.0	2.6	+	–	+	+	–	+	+	Alcohol
5	55	M	10	–	+	+	–	40	36	42	44	3.8	2.6	+	+	+	–	+	+	+	Alcohol, HBV carrier, dead
6	53	F	6	+15	±	–	–	28	30	74	80	4.1	3.6	–	–	–	–	–	–	–	Non-A non-B type hepatitis
7	42	M	8	–	+	–	–	24	16	62	68	4.0	3.8	+	–	–	–	–	–	–	Alcohol
8	55	M	6	–	–	+	–	40	42	58	54	3.8	3.1	+	–	–	–	–	–	–	HBV carrier
9	67	M	9	–	+	–	–	28	36	62	70	4.2	2.8	+	+	+	–	+	+	+	Alcohol, dead
10	59	M	11	+33	+	–	–	41	46	44	38	4.0	2.6	+	–	+	–	+	+	+	Alcohol, dead
11	63	F	12	–	–	–	–	54	48	44	35	4.0	2.6	+	+	+	–	–	+	–	Non-A non-B type hepatitis
12	61	M	6	+28	±	–	–	44	46	41	40	4.1	2.6	+	+	+	–	+	+	+	Non-A non-B type hepatitis, dead
13	56	M	7	–	+	+	–	38	42	52	35	3.8	3.0	+	+	+	–	+	+	+	HBV carrier, dead
14	66	F		+22	–	–	–	28	26	74	72	4.4	4.1	–	+	–	–	–	–	–	Non-A non-B type hepatitis
15	48	M	5	–	±	+	–	30	32	66	70	4.1	3.6	+	+	–	–	–	–	–	HBV carrier
16	51	M	4	–	–	–	–	28	26	74	72	4.0	4.0	+	–	–	–	–	–	–	Non-A non-B type hepatitis
17	59	M	12	–	+	–	–	36	54	60	35	4.1	2.4	+	–	+	+	+	+	+	Alcohol, dead
18	64	M	15	–	+	–	–	40	46	48	40	4.2	2.8	+	–	+	–	–	–	+	Alcohol
19	32	F	2	+9	–	–	–	32	28	72	78	4.1	3.9	+	–	–	–	–	–	–	Non-A non-B type hepatitis
20	56	M	7	+22	–	–	–	36	40	52	46	3.9	4.1	–	+	–	–	–	–	–	Non-A non-B type hepatitis

This group consisted of 14 males and 6 females between 32–69 years of age. The time elapsed since the initial diagnosis of cirrhosis ranged from 2–15 years (mean 8.1 years). The patients' history regarding blood transfusions, alcohol consumption, and HBs antigen/antibody titer were taken into consideration. Five patients were diagnosed as hepatitis B carriers, 8 patients as non-A, non-B hepatitis carriers, and 8 cases were caused by alcohol consumption. In one case, the patient was diagnosed as being a hepatitis B carrier in association with heavy alcohol consumption. In these 20 patients, 10 developed HCC. The mean age of the three hepatitis B carriers was relatively young at 52 years. One had been diagnosed with cirrhosis for over 10 years, and another had associated HCC appearing within the last 1–2 years. It is remarkable that the hepatitis B carriers developed HCC at a relatively young age [3, 4]. However, 5 patients out of the 8 non-A, non-B hepatitis carriers with a history of blood transfusion were diagnosed with HCC. In this group, 4 patients were over 60 years old, with the mean age being 63 years old.

A difference of ten years has been reported between the onset of cirrhosis caused by the hepatitis B virus and cirrhosis caused by non-A, non-B hepatitis in patients with a history of blood transfusion. This tendency was also noted in the 20 cases reported in this paper.

Of the patients with cirrhosis caused by non-A, non-B-type hepatitis, three were diagnosed without HCC, but the patients were relatively young (50, 51, and 32 years old). However, the chances of being diagnosed with HCC within the next 10 years are quite high.

The 8 alcoholic cirrhosis patients were 42–67 years of age, and the mean age was 56 years. It is difficult to discuss the incidence of HCC in patients with alcoholic cirrhosis because there are many variables involved, such as the duration of drinking history, as well as the quantity of alcohol consumed. However, cirrhosis can occur at a relatively young age when associated with a high alcohol intake.

It is said that HCC is seldom caused by alcoholic cirrhosis. In these eight patients, only one was diagnosed with HCC. The details of this case with HCC are unknown, but a link with non-A, non-B hepatitis cannot be ignored.

Cases of alcoholic cirrhosis with associated HCC must be examined, including a test for the hepatitis C antibody as well as hepatitis B and non-A, non-B hepatitis virus carrier status.

4 Progression of HCC and deterioration of liver function

Although the natural progression of liver cirrhosis is ultimately fatal, it is interesting to study how liver function changes during progression of the disease. A comparison of the results of a blood examination of the patients with fatal cases of liver cirrhosis with associated HCC (13 males, 2 females), and the 9 patients with liver cirrhosis but without HCC (6 males, 3 females) at 1 month, 1 year, and 2 years prior to each death was performed. The mean age was 60 years old. In the patients having cirrhosis with HCC, the mean time from the diagnosis of cirrhosis to death was 4 years and 11 months, and from diagnosis of HCC to death was over 1 year and 8 months. For cirrhosis without HCC, the mean time from diagnosis to death was 3 years and 10 months.

As for viral markers, five of the patients with HCC were positive for HBs antigen, three were positive for HBe antigen, four were positive for antibody, and two were positive for hepatitis C antibody. Of the cases without HCC, two were HBs antigen positive, one HBe antigen postive, and one was antibody positive.

With regard to the cause of death in the HCC-diagnosed patients, 11 suffered hepatic failure caused by enlargement of the HCC, 2 suffered respiratory failure caused by metastasis to the lung, and 2 had rupture of esophageal varices. In the fatal cirrhosis cases without HCC, 5 suffered rupture of esophageal varices, 2 died from sepsis, one from cerebral bleeding and one from pneumonia.

Figures 3 and 4 show the blood test factors, coagulation factors, and the liver function test results from the fatal cases of cirrhosis with and without HCC. No significant difference was found in the results of the blood and coagulation tests between the cirrhosis cases with and without HCC. However, the biliary enzymes lactate dehydrogenase (LDH), leucine aminopeptidase (LAP) and, γ-glutamyl transpeptidase (γ-GTP) increased significantly in each stage of cirrhosis with associated HCC compared to those cases without HCC (Figs. 5 and 6). This may suggest that in cirrhosis with HCC, the biliary enzymes increase in the early stages due to the presence of the tumor. However, it was clearly indicated that impairment of hepatocytes and coagulation factors were not strongly correlated to the presence of HCC.

There was no difference in the NH_3 value, an indicator for liver failure, between cases of

Fig. 3. Peripheral blood tests. *Hb*, hemoglobin; *Ht*, hematocrit; *PLT*, platelet; *light shading*, liver cirrhosis with hepatoma; *dark shading*, liver cirrhosis without hepatoma

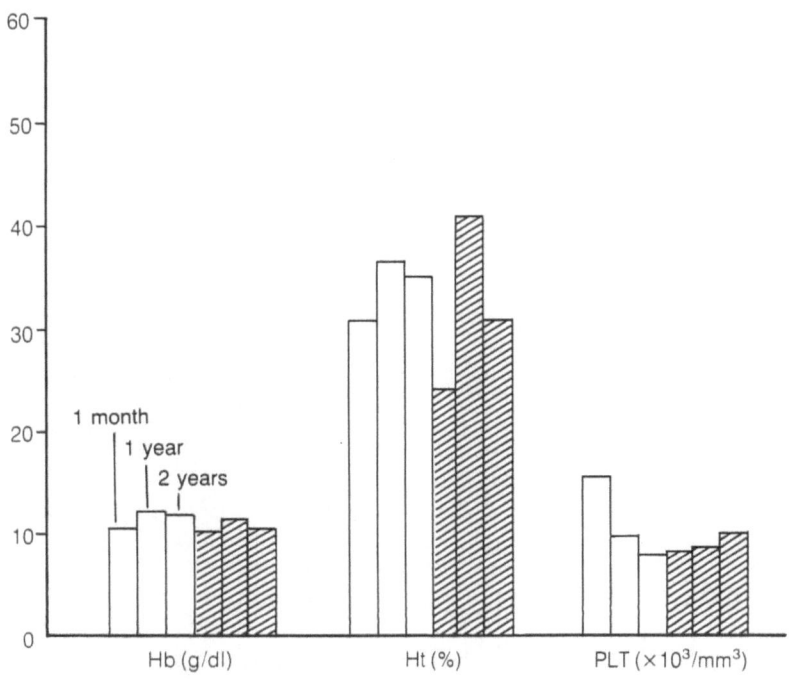

Fig. 4. Blood coagulation tests. *HPT*, hepaplastin test; *TT*, thrombo test; *Light shading*, Liver cirrhosis with hepatoma; *Dark shading*, Liver cirrhosis without hepatoma

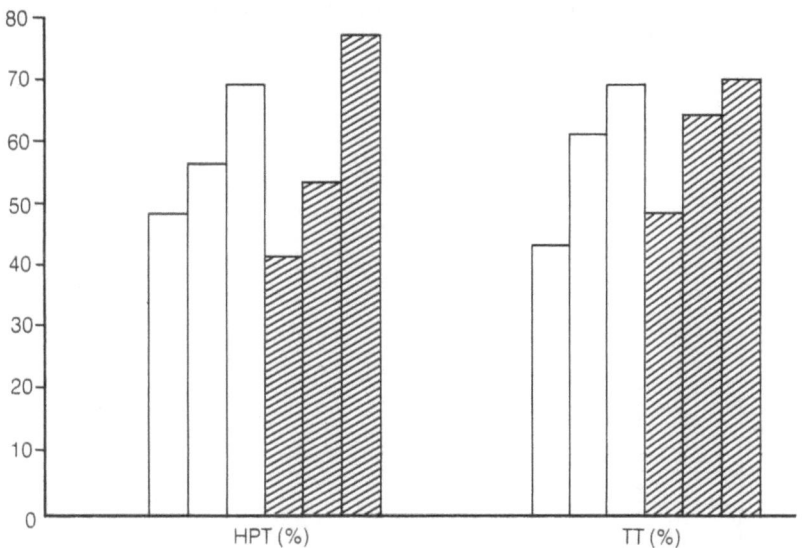

cirrhosis with and without HCC. The tumor marker alpha fetoprotein (AFP), demonstrates a clear difference between cases of cirrhosis with and without HCC, but it was remarkable that almost every case with HCC showed near normal values even one month prior to death [5, 6]. The values of NH_3 were 270 ± 616, $256 \pm 2,818$ and $6,124 \pm 164,261$ ng/dl at 2 years, 1 year and 1 month prior to death, respectively.

The stagnation rate of $ICGR_{15}$, which is thought to be an indicator of reserve liver function, also increased to $35 \pm 9\%$, $30 \pm 1\%$, and $11 \pm 17\%$ at 2 years, 1 year, and 1 month before death, respectively [7]. Tables 2 and 3 show the

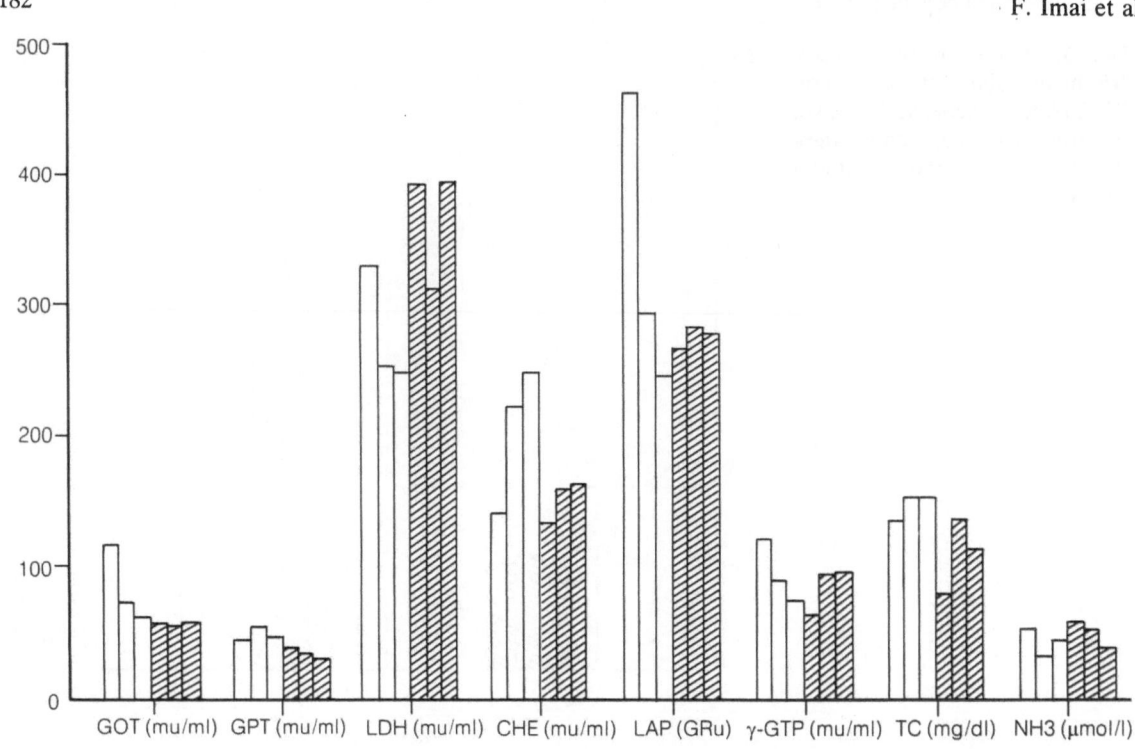

Fig. 5. Biochemistry(I) *GOT*, glutamic oxaloacetate transaminase; *GPT*, glutamate pyruvate transaminase; *LDH*, lactate dehydrogenase; *CHE*, cholinesterase; *LAP*, leucine aminopeptidase; γ-*GTP*, gamma-glutamyl transpeptidase; *TC*, total cholesterol; *light shading*, liver cirrhosis with hepatoma; *dark shading*, liver cirrhosis without hepatoma

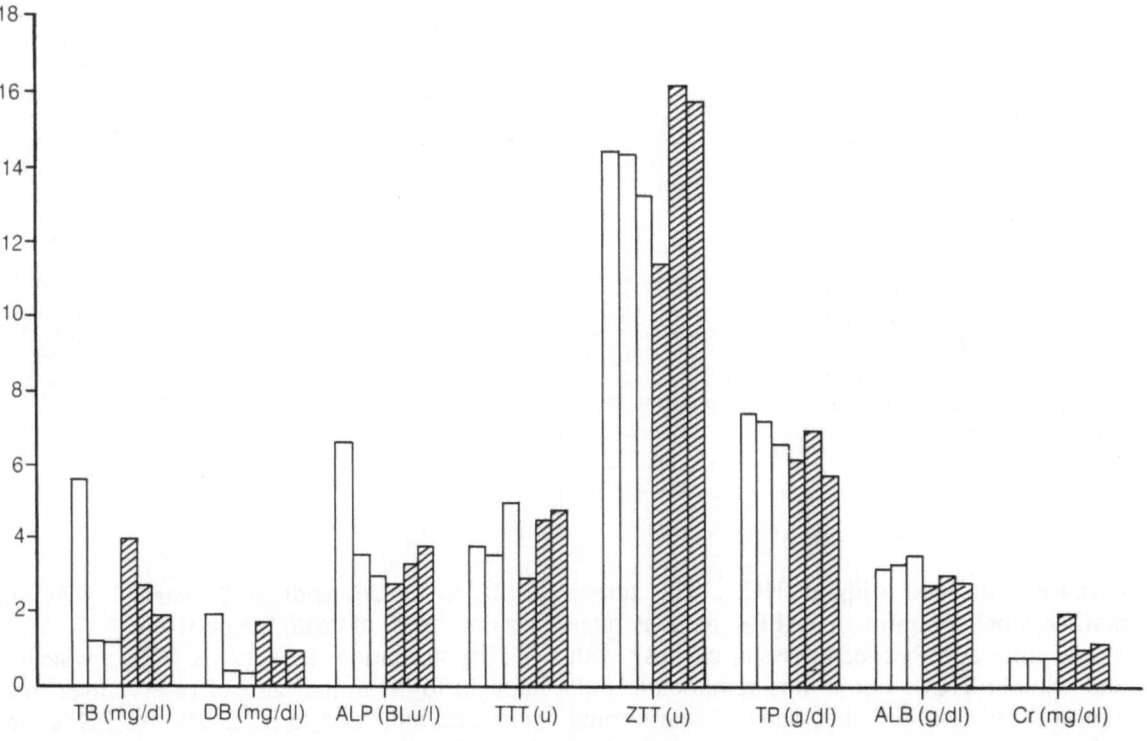

Fig. 6. Biochemistry(II) *TB*, total bilirubin; *DB*, direct bilirubin; *TTT*, thymol turbidity test; *ZTT*, zinc turbidity test; *TP*, total protein; *ALB*, albumin; *Cr*, creatinine; *Light shading*, Liver cirrhosis with hepatoma; *Dark shading*, Liver cirrhosis without hepatoma

Table 2. Tumor marters and ICG-R$_{15}$ (LC with HCC)

	AFP (ng/ml)	CEA (ng/ml)	CA 19-9 (U/ml)	PIVKA-II (AU/ml)	ICGR$_{15}$ (%)
1 month before death	6,124 ± 164,261	4 ± 3	59 ± 43	1 ± 2	41 ± 17
1 year before death	1,256 ± 2,818	4 ± 6	38 ± 31	0 ± 0	30 ± 1
2 years before death	270 ± 616	1 ± 1	39 ± 24	9 ± 9	35 ± 9

AFP, alpha fetoprotein; CEA, carcinoembryonic antigen; CA19-9, carbohydrate antigen 19-9; PIVKA-II, protein induced by vitamin K absence-II; ICGR$_{15}$, indocyanine green reduction

Table 3. Tumor marker and ICG-R$_{15}$ (LC withoit HCC)

	AFP (ng/ml)	CEA (ng/ml)	CA 19-9 (U/ml)	PIVKA-II (AU/ml)	ICGR$_{15}$ (%)
1 month before death	38 ± 83	2 ± 1	62 ± 38	0 ± 0	40 ± 31
1 year before death	19 ± 10	2 ± 1	44 ± 19	—	37 ± 20
2 years before death	7 ± 6	—	—	—	7 ± 7

See Table 2 for definitions

clinically observed values for various tumor markers and their relation to cirrhosis cases both with and without HCC.

5 Conclusion

Most cases of primary HCC observed in our department occurred during the observation period of cirrhosis. Better therapy for cirrhosis and the concomitant prolongation of life expectancy of cirrhotic patients has lead to an increase of cirrhosis with associated HCC. Comparing cirrhosis cases with HCC in the last decade before death and the previous decade, it has been confirmed by our clinical experience and by autopsy cases in our department. To elucidate the changes in liver function caused by HCC, liver function test results, NH$_3$, tumor markers, and ICGR$_{15}$ were studied, and a comparison of cirrhotic patients with and without HCC was carried out. Significant differences were found in the biliary enzymes, tumor markers, and ICGR$_{15}$ values.

References

1. Tanikawa K, Tanaka M (1990) Liver function in hepatocellular carcinoma. Jpn J Clin Exp Med 67:88–92
2. Imai F, Kameda H (1990) Natural history of liver cirrhosis. Geka Shinryo 32:173–182
3. Kiyosawa K (1991) Occurrence of hepatocellular carcinoma in association with clinical progress. Jpn J Cancer Dig Organs 1:43–51
4. Kiyosawa K, Akahane Y, Nagata A, et al. (1984) Hepatocellular carcinoma after non-A, non-B post-transfusion hepatitis. Am J Gastroenterol 79:777–781
5. Endo Y (1987) Subtype AFP (in Japanese). Kan Tan Sui 14:767–774
6. Okuda K (1988) Symptomatology and test results of primary hepatocellular carcinoma. Jpn J Clin Med 574:60–66
7. Takase S (1982) Total functioning hepatic cell mass for assessment of prognosis in liver cirrhosis. Jpn J Gastroenterol 79:1589–1596

CHAPTER 18

Hepatic functional reserve and surgical indication in primary liver cancer

Ryuji Mizumoto and Takashi Noguchi[1]

1 Introduction

Radical hepatectomy is the most effective means of treatment for hepatocellular carcinoma (HCC), however a number of HCC patients who also have cirrhosis show a deterioration of hepatic function after hepatectomy, some developing postoperative hepatic insufficiency [1, 2, 3]. Approximately 20 years ago, one of us pointed out that the indication of hepatectomy for HCC associated with cirrhosis was remarkably limited and its determination should be based on a preoperative estimation of hepatic functional reserve [4]. Since then, hepatectomy has been successfully performed even on cirrhotic patients in accordance with their individual preoperative risk factors at various medical institutions in Japan. This has resulted in longer survival as well as decreased mortality and morbidity after surgery.

In this report, we describe selection of the most suitable surgical procedure considering the preoperative risk for HCC patients with cirrhosis in our department, and also our clinical trials to extend the hepatic resectability for patients of critical risk.

2 Review of HCC patients treated surgically in our department

2.1 Types of surgical treatment

From the begining of October 1976 to the end of December 1990, 189 adult patients with primary liver cancer were treated surgically in our depart-

ment. These comprised 157 HCCs, 26 cholangiocellular carcinomas, 4 cystic adenocarcinomas and 2 malignant mixed tumors. Out of the 157 patients with HCC, 134 (85.4%) were associated with liver cirrhosis. One hundred fifty-eight (83.6%) of 189 operated patients with primary liver cancer underwent hepatic resection. This included one hundred thirty-five (86.0%) of the 157 HCCs patients, 115 (85.8%) of the 134 cirrhotic patients, 18 (69.2%) of the 26 with cholangiocellular carcinoma, all 4 with cystic adenocarcinoma and one (50%) of the 2 with malignant mixed tumor. We have always attempted, whenever possible, to perform radical hepatectomy for liver cancer, even for patients with cirrhosis. Among the 135 hepatectomy patients with HCC, the extent of hepatic resection was as follows: according to Healey's classification of the liver segments [5], 5 underwent resection of 3 segments; 11 underwent resection of over 2 segments, such as extended lobectomy; 26 underwent resection of 2 segments; 35 underwent resection of one segment, and 58 underwent subsegment or partial resection. The remaining 22 patients with unresectable HCC underwent palliative operations: 17 had ligation of the hepatic artery or portal vein branch, and 5 had continuous infusion of anti-cancer drugs through a catheter in the hepatic artery. On the other hand, during the same period, we experienced 30 non-operated HCCs associated with cirrhosis which were treated with transcatheter arterial embolization (TAE) [6] because of poor hepatic functional reserve and/or extensive intrahepatic metastases.

2.2 Operative results and postoperative course

As defined in our previous report [7], patients with intractable ascites, jaundice, or a tendency

[1] 1st Department of Surgery, Mie University School of Medicine, Tsushi, Mie, 514 Japan

Table 1. Operative results and postoperative course in hepatocellular carcinoma patients, including patients treated with transcatheter arterial embolization (TAE)

	No. of patients	No. of patients with severe liver dysfunction and hepatic insufficiency after treatment	No. of patients who died because of hepatic insufficiency after operation or TAE[b]	
			within one month	within 1–6 months
Operation				
Hepatectomy	135	26 (19.3)	5 (3.7)	8 (5.9)
[with cirrhosis]	[115]	[23 (20.0)]	[5 (4.3)]	[7 (6.1)]
Nonhepatectomy	22	6 (27.2)	2 (9.1)	2 (9.1)
[with cirrhosis]	[19]	[5 (26.3)]	[2 (10.5)]	[2 (10.5)]
Total	157	32 (20.4)	7 (4.5)	10 (6.4)
[with cirrhosis]	[134]	[28 (20.9)]	[7 (5.2)]	[9 (6.7)]
No operation (TAE[a])	30	7 (23.3)	2 (6.7)	3 (10.0)

Figures in parentheses represents the percentage
[a] All patients were associated with cirrhosis
[b] In operated patients or in TAE patients

to bleed after surgery and who showed no improvement after more than one moth, were judged to have severe liver dysfunction. In particular, these included patients with postoperative hepatic insufficiency associated with a hepatic coma of grade II or worse according to the classifications of the Japanese Fulminant Hepatitis Association. Grade II insuffiency requires that 4 or more out of the following 6 blood chemistry items are met: total bilirubin (T-Bil) above 10 mg/dl; transaminase (GOT or GPT) over 200 U/L; ammonia over 100 μg/ml; hepaplastin test (HPT) below 40%, which is also called normotest; lecithin cholesterol acyltransferase (LCAT) below 10 nmol/ml/h; and fibronectin below 150 μg/ml. Among 32 operated patients with primary liver cancer other than HCC, no postoperative severe liver dysfunction or hepatic insufficiency after liver surgery was recognized even in extended hepatectomy. However, among the 157 operated patients with HCC, these complications were recognized in 26 (19.3%) out of 135 hepatectomy patients, including 5 (3.7%) cirrhotic patients with operative death within one month, and in 6 (27.2%) out of 22 nonhepatectomy patients, including 2 (9.1%) patients with operative death. Among these 32 patients with poor postoperative course, 28 (87.5%) were associated with cirrhosis, 17 dying of hepatic insufficiency within 6 months after surgery, including 7 patients with operative death. Also, 4 of the 115 hepatectomy patients with cirrhosis developed disseminated intravascular coagulation syndrome (DIC) after surgery, which led to severe liver dysfunction. Further,

among 30 patients with cirrhosis treated with TAE, severe liver dysfunction even after TAE was recognized in 7 (23.3%), including 2 patients (6.7%) with hepatic insufficiency who died within one month (Table 1). On the other hand, since we established the preoperative risk evaluation of hepatic resectability at the end of December, 1986 [7], operative death has not been experienced and cases with severe liver dysfunction after surgery have been remarkably decreasing over the past 4 years.

2.3 Long-term prognosis

2.3.1 Survival rates

Cumulative survival rates of HCC patients with resection or TAE are shown in Fig. 1, excluding postoperative death within 1 month. Survival rates after hepatectomy were calculated according to curability as defined by the general rules of the Liver Cancer Study Group of Japan [8]. Comparing the 5-year survival rates among types of resection, we found 100% in the absolute curative resection, 59.1% in the relative curative resection, 10.9% in the relative noncurative resection and no survivors of more than 4 years in the absolute noncurative resection. In the cirrhotic patients, the main causes of death were hepatic insufficiency and tumor recurrence. In the noncirrhotic patients, cancers were generally more advanced, and most died of tumor recurrence within 2 years. Conversely, only one out of 22 unresectable patients survived 3 years and 2 months after hepatic artery ligation. Moreover,

Fig. 1. Cumulative survival rate after resection or TAE for hepatocellular carcinoma (Kaplan-Meier's method), excluding patients who died within 1 month. *Open squares*, absolute curative resection (n = 11); *solid circles*, absolute non-curative resection (n = 12); *open circles*, relative curative resection (n = 39); *thin line*, TAE (n = 28); *thick line*, all resected patients (n = 130); *dotted line*, palliative operation (n = 20); *open triangles* relative non-curative resection (n = 68)

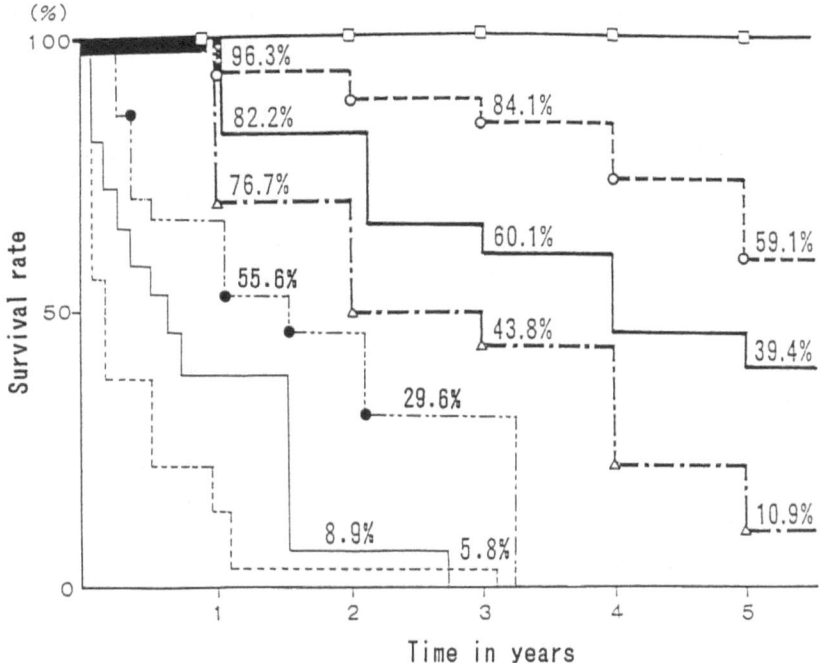

Table 2. Extent of hepatic resection and prognosis of patients with hepatocellular carcinoma—cumulative 1-year and 3-year survival rates, excluding death from hepatic insufficiency within 6 months after hepatectomy. 115 (85.2%) of all 135 resected patients were associated with liver cirrhosis

		Extent of hepatic resection					
		3 segments	2–3 segments	2 segments	1 segment	subsegment	less than a subsegment
Tumor presented segment	H_3	100 → 0	67 → 0				
	H_2		100 → 100	67 → 33	40 → 0		
	H_1			100 → 100	88 → 33	60 → 0	
	H_s			100 → 100	100 → 75	100 → 44	50 → 25
	H_0				100 → 100	100 → 100	100

H_3, H_2, H_1, and H_s, tumor located in 3 segments, 2 segments, 1 segment, and subsegment, respectively; H_0, a single tumor of 2 cm or less at its greatest dimension without vascular invasion and located within one subsegment; *hatched area*, cumulative 1-year survival rate; *dotted area*, cumulative 3-year survival rate

R. Mizumoto and T. Noguchi

Table 3. Extent of hepatic resection and prognosis of patients with hepatocellular carcinoma—rate of development of hepatic insufficiency within 6 months after hepatectomy. 13 (9.6%) of all 135 resected patients developed hepatic insufficiency

		Extent of hepatic resection					
		3 segments	2–3 segments	2 segments	1 segment	subsegment	less than a subsegment
Tumor presented segment	H_3	50%	33%				
	H_2		67%	38%	0%		
	H_1			67%	13%	0%	
	H_s, H_0			50%	50%	23%	25%

H_3, H_2, H_1, H_s, H_0, see Table 2

among the 30 patients with TAE, there were no survivors longer than 3 years (Fig. 1).

2.3.2 Prognosis in relation to the HCC presented segment and extent of hepatectomy

Regarding the one-year and three-year survival rates, excluding deaths from hepatic insufficiency within 6 months after hepatectomy, all patients in whom the extent of hepatectomy was wider than the tumor presented segment (H) survived for over 3 years, as indicated on the left side of the heavy line in Table 2. The only exception is the patients with one segmentectomy for Hs whose 3-year survival rate was 75%. However, the three-year survival rate was very low for patients in whom the extent of hepatectomy was approximately equal to the tumor presented segment, as indicated on the right side of the heavy line in the same table. These results suggest the necessity of extensive hepatectomy beyond the tumor presented segment in order to prolong survival. On the other hand, Table 3 shows the incidence of deaths due to hepatic insufficiency within 6 months after hepatectomy. Postoperative death due to hepatic insufficiency occurred in more than half of the patients in whom the extent of hepatectomy was wider than the tumor presented segment. However, the postoperative mortality due to hepatic insufficiency was lower in patients in whom the extent of hepatectomy was approximately equal to the tumor presented segment (Table 3). These results indicate that extensive hepatectomy is required to prevent cancer recurrence, but that the extent of hepatectomy has to be minimized to prevent postoperative hepatic insufficiency. Hepatic surgeons must select a suitable operative method based on the functional resectability of the liver, taking into accout the pathological characteristics of HCC [3, 7, 9, 10]

3 Preoperative estimation of surgical risk based on hepatic cell function

3.1 Overall evaluation of the results of various liver function tests

Because the liver has many and varied functions, it is too difficult to completely evaluate the hepatic function with a single test, even a very sensitive test. Therefore, preoperative estimation of surgical risk must be assessed by taking into account the distinctive character of each hepatic function test.

3.1.1 Clinical stage of HCC patients according to the general rules by Liver Cancer Study Group of Japan [8]

The parameters of this clinical stage comprise 2 liver function tests, including indocyanine green retention rate at 15 min ($ICGR_{15}$), prothrombin activity (PT), and items of Child's criteria [11]. Three stages are defined for the degree of liver function. This classification refers to one I defined

Table 4. Various parameters for preoperative risk estimation in cirrhotic patients at the leading medical institutions in Japan

	T-Bil	ICG R_{max}	K	R_{15}	Alb	Ch-E	LCAT	PT	PTT	HPT	GOT	GPT	OGTT	AKBR	WHVP	Ascites	Age	Other[a]
1st Dept. of Surgery, Hokkaido University	●	●			●	●		●	●	●			●			●		●
1st Dept. of Surgery, Tohoku University			●	●	●			●			●					●		●
1st Dept. of Surgery, Tokyo University		●		●	●			●					●			●		●
National Cancer Center Hospital	●			●												●		
Tokyo Women's Medical College				●														
2nd Dept. of Surgery, Juntendo University	●		●	●	●			●		●								
1st Dept. of Surgery, Niigata University	●		●		●	●		●								●		●
1st Dept. of Surgery, Yamanashi Medical College													●	●				
1st Dept. of Surgery, Aichi Medical University		●	●							●					●			
1st Dept. of Surgery, Mie University	●	●	●		●	●	●	●		●	●		●					●
2nd Dept. of Surgery, Kyoto University	●		●										●	●				
1st Dept. of Surgery, Kobe University		●																●
1st Dept. of Surgery, Hyogo College of Medicine		●		●													●	
1st Dept. of Surgery, Okayama University																		●
2nd Dept. of Surgery, Hiroshima University	●		●		●	●		●			●	●				●		
2nd Dept. of Surgery, Ehime University	●		●		●			●			●							
2nd Dept. of Surgery, Kyushu University				●														
2nd Dept. of Surgery, Nagasaki University	●	●	●	●	●	●		●	●	●	●	●				●		●
1st Dept. of Surgery, Kumamoto University	●	●	●								●							●
Total 19 institutions (%)	10 (52.6)	8 (42.1)	10 (52.6)	8 (42.1)	9 (47.4)	5 (26.3)	1 (5.3)	9 (47.4)	2 (10.5)	5 (26.3)	6 (31.6)	2 (10.5)	5 (26.3)	2 (10.5)	1 (5.3)	7 (36.8)	1 (5.3)	9 (47.4)

ICG, indocyanine green; T-Bil, serum total bilirubin; R_{max}, ICG maximal removal rate; K, disappearance rate; R_{15}, ICG retention rate at 15 mins; Alb, serum albumin; Ch-E, cholinesterase; LCAT, lecithin cholesterol acyltransferase; PT, prothrombin time; PTT, partial thromboplastin time; HPT, hepaplastin test; GOT, glutamic oxaloacetic transaminase; GPT, glutamate-pyruvate transaminase; OGTT, oral glucose tolerance test; AKBR, arterial ketone body ratio; WHVP, wedged hepatic venous pressure; Shading, more than 40%
[a] Including ALP, γ-globulin, mental confusion, nutritional assessment, and so on

20 years ago [4]. Although these parameters are clinically easy to use for estimating operability, they are not sufficient to select the most suitable operative procedure.

3.1.2 Preoperative risk evaluation in the leading institutions in Japan

Various parameters, two or more, are being used at each institution to evaluate risk. Among 19 institutions, 10 (52.6%) are using total serum bilirubin (T-Bil) and ICG disappearance rate (K_{ICG}); 9 (47.4%) are using the serum albumin (Alb) and prothrombin time (PT); 8 (42.1%) use the ICG maximal removal rate (R_{max}) and $ICGR_{15}$; 7 (36.8%) use the degree of ascites; and more than 2 institutions are using other parameters such as GOT, HPT, also called normotest, and so on (Table 4). Risk evaluation among the main institutions is as follows:

1. *Hokkadio University* (1st Dept. of Surgery) [12]: Operative risk is estimated from overall

results of several parameters such as $ICGR_{max}$, blood sugar curve of oral glucose tolerance test (OGTT), HPT and routine liver function tests selected by the chi-square statistical test. In addition to these parameters, hepatic functional reserve is evaluated by the response of plasma cyclic-AMP in the glucagon tolerance test.

2. *Tokyo University* (1st Dept. of Surgery) [13]: Operative risk is estimated by calculating the weight of individual parameters. The weight of liver function tests are added to the degree of ascites and the age of patients using linear discrimination. In particular, $ICGR_{max}$, prothrombin time and the linearity index in OGTT are important parameters for estimation of the extent of hepatectomy.

3. *Kyoto University* (2nd Dept. of Surgery): Ozawa utilized the pattern of the blood sugar curve after an OGTT [14] and more recently measured the ratio of ketones in arterial blood (AKBR), further developing the Redox theory [15]. The measurement of AKBR in the perioperative stage is very useful to estimate the postoperative course of hepatectomy or liver transplantation.

4. *Hyogo Medical School* (1st Dept. of Surgery) [16]: Prognostic score for operability is estimated based on the reliability of each risk factor in hepatectomy using multivariate analysis. Important risk factors are the hepatic resection rate calculated by X-ray computed tomography, $ICGR_{15}$, age of patient, and $ICGR_{max}$.

3.1.3 Total risk and the results of hepatic surgery in our department

In order to estimate heaptic functional reserve accurately, it is necessary to evaluate the overall results of various hepatic function tests, but the results of these different tests do not all indicate the same grade for any given patient. Therefore, to estimate the liver function in determining operability before surgery, we use total risk employing multivariate analysis. As indicated in our previous reports [3, 7], the following 10 tests were found to be highly reliable for estimating surgical risk: Serum albumin (Alb), GOT, T-Bil, cholinesterase (Ch-E), PT, K_{ICG}, $ICGR_{max}$, 75 g OGTT, HPT and LCAT. The results of these tests were classified into grades I to V (low to high risk), and also the predictive reliability of each test in terms of surgical risk was expressed as a weight in the statistics (Table 5). Therefore, the total risk could be calculated from the grade and weight of each test using a load mean method as expressed in the following formula:

Total risk
$$= \frac{\Sigma a_n \cdot G_n(a_1 \cdot G_1 + a_2 \cdot G_2 + \ldots + a_n \cdot G_n)}{\Sigma a_n(a_1 + a_2 + \ldots + a_n)}$$

where a_{1-n} is the predictive reliability-weight of each test and G_{1-n} is the grade of each test.

Table 5. Grade of hepatic function and predictive reliability—Weight of each test

hepatic function test \ Grade	I	II	III	IV	V	Weight
Alb (g/dl)	~4.0	~3.5	~3.0	~2.5	2.5~	16
GOT (U/L)	~50	~100	~200	~300	300~	11
[a] T-Bil (mg/dl)	~0.5	~1.0	~2.0	~3.0	3.0~	21
Ch-E (Δ pH)	~1.0	~0.8	~0.5	~0.3	0.3~	25
PT (%)	~100	~80	~60	~40	40~	15
K_{ICG} (/min)	~0.15	~0.10	~0.06	~0.03	0.03~	32
$ICGR_{max}$ (mg/kg/min)	~2.0	~1.0	~0.4	~0.2	0.2~	37
[b] OGTT	N	B—P	D—P	P—L	L	20
HPT (%)	~100	~70	~50	~30	30~	30
LCAT (n mol/ml/hr)	~80	~60	~40	~20	20~	36

N, normal type; B—P, parabolic type in the cases with the impaired glucose tolerance; D—P, parabolic type in the cases with type of diabetes mellitus; P—L, transient type from parabolic type to linear type; L, linear type
[a] the cases with obstructive jaundice are excluded
[b] the cases with disturbance of pancreatic endocrine function are excluded

Table 6. Relationship between total risk measured by multivariate analysis preoperatively and postoperative course of hepatocellular carcinoma

operative method \ total risk	1	2	3	4	5
tri-segmentectomy	○ ○ △	△ ⊗			
2~3 segmentectomy	○○○○ ○ ○ △	⊗ ⊗ △	⊗		
2 segmentectomy	○ ○ ○	○○○○○ ○○○○○ ○○○	⊗ ⊗	⊗	
1 segmentectomy	○ ○	○○○○○ ○○○○○	○○○○△○ ○○○○ ○	○ △ △ ⊗	
sub-segmentectomy or partial resection	○ ○ ○	○○○○○ ○○○○○ ○○○○○	○○○○○△ ○○○○○○ ○○○○○○	○ △ △ ⊗ ⊗ ○○○ △ △ ○○○○ ⊗	⊗ ⊗
ligation of hepatic artery or portal vein branch	○○○	○○○○	○○○○	○○○⊗⊗	⊗
hepatic artery catheterization for infusion chemotherapy			○	○	⊗ ⊗ ⊗
transcatheter arterial embolization (TAE)		○ ○ ○ ○ ○	○○○○ ○○○○	○ ○○△ ○○△	○ ⊗ ⊗ ⊗ ○○ ⊗ ○○⊗

For the postoperative course, *open circles* signify the patient is well, *triangles* signify the patient has severe liver dysfunction without improvement more than 1 month after surgery, and crossed circles indicate death due to hepatic insufficiency within 6 months after surgery

Furthermore, the total risk was classified into 5 levels. Table 6 shows the relationship between the postoperative course of 192 HCC patients including 30 patients with TAE and their total risk.

In the results of each operation according to total risk, unfavorable cases with severe liver dysfunction after surgery are shown mainly on the right side of the central heavy line in Table 6. It was found that the evaluation of total risk was very important for selection of the safest surgery. Thus, as shown in Table 6, with total risk of 1, resection of more than 2 segments, such as tri-segmentectomy or extended hepatic lobectomy, may be well tolerated; while with total risk 2, hepatic lobectomy may be tolerated; and with total risk 3, segmentectomy is possible. However, if the total risk is 4, liver surgery is limited to subsegmentectomy or partial resection of the liver and ligation of the hepatic artery or portal vein branch. Total risk 5 indicates that any type of surgery is dangerous. In hepatic partial resection or subsegmentectomy, our success rate in

total risk 4 was 50%, while the other 50% of cases had a poor prognois (Fig. 4). Our total risk gradation enabled us to select the most suitable of various operative methods, and its usefulness was confirmed by the prospective study, as shown in detail in our previous paper [7]. However, when using total risk, the characteristics of each hepatic function test must be kept in mind. For instance, the highly sensitive $ICGR_{max}$ test is a very good way to detect changes in hepatic functional reserve, and is extremely useful for estimating liver pathogenesis before and after surgery [17]. On the other hand, if total risk is estimated as 5, TAE may be selected for treatment of HCC. Regardless, we experienced 2 out of 5 patients with total risk 5 who died of hepatic insufficiency within 1 month after TAE. As shown in Fig. 2, TAE is indicated from the viewpoint of liver function when $ICGR_{max}$ was above 0.2 mg/kg/min, K_{ICG} was above 0.04/min, $ICGR_{15}$ was below 50%, LCAT was above 10 nmol/ml/hr, HPT was above 50%, and T-Bil was below 3.0 mg/dl.

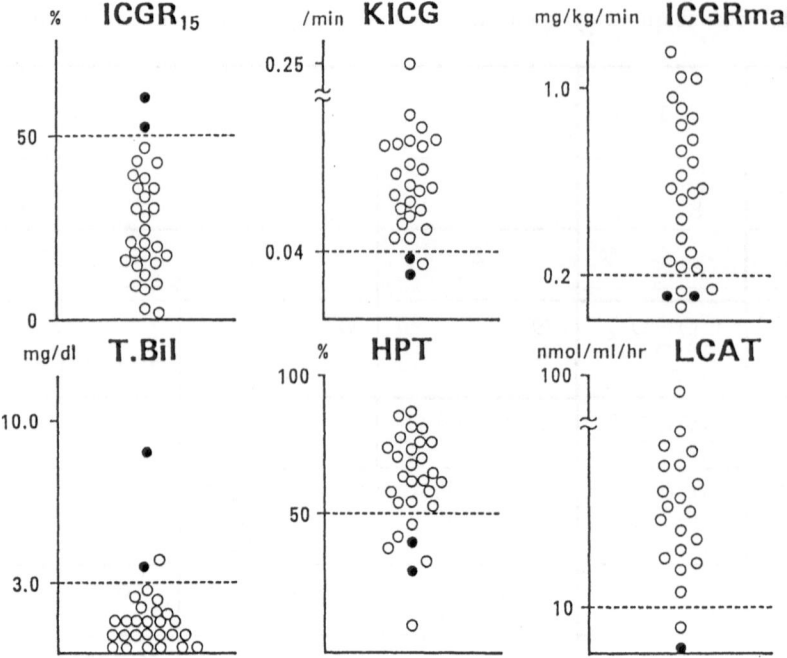

Fig. 2. Functional indication of TAE for hepatocellular carcinoma. *Open circle*, alive more than 1 month after TAE; *solid circle*, dead within 1 month after TAE; *dotted line*, critical level. See Table 4 for other definitions

3.2 Functional reserve of the remnant liver after hepatectomy

The results of our total risk evaluation reflect whole liver function which may well diminish after hepatectomy. Because hepatectomy includes resection not only of tumor but also of functional liver parenchyma, prognosis will obviously be poor if, as a result of extensive resection, the remnant liver function drops below a critical level. Therefore, if the remnant liver function following hepatectomy could be predicted prior to surgery, it would be very useful for estimating the operability of the liver.

3.2.1 Measurement of remnant liver function
Takasaki [18] evaluated every liver segment function by measuring the extraction rate of ICG in each segment using hepatic vein catheterization, and pointed out that hepatectomy could be performed if the extraction rate of ICG in the remnant liver was below 40%. Mimura et al. [19] developed the estimation method of expected residual hepatic blood flow index ($K_{L_{AU}}$) after hepatectomy from hepatic clearance of ^{198}Au-colloid and indicated the functional limited value of $K_{L_{AU}}$ in hepatectomy. Alternatively, the resection rate of the liver has been calculated from measurement of liver volume using X-ray computed tomography. However, the calculated resection rate may differ from the actual rate

when tumor or compensatory hypertrophy are present in the liver, and this result also does not take into account the functional aspect. We have been evaluating the functional liver volume in accordance with the degree of hepatocyte uptake of radioisotope.

3.2.2 ICGR$_{max}$ of the remnant liver in our department
As shown in our previous reports [3, 7, 20, 21], the effective liver volume rate (ELVR) of the remnant liver is measured preoperatively as a ratio of the uptake in the expected remnant area to that in the whole liver on liver scintigraphy using ^{99m}technetium-N-pyridoxyl-5-methyl-tryptophan (^{99m}Tc-PMT). Recently, we have been measuring ELVR by single photon emission computed tomography in order to estimate the functional reserve of the remnant liver. The ELVR is multiplied by ICGR$_{max}$, to quantitatively evaluate hepatic function (on the left in Fig. 3). Most of the patients in which the preoperative ICGR$_{max}$ of the remnant liver was above 0.4 mg/kg/min, had a good postoperative course in terms of functional reserve, irrespective of the type of hepatectomy. In patients with an ICGR$_{max}$ of the remnant liver between 0.4 and 0.2 mg/kg/min, postoperative severe liver dysfunction occurred in about 50% of the patients. In all the patients with this value below 0.2 mg/kg/min, the prognosis was hopeless, so hepatectomy should not be considered in such cases

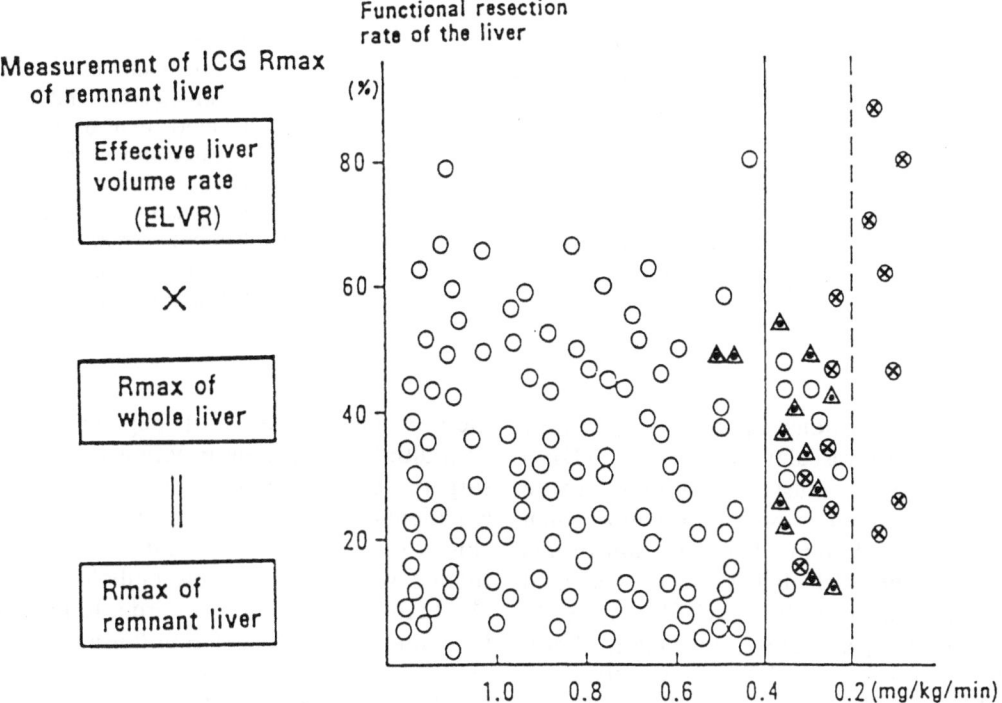

Fig. 3. Relationship between $ICGR_{max}$ or remnant liver estimated preoperatively and postoperative course of hepatocellular carcinoma patients. For the postoperative course, *open circles* indicate the patient is well, *triangles* indicate severe liver dysfunction without improvement more than 1 month after surgery, and *crossed circle* indicate death due to hepatic insufficiency within 6 months after surgery. *Solid line*, critical level; *dotted line*, dangerous level

(Fig. 3). These clear-cut results were confirmed both retrospectively and prospectively in our previous study [7].

3.3 Preoperative estimation of long-term prognosis after hepatectomy in terms of hepatic regenerative capacity

It has been pointed out the there is a discrepancy between the morphological regeneration and functional restoration of the liver after hepatectomy. We evaluated the relationship between the occurrence of postoperative hepatic insufficiency and $ICGR_{max}$ per unit hepatic volume which was calculated by dividing $ICGR_{max}$ of the remnant liver by the remnant liver volume measured on X-ray computed tomography. Patients with $ICGR_{max}$ per unit hepatic volume of the remnant liver of more than $0.8 \mu g/kg/min/cm^3$ survived an average of more than 6 months (Fig. 4) and long-term prognosis was good, showing good functional recovery measured by $ICGR_{max}$ and good morphological

regeneration of the remnant liver examined by X-ray computed tomography after hepatectomy. Half of the patients with values from $0.8-0.5 \mu g/kg/min/cm^3$ died of hepatic insufficiency within 6 months, but survivors had moderate morphological regeneration without functional recovery. All patients below $0.5 \mu g/kg/min/cm^3$ died within 6 months. The usefulness of this parameter was confirmed both retrospectively and prospectively in our previous study [7].

4 Preoperative risk evaluations except for hepatic cell function and extention of hepatic resectability

4.1 DIC risk

We have encountered 4 patients with cirrhosis that developed DIC following hepatectomy, most of them with a critical preoperative total risk and/or remnant hepatic reserve [3, 7, 21]. As

ICGRmax per unit volume of the remnant liver

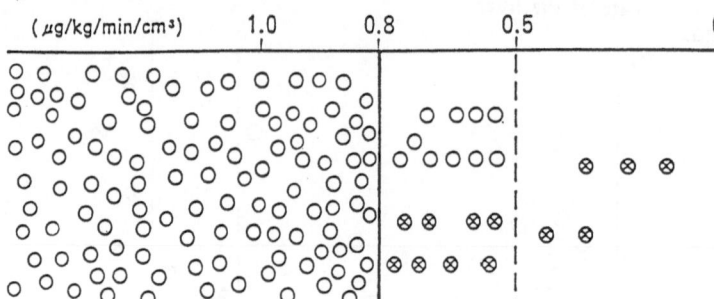

Fig. 4. Relationship between ICGR$_{max}$ per unit volume of remnant liver estimated preoperatively and prognosis at more than 6 months after hepatectomy for hepatocellular carcinoma patients. *Open circle*, alive more than 6 months; *crossed circle*, death due to hepatic insufficiency within 6 months

described in our previous report, a preoperative disseminated intravascular coagulation (DIC) risk in hepatectomy must be considered to be present if the patient is positive for more than 5 of the following 8 items: Platelet count of less than 60,000/mm³, PT below 70%, activated partial thromboplastin time (APTT) above 40 seconds, fibrinogen below 150 mg/dl, fibrin degradation products (FDP) above 10 µg/ml, maximal amplitude (ma) below 30 mm and a thrombodynamic index [ma/Koagulation (K)] less than 2.0 in thromboelastogram, as well as antithrombin (ATIII) below 50%. Out of 113 hepatectomies for HCC patients with cirrhosis, 15 (13.3%) were considered preoperatively to be at DIC risk. Nine patients of these 15, excluding the 6 most recent ones, had a blood loss of more than 3,000 ml during operation and considerable bleeding after hepatectomy. Consequently, 4 of

these 9 patients died of hepatic insufficiency or multiple organ failure within 6 months after surgery. On the other hand, the most recent 6 patients with DIC risk and 7 other patients close to critical total risk and/or DIC risk were treated with partial splenic embolization (PSE) [22] before hepatectomy, in order to improve the function of the coagulation-fibrinolysis system and reduce the amount of intraoperative bleeding. In these 13 patients, the average item number of criteria for DIC risk decreased from 3.6 to 1.0 within 4 weeks after PSE, indicating marked improvement in the function of the coagulation-fibrinolysis system. Improvement of total risk from 4 to 3 was recognized in 2 patients. All patients had an uneventful course after hepatectomy with well maintained function of the coagulation-fibrinolysis system, and they are still alive at present (Table 7). Therefore, preoper-

Table 7. Results of hepatectomy for HCC with cirrhosis after PSE

Case	Age	Sex	Total risk			Positive number of 8 items in the potential DIC risk			Hepatic resection	Prognosis after sugery	
			before PSE	→	after PSE	before PSE	→	after PSE			
1	53	F	4	→	4	7	→	2	S_7	5Y3M	alive
2	39	M	4	→	3	5	→	1	$S_5 + S_8$	3Y10M	alive
3	58	M	4	→	3	6	→	1	$S_5 + S_8$	3Y6M	alive
4	65	F	4	→	4	5	→	1	partial	2Y19M	alive
5	56	M	3	→	3	4	→	1	$S_5 + S_8$	2Y3M	alive
6	53	M	4	→	4	6	→	2	partial	2Y1M	alive
7	51	M	4	→	4	6	→	2	S_8	1Y	alive
8	51	M	4	→	4	0	→	0	S_8	1Y8M	alive
9	66	F	4	→	4	3[a]	→	2[a]	partial	1Y6M	alive
10	55	M	2	→	2	3	→	2	$S_5 + S_6 + S_7 + S_8$	8M	alive
11	57	M	2	→	2	1[a]	→	0	S_3	5M	alive
12	50	M	3	→	3	3	→	0	S_8	4M	alive
13	60	F	3	→	3	1[a]	→	0	S_8	4M	alive
	Average		3.4 ± 0.8		3.2 ± 0.8	3.6 ± 2.2		1.0 ± 0.8			
				—NS—			—$P < 0.01$—				

[a] critical level

Fig. 5. Relationship between total risk and Prognostic Nutritional Index for Surgery (*PNI-s*), preoperatively, with regard to long-term prognosis after operation for hepatocellular carcinoma patients. *Open circle*, good prognosis; *solid circle*, unfavorable long-term prognosis (including severe liver dysfunction and hepatic insufficiency); *bars*, mean PNI-s value; *dotted area*, critical level

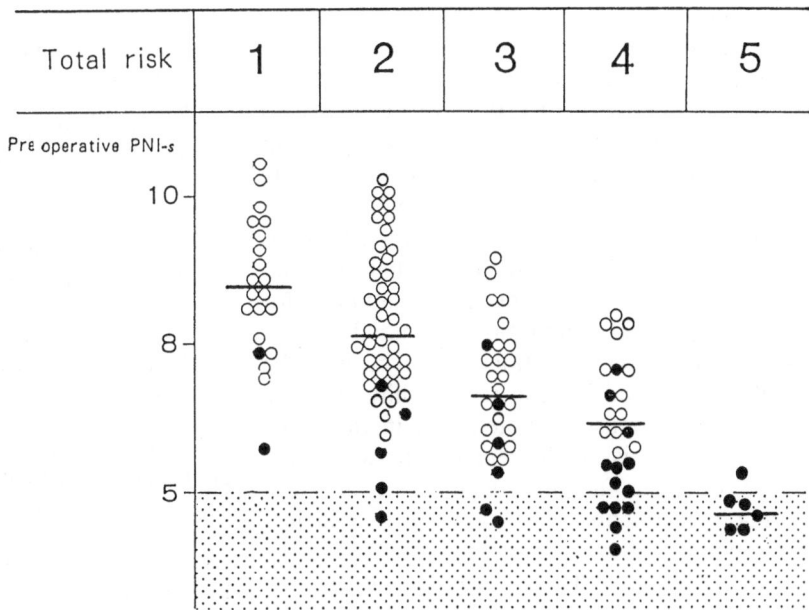

ative PSE contributes to extending the hepatic resectability of high risk patients.

4.2 Function of the reticulo endothelial system

The incidence of postoperative complication was markedly high in cirrhotic patients with poor preoperative reticuloendothelial function such as lipid emulsion test ($T_{1/2}$ over 15 min), fibrinogen degradation products in the serum over 10 mg/ml, blood endotoxin measured by Toxicolor method over 40 ng/ml, and plasma fibronectin below 150 µg/ml. Improvement in the prognosis of these high risk patients after hepatectomy was obviously the result of clearing out colonic flora to prevent endogenous endotoxemia or the administration of fresh plasma to increase plasma fibronectin level [3, 23].

4.3 Nutritional assessment

In order to improve the operative risk and long-term prognosis after hepatectomy, it is extremely important to assess the nutritional status quantitatively. We have had good results in pre- and postoperative nutritional support for hepatectomy patients with cirrhosis according to our original Prognostic Nutritional Index for surgery (PNI-s) [3, 24]. It is calculated by the following

formula: PNI-s = ($-0.014 \times$ percent body weight loss) + ($0.046 \times$ weight/height ratio) + ($0.010 \times$ skinfold thickness at the triceps muscle) + ($0.051 \times$ HPT). When the PNI-s is below 5, the prognosis will be poor, but when it is over 10 the prognosis will be satisfactory. Values ranging from 5 to 10 show the transitional zone. Although PNI-s estimated preoperatively was corelated with our total risk, subsegmentectomy for critical patients with total risk 4 was safe if their PNI-s could be improved to 8 or above (Fig. 5). Further, the long-term prognosis of critical patients could be improved by administration of both calories, over 40 kcal/kg/day, and branched-chain amino acid according to serum aminogram.

5 Conclusion

Hepatic surgeons always face a dilemma in deciding the extent of the resection to be performed when HCC is associated with cirrhosis because an extended hepatectomy should be performed to prevent tumor recurrence and a limited hepatectomy [25] to avoid postoperative hepatic failure. Therefore, in order to improve the results of radical hepatectomy in cirrhotic patients, the functional resectability of the liver must be accurately evaluated before surgery according to hepatic cell function. Further, preoperative estimation of surgical risk should take into consideration regeneration of the remnant liver and recovery of liver function, as well as selection of an appropriate surgical technique. Total risk, $ICGR_{max}$ of the expected remnant liver and $ICGR_{max}$ of the liver per unit liver volume in our department are extremely useful for risk evaluation. In addition to these considerations, it is also very important to evaluate DIC risk, reticuloendothelial function and nutritional status. Specific treatments for severely impaired conditions, estimated by the several parameters mentioned above, may be possible to extend hepatic resectability. On the other hand, it must be noted that in the some patients there is a discrepancy between the degree of liver function disturbance and the morphological abnormality of the liver, which is often seen in patients positive for HBsAg [3, 21], because these patients have a high rate of post-operative complications. Further, patients with cirrhosis often display hyperdynamic hemo-dynamics prior to surgery and a reduction in the effective circulating blood volume of the liver, as well as an increased number of intrapulmonary shunts and a decrease in free water clearance [3, 23]. Since these factors can easily lead to post-operative complications involving the heart, lung, and kidney, surgery for patients with cirrhosis requires, both before and after surgery, adequate management and treatment not only of the liver function, but also of all the main vital organs.

References

1. Honjo I, Mizumoto R (1974) Primary carcinoma of the liver. Am J Surg 128:31–36
2. Lin TY, Chen CC (1979) Metabolic function and regeneration of cirrhotic and non-cirrhotic livers after hepatic lobectomy in men. Ann Surg 190:959–972
3. Mizumoto R (1986) Primary carcinoma of the liver associated with cirrhosis. Asian Med J 29:323–332
4. Mizumoto R, Ohsawa J, Kohno A, Yokota T, Honjo I (1972) Operability of primary cancer of the liver with cirrhosis (in Japanese). The Saishin-Igaku 27:553–556
5. Healey JE Jr, Schroy PC (1953) Anatomy of the biliary ducts within the human liver: Analysis of the prevailing pattern of branching and the major variations of biliary ducts. Arch Surg 66:599–616
6. Yamada R, Sato M, Kawabata M, Nakatsuka H, Nakamura K, Takashima S (1983) Hepatic artery embolization in 120 patients with unresectable hepatoma. Radiology 148:397–401
7. Noguchi T, Imai T, Mizumoto R (1990) Pre-operative estimation of surgical risk of hepa-tectomy in cirrhotic patients. Hepatogastro-enterology 37:165–171
8. The Liver Cancer Study Group of Japan (1989) The general rules for the clinical and pathological study of primary liver cancer. Jpn J Surg 19:98–129
9. Okamoto E, Tanaka N, Yamanaka N, Toyosaka A (1984) Results of surgical treatments of primary hepatocellular carcinoma: Some aspects to im-prove long-term survival. World J Surg 8:360–366
10. Yamazaki S, Hasegawa H, Mukuuchi M (1981) Clinicopathological observation of minute liver cancer and the new method of hepatectomy: Analysis of 27 resected cases. Acta Hepatol Jpn 22:1714–1724
11. Child CG, Turcotte JG (1964) Surgery in portal hypertension. In: Child CG (ed) Major problems in clinical surgery: The liver and portal hyper-tension. WB Saunders, Philadelphia, pp 1–85
12. Nakanishi Y, Sano H, Kasai Y (1984) Indication of minimized regional operation for primary liver cancer (in Japanese). Gan No Rinsho 30:1087–91
13. Nagao T, Inoue S, Goto S, Mizuta T, Omori Y, Kawano N, Morioka Y (1987) Hepatic resection for hepatocellular carcinoma: Clinical features and long-term prognosis. Ann Surg 205:33–40
14. Ozawa K, Ida T, Yamada T, Honjo I (1976) Significance of glucose tolerance as prognostic sign in hepatectomized patients. Am J Surg 131:541–546
15. Ozawa K (1983) Biological significance of mitochondrial redox potential in shock and multiple organ failure -Redox theory-. In: Lefer AM and Schumer W (eds) Molecular and Cellular Aspects of Shock and Trauma. p 39–66 Alan R. Liss, New York
16. Yamanaka N, Okamoto E, Kuwata K, Tanaka N (1984) A multiple regression equation for predic-tion of posthepatectomy liver failure. Ann Surg 200:658–663
17. Moody FG, Rikkers LF, Aldrete JS (1974) Estimation of the functional reserve of human liver. Ann Surg 180:592–598
18. Takasaki T (1978) Development of a method of estimating postoperative hepatic functions upon hepatectomy before the operation (in Japanese). Jpn J Surg 79:1526–1534
19. Mimura H, Takakura N, Ohno Y, Matsuda T, Kin H, Hamazaki K, Tsumura M, Toda S, Hiraki Y (1986) Determination of the extent of feasible hepatic resection from hepatic blood flow. World J Surg 10:302–310
20. Mizumoto R, Kawarada Y, Noguchi T (1979) Preoperative estimation of operative risk in liver surgery, with special reference to functional reserve of the remnant liver following major hepatic resection. Jpn J Surg 9:343–349
21. Mizumoto R, Noguchi T (1981) Estimation of functional reserve of the liver in hepatectomy. Asian Med J 24:293–312

22. Spigos DG, Jonassan O, Mozes M, Mozes M, Capek V (1979) Partial splenic embolization in treatment of hypersplenism. Am J Roentgenol 132:777–782
23. Kawarada Y, Mizumoto R (1985) Importance of intensive care of various vital organs in radical hepatectomy for primary liver cancer associated with cirrhosis. Asian Med J 28:205–217
24. Higashiguchi T, Noguchi T, Mizumoto R (1989) Primary liver cancer—nutritional assessment (in Japanese). Kan Tan Sui 19:49–57
25. Kanematsu T, Takenaka K, Matsumata T, Furita T, Sugimachi K, Inokuchi K (1984) Limited hepatic resection effective for selected cirrhotic patients with primary liver cancer. Ann Surg 199:51–6

CHAPTER 19

Mass survey of hepatocellular carcinoma by ultrasound

Kenichiro Hirata, Morimichi Fukuda[1] and Satoaki Mima[2]

1 Introduction

Hepatocellular carcinoma (HCC) is rather rare in the Western Hemisphere and in Europe, however, it is far more prevalent in the Orient and Africa and is indeed one of the most common causes of cancer death in these areas [1–3].

In spite of remarkable advances in the diagnosis and treatment of HCC, prognosis for patients with this disease remains poor. Early detection is the best solution available to cope with the disease at present.

It is already well documented that use of the alphafetoprotein (AFP) assay is effective in detecting primary liver cancer, however, because of the limited sensitivity of the test in detecting small HCC, AFP is mostly used in the differential diagnosis of liver tumors or evaluation of disease activity such as the indices of therapeutic responses of HCC [4–6].

The rapid development of imaging modalities including ultrasound, X-ray computed tomography (CT) and magnetic resonance imaging (MRI), on the other hand, has revolutionized cancer detection by shifting the emphasis from laboratory tests to the direct visualization of the masses caused by malignant neoplastic growth.

The recent advance in ultrasound technology, especially of real-time ultrasound, has amply demonstrated its usefulness as one of the screening measures for HCC because of its non-invasiveness, economy, reproducibility of diagnostic results and transportability of the equipment to the remote examination sites where it is used for mass survey of HCC and related conditions [7–10]. In fact, realtime ultrasonic imaging has

shown remarkable improvement in terms of spatial and contrast resolution so that detection of masses as small as 1 cm in diameter can be accomplished provided high performance equipment is used. Furthermore, the recording media of images has shown considerable progress over the previous formats in terms of image quality and cost effectiveness. Ultrasound mass survey of HCC is fast becoming a viable means of obtaining statistical data.

In this chapter, recent progress in ultrasonic imaging will be described together with some of our studies on mass survey of HCC on high risk groups carried out in last 9 years.

2 Ultrasonic diagnostic criteria for HCC

A number of ultrasonographic criteria were described to facilitate differential diagnosis of HCC in the past [11–17].

Though ultrasound examination by a high quality contact compound scanner effectively characterized HCC and metastatic liver tumors to certain extents, smaller masses were extremely difficult to diagnose even by an experienced examiner.

Because of rapid improvement in ultrasonography with realtime machines, the ease of handling, and non-invasiveness of the examination, the method has established itself as on of the primary diagnostic tools for HCC in addition to X-ray CT and MRI.

In 1986, the Japan Society of Ultrasonics in Medicine publicised ultrasonic diagnostic criteria for liver masses, especially of HCC, after a year-long cooperative effort among committee members [18]. Subsequently, the criteria were unanimously supported by a number of investi-

[1] Department of Ultrasound and Medical Electronics, Sapporo Medical College Sapporo, 060 Japan
[2] Kin-ikyo Hospital Sapporo, 060 Japan

Table 1. Diagnostic criteria of hepatic mass lesions

Finding			Marginal hypoechoic zone			Internal echoes			
Tumor	Shape	Boundary	Presence	Thickness	Internal side	Whole arrangement	Anechoic area	Posterior echo	Lateral shadows
Hepatocellular carcinoma	round	sharp and smooth	present	thin	sharp	mosaic	starry	enhanced	present occasionally
Hemangioma	round or infinitive	finely irregular	absent	—	—	echogenic and infinitive	round	even ~ enhanced	absent
Metastatic carcinoma or cholangiocellular carcinoma	potato-or cauliflower-shape	coarsely irregular	present	thick	blurred	target-like distribution	observed at the center. convexed to the outside	attenuated ~ even	absent
Metastatic sarcoma or carcinoid	round	sharp and smooth	almost absent	—	—	uniform	round and scattered	even ~ enhanced	rarely paesent

gators and they were recognized as adequate not only for HCC but also in diagnosing metastatic tumors of the liver [19, 20]. The criteria are described below.

Existence of mass lesions
1. Definitive
   a) Marked difference of echo levels from those of the surrounding liver tissue
   b) The lesion is demonstrated on two different scan plane
2. Suspected
   a) Marked difference of echo levels from those of the surrounding liver tissue
   b) The lesion is demonstrated on one scan plane
3. Further examination recommended
   a) Slight difference of echo levels from those of the surrounding liver tissue
   b) The lesion is demonstrated on two different scan planes
4. Follow-up observation recommended
   a) Slight difference of echo levels from those of the surrounding liver tissue
   b) The lesion is demonstrated on one scan plane

Location of mass lesions
1. Location of a small mass in the liver is designated according to the segmentation as defined by Couinaud
2. Location of a large mass in the liver is designated according to the segmentation as defined by Healey
3. If a mass exists on the intersegmental plane designated according to Healey, a three dimensional relationship with the hepatic

veins or the umbilical portion of the left portal vein should be described
4. When it is difficult to estimate whether a mass belongs to the superior or inferior segment according to Couinaud, which portal venous branch of the Healey's segmental portal vein should be described

Differentiation of mass lesions by echo pattern characteristics
The echo pattern characteristics are shown in Table 1.

1. Typical sonographic patterns are described. Criteria for metastatic carcinomas indicated

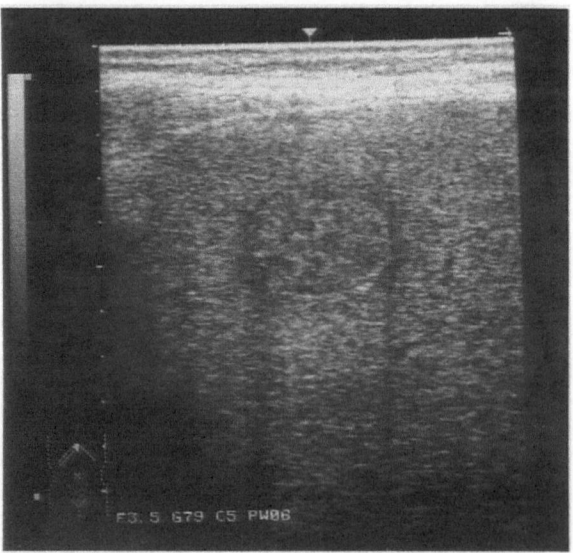

Fig. 1. Typical tumor of hepatocellular carcinoma exhibiting halo sign and mosaic pattern

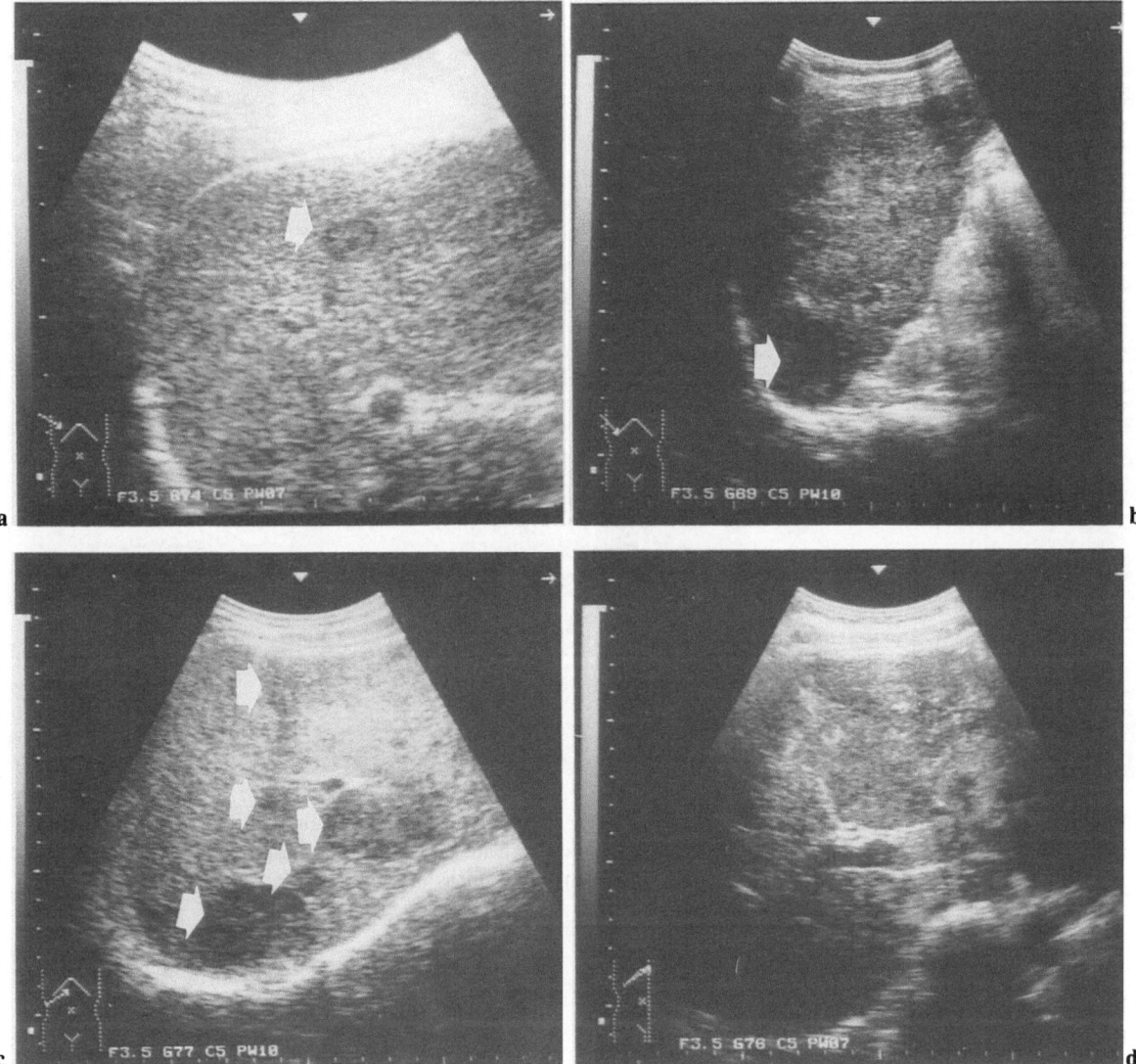

Fig. 2. Real-time ultrasonograms of hepatocelluar carcinoma. **a** Solitary small tumor in the right lobe of the liver (*arrow*). **b** A medium-sized hypoechoic mass of HCC in S6 segment (*arrow*). **c** Multiple masses of HCC (*arrows*). **d** Diffuse type HCC with tumor thrombi in the portal vein trunk.

are mainly based on typical sonograms of metastasis from gastric or colonic cancer.

2. Many small nodules of similar size scattered in all parts of the liver suggest a metastatic tumor, and nodules of different size are frequently seen in primary liver tumor. However, as the number and size of nodules are merely indirect findings, these should be omitted from this criteria.

3. Tumor thrombus is frequently associated with hepatocellular carcinoma and the finding of liver cirrhosis is helpful for the diagnosis of hepatocellular carcinoma. However, these are also indirect findings, and, as such, are omitted.

4. Findings mentioned in 2 and 3 should be described because they are potentially meaningful.

5. These criteria are not applicable to small tumors.

The main sonographic features characteristic of HCC include: a) appearance of round tumor mass circumscribed by thin capsular echoes which cast bilateral shadows, b) a thin and discrete halo around the mass, c) complex internal structures described as the mosaic pattern or tumors within tumors and, d) posterior echo enhancement reflecting less attenuation by hepatoma tissues (Figs. 1–3).

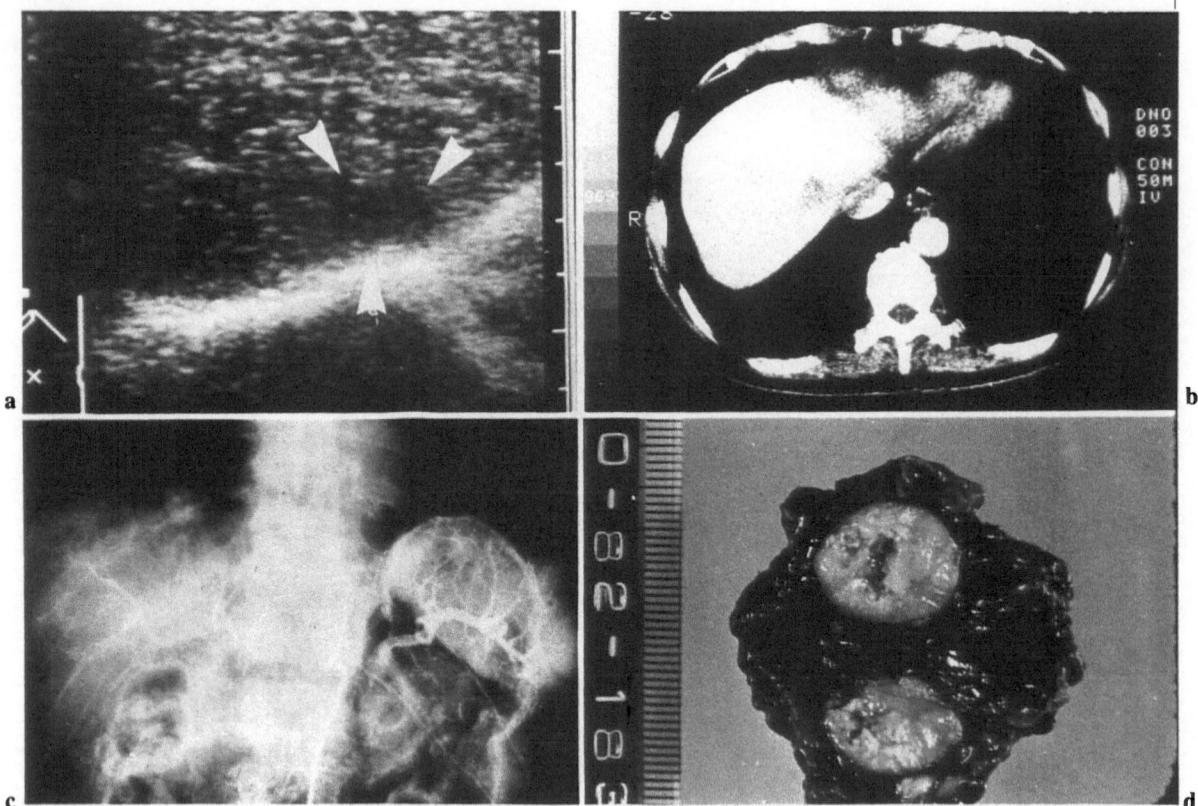

Fig. 3. Small hepatocellular carcinoma of Segment 8 detected by US mass survey and identified through X-ray CT and angiography. **a** Real-time ultrasound image. *Arrows* indicate a hypoechoic mass of HCC. **b** X-ray CT. **c** Angiography of the liver. **d** Resected specimen indicating small mass of HCC with incomplete encapsulation

These sonographic findings are characteristic of HCC with solid masses, however, they may not be applicable for diffuse type HCC [18]. Furthermore, lesions smaller than 2 cm in diameter frequently exhibit small hypoechoic nodules devoid of any other signs suggestive of the diagnosis of HCC.

Problems still remain, however, since certain benign focal lesions, small hemangiomas, focal nodular hyperplasia (FNH), adenomatous hyperplasia (AH), and regenerative nodules in cirrhotic liver may not be distinguishable from HCC simply based on image parameters if the size of HCC is very small [21].

3　Mass survey of HCC by ultrasound

Due to the rapid development of realtime ultrasound, a number of attempts were made to utilize ultrasound the method of first choice for early detection of HCC in clinical routine as well as for procedure of mass screening for HCC [10, 22–24].

It is well established that patients suffering from B-type chronic hepatitis or liver cirrhosis are more prone to develop HCC at a much higher rate than those without these afflictions. It is therefore advisable for afflicted patients to have regular check-ups at 3 to 6 month intervals by realtime ultrasound [7]. In fact, frequent clinical follow-up of high-risk groups by ultrasound has resulted in early detection of a significant number of HCC cases.

Because of the total absence of subjective symptoms in the early stages of HCC, it is seldom possible to diagnose small HCCs in routine clinical investigations. It is necessary, therefore, to perform a field mass survey to detect and treat HCC in the subclinical, curable stage.

To date, a number of pilot studies were made to investigate an ideal protocol for HCC mass survey including ultrasound examination.

From 1983 to 1988, the Japanese Society of Gastroenterological Mass Survey filed approxi-

Table 2. Accumulated data on mass survey of hepatobiliary diseases in Japan (1983–1988)

Year	1983	1984	1985	1986	1987	1988
Total	76,784	111,764	168,499	185,186	281,139	295,735
Male	46,575	56,868	95,097	110,770	149,261	168,413
Female	26,500	33,126	59,042	65,100	106,486	120,471
Sex not known	3,700	21,752	14,360	9,326	25,392	6,851

Diseases	1983	1984	1985	1986	1987	1988
HCC	16 (0.02%)	11 (0.01%)	25 (0.01%)	27 (0.01%)	65 (0.02%)	64 (0.02%)
Metabolic liver cancer	0	2 (0.002%)	7 (0.004%)	4 (0.002%)	4 (0.001%)	6 (0.002%)
Liver cirrhosis	61 (0.08%)	91 (0.08%)	88 (0.05%)	153 (0.08%)	136 (0.05%)	188 (0.06%)
Gallbladder cancer	6 (0.008%)	2 (0.002%)	12 (0.007%)	22 (0.01%)	26 (0.01%)	29 (0.01%)
Gallbladder polyp	0	1,760 (1.6%)	3,236 (1.9%)	5,480 (3%)	8,254 (2.9%)	12,023 (4.1%)
Gallbladder stone	2,939 (3.8%)	3,138 (2.8%)	3,733 (2.2%)	5,232 (2.8%)	7,109 (2.5%)	8,264 (2.8%)
Pancreatic cancer	3 (0.004%)	3 (0.003%)	6 (0.004%)	5 (0.003%)	5 (0.002%)	14 (0.005%)
Pancreatic stone	13 (0.02%)	6 (0.005%)	4 (0.002%)	5 (0.003%)	20 (0.01%)	19 (0.06%)
Pancreatic cyst	9 (0.01%)	12 (0.01%)	44 (0.03%)	64 (0.03%)	129 (0.05%)	188 (0.06%)

(%), the percentage of cases against the total number examined during the respectice year

Table 3. Method of HCC screening by institution and by combination of screening method used

HCC screening method	1984	1985	1986	1987	1988
Direct GI Series	11[a] (29.7%)	16 (39%)	21 (40%)	26 (43%)	21 (33%)
Age factor	9 (24.3%)	13 (32%)	16 (31%)	18 (30%)	21 (33%)
Indirect GI Series	7 (18.9%)	3 (7%)	7 (13%)	16 (27%)	17 (27%)
Subjective symptoms	1 (2.7%)	3 (7%)	2 (4%)	4 (7%)	5 (8%)
Others	15 (40.5%)	12 (29%)	20 (38%)	19 (32%)	26 (41%)

Combined methods	1984	1985	1986	1987	1988
US + liver Functions	18 (48.6%)	14 (38%)	20 (38%)	33 (50%)	29 (45%)
US only	14 (37.8%)	16 (39%)	20 (38%)	20 (33%)	27 (42%)
Liver functions only	4 (10%)	4 (10%)	6 (12%)	7 (12%)	4 (6%)
Other methods	1 (2.8%)	3 (7%)	4 (8%)	0 (0)	4 (7%)

[a] Number denotes number of institutions with similar program

mately 111,000–295,000 ultrasound examinations annually which were performed as part of a mass survey. The most common protocol combination was the hepatobiliary check-up with the routine mass survey of gastric cancer. The overall detection rate for HCC was, however, extremely low and it is reasonable to assume that using the age factor as the sole criteria in selecting candidates for HCC is seriously questioned (Tables 2, 3).

Fukuda et al., on the other hand, carried out studies on ultrasound screening of HCC over the last 9 years according to the format described in the followings. High risk groups for liver cancer [2, 3, 25, 26] were selected for the ultrasonic mass survey from the resident population in Hokkaido, where the frequency of HBs antigen is slightly less than the mean value for the whole of Japan. The high-risk groups include individuals with a previous history of liver disease; a family history of liver diseases, with or without liver cancer; those with previous blood transfusions; and HBs carriers [23, 25, 26]. The procedure for carrying out the mass survey is as follows:

1. Define high-risk groups for HCC mass survey
   a) Patients with viral hepatitis
   b) Persons with previous history of liver diseases, family history of HCC, history of blood transfusion
   c) HBs carriers
2. Take history and carry out venipuncture for liver functions, HBs and AFP
3. Ultrasound examination using realtime equipment, and double checking
4. Report data, with advice to recipient
5. Follow-up and re-examination of suspected cases of HCC using X-ray CT, angiography, laparoscopic ultrasound, etc.

The serum battery tests including alanine aminotransferase (GOT), glutamic pyruvic transaminase (GPT), alkaline phosphatase (ALP), cholinesterase, gamma-glutamyl transferase (GTP), HBs, HBe antigens, antibodies, and AFP were carried out concurrently with the ultrasound examination. The survey covered 5 major cities on 32 occasions and the total number of cases examined by the end of 1988 was 8,244.

An analysis of this population revealed 1,241 case (20.3%) of chronic hepatitis, based on the liver function profiles and sonographic findings, 353 cases (5.8%) of liver cirrhosis, 811 cases (13.3%) with fatty liver and 221 cases (3.6%) with alcoholic liver disease. The HBs antigen was present in 1,381 cases (22.6%), higher than the average for the population of Hokkaido.

Out of the total true number of 6,104 cases examined, 64 HCC cases (1.05%) were detected (Table 4). Of these 64, 59 (96%) were correctly diagnosed by ultrasound alone. Ultrasound negative with AFP levels higher than 100 ng/ml were

Table 4. List of diseases detected by mass survey for hepatocellular carcinoma

Disease	No. of cases	Percent of true numbers examined (%)
Hepatocellular carcinoma	64	1.05
Liver echinococcosis	4	
Gallbladder cancer	1	
Metastatic liver cancer	3	
Stomach cancer	1	
Leiomyosarcoma	1	
Renal cancer	2	
Pancreatic cancer	1	
Focal nodular hyperplasia	1	
Gallstone	324	5.4
Liver hemangioma	153	2.55
Liver cyst	390	6.5

reexamined and 5 additional cases with HCC were found. Of the 59, 34 cases (57.6%) of HCC diagnosed by ultrasound alone were found to have alpha-fetoprotein (AFP) levels lower than 100 ng/ml.

These data support the previous findings that even though AFP positivity may suggest the presence of HCC, the biochemical data alone may not be sufficient to serve as a screening measure for early detection of hepatocellular carcinoma.

Therefore, the study clearly demonstrated that AFP determination in conjunction with ultrasound is a good safeguard to avoid overlooking HCC cases by one modality alone.

The sonographic patterns of HCC detected by mass survey were generally in good agreement with the ultrasonic diagnostic criteria for HCC (Fig. 4) [18]. The most frequent echo pattern of HCC encountered during mass survey was a iso- or hypoechoic small round tumor surrounded by a thin hypoechoic halo accompanied by an acoustic enhancement posterior to the tumor mass. Tumors larger than 3 cm in diameter tend to show a characteristic mosaic pattern or a tumor within a tumor indicating multiple tumor nodules with altered echogenicity being encapsulated to form a single tumor mass. Multiple tumors exist are frequently detected, and, to a lesser extent, nodular HCC with echo patterns quite indistinguishable from benign cavernous hemangioma showing hyperechoic or marginated pattern appearance. These echo patterns are mostly due to variable degrees of fatty metamorphosis of the HCC nodules. In a small percentage of cases, the tumors also have shown a diffusely infiltrating echo pattern in which tumor tissue is poorly marginated and the echogenicity from the surrounding liver tissue most closely resembles the tumor itself.

As a rule, however, mass HCC lesions were invariably accompanied by the parenchymal echo pattern characteristic of liver cirrhosis, the coarse texture or macron dular changes of the liver parenchyma, shrunken liver lobes with rounding and thickening of the lower hepatic angle, increased size of the caudate lobe, and medium to extensive degrees of splenomegaly. These sonomorphological changes frequently coexist in small HCC cases found during the present mass survey. This strongly suggests that the basic changes responsible for the evolution of HCC may exist as a precancerous states in the liver.

Occasionally, the small hypoechoic lesions of adenomatous hyperplasia, which resemble closely

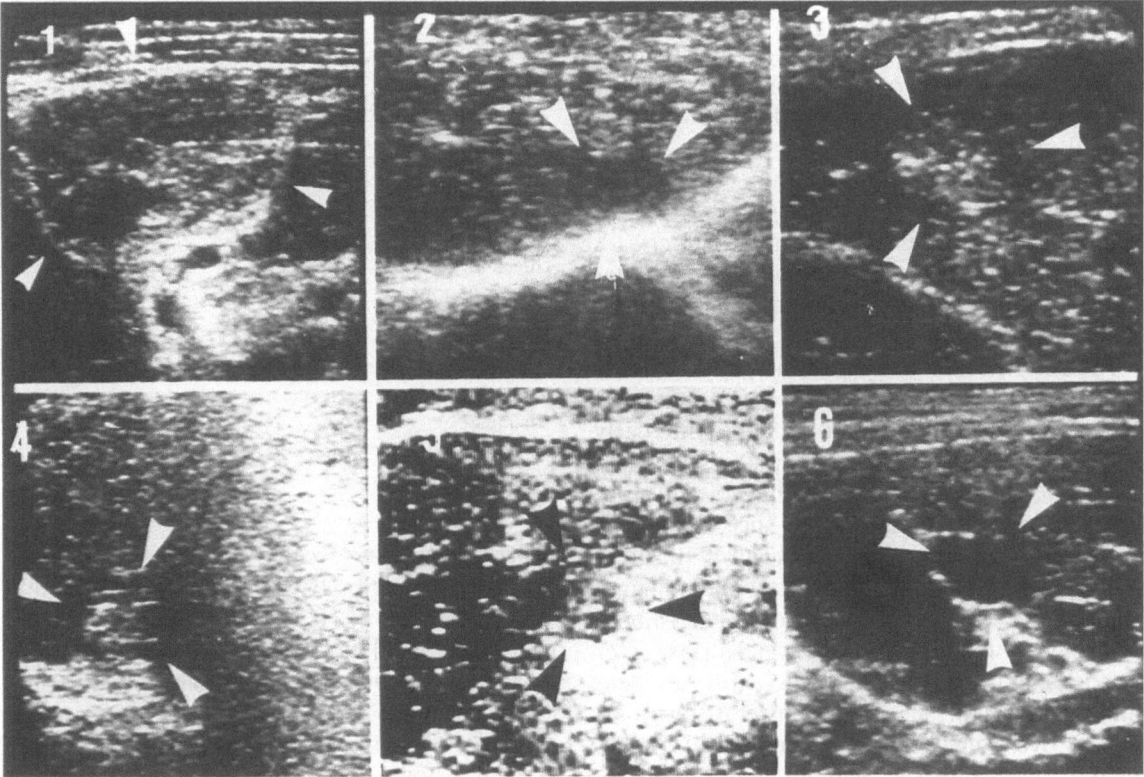

Fig. 4. Examples of tumors detected by mass survey for hepatocellular carcinoma. **1** Marginal type cavernous hemangioma of the liver. **2–5** Small hepatocellular carcinoma. **6** Regenerative nodule

those of HCC, eventually develop into HCC during prolonged observations. Similar observation supporting the above view were obtained by us through statistical analyses of biochemical laboratory data profiles of HCC cases in this study using multi-variate analysis [27].

HCC cases detected by ultrasound mass survey includes both single and multiple tumor types. Of the total HCC cases detected, 23 cases (35.9%) had a single mass lesion smaller than 3 cm in diameter, and were considered candidates for radical resection. There were 11 cases, (17.1%) with single tumors 2 cm in diameter or less, coinciding to T1 tumor of TNM classification. Consequently, the remaining cases were treated either by transarterial embolization (TAE) followed by surgical resection, chemical embolization, or by cancer chemotherapy alone.

Relatively few cases with small tumors were also treated by percutaneous ethanol injection (PEI) treatment.

Forty six of the cases received treatment: surgical resection of the tumor mass in 23 cases, TAE in 22 cases, and PEI in one case. Among the 46 cases treated by any kind of active treat-

ment, the cumulative survival rates calculated by the Kaplan-Meier method were: one year 95.0%, 3 years 51.5%, and 5 years 29.7%. These results are significantly better than the data accumulated by the Japanese Assessment Group Data on Therapeutic Results on Hepatocellular Carcinoma [28], of which reflected the following survival rates: one year 67.1%, 3 years 39.6%, and 5 years 28.5%. The survival rates of the nontreated group were: one year 59.6%, 3 years 22.7%, and 5 years 0%. As these figures indicate, there still remained a significant number of cases who refused active treatment for HCC. One exceptional case in this group who had a small HCC and refused any active treatment survived about 4 years following initial examination: the remainder terminated rather shortly.

4 Discussion

For maximal efficacy of the mass survey of hepatocellular carcinoma by ultrasound, it is evident that the prior determination of high-risk groups is of prime importance. If a mass survey using ultrasonography, a non-invasive yet labor-intensive and individual-dependent imaging method, were carried out based on age as the only criteria, a tremendous number of cases would be normal.

Evidently, ultrasound screening plus serum biochemical determinations including AFP can efficiently screen the HCC cases from high-risk groups with the least burden on the examiner and still ensure a reasonable rate of detection of HCC at an early stage.

The survival rate analysis of the patients based on the mass survey data has clearly demonstrated the usefulness of the method in identifying early stage HCC cases to be treated operatively. Mass surveys also enable us to exclude normal cases from further examination during successive years by virtue of the complete check-up of the liver function profiles and detailed ultrasound imaging. Individuals with the following conditions should be excluded from future surveys: Normal liver function and negative hepatitis virus antigen, minor abnormality in aminotransferase attributable to overweight or fatty liver, and alcoholic-related liver diseases without any abnormal findings on ultrasound. Conversely, individuals with positive viral antigens, with or without liver dysfunction, require continued observation. This policy is extremely important to keep the system functioning properly in subsequent years if mass surveys are to be carried out on an annual basis for long periods of time.

Because of the limited number of HCC cases in the present report, it is premature to interpret the prognostic aspects of HCC cases detected by mass survey. However, because of the thoroughness of the observations from the screening steps to the final treatment over 9 years based on a complete database registering the population surveyed, it is believed to be worthwhile to evaluate the overall effectiveness of the mass survey based on the survival rate analysis.

It is clear that the present system of mass survey detects a significant number of HCC cases in the T1 stage of TNM classification as shown in Table 5.

The life expectancy of HCC patients who undergo resection, in general, has been mostly limited compared to carcinomas at other sites. The survival rate analysis of the present series of HCC detected by mass survey, also suffers limited life expectancy as a whole, however, HCC classified as small liver cancer or T1 stage tumor of TNM classification apparently has

Table 5. Prognosis of HCC cases diagnosed by the mass survey

Tumor size and nodule number	No. of cases	Survival (years)	Cumulative survival ratio (%)
Solitary tumor less than 2 cm in diameter	11	1	100
		3	76.2
		5	50.8
Solitary tumor 2.1–5 cm in diameter	23	1	90.6
		3	55.7
		5	31.8
Multiple tumors or Solitary tumor larger than 5.1 cm in diameter	27	1	72.3
		3	14.5

shown encouraging results. This seemed to imply that even though HCC cannot be completely cured, detection of HCC cases at the stage of T1 or solitary small tumors have better chance of survival provided all the possible therapeutic efforts are made.

Successful mass survey of HCC by ultrasound imaging, however, requires several factors: Availability of diagnostic expertise and high quality equipment, cost efficacy, education of both the examiners and the recipients, and finally financial support of the program. Certain objective evaluations also have to be carried out based on rigid statistical analysis on the accuracy of the system to ensure quality control. Without these strict measures for qualification, a mass survey system for liver cancer detection should not be undertaken. Furthermore, in light of the high incidence of liver cancer in certain areas of the world and misery associated with the disease, a mass survey system should be instituted as soon as possible by the government just as they have done successfully in the screening of stomach cancer in this country.

5 Summary

1. Ultrasound mass survey combined with serum battery tests on high-risk populations of HCC has proven to be very effective in detecting asymptomatic subclinical HCC. Small solitary masses less than 3 cm in diameter amenable for radical treatment constituted one third of the HCC detected.

2. Serum biochemical analysis carried out concurrently with ultrasound consistently detected even minimal hepatic dysfunction in HCC, and AFP determinations were relatively insensitive for detections of small HCCs. AFP assays, however, were found to be useful as a safeguard in avoiding false negatives by ultrasound.

3. Detection rates of HCC in the general population as high as 1% and normal incidence of carcinomas at other sites definitely support the view that patients with liver cirrhosis, chronic hepatitis, blood transfusions, or HBs antigen, all of which are related to infection by hepatitis viruses, may have a strong correlation with HCC.

4. Survival rate analysis of HCC using the Kaplan-Meier method has revealed significant improvement in postoperative survival in T1 cases, and solitary liver tumors less than 2 cm in diameter, thus reiterating the importance of early detection of HCC by mass survey or by equivalent procedures.

References

1. Higginson DA Jr (1976) The geographic pathology of liver cell cancer In: Cameron HM, Linsel DA, Warwick GP, (eds) Liver Cell Cancer, Elsevier, Amsterdam, pp 1–16

2. Kurihara M, Aoki K, Hisamichi S (1990) UICC Cancer Mortality Statistics in the World, 1950–1985. University of Nagoya Press

3. Beasley RP, Hwang LY, Lin CC, Chien CS (1981) Hepatocellular carcinoma and hepatitis B virus. Lancet 2:1129–1133

4. Abelev GI, Perova SD, Khramkova NI (1963) Production of embryonal alpha-globulin by transplantable mouse hepatoma. Transplantation 1:174–180

5. Okuda K, Kubota K, Obata H (1975) Clinical observations and diagnosis of relatively early stage of hepatocellular carcinoma with special referece to serum alphafetoprotein levels. Gastroenterology 69:226–234

6. Zhao-you T, Bing-hui Y (1985) Early detection of subclinical hepatocellular carcinoma, In: Zhao-you T (ed) Subclinical Hepatocellular Carcinoma. China Academic Publishers Beijing and Springer-Verlag, Berlin, pp 12–21

7. Taylor KJW, Ramos I, Morse SS et al. (1987) Fortune KL, Hammer SL, Taylor CR Focal liver masses, differential diagnosis with pulsed Doppler US. Radiology 164:643–647

8. Taylor KJW, Burns PN, Wells PNT (eds) (1988) Clinical Application of Doppler Ultrasound. Raven Press, New York.

9. Fukuda M (1984) Intraluminal scanning: Use of the echoendoscope and echo-laparoscope in the diagnosis of intra-abdominal cancer, In: Kossoff G, Fukuda M (eds) Ultrasonic Differential Diagnosis of Tumors, Igakushoin, New York-Tokyo, pp 186–199

10. Fukuda M (1989) Ultrasonic screening for hepatocarcinoma. In: Bigot JM (ed) Radiodiagnostics, ICR89, International Congress Series 876, Elsevier, Amsterdam pp 279–284

11. Fukuda M (1977) Evaluation of sensitivity graded ultrasonotomography in diagnosis of malignant tumors of upper abdominal organs. In: White DN, Brown R (eds) Ultrasound in Medicine, New York, Plenum Press, vol 3A, pp 303–314

12. Green B, Bree RL, Goldstein M, Stanley C (1977) Gray scale ultrasound evaluation of hepatic neoplasms: Patterns and correlations. Radiology 124:203–208

13. Kamin PD, Bernadino ME, Green B (1979): Ultrasound manifestations of hepatocellular carcinoma. Radiology 131:459–461

14. Dubbins PA, Oriordan D, Melia WM (1981) Ultrasound in hepatoma. Can specific diagnosis be made? Br J Radiol 54:307–311

15. Broderick TW, Gosink B, Menuck L, Harris R, Wilcox J (1980) Echographic and radionuclide detection of hepatoma. Radiology 135:149–151

16. Hillman BJ, Smith EH, Gammelgaard J, Holm HH (1979) Ultrasonographic-pathologic correlation of malignant hepatic masses. Gastrointest Radiol 4:361–365

17. Calder JF (1981) Ultrasound in Hepatoma. Br J Radiol 54:819

18. Makuuchi M, Akimoto S et al. (1986) Diagnostic criteria of liver tumors. In: Fukuda M et al. (eds) Diagnostic Ultrasound, Principles and Clinical Applications. Igakushoin, Tokyo, pp 754–757

19. Yoshida T, Matsue H, Okazaki N, Yoshino M (1987) Ultrasonographic differentiation of hepatocellular carcinoma from metastatic liver cancer, JCU 15:431–437

20. Gibo Y, Furuta K, Uemura K, et al. (1990) Examination of the usefulness of ultrasonic diagnostic criteria for hepatocellular carcinoma and metastatic liver cancer (in Japanese). Jap J Med Ultrasonics 17:160–167

21. Fukuda M (1987) Laparoscopic sonography. In: Rifkin MD (ed) Clinics in Diagnostic Ultrasound, 22. Endoscopic and Intraoperative Sonography. Churchill Livingstone, New York pp 151–166

22. Ebara M, et al. (1989) Strategy for early diagnosis of hepatocellular carcinoma (HCC). Ann Acad Med Singapore 18:83–89

23. Itaya H, Fukuda M, Mima S (1985) Studies on early detection of hepatocellular carcinoma-HCC cases detected by ultrasound mass survey with

subsequent therapeutic results. In: Hepatocellular Carcinoma in Asia. Kobe University Press, Kobe, pp 183–195

24. Ohto M, Ebara M (1986) Ultrasound diagnosis of hepatocellular carcinoma (in Japanese). Gan no Rinsho 32:1262–1266

25. Sakuma K, Takahashi T, Okuda K et al. (1982) Prognosis of hepatitis B virus surface antigen carriers in relation to routine liver function tests: A prospective study. Gastroenterology 83:144–147

26. Di Bisceglie A, Rustgi VK, Hoofnagle JH, Disheiko GM, Lotze MT (1988) NIH Conference: Hepatocellular carcinoma. Ann Intern Med 108: 390–401

27. Hirata K, Fukuda M, Mima S (1985) Correlation between liver function profile and pathology with special reference to mass survey of liver cancer (in Japanese). Jap J Clin Pathol 33:239–248

28. Japanese Working Group for Liver Cancer (1986) Follow-up study of HCC cases, VII (in Japanese). Jap J Hepatology 27:1161–1169

Part 7. Treatment

Section 1
Surgical Treatment

CHAPTER 20

Improving survival after resection of hepatocellular carcinoma: Characteristics and current status of surgical treatment of primary liver cancer in Japan

Takayoshi Tobe and Shigeki Arii[1]

1 Characteristics of primary liver cancer in Japan and recent advances in diagnosis

1.1 Characteristics of primary liver cancer in Japan

The Liver Cancer Study Group of Japan has been conducting a follow up study of primary liver cancer since 1965 [1–7]. The records of 38,255 patients show that primary liver cancer in Japan has the following characteristics:

1. Over 90% of all microscopically proven liver cancers are hepatocellular carcinomas
2. The incidence of primary liver cancer is highest in the sixth decade of life
3. Primary liver cancer is more common in men than in women
4. Many patients have a past history of hepatitis and frequently have hepatic cirrhosis; however, the number of carriers of HBs antigen has been decreasing (40% in 1970, 22.5% in 1987)
5. About half of the hepatocellular carcinoma patients have high blood levels of AFP

1.2 Clues for diagnosis of liver cancer

On the basis of the above characteristics of primary liver cancer, the following three points are important in the diagnosis of the early stage of liver cancer: 1) follow-up studies of high risk groups, 2) AFP screening, and 3) greater use of ultrasonography (US) or computerized tomography (CT) for lesions suspected of being malignant.

High risk patients are men in the sixth decade of life with a past history of blood transfusion or hepatitis, patients with hepatic cirrhosis caused by blood transfusion or hepatitis, and HBs antigen carriers. Regular screening for AFP in these high risk patients is important. If the serum AFP level is more than 200 ng/ml, and especially if the AFP value increases considerably in 3–4 weeks, hepatocellular carcinoma is definitely suspected. Use of US or CT is safe and quite effective in the diagnosis of primary liver cancer.

1.3 Recent advances in diagnosis and important findings

Recent advances in diagnostic imaging have made it possible to detect small liver cancers (less than 2 cm in diameter) in 10% of cases.

One of the important findings in this follow up study is the gradual but definite change in the number of HBs antigen carriers, which decreased from 40% in 1970 to 22.5% in 1987. The percentage of resectability of HCC patients in Japan is shown in the Fig. 1. The resectability is gradually but definitely increasing. The recent resectability of hepatocellular carcinoma in Japan is approximately 20%.

2 Current status of surgical treatment for liver cancer

2.1 Change of surgical procedures

Figure 2 shows the types of surgery in each report. The 4th report was a summary of the 10 years from 1968 to 1977 [4]. After 1977, the Liver Cancer Study Group published a report every 2 years. Reports 5–9 cover the last 10 years.

---

[1] 1st Department of Surgery, Kyoto University Faculty of Medicine, Sakyo-ku, Kyoto, 606 Japan

215

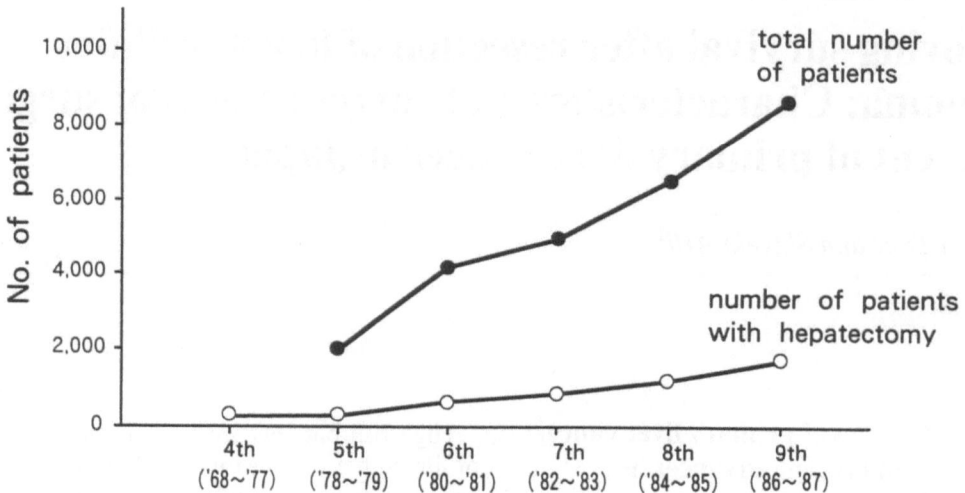

Fig. 1. Resectability of HCC patients in Japan

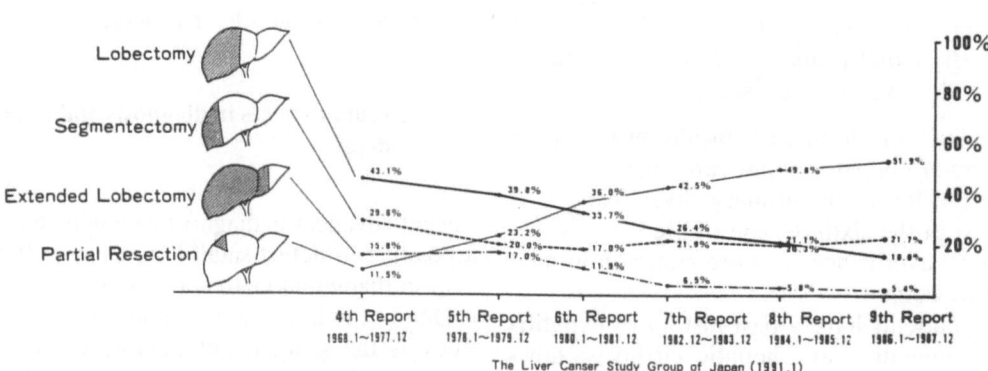

Fig. 2. Changes in methods of resection of HCC in Japan

In the earlier 10-year period, Japanese surgeons tried to resect widely to cure the cancer, so the extent of resection was large. Trisegmentectomy and lobectomy were commonly performed. During this period, complications and postoperative deaths due to multiple organ failure were numerous after hepatic insufficiency because of limited reserve function in cirrhotic livers.

Gradually but definitely the extent of resection has become smaller. Limited but anatomically precise hepatectomies for hepatocellular carcinoma in cirrhotic livers are now the rule in Japan.

2.2 Surgical procedures for liver cancer associated with hepatic cirrhosis

When a high degree of hepatic cirrhosis is detected, resection of the liver should be limited. However, it is well known that hepatocellular carcinoma metastasizes easily through the portal vein to form multiple daughter nodules in other portions of the liver. Therefore, segmental resection of the liver is much better than enucleation of the tumor. This procedure was developed in Japan by Dr. Makuuchi, Dr. Hasegawa, and their associates in the National Cancer Research

Fig. 3. Operative death rate and limited resection. Subsegmentectomy includes partial resection smaller than subsegmentectomy

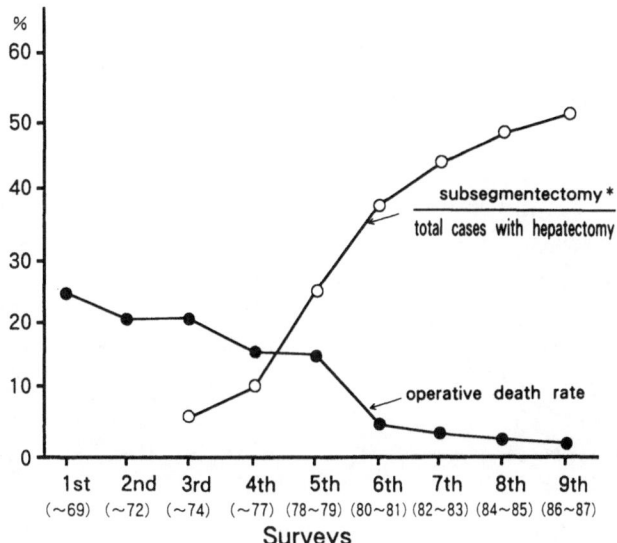

Institute, Tokyo [8]. This approach will be introduced by Dr. Makuuchi in detail, and briefly here.

After mobilization of the liver, an ultrasound probe is placed on the surface of the liver, and the location of the tumor and its relationship with the vessels are determined. Under ultrasonographic guidance, a 22-gauge percutaneous transhepatic cholangiography (PTC) needle is inserted into the liver and the tip of the needle is placed in the portal vein, which supplies the hepatic tumor. After ascertainment of the location of the needle, indigo carmine or indocyanine green (ICG) is injected through the PTC needle until the surface of the liver is clearly stained. On the ultrasonogram, the flow of the staining solution can be demonstrated clearly as a tiny echogenic spot in the portal vein. When the subsegmental region has been made clearly visible by this technique, subsegmental resection can be performed.

With the use of this limited resection, intraoperative mortality and postoperative complications have greatly decreased in Japan (Fig. 3). Recent reports indicate that postoperative complications after hepatectomy in Japan are 3%–4%.

2.3 Surgical procedures for liver cancer without cirrhosis

When hepatic cirrhosis is minimum or not evident and good functional reserve of the liver can be

predicted, extended hepatectomy can be performed. One of the types of extended resection is trisegmentectomy for large tumors with combined partial resection of the inferior vena cava. One of these cases will be described here by Professor Ozawa.

Figure 4 shows a CT scan of a huge liver tumor and Fig. 5 shows a MR image of a huge liver malignancy infiltrating the inferior vena cava—a cholangiocellular carcinoma. Because no definite chemotherapy or irradiation was feasible for this large cancer, it was resected with combined partial resection of the diaphragm and inferior vena cava after a venous shunt had been formed. An artificial dacron vein graft was inserted (Fig. 6). The postoperative course was uneventful, and the patient's quality of life after surgery was adequate and enjoyable.

2.4 The role and objective of surgery

The role and the objective of surgery in the treatment of primary liver cancer are as follows:

1. Absolute cure of malignancy in the early stage
2. Prolonged survival and improved quality of life by reduction surgery in the advanced stage

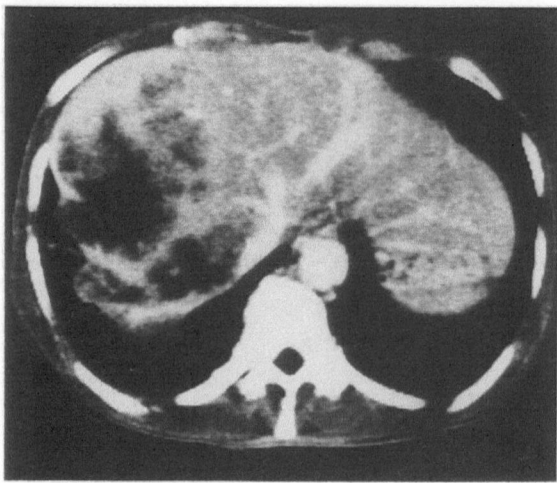

Fig. 4. CT scan of huge liver tumor

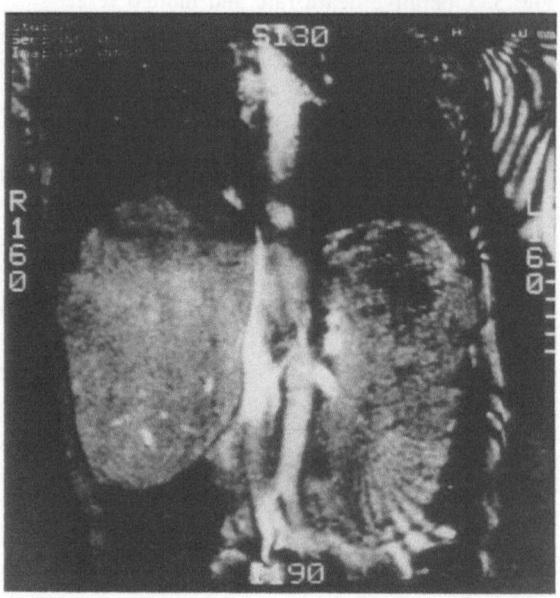

Fig. 5. MRI of huge liver tumor, showing infiltration to the inferior vena cava

3 Survival rates after hepatic resection in relation to various backgrounds and factors influencing the survival rate

Survival rates after hepatic resection in relation to various backgrounds and factors influencing the survival rate are now being clarified. The results of hepatic resection in 4,152 patients from 1978–1987 were analyzed by computer. The 1-year survival rate was 71.9%, and the 5-year survival rate was 30.9%.

3.1 Cumulative survival of HCC patients after surgery

The cumulative survival of HCC patients treated with curative resection were 77.4% at 1 year, 55.0% at 3 years, and 36.6% at 5 years. Curative resection refers to surgery which removes the tumor completely so that a cure can be expected. These results will be described by Dr. Arii in detail, and introduced here briefly.

Cumulative survival of HCC patients in relation to the number of tumors showed that those with solitary tumors had good survival rates. Cumulative survival of HCC patients treated with hepatic resection in relation to the extent of tumor showed that the survival rate was relatively high in patients with tumors located in a subsegment or single segment. Survival rates in relation to tumor diameters showed that the patients with smaller tumors tend to have better survival rates. Those with HCC less than 2 cm in diameter have the best survival rates.

The survival rate was not affected by the presence of a macroscopic capsule, i.e., there is no significant difference between HCC patients with and without macroscopic capsular formation around the tumor. This is possibly because more small tumors than large tumors have no capsule. However, there is a significant difference between patients with and without histological evidence of infiltration of cancer cells into or beyond the tumor capsule. Survival rates in relation to the growth patterns of tumors show that patients with tumors with an expanding growth pattern survived longer than did those with tumors with an infiltrating pattern. Survival rates in relation to the degree of portal invasion by the tumor show that patients with tumors with no portal invasion (Vpo) had the best survival rates. A significant difference was noted between those with and those without portal invasion.

Fig. 6. After the combined resection of IVC and diaphragm, an artificial dacron vein graft and diaphragma were inserted

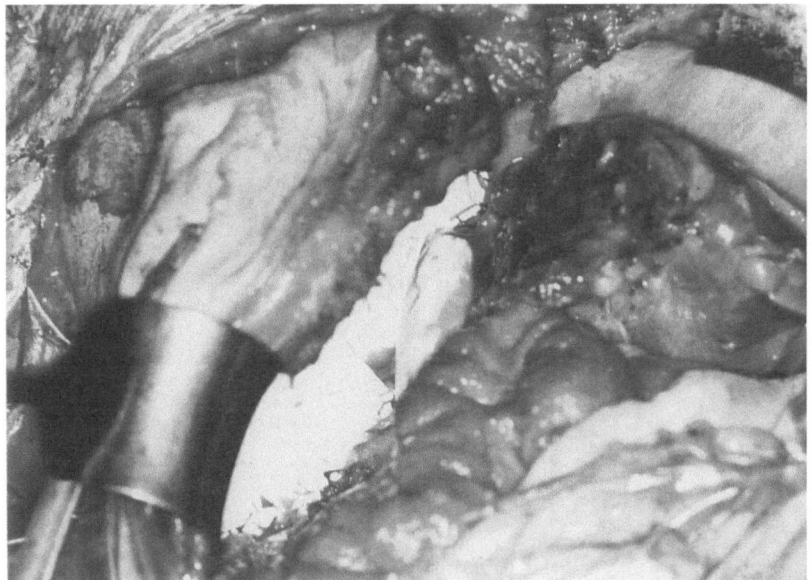

3.2 HCC patients with good survival rates after surgery

These results indicated that the factors in hepatocellular carcinoma patients which promote good survival rates after surgery are:

1. Solitary tumor
2. Location in one segment or two adjacent segments
3. Small size
4. Expanding growth pattern
5. No infiltration into or beyond the capsule
6. No portal invasion
7. No hepatic vein invasion
8. Curative resection

3.3 The most important risk factors for intrahepatic recurrence

The most important risk factors predicting intrahepatic recurrence after hepatic resection are:

1. Microscopic intrahepatic metastasis, −im(+)
2. Cancerous invasion in the portal vein, −Pv(+)
3. Infiltration into or beyond the capsule, −Fc inf(+)

Adjuvant therapy should be performed after surgery.

4 Conclusion

The factors influencing the prognosis in hepatocellular carcinoma patients after surgical resection were derived from the survival rates analyzed by the Liver Cancer Study Group of Japan. Many of these factors can now be demonstrated preoperatively by the combination of CT scans, US, and angiography.

Appropriate surgical indications have now been clarified by the present study and the development of promising adjuvant therapy for the recurrence and for advanced disease as well as the further progress of surgical treatment can be expected in near future.

References

1. Murakami F, Okamura T, Ohta M, et al. (1970) Liver disease and surgical treatment, particularly hepatic resection and transplantation. Shinryo 23: 265–277
2. Ishikawa K, Kosaka K (1973) Results of hepatic resection for primary liver cancer. Acta Hepatol Jpn 14:409–410
3. Ishikawa K (1976) Follow-up study of patients with primary liver cancer: Report 3. Acta Hepatol Jpn 17:460–465

4. Okuda K and The Liver Cancer Study Group of Japan (1980). Primary liver cancer. Cancer 45: 2663–2669
5. The Liver Cancer Study Group of Japan (1984) Primary liver cancer in Japan. Cancer 54:1747–1755
6. The Liver Cancer Study Group of Japan (1987) Primary liver cancer in Japan. Cancer 60:1400–1411
7. The Liver Cancer Study Group of Japan (1990) Primary liver cancer in Japan: Clinicopathologic features and results of surgical treatment Ann Surg 211:277–287
8. Makuuchi M, Hasegawa H, Yamazaki S (1985) Ultrasonically guided subsegmentectomy. Surg Gynecol Obstet 161:346–350

CHAPTER 21

Extended surgery for malignant liver tumors

Yoshio Yamaoka, Kaoru Kumada, Takashi Takayasu, Keiichi Ino, Yasuyuki Shimahara,
Taisuke Morimoto, Akira Tanaka, Keiichiro Mori, and Kazue Ozawa[1]

1 Introduction

Even though recent advances in imaging technology has allowed detection of small liver tumors, only 20% of patients with liver tumors benefit from surgical resection. The reason for this low incidence of resectability in our country is mainly due to decreased liver functional reserve caused by coexisting chronic liver diseases such as cirrhosis or chronic hepatitis [1]. Therefore, even when the tumor is small, and is located in the center of one lobe, wide resection may not be advisable. In the last five years, we have reformed the operative procedures and postoperative management according to the redox theory, which involves measurement of the arterial ketone body ratio (AKBR), improving in operative mortality and morbidity [2–7]. In this paper, some of the operative procedures will be presented such as liver resection under hepatic vascular exclusion (HVE) using veno-venous bypass, and hepatic resection using a technique for living related liver transplantation which we have performed in 14 cases in the last 10 months.

Another problem in the treatment of hepatocellular carcinoma (HCC) is tumor thrombi in the main portal vein which had been considered as a contraindication for liver resection. We had also treated these patients conservatively in the early experience of our work. Most of these patients, however, died of rupture of the esophageal varices or liver failure soon after the diagnoses was made. These appalling consequences of the tumor thrombus cases prompted us to perform tumor thrombectomy with hepatic resection as an emergency operation to decompress the portal

vein pressure. In this paper, the outcome of this type of operation will be also introduced.

2 Hepatic vascular exclusion for liver resection using veno-venous bypass

The utility and safety of HVE for hepatic resection have been well documented by Delva et al. [8], Bismuth et al. [9] and others [10] that a noncirrhotic human liver can tolerate HVE for up to 90 minutes. HCC in Japan, however, is commonly associated with cirrhosis and, in our own experience with 308 patients operated on for HCC, 78% of the cases were accompanied by cirrhosis. Huge's report included discouraging results for the application of HVE in cirrhotics [11]. There are some inherent problems with HVE that contribute to such a high mortality rate. One is decreased blood return to the heart resulting in decreased cardiac index or arrhythmia [12, 13]. Another is recirculation injury to the ischemic liver related to portal congestion, especially in cirrhotics [14, 15]. The introduction of the double veno-venous bypass concept is expected to solve these problems. In this section, the operative procedures and the results will be discussed.

2.1 Patients

Between January 1985 and April 1990, 520 patients underwent liver resection in our clinic. Liver resection with the HVE technique using veno-venous bypass was decided upon for 26 patients. Twenty of these 26 patients eventually underwent hepatic resection with this method. The mean age of patients (of which 17 were male

---

[1] The Second Department of Surgery, Kyoto University Faculty of Medicine, Sakyo, Kyoto, 606 Japan

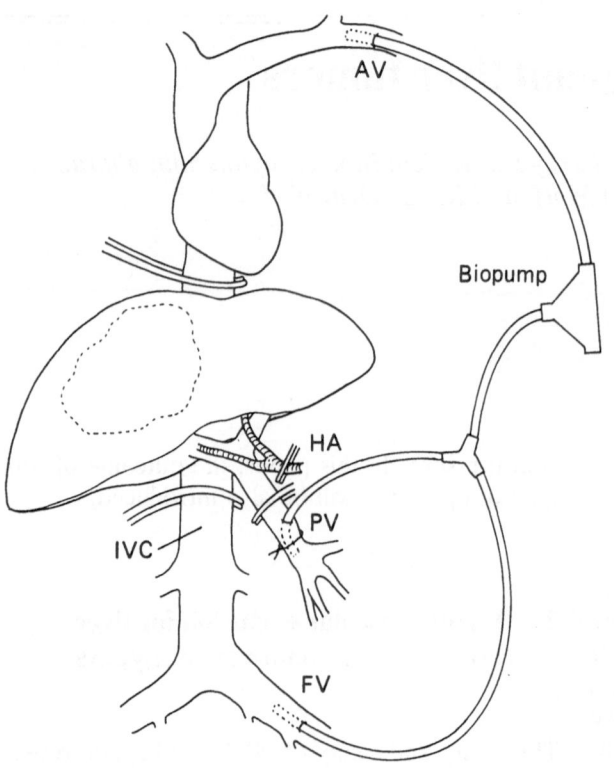

Fig. 1. The combined technique of HVE and veno-venous bypass using Biopump. *AV*, axillar vein; *PV*, portal vein; *IVC*, inferior vena cava; *FV*, femoral vein; *HA*, hepatic artery

and 3 were female) was 56.6 ± 2.2 years (range 36–72). Indications for liver resection were HCC in 12 cases and metastatic cancer in 8 cases. The other 6 cases who were initially scheduled for hepatectomy with HVE prior to surgery, however, ended up receiving a simple bypass from the inferior vena cava (IVC) to the axillary vein, since it was possible to isolate the retrohepatic IVC below the orifice of the hepatic vein and to place a clamp on the IVC just below the hepatic vein of the non-invaded lobe. The latter 6 patients, therefore, have no period of warm ischemia.

2.2 Operative procedure

Operative procedures consisted of the combined technique of HVE [8–10] and veno-venous bypass using an active centrifugal force pump (Biopump; Bio-medicus Inc., Minetonka, MN) [16] as illustrated in Fig. 1. The femoral and portal vein cannulae come together at the Y-connector, the other end of which leads to the conical head of the centrifugal force pump. The return flow is to the axillar vein. Vascular exclusion is obtained by applying a vascular clamp to the hepatic pedicle to occlude inflow, after which the IVC is first clamped below and then

Table 1. Types of resections

Right trisegmentectomy	5
Extended right lobectomy	7
Right lobectomy	6
Left lobectomy	2
Total	20

above the liver. Since the liver is now bloodless, it can be resected with a knife or scissors.

2.3 Results

Liver resection with HVE technique using veno-venous bypass was performed in 20 patients. The types of liver resections are shown in Table 1. Massive liver resection was performed in most of the cases. Liver cirrhosis was coexistent in 8 of them.

Many advanced HCC cases which had formerly been considered inoperable were treated in this series including removal of portal thrombi in the main trunk or its bifurcation in 6 cases, and removal of hepatic vein and/or IVC thrombi in 5 cases. Additional operative procedures to the retrohepatic IVC (8 patients) included segmental

Fig. 2. Changes in AKBR during the liver resection using the HVE method and active veno-venous bypass. *HVE*, the period of HVE

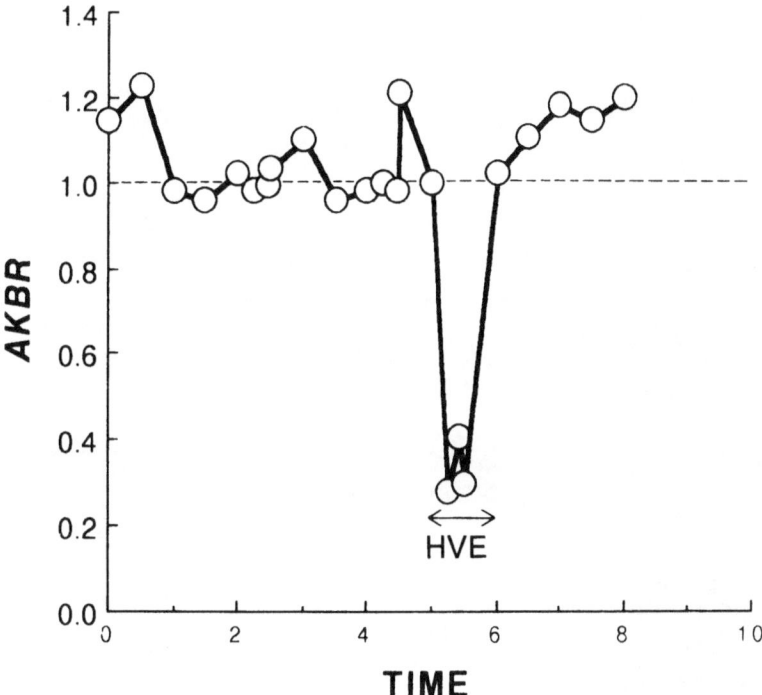

resection and reconstruction with artificial vein grafts (EPTFE) in 4 cases, partial resection followed by simple closure in 3, and replacement of vessel wall with an EPTFE patch in one. Blood loss during operation was 5,743 ± 393 ml (range 2,230–9,000 ml). When the surrounding tissues were being dissected from the liver, unexpected collaterals into the liver were anchored, and massive bleeding occurred in some cases. Duration of Biopump operation was 56.1 ± 3.4 minutes (range 23–80 minutes) and the period of warm ischemia was 36.9 ± 3.5 minutes (range 13–70 minutes).

The postoperative changes in hepatic and renal function tests such as transaminase, prothrombin time, creatinine and bilirubin levels were not so drastic. Gastrointestinal bleeding was observed in 2 patients as a postoperative complication. Ten of 20 patients developed pleural effusion, three of which necessitated drainage. Bilirubin levels were below 5.0 mg/dl in all but 3 cases. Postoperative renal insufficiency was not observed in this series.

Postoperative death within 30 days after operation occurred in one cirrhotic patient, who under-went right lobectomy associated with IVC reconstruction. In this patient, in whom the period of warm ischemia was 70 minutes, transaminase increased to 788 Glutamic-pyruvic transaminase (GPT) and 633 Glutamic-oxaloacetic transaminase (GOT), and total

bilirubin increased to 6.2 mg/dl on the 2nd day postoperatively, maximally to 21.2 mg/dl on the 10th day. Massive bleeding from a stomach ulcer occurred on the 11th day which necessitated gastrectomy. Finally, the patient died of liver insufficiency on the 16th day.

Decreasing period of AKBR to below 0.4 was limited only during the warm ischemic time in each case (Fig. 2) and the recovery tendency of AKBR after reflow to the liver was sharp in all but the one case whose ischemic time was 70 minutes.

2.4 Discussion

Delva et al. emphasized that a non-cirrhotic human liver can tolerate HVE for up to 90 minutes [8]. Bismuth et al. applied HVE for 46.5 ± 5.0 minutes to major hepatic resection with an operative mortality rate of 2.0% [9]. Although their results are excellent, their series did not include cirrhotic cases. Since a great number of HCC cases are cirrhotic, it remained unclear whether HVE could be applied in these cases. As reported by Bismuth et al., fluid preloading before clamping is necessary to obtain hemodynamic stability during HVE [9]. Cirrhotic patients who are scheduled to undergo hepatic

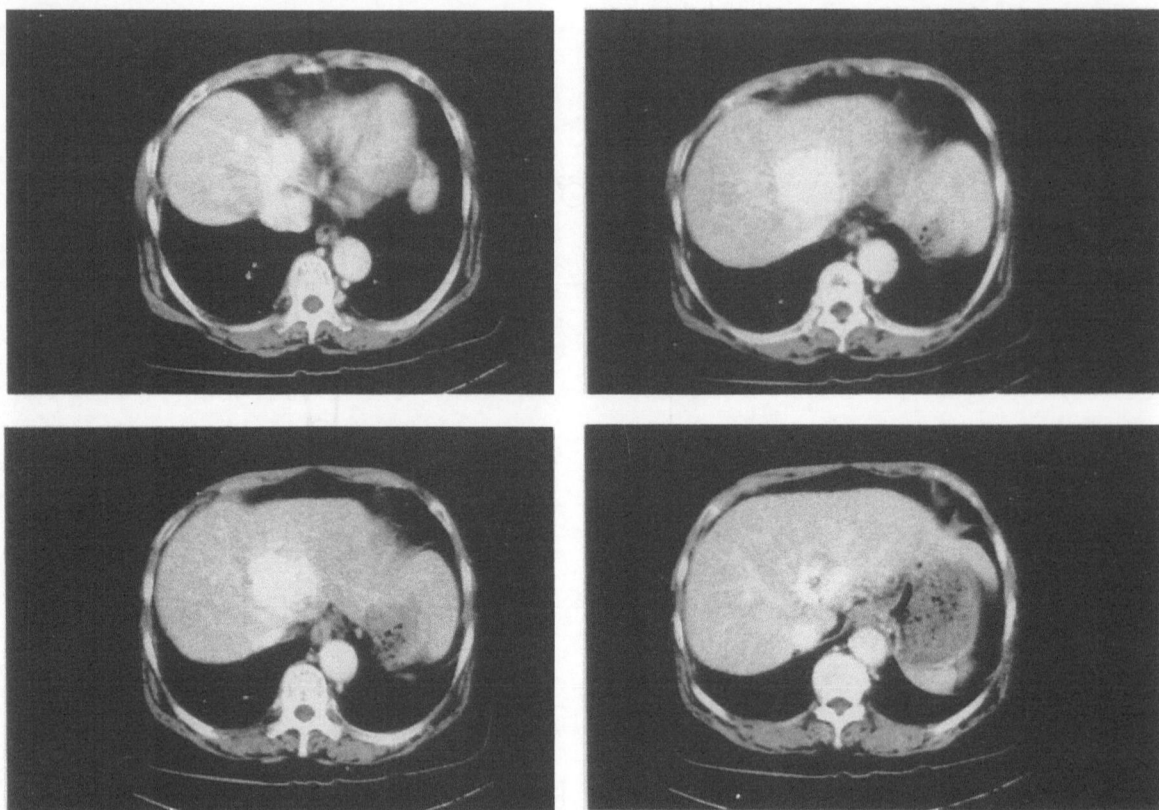

Fig. 3. CT images of a 68-year-old female. The tumor is located between the middle and the left hepatic veins

resection are usually kept relatively dehydrated to control ascites and to prevent postoperative pulmonary complications. Thus, the test clamping of the IVC performed to evaluate hemodynamic stability sometimes results in severe hypotension. Hence, we routinely apply HVE to liver resection in combination with active veno-venous shunting. In our series, no patients developed hypotension, even during HVE, since the use of Biopump contributed greatly to the maintenance of intra-operative hemodynamics.

We have previously reported that the recovery of AKBR after reperfusion reflects the extent of hepatic mitochondrial damage [14], and the recovery tendency of AKBR after reperfusion predicts the viability of the liver after hepatectomy [17] and liver graft after transplantation [18, 19]. In the cirrhotics, the redox state of the hepatic mitochondria, which had been reduced by HVE, was oxidized immediately after reperfusion except for one case whose liver was exposed to warm ischemia exceeding 70 minutes. Hence, it may be conjectured that the application of the active veno-venous bypass has a major advantage

in the recovery of the hepatic energy metabolism by achieving complete decompression of the portal system and hemodynamic stabilization during operation. Judging from these data, the early recovery of AKBR after recirculation observed in the cirrhotic patients in our series clearly demonstrates the fact that even a cirrhotic liver can tolerate prolonged ischemia when portal congestion is neutralized.

3 Hepatic resection using the technique for living related liver transplantation

The hepatic resection of the left lobe (Segments 2, 3 and 4) is indicated for the treatment of a tumor located between the middle and left hepatic veins. When a patient has severe cirrhosis, however, it will be difficult to determine whether or not to go ahead with surgery. Based on our belief that surgical resection is the best treatment now available for HCC, the tumor was

Fig. 4. Changes in AKBR during liver resection using the technique for living related liver transplantation. *1*, left lobectomy; *2*, reconstruction of the left portal vein; *3*, reconstruction of the left hepatic artery

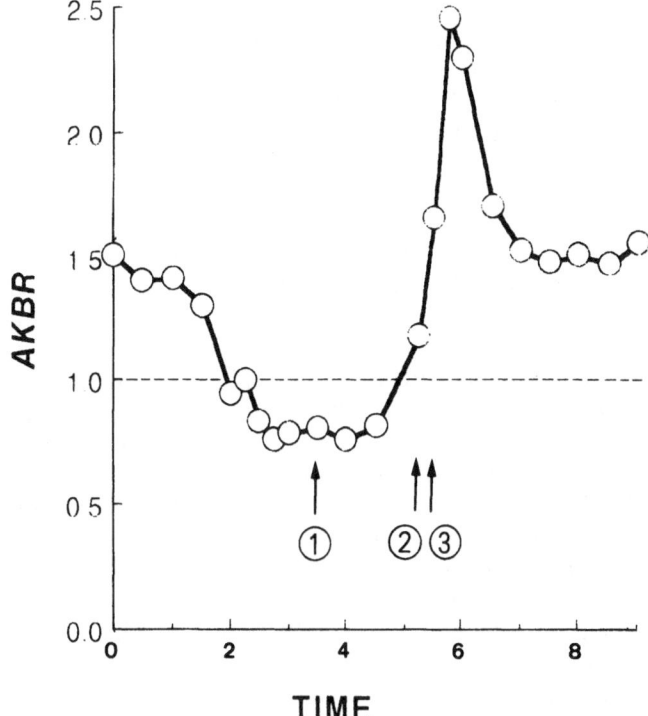

removed on the back table. The following is a case report.

3.1 Patient

A 68-year-old female was admitted with diagnoses of HCC with liver cirrhosis and diabetes mellitus. The tumor was 6 cm in diameter located adherent to the bifurcation of the left hepatic and middle hepatic veins (Fig. 3). The volumetric analysis from the CT image showed that the right lobe had only 42% of the whole volume and the left lobe 45%.

3.2 Operative procedure

The left lobe was resected under maintaining blood flow to both lobes using the operative procedure for harvesting of liver graft from living donor [20]. After the left lobe was perfused with the University of Wisconsin (UW) solution in situ following wash out of blood, it was transported on the back table. The tumor and most of medial segment (S4) was removed and the middle hepatic vein was resected. Many holes and laceration on the left hepatic vein were reconstructed to make it possible to anastomose with the orifice of

the left hepatic vein on the IVC. The left caudate lobe was resected while the tumor was resected on the back table. The remaining lateral segment was put in the bowel cavity again for auto-transplantation. Vascular anastomoses were performed at the left hepatic vein, the left portal vein and the left hepatic artery. The biliary duct was anastomosed to the jejunal loop of Roux-en Y limb. Cold ischemic time was 113 minutes. Bile flow was obtained with a bilioenteroanastomosis.

The patients is now alive some 8 months after the operation and works as a housewife.

3.3 Discussion

When resection of the medial segment is scheduled, hazardous bleeding from hepatic veins could occur, and the lack of hilar control would deteriorate the liver functions. Left lobectomy is risky due to the possibility of postoperative liver failure. Figure 4 shows that AKBR decreased to 0.7 when the left lobe was removed, increased to more than 1.0 with portal reflow, reached 2.0 after arterial reflow, then maintained a level of 1.5 afterward. These changes will be different from the so-called bench surgery (ex situ) [21] where the whole liver is removed, when the transplanted liver will be stressed during the anhepatic period. On the other hand, the intraoperative stress will be loaded and metabolized in the remnant cirrhotic liver in this revised partial liver transplantation. The lateral segment implanted would work as additional salvage.

4 Liver resection and removal of tumor thrombi in the main portal vein

In many patients with portal thrombi from advanced HCC, death results from rupture of the esophageal varices or hepatic failure. We performed tumor thrombectomy with hepatic resection as an emergency operation to decompress the portal vein pressure. Since portal flow was maintained to the remnant liver by this procedure, this further enabled us to perform transcatheter arterial embolization (TAE) or percutaneous ethanol injection therapy (PEIT). In this report, the clinical outcome will be presented.

4.1 Patients

Among 298 liver resections with HCC, there were 29 portal thrombi cases treated by direct removal with liver resection during the past 5 years. In the present study, 76% of them had some form of underlying chronic liver disease. In 16 patients, the main tumors were located in the right lobe and 13 in the left lobe.

4.2 Operative procedures [4]

4.2.1 Hepatectomy
If the tumor thrombi were confined to the first branch of the portal vein, they were automatically removed by conventional hemihepatectomy.

4.2.2 Simple thrombectomy
Balloon catheter, suction and a spatula were used for removal.

4.2.3 Bypass
From the umbilical portion to the main trunk of the portal vein, bypass anastomosis was performed with a vein graft to obtain the portal flow to the remnant liver during the liver resection. Tumor thrombi were contained inside the removed portal vein segment.

4.2.4 Open method
Under HVE using veno-venou bypass [17], the portal vein was incised to directly remove the portal thrombi, and then closed with running suture of the vein.

4.3 Results

Three patients died within 30 days after operation (mortality, 11%). Postoperative complications included respiratory problems in 6 cases requiring mechanical ventilation, liver insufficiency in 2, and postoperative bleeding necessitating relaparotomy in 2.

Although improved patient survival was not the primary goal of this emergency operation, half of the patients had the unexpectedly high survival rate of 1 year, 52.2%; 2 years, 23.2%; and 3 years, 11.6%

4.4 Discussion

HCC has a noted propensity to invade the portal vein [22]. The early intrahepatic spread of HCC via the portal vein has been a major limiting factor in its indication and curability by resection [1, 23, 24]. Any attempt to remove the tumor thrombus or to resect the liver has generally been thought to be futile in such cases. Our attempt to remove the tumor thrombus was based on the assumption that if we could relieve the portal pressure, we would be able to prevent the fatal rupture of the esophageal varices. Since no variceal bleeding was encountered postoperatively, we were satisfied that we attained our primary goal. When we did a follow-up study of our patients treated with TAE and PEIT as postoperative adjuvant therapies, we noted an unexpectedly large number of long term survivors.

In order for the proposed operation to be accepted as a form of surgical treatment for HCC, not merely as an emergency life saving procedure, it is necessary to establish a preoperative standard by which surgeons can distinguish between patients with the early recurrence type of HCC and those with the long-term survivor type.

References

1. The Liver Cancer Study Group of Japan (1990) Primary liver cancer in Japan, clinicopathologic

features and results of surgical treatment. Ann Surg 211:277–287

2. Ozawa K (1990) Hepatic function and liver resection. J Gastroenterol Hepatol 5:296–309

3. Yamaoka Y, Ozawa K, Shimahara Y, Nakatani T, Mori K, Kobayashi N, Kumada K (1988) A simple and direct approach to the portal triad structures for a left lobectomy or a left lateral segmentectomy. Surg Gynecol Obstet 166:78–80

4. Kumada K, Ozawa K, Okamoto R, Takayasu T, Yamaguchi M, Yamamoto Y, Higashiyama H, Morikawa S, Sasaki Y, Shimahara Y, Yamaoka Y, Takeuchi E (1990) Hepatic resection for advanced hepatocellular carcinoma with removal of portal vein tumor thrombi. Surgery 108:821–827

5. Mori K, Ozawa K, Yamamoto Y, Maki A, Shimahara Y, Kobayashi N, Yamaoka Y, Kumada K (1990) Response of hepatic mitochondrial redox state to oral glucose load—redox tolerance test as a new predictor of surgical risk in hepatectomy. Ann Surg 211:438–446

6. Kiuchi T, Shimahara Y, Wakashiro S, Tokunaga Y, Ozaki N, Takayasu T, Mori K, Kobayashi N, Yamaoka Y, Ozawa K (1990) Reduced arterial ketone body ratio during laparotomy: An evaluation of operative stress through the changes in hepatic mitochondrial redox potential. J Lab Clin Med 115:433–440

7. Shimahara Y, Kiuchi T, Yamamoto Y, Yamaguchi T, Takada Y, Yamauchi A, Higashiyama H, Kobayashi N, Mori K, Yamaoka Y, Kumada K, Ozawa K (1990) Hepatic mitochondrial redox potential and nutritional support in liver insufficiency. In: Tanaka T and Okada A (eds) Nutritional support in organ failure. Elsevier, Amsterdam, pp 295–307

8. Delva E, Camus Y, Nordlinger B, Hannoun L, Parc R, Deriaz H, Lienhart A, Huge C (1989) Vascular occlusion for liver resections. Operative management and tolerance to hepatic ischemia: 142 cases. Am J Surg 209:211–218

9. Bismuth H, Castaing D, Garden J (1989) Major hepatic resection under total vascular exclusion. Ann Surg 210:13–19

10. Fortner GF, Shiu MH, Howland WS, Gaston JP, Kunlin A, Kawano N, Hattori T, Beattie EJ (1971) A new concept for hepatic lobectomy: Experimental studies and clinical application. Arch Surg 102:312–315

11. Huget C, Nordlinger B, Bloch P, Conard J (1978) Tolerance of the human liver to prolonged normothermic ischemia: A biological study of 20 patients submitted to extensive hepatectomy. Arch Surg 113:1448–1451

12. Howland WS, Schweizer OS, Fortner J, Shiu MH, Ragasa JP, Wightman AE, Gould P (1975) Intraoperative physiologic monitoring and management during hepatic lobectomy using the liver isolation-perfusion technique. Am J Surg 129:608–615

13. Delva E, Barberousse JP, Nordlinger B, Olliver JM, Vacher B, Guilmet C, Huget C (1984) Hemodynamic and biochemical monitoring during major liver resection with use of hepatic vascular exclusion. Surgery 95:309–318

14. Yamaoka Y, Shimahara Y, Nakatani T, Mori K, Kobayashi N, Maki A, Nitta N, Yamamoto S, Ozawa K (1988) Clinical role of blood ketone body ratio as an indicator evaluating hepatic tolerance for portal triad cross-clamping in cirrhotic liver resection. Surg Res Comm 3:87–93

15. Nitta N, Yamamoto S, Yamaoka Y, Ozawa K (1988) Arterial blood ketone body ratio as an indicator of the no-return point in hepatic inflow occlusion without venous shunt in dogs. Life Sci 42:1973–1979

16. Shaw BW, Martin D, Marquez JM, Kang YG, Bugbee AC, Iwatsuki S, Griffith BP, Hardesty RL, Bahnson HT, Starzl TS (1984) Venous bypass in clinical liver transplantation. Ann Surg 200:524–532

17. Yamaoka Y, Ozawa K, Kumada K, Shimahara Y, Tanaka K, Mori K, Takayasu T, Okamoto R, Kobayashi N, Konishi Y, Egawa H (to be published) (1991) Total vascular exclusion for hepatic resection in cirrhotic patients: Application of veno-venous bypass. Arch Surg

18. Taki Y, Gubernatis G, Yamaoka Y, Oellerich M, Yamamoto Y, Ringe B, Okamoto R, Bunzendahl H, Beneking M, Burdelski M, Bornscheuer A, Ozawa K, Pichlmayr R (1990) Significance of arterial ketone body ratio measurement in human liver transplantation. Transplantation 49:535–539

19. Asonuma K, Takaya S, Selby R, Okamoto R, Yamamoto Y, Yokoyama T, Todo S, Ozawa K, Starzl TE (1991) The clinical significance of the arterial ketone body ratio as an early indicator of graft viability in human liver transplantation. Transplantation 51:164–171

20. Yamaoka Y, Ozawa K, Tanaka A, Mori K, Morimoto T, Shimahara Y, Zaima M, Tanaka K, Kumada K (to be published) (1991) New devices for harvesting the hepatic graft from the living donor. Transplantation 52:157–160

21. Pichlmayr R, Grosse H, Hauss J, Gubernatis G, Lamesch P, Bretschneider HJ (1990) Technique and preliminary results of extracorporeal liver surgery (bench procedure) and of surgery on the in situ perfused liver. Br J Surg 77:21–26

22. Kishi K, Shikata T, Hirohashi S, Hasegawa H, Yamazaki S, Makuuchi M (1983) Hepatocellular carcinoma: A clinical and pathologic analysis of 57 hepatectomy cases. Cancer 51:542–548

23. Nagasue N, Yukaya H, Ogawa Y, Sasaki Y, Chang YC, Niimi K (1986) Clinical experience with 118 hepatic resections for hepatocellular carcinoma. Surgery 99:694–702

24. Yamanaka N, Okamoto E, Toyosaka A (1990) Prognostic factors after hepatectomy for hepatocellular carcinomas. Cancer 65:1104–1110

Anatomical resection of the right hepatic subsegments preceded by suprahilar ligation of the portal pedicles

Eizo Okamoto and Naoki Yamanaka[1]

1 Introduction

In recent years, with the rapid increase of cirrhotic patients with smaller hepatocellular carcinomas, limited hepatectomies of less than one segment tend to greatly outnumber the regular and extended lobectomies. In view of the early intrahepatic spread of this cancer through portal blood stream [1], an anatomical segmental or subsegmental resection which is preceded by initial ligation of Glisson's pedicles at the liver hilum is highly desirable even in such a limited hepatectomy.

Fortunately for liver surgeons, the portal triads including portal vein, hepatic artery and bile duct are encased together in the thick Glisson's sheath as they enter the liver and take the same course through the hepatic segment and subsegment, requiring no separate maneuver to isolate. In addition, bifurcations of these triads for each segment or subsegment are located so close to the porta hepatis that their roots can be readily accessed without cutting much liver parenchyma.

Based on these anatomical facts, we reported a new device of an anatomical resection of the right hepatic subsegments preceded by suprahilar ligation in 1986 [2] and have been trying to improve the technique. In this paper, the most recent achievement of our technique will be described.

2 Details of the technique

Fundamentally, the procedure is divided into the following steps: 1) detachment and dislocation of the right portal pedicle, 2) dissection and isolation of segmental and subsequent subsegmental pedicles, encircling each with snaring tapes. 3) temporary occlusion of pedicles delineating the discolored segmental or subsegmental territories by electrocautery, 4) resection of the target area (Fig. 1).

2.1 Detachment and dislocation of the right portal pedicle

Cholecystectomy is performed in the usual fashion. The posterior extremity of the cystic plate is devided from the hilar plate by electrocautery. This is important to mobilize widely the right portal pedicle afterwards. The hepatic capsule is transversely incised with electrocautery between the posterior margin of the quadrate process and the hilar plate. The hilar plate is then gently detached from the liver using a pair of spatulas applied oppositely (Fig. 2). Detachment is further continued until only a sheet of peritoneum remains between the surgeons finger posteriorly and the dissecting spatula anteriorly (Fig. 3). A pair of strongly curved Kelly's forceps is introduced behind the right portal pedicle and sticks its tip posteriorly through the peritoneum to bite one end of a tape and to pull it out anteriorly, thus the right portal pedicle can be encircled safely. By manipulating the tape, the whole length and width of the right portal pedicle is carefully mobilized with attention not to injure the caudate branches which are located posteriorly and centrally in the hilar plate.

Tiny vascular bridges which are often encountered during detachment may be cauterized without trouble. Most caution must be paid not to injure the terminal branches of the middle hepatic vein which are often barely exposed over the undersurface of the detached quadrate lobe. If

[1] The First Department of Surgery, Hyogo College of Medicine, Nishinomiya, Hyogo, 663 Japan

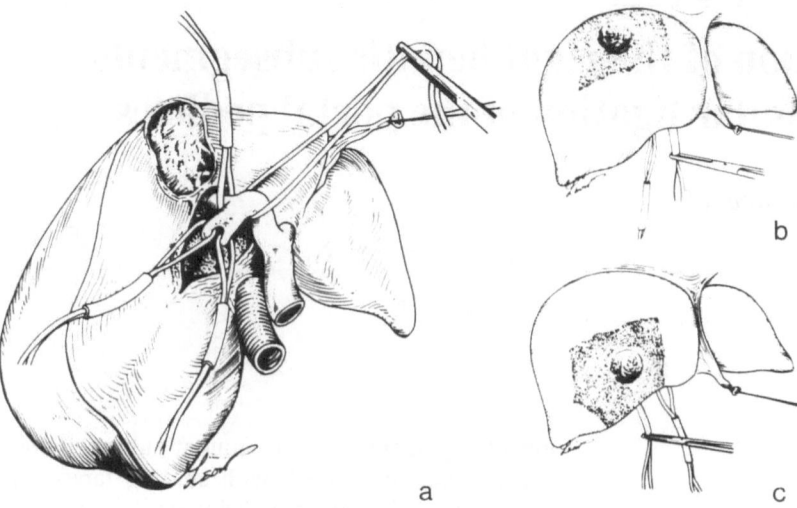

Fig.   1a–c. Fundamental steps. **a** Detachment and dislocation of the right portal pedicle and subsequent isolation of segmental and subsegmental pedicles. Each pedicle is encircled with a tourniquet. After test occlusion, the subsegment to be resected is decided. **b** The discolored anterior superior subsegment (S8), **c** The discolored anterior interior subsegment (S5)

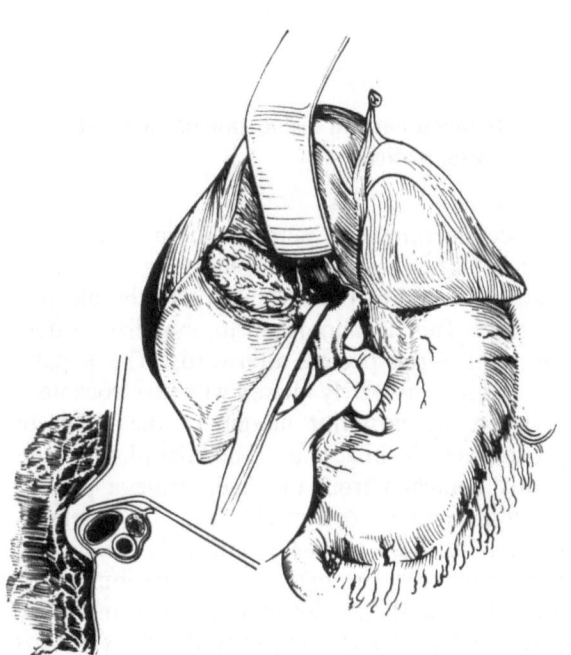

Fig. 2. Detachment of the right portal pedicle from the undersurface of the quadrate lobe

torn, a thin sheet of Oxycel Cotton^R is put on the liver surface and pressed down by an assistant's hand with a spatula without discontinuing the operation.

2.2 Isolation of the right segmental pedicles

At the right corner of the transverse fissure, the right anterior segmental pedicle enters the liver

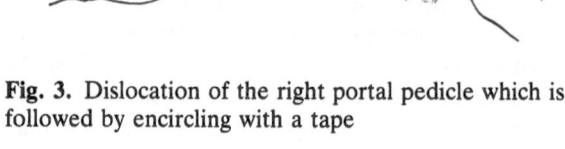

Fig. 3. Dislocation of the right portal pedicle which is followed by encircling with a tape

usually through the plane of the main lobar fissure (Cantlie's line) and the right posterior segmental pedicle through the plane of the right lobar fissure. Keeping this anatomy in mind, it is not difficult to identify the roots of both pedicles. With traction being kept on both anterior and posterior pedicles by pulling up the tape placed around the right portal pedicle, a pair of curved Kelly's forceps is introduced posteriorly through the crotch formed by the two segmental pedicles and stick out its tip above or below the dislocated right portal pedicle. Using this forceps, a tape is passed from below to encircle the posterior pedicle and from above for the anterior pedicle (Fig. 4). Each tape is passed through a

Fig. 4a,b. a Encircling of the right posterior segment with a tape. **b** The same of the anterior segmental pedicle

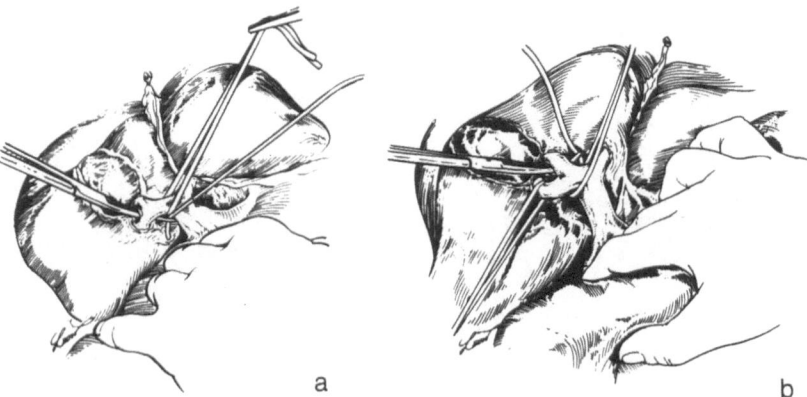

a   b

short length of Nelaton tube to function as a tourniquet.

The forceps should be introduced as close to the Glisson's sheath as possible unless it may injure the sheath. If any resistance is felt at the tip of the forceps, take it back and try again taking a little roundabout route until it passes safely.

Each tourniquet is alternately and temporarily snugged down and the darkly discolored areas are delineated exactly on the liver surface by cautery. The boundaries of both anterior and posterior segments are thus clearly mapped on the right lobe of the liver. If resection of either the anterior or posterior segment is attempted, the corresponding pedicle is left to be snugged down or permanently ligated by a thick silk string and the discolored segment is dissected out and removed.

2.3 Isolation of the subsegmental pedicles

The sites of ramification of each segmental pedicle into the subsegmental pedicles vary considerably on a case by case basis. On a rare occasion, the sites of ramification are located so close to the hilum that all of the four subsegmental pedicles can be individually isolated and taped without dividing the liver. In most cases, however, division of the liver through an appropriate plane is necessary to get access safely to the pedicles.

2.3.1 Anterior inferior (V) and superior (VIII) subsegments

In order to explore these subsegmental pedicles, the liver should be entered through the plane of the main lobar fissure that has been delineated with cautery as described above. Dissection is carried out bluntly both of the dissected liver edges being retracted and opened, and is con-

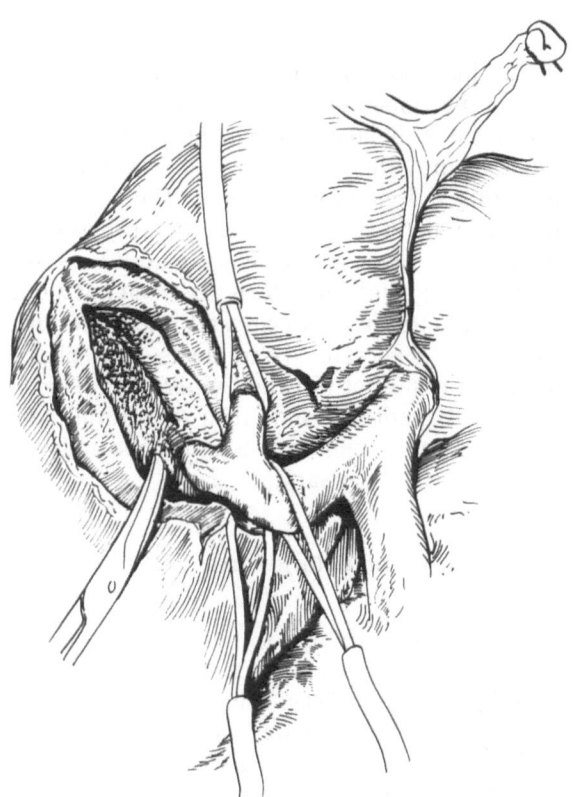

Fig. 5. Isolation of the subsegmental pedicles. The pedicle for the right anterior superior subsegment (S8) is encircled with a tourniquet

tinued to expose the right segmental pedicle and its subsegmental tributaries consecutively.

When the two subsegmental pedicles bifurcate regularly, the fork of these pedicles is generally found within one to two cm in depth. Each of these is separately encircled by a tourniquet (Fig. 5). After alternative occlusion test, the areas of the inferior (S5) and superior (S8) subsegments are identified by discoloration and mapped on the liver surface using cautery.

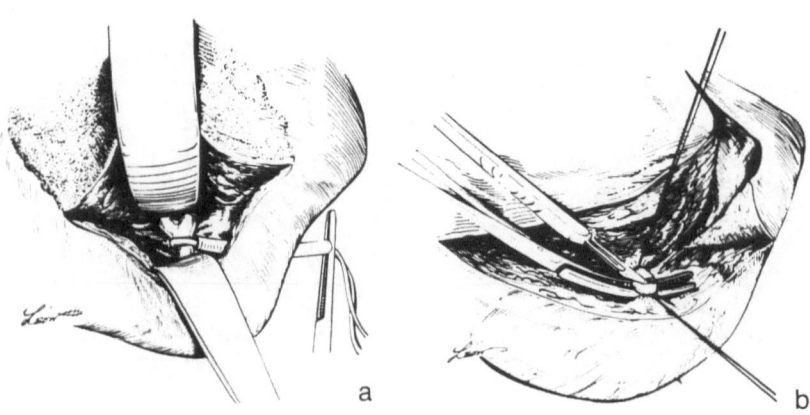

Fig. 6a,b. Resection of the discolored subsegment. **a** The liver parenchyma is being dissected through the borderline between the discolored anterior superior subsegment (S8) and the inferior subsegment (S5) splitting the liver with two spatulas applied oppositely. **b** The pedicle for the anterior superior subsegment is doubly ligated and divided

2.3.2 Posterior inferior (VI) and superior (VII) subsegments

The liver is divided through the plane of right lobar fissure, the borderline between the right posterior and anterior segments. The borderline has been delineated with cautery as described above. The liver parenchyma anterior to the posterior segmental pedicle is dissected out along this line until its subsegmental tributaries are sufficiently exposed. Tourniquets are placed around the inferior (VI) and superior (VII) subsegmental pedicles and their territories are identified after occlusion tests and delineated with cautery on the liver surface.

2.4 Resection of the target area

The subsegment or area to be resected is finally decided after repeated occlusion tests using a tourniquet. The pedicles going to the target subsegment or area are ligated with thick silk string and divided. The discolored liver parenchyma is dissected out and removed (Fig. 6).

The dissection is carried out exactly through the plane of discolored borderline and always directed toward the liver hilum or the root of the ligated pedicle. We do not use finger fracture technique but use "split the liver technique", ligating and dividing hepatic vein branches bridging between the split liver edges.

3 Discussion

In 1985 when this method was started in our clinic, the process of deroofing by mobilizing a part of the quadrate lobe was considered to be

necessary to open the hilar plate widely, especially in selective resection of the right segment and its two subsegments. With the rapid accumulation of experience, however, this process soon became unnecessary. Takasaki and his associates [3] independently arrived at a method similar to the one described in this paper, and it was reported also in 1986. They used dye injection to identify the small area to be resected.

Several years after we published this method, we became aware that Couinaud had already proposed the concept of this type of hepatectomy named "extrafascial portal approach" based on his vast anatomical and technical studies using autopsy liver [Couinaud C (1981) Controlled hepatectomies and exposure of the intrahepatic bile ducts: Anatomical and technical study. Paris, personal edition]. He reported [4] his own clinical case of left hepatectomy applying this concept, however, no report of clinical experience is seen concerning the right hepatic segments or subsegments. It may thus be said that the concept proposed by Couinaud has been first realized by Japanese surgeons in clinical practice.

In this chapter, we have described the fundamental and typical procedure of our suprahilar subsegmentectomy. The neoplastic lesions that need hepatic resection, however, do not always exist in the center of a hepatic segment or subsegment. In these instances, the area of resection is designed previously considering the location of tumor and the related subsegmental pedicular distribution, and this technique is applied. It is not difficult to resect a part of the adjacent subsegment in this technique.

Either the subsegmental pedicles do not always bifurcate so regularly as in a textbook, but sometimes three or more subsegmental pedicles arise from the extremity of one segmental pedicle. In

Table 1. Types of right hepatic subsegmentectomy (1985–1990)

Single		
	S5	8
	S6	7
	S7	4
	S8	8
		29
Two		
	S5 + S4	7
	S5 + S6	15
	S5 + S8	8
	S6 + S7	20
	S6 + S8	1
	S7 + S8	11
	S8 + S4	5
		67
Three		
	S3 + S6 + S8	1
	S4 + S5 + S6	1
	S5 + S6 + S7	5
	S5 + S6 + S8	1
	S4 + S7 + S8	1
		9

these cases, the pedicles that are encountered during dissection are taped in order and decide exactly the resecting area after repeated occlusion tests.

The dissection should be carried out through the discolored border, namely, the intersegmental or intersubsegmental plane, which is essentially avascular except for hepatic vein branches, and this provides the best route for splitting the liver and controlling the hepatic vein branches.

In the last six years from 1985 through 1990, this type of subsegmentectomy has been carried out in 105 patients. The underlying hepatic lesions were hepatocellular carcinoma (93), cholangiocellular carcinoma (2), metastatic cancer (4), intrahepatic caliculi (3), angiomyolipoma (1) and cyst (2). The resected areas are listed in

Table 1 according to Couinaud's designation of the liver segments.

Three of 105 patients (3.2%) with hepatocellular carcinoma died of postoperative liver failure. All of these three were associated with severe liver cirrhosis. As postoperative complications, postoperative bleeding was seen in three patients who required relaparotomy. Bile leakage and abscess was seen in 7 patients who were treated with ultrasound-guided drainage. There was no specific complication which is responsible to this technique itself.

Finally, the merits of this method are summarized as follows: 1) en bloc ligation of portal triads facilitates a safe and anatomic resection of the hepatic subsegment, 2) favorable to secure a wide surgical margin in cases where the tumor is located deeply, 3) favorable for tumor located very close to the hilum, and 4) protects transportal dissemination of cancer cells during surgical manipulation of the liver.

References

1. Okamoto E, Yamanaka N, Toyosaka A, Tanaka N, Yabuki K (1987) Current status of hepatic resection in the treatment of hepatocellular carcinoma. In: Okuda K, Ishak KG (eds) Neoplasm of the liver. Springer-Verlag, Tokyo pp 354–365
2. Okamoto E (1986) Hepatic resection for primary hepatocellular carcinoma: New trials for controlled anatomic subsegmentectomies by an initial suprahilar Glissonian pedicular ligation method (in Japanese). Shokakigeka Seminar 23:229–241
3. Takasaki K, Kobayashi S, Tanaka S, Muto H, Saiyo T, Saito A, Ueda T, Shimada Y, Tanaka T, Honda H (1986) A new method of systmatic hepatectomy by en bloc ligation of Glissonian pedicles (in Japanese). Operation 40:7–14
4. Couinaud C (1985) A simplified method for controlled left hepatectomy. Surgery 97:358–361

CHAPTER 23

Systematic subsegmentectomy for hepatocellular carcinoma

Seiji Kawasaki, Masatoshi Makuuchi[1], Tomoo Kosuge, and Tadatoshi Takayama[2]

1 Introduction

According to the eighth report published by the Liver Cancer Study Group of Japan in 1988 [1], surgical treatment and its outcome for patients with hepatocellular carcinoma had improved remarkably since the report issued in 1979 [2]. Two major reasons for the decreased operative mortality and improved long-term survival rate following hepatectomy are early detection with various diagnostic modalities for high-risk patients and advances in surgical treatment based on an understanding of the clinicopathological features of hepatocellular carcinoma.

Ultrasonically guided subsegmentectomy devised by Makuuchi [3] is representative of recent advances in treatment for small hepatocellular carcinomas in Japan. This surgical procedure and its results are summarized and reported herein.

2 Clinicopathological features of hepatocellular carcinoma necessitating systematic subsegmentectomy

Hepatocellular carcinoma tends to invade the portal venous pedicles, and tumor cells spread through the portal vein into the distal part of the liver as a result of portal venous flow. Tumor cells in the portal veins may grow into tumor thrombi, which become a source of wider tumor spread (Fig. 1). Major hepatectomy is indicated for patients with hepatocellular carcinoma but having normal liver function, and complete regeneration of the remnant liver can be expected.

However, hepatocellular carcinoma is associated with liver cirrhosis in the majority of cases and this is the main obstacle to substantial hepatic resection. Therefore, complete resection confined to the portal unit containing the tumor appears to be the only practical choice for patients with poor hepatic functional reserve in order to avoid poor surgical outcomes such as immediate postoperative liver failure or early tumor recurrence.

Subsegmental (Couinaud's segmental) resection has been performed by others [4–6] based on knowledge of liver anatomy. However, there are wide variations in the ramification pattern of the portal vein and hepatic artery, and the volume of each subsegment differs from patient to patient, especially in cirrhotic livers. Furthermore, no landmarks exist on the liver surface to aid the identification of each subsegment, and subsegmental branches of the portal vein and hepatic artery supplying the right lobe cannot be readily exposed in the hepatic hilum.

Ultrasonically guided subsegmentectomy, which enables each subsegmental area with its feeding vessels to be precisely identified, was developed with the above problems in mind.

3 Patient selection criteria

Mortality and morbidity associated with hepatic resection including systematic subsegmentectomy is dictated mainly by whether the patient has sufficient hepatic functional reserve to tolerate this procedure. Selection criteria for patients in whom systematic subsegmentectomy is indicated in terms of hepatic reserve are listed in Table 1.

---

[1] First Department of Surgery, Shinshu University School of Medicine, Matsumoto, 390 Japan
[2] National Cancer Center Hospital, Tokyo, Japan

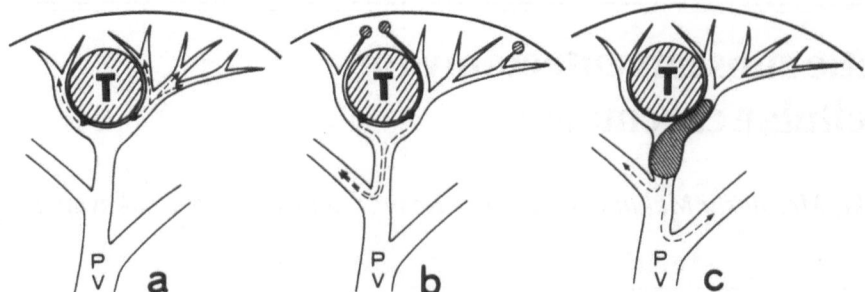

Fig. 1a–c. Intrahepatic extension and invasion of hepatocellular carcinoma. **a** Tumor invades the portal venous branches, and tumor cells are carried to the distal part of the liver by portal venous flow. **b** These cells grow into microscopic tumor thrombi and then into daughter nodules. **c** Tumor thrombus is in turn a source of wide tumor spread. T, tumor; PV, portal venous branch. (From [3] with permission of Surgery, Gynecology and Obstetrics.)

Table 1. Selection criteria on the basis of hepatic reserve for systematic subsegmentectomy

Ascites	None or Controllable
Serum bilirubin	$\leqq 1.0$ mg/dl
ICG[a] 15-min retention rate	<30%

[a] indocyanine green

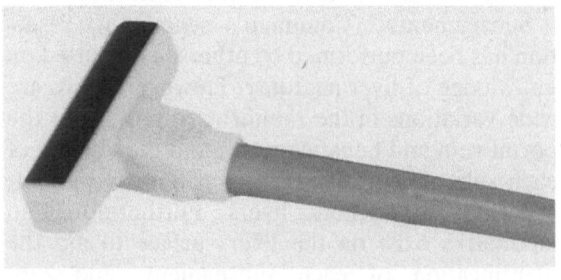

Fig. 2. T-shaped linear-array 7.5-MHz probe for intra-operative ultrasound during liver surgery

The presence of ascites is a clinical manifestation of poor hepatic functional status. If ascites are not controlled with diuretics preoperatively, no form of hepatectomy, including subsegmentectomy, is indicated since portal pressure tends to be elevated following liver resection which would, in turn, cause a further increase of ascites. As bacterial growth in ascites is frequent, peritonitis and intra-abdominal abscesses may result.

If the patient has a persistently elevated serum bilirubin level, we are reluctant to carry out systematic subsegmentectomy, and instead other types of hepatectomy such as limited resection or enucleation would be indicated. These less extensive procedures spare the non-cancerous

liver parenchyma as much as possible. Considering that cirrhotic liver has little ability to regenerate, significant long-term survival would not be expected following systematic subsegmentectomy in patients with a high serum bilirubin level, even though immediate postoperative hepatic failure may be unlikely.

4 Intraoperative ultrasonography

Intraoperative ultrasonography (IOUS) is *sine qua non* for systematic subsegmentectomy.

IOUS has been performed by Makuuchi in hepatic surgery since 1979 using a specially designed apparatus with various probes [7, 8]. A T-shaped linear-array probe of 7.5 MHz is now used most often for liver surgery [8] (Fig. 2).

With regard to IOUS, special emphasis should be placed on the following characteristics.

1. Hepatocellular carcinoma is frequently invisible and non-palpable from the liver surface. More than 50% of patients with small hepatocellular carcinomas (less than 5 cm in diameter) have a main tumor that is neither visible nor palpable [3, 9]. Precise liver resection is not possible without IOUS in these cases, even though preoperative diagnostic methods can indicate the segment in which the tumor is located.

2. Accurate localization of the tumor is determined in relation to the intrahepatic vessels. The feeding portal venous branches and the draining hepatic venous branches of the tumor can be identified.

Fig. 3. Sonogram obtained during staining of subsegment. The tip of the puncture needle is clearly seen and the injected dye is recognizable as moving echoes

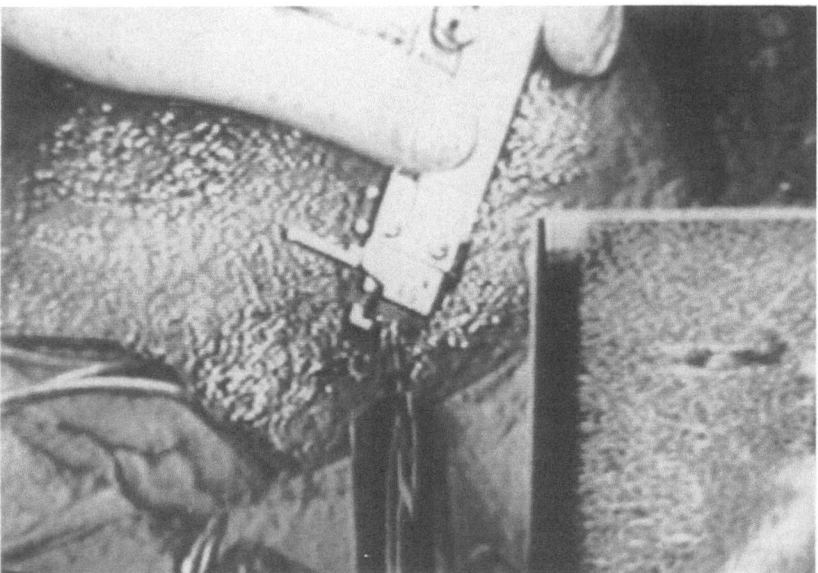

3. IOUS facilitates identification of smaller hepatic lesions than is possible with preoperative ultrasonography, since a higher-frequency transducer (7.5 MHz) can be used. Therefore, small daughter nodules or tumor thrombi in the portal or hepatic venous branch, which cannot be detected preoperatively, are frequently identified using IOUS.

4. Multiple images from almost all directions can be obtained without interference from ribs or bowel gas.

5. Needle biopsy can be performed for suspected lesions via the optimum route under ultrasonic guidance and the specimen submitted for immediate histological examination.

6. IOUS is indispensable for the key steps of systematic subsegmentectomy such as "staining" and "tattooing", which are described later.

7. The transection line can be recognized as an echogenic line during liver parenchymal resection, allowing accurate excision.

5 Surgical technique

A J-shaped or inverted T-shaped incision is made and the abdominal cavity is entered. A right thoracotomy is usually added through either the 8th or 9th intercostal space, and the diaphragm divided, if the tumor is located in the upper part of the right lobe. After the liver has been mobilized, intraoperative ultrasonography is per-

formed to determine the size and location of the tumor together with its relationship to the intrahepatic vessels. Ultrasonography can also demonstrate small daughter nodules or unexpected lesions within the liver, allowing appropriate decision-making about liver resection.

Following cholecystectomy, the right and left hepatic arteries, common bile duct, and the right and left portal venous trunks are dissected and encircled with vessel loops in the hepatic hilum in order to carry out hemihepatic vascular occlusion [10] later during transection of the liver parenchyma. The area of tumor involvement is scanned again by ultrasound and the ligation point of the portal venous branch which supplies the area containing the tumor is determined. In order to accurately define the tumor-bearing subsegment to be resected, the corresponding portal venous branches are punctured and 5 ml of indigocarmine is injected about 1 to 2 cm distal to the ligation point, which prevents dye regurgitation into the other portal branches. The tip of the puncture needle is clearly seen by ultrasonography, and dye injected into the portal venous branch can be identified as moving echoes (Fig. 3). The stained area of the liver surface is then marked by electrocautery (Fig. 4). Parenchymal division can be performed along this landmark.

One to two ml of patent blue is injected into the parenchyma adjacent to the ligation point of the vessels just prior to parenchymal transection. The injected dye is recognized as an echogenic spot by ultrasonography. This procedure, known as

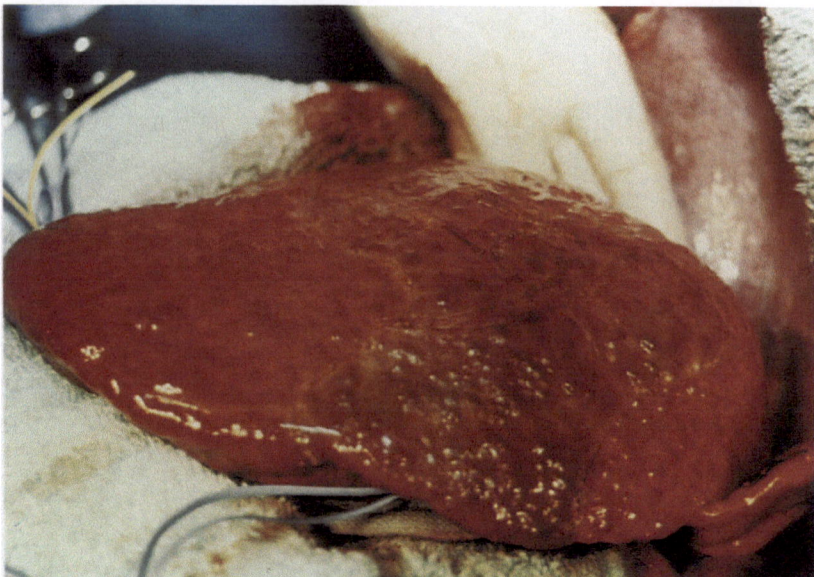

Fig. 4. The liver surface of segment 5 stained following injection of indigocarmine. The stained area is marked by electrocautery

"tattooing", which is helpful for identifying the ligation point during transection of the liver parenchyma.

To minimize intraoperative blood loss during division of the liver parenchyma, the hemihepatic vascular occlusion technique [10] is used, which causes less severe hemodynamic and biochemical changes than does total compression of the hepatoduodenal ligament (Pringle's maneuver). With this technique, lobar afferent vessels are occluded, and perfusion to the opposite lobe is preserved. Thirty minutes of occlusion is alternated with 5 min of perfusion. During the 5-min declamping period, parenchymal transection is discontinued and the divided surfaces of the liver are put together into their natural position with gentle compression in order to minimize bleeding. Intraoperative ultrasound is frequently performed during declamping to confirm the plane of transection, which can be seen as an echogenic line, and its relationship to the tumor and vessels. For liver resection of right anterosuperior area (Couinaud's subsegment 8), the blood supply to the right lobe is occluded during transection of the plane between segments 8 and 5 or between segments 8 and 7, whereas the inflow to the left lobe is interrupted during division of the plane between segments 8 and 4.

A Kelly clamp is used to crush the liver tissue without damaging the vessels or ducts. A pediatric Kelly forceps is then passed through these vessels and ducts, which are subsequently ligated on the side of the remaining parenchyma

and divided with scissors. The steps of systematic subsegmentectomy are illustrated in Fig. 5.

The areas resected by systematic subsegmentectomy do not always coincide with Couinaud's segment. The area of resection should be extended to two Couinaud's segments if the tumor is located in the intersegmental plane and the patient is considered capable of tolerating the procedure. On the other hand, the liver resection can be reasonably confined to one-half or two-thirds of a subsegment if the tumor is very small and located near the liver surface and if only one portal venous branch, which is smaller than the main subsegmental branch, is feeding the area containing the tumor. The ramification pattern of the portal venous pedicle is variable, and there are some cases where the posterior segment of the right lobe appears to comprise three subsegments (posterosuperior area, posteroinferior area, and one between these two). If the tumor is located in the "subsegment" between segments 7 and 6, total resection of that area may be indicated.

6 Operative procedure for each subsegment

6.1 Segment 8 (anterosuperior area)

The portal venous branches supplying the anterosuperior area usually consist of two main branches, i.e., a dorsal branch and a ventral one.

Fig. 5. Operative procedure for systematic subsegmentectomy. (From [3] with permission of Surgery, Gynecology and Obstetrics.)

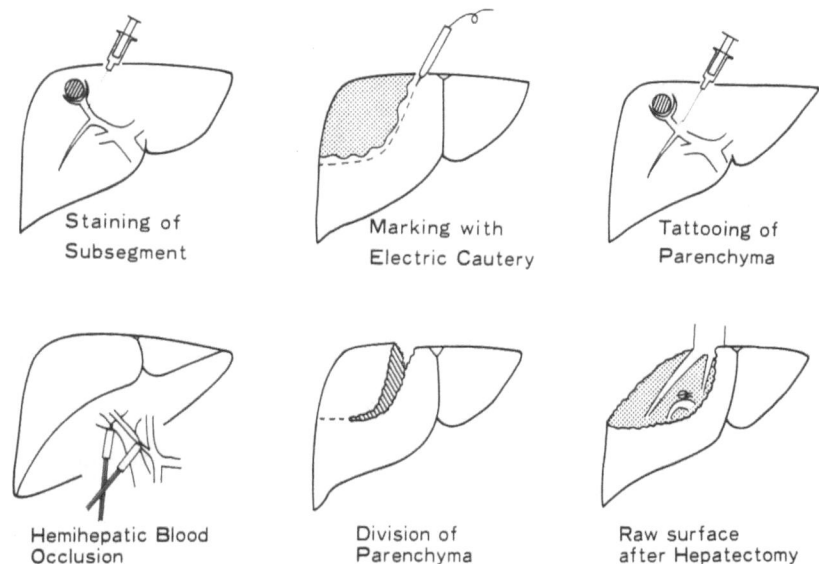

Both branches, therefore, need to be ligated in order to accomplish the complete resection of segment 8. A large branch of the middle hepatic vein is identified between the ventral and dorsal branches of the anterosuperior area in the majority of cases, whereas a branch of the right hepatic vein drains that area in a smaller number of cases.

After segment 8 has been identified on the liver surface by injection of indigocarmine into both the dorsal and ventral portal venous branches, division of the liver parenchyma is started about 1 cm left of Cantlie's line under hemihepatic vascular occlusion of the left lobe. The occlusion is declamped when two-thirds of the right side of the middle hepatic vein is exposed. Vascular occlusion of the right lobe is then performed, and parenchymal transections between segments 8 and 5, and between segments 8 and 7 are carried out following tattooing adjacent to the bifurcation of the anteroinferior and anterosuperior portal venous branches. The line of transection between segments 8 and 5 is 1 to 2 cm caudal to the stained area. The Glissonean sheath including the antero-inferior portal venous branch is exposed, and parenchymal division is continued proximally along the Glissonean sheath until the dye (tattoo) on the raw surface is identified. The ventral branch of the anterosuperior area is exposed close to the "tattoo", ligated and divided. Transection of the liver parenchyma is continued proximally, and the dorsal branch of the anterosuperior area is then exposed and divided. When these procedures are completed, parenchymal division is

performed along the proximal one-third of the middle hepatic vein. Care must be taken near its confluence with the inferior vena cava, where large branches of the middle hepatic vein draining segment 8 frequently exist. The parenchymal division next proceeds along the right hepatic vein, which is located between segments 8 and 7. The distal portion of the right hepatic vein is located 1 to 2 cm dorsolateral to the ligature of the dorsal portal branch of the anterosuperior area. If the right hepatic vein is not identified, IOUS can show the direction of the parenchymal transection. The main trunk of the right hepatic vein is exposed in a distal to proximal direction during parenchymal transection. If bleeding starts from the right hepatic vein or its tributaries, the surgeon's left index finger is inserted behind the liver to compress the bleeding point with the liver lifted ventrally. This maneuver makes it possible to minimize the bleeding and to safely suture or ligate the bleeding point. After the right hepatic vein has been exposed to its juncture with the vena cava, the cranial or diaphragmatic side of the liver transection is completed. The main trunks of the middle and right hepatic veins, stumps of the anterosuperior portal venous tributary are exposed on the raw surface of the liver following total resection of segment 8.

6.2 Segment 5 (anteroinferior area)

Since the anteroinferior area is small in comparison with each of the other three subsegments in the right lobe (segments 6, 7, 8), resection

240 S. Kawasaki et al.

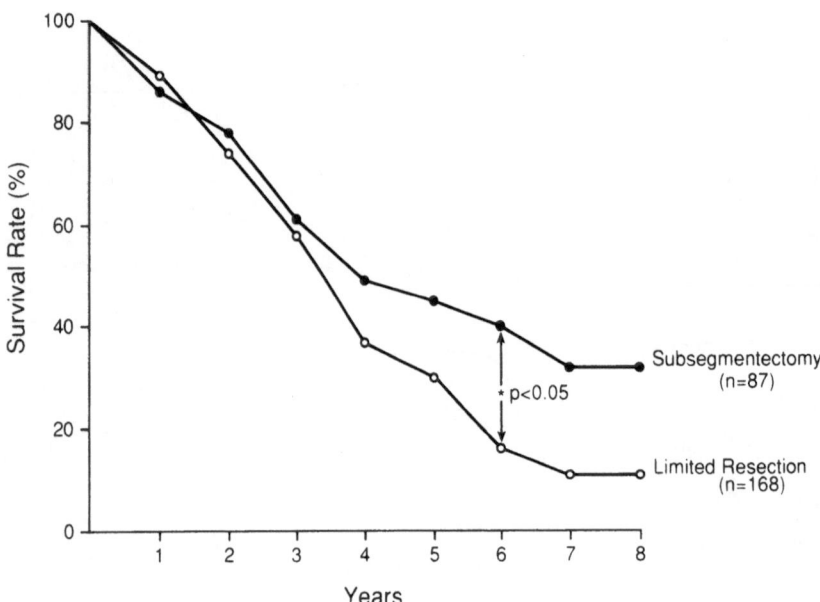

Fig. 6. Cumulative survival rates for systematic subsegmentectomy (*solid circle*) and non-anatomical limited resection (*open circle*) for hepatocellular carcinomas less than 5 cm in diameter. Survival is significantly better at 6 years for the subsegmentectomy group

limited to this area is rarely indicated. There are three to five portal venous branches feeding segment 5. Indigocarmine is injected into the ventral branches of the anterosuperior and posteroinferior areas instead of those three to five branches supplying segment 5 (counterstaining method) [11]. The cranial and right lateral margins of segment 5 on the liver surface are identified by this technique. The left margin of segment 5 can be recognized by hemihepatic vascular occlusion. Liver parenchymal transection is initiated from the left border of this segment. The right branch of the middle hepatic vein is exposed, ligated and divided. The cranial margin of this area is then transected, and each of the portal venous branches supplying segment 5 is identified, ligated and divided serially until the main trunk of the anterior portal triad is exposed. Following parenchymal division along the right lateral border of segment 5, total resection of this area is completed.

6.3 Segment 7 (posterosuperior area)

The thoracoabdominal approach through the 7th intercostal space is indicated for this resection. The bare area is dissected completely and the inferior vena cava is exposed including its juncture with the right hepatic vein. There is usually only one main portal venous branch supplying segment 7, to which staining is applied. The hepatic parenchyma is transected between segments 7 and 8 from the diaphragmatic surface and then from the visceral surface under hemihepatic vascular occlusion of the right lobe. The main portal triad of the posterosuperior area is identified, ligated and divided. Parenchymal transection is continued along the right hepatic vein to its confluence with the vena cava. After transection has been completed, the main trunk of the right hepatic vein and the stump of the posterosuperior portal venous branch are seen on the raw surface.

6.4 Segment 6 (posteroinferior area)

This area is located in the right lateral and most caudal part of the liver. Total resection of segment 6 is technically easy in comparison with the other types of subsegmentectomy. Parenchymal transection is performed with hemihepatic vascular occlusion of the right lobe. There is no significant risk of massive bleeding during transection.

6.5 Subsegments in the left lobe

Each subsegment in the left lobe (segments 2, 3, 4) can be resected with conventional hilar dissection around the umbilical portion of the left lobe. Staining is rarely applied, since ligation of the subsegmental portal venous branches prior to

Fig. 7. Cumulative survival rates for systematic subsegmentectomy (*solid circle*) and non-anatomical limited resection (*open circle*) for solitary hepatocellular carcinomas less than 2 cm in diameter. Survival is significantly better at 7 years for the subsegmentectomy group

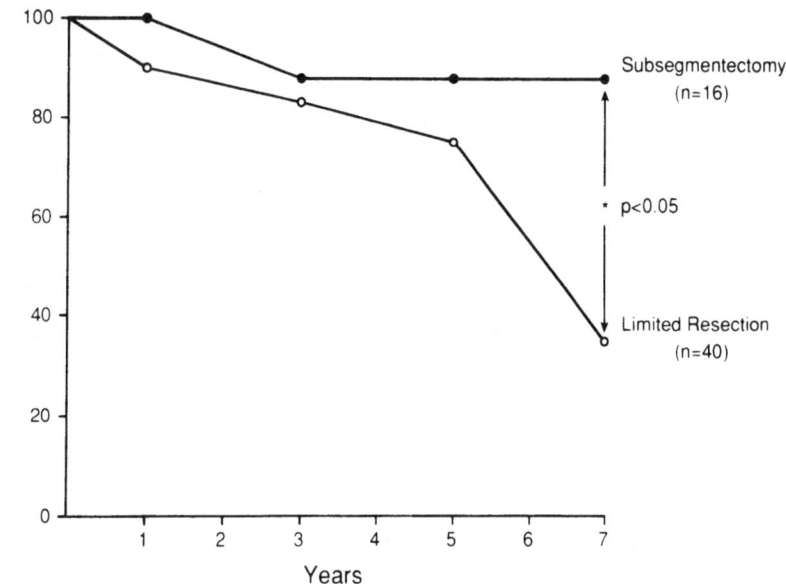

parenchymal division produces an ischemic color change in the corresponding area of the liver surface. As each subsegment in the left lobe is relatively small, any two of the subsegments can also be resected *en bloc* or separately.

7   Results of subsegmentectomy

Cumulative survival rates during eight years following systematic subsegmentectomy in 87 patients with small hepatocellular carcinomas less than 5 cm in diameter were 86%, 78%, 61%, 49%, 45%, 40%, 32%, and 32%, respectively, whereas those for non-anatomical limited liver resections in 168 patients were 89%, 74%, 58%, 37%, 30%, 16%, 11% and 11%, respectively. The survival rates for systematic subsegmentectomy were significantly better than those for limited resection at 6 years ($P < 0.05$) (Fig. 6). In cases where the HCC was solitary and less than 2 cm in diameter, cumulative survival rates following systematic subsegmentectomy (16 cases) were 100%, 88%, 88%, and 88% at 1, 3, 5, and 7 years, respectively, whereas those for limited resection (40 cases) were 90%, 83%, 75%, and 35%, respectively, showing a significant difference at 7 years between the two groups (Fig. 7).

These results indicate that systematic subsegmentectomy may be superior to non-anatomical limited resection in terms of radicality and curability, which we had assumed from the outset.

8   Discussion

With the advances in various diagnostic modalities, small hepatocellular carcinomas have been detected with increasing frequency since the late 1970s. However, hepatocellular carcinoma shows a strong tendency for intraportal metastasis, and liver cirrhosis coexists in approximately 80% of all patients with hepatocellular carcinoma in Japan. These clinicopathological features of hepatocellular carcinoma made it necessary to devise a radical but less extensive type of liver resection for patients with hepatocellular carcinoma and poor hepatic functional reserve.

In 1981, Makuuchi et al. first reported the technique of systematic subsegmentectomy [7, 12, 13], which makes it possible to remove the entire portal bed of a tumor, while sparing as much of the functional hepatic mass as possible. The essential points of this surgical procedure are as follows: 1) Injection of dye (indigocarmine) into the portal venous branches feeding the tumor-bearing area to be resected (staining). 2) Injection of dye (patent blue) into the liver parenchyma close to the portal pedicle, which must be ligated (tattooing). 3) Hemihepatic vascular occlusion in the hilum in order to prevent significant blood loss. Intraoperative ultrasonography is indispensable for performing both "staining" and "tattooing".

Long-term survival rates following systematic subsegmentectomy were significantly better than those after non-anatomical limited resection.

Considering that even small liver cancers less than 5 cm in diameter frequently have tumor thrombi in the portal venous branches or intrahepatic metastases, systematic subsegmentectomy will be the future treatment of choice in many more patients with hepatocellular carcinoma and should contribute to the improvement of patient survival.

References

1. Liver Cancer Study Group of Japan (1988) Survey and follow up study of primary liver cancer in Japan—Report 8 (in Japanese). Acta Hepatol Jpn 29:1619–1626
2. Liver Cancer Study Group of Japan (1979) Survey and follow up study of primary liver cancer in Japan—Report 4 (in Japanese). Acta Hepatol Jpn 20:443–441
3. Makuuchi M, Hasegawa H, Yamazaki S (1985) Ultrasonically guided subsegmentectomy. Surg Gynecol Obstet 161:346–350
4. Tung TT (1979) Les résections majeures et mineures du foie. Masson et Cie, Paris
5. Couinaud C (1957) Le foie, études anatomiques et chirurgicales. Masson et Cie, Paris
6. Bismuth H, Houssin D, Castaing D (1982) Major and minor segmentectomies "réglées" in liver surgery. World J Surg 6:10–24
7. Makuuchi M, Hasegawa H, Yamazaki S (1981) Intraoperative ultrasonic examination for hepatectomy. Jpn J Clin Oncol 11:367–390
8. Makuuchi M, Hasegawa H, Yamazaki S, et al. (1987) The use of operative ultrasound as an aid to liver resection in patients with hepatocellular carcinoma. World J Surg 11:615–621
9. Shanghai Coordinating Group for Research on Liver Cancer (1979) Diagnosis and treatment of primary hepatocellular carcinoma in early stage, report of 134 cases. Clin Med J 92:801–810
10. Makuuchi M, Mori T, Gunvén P, et al. (1987) Safety of hemihepatic occlusion during resection of the liver. Surg Gynecol Obstet 164:155–158
11. Takayama T, Makuuchi M, Watanabe K, et al. (1991) A new method for mapping hepatic subsegment: Counterstaining identification technique. Surgery: 109:226–229
12. Tobe T (1984) Hepatectomy in patients with cirrhotic liver: Clinical and basic observations. In: Nyhus LM (ed) Surgery annual. Appleton-Century-Crofts, Connecticut, pp 177–202
13. Makuuchi M (1987) Intraoperative ultrasonography for hepatic surgery: Application of intraoperative ultrasonography to hepatectomy. In: Makuuchi M (ed) Abdominal intraoperative ultrasonography. Igaku-shoin, Tokyo New York, pp 89–123

Results of surgical treatment: Follow up study by Liver Cancer Study Group of Japan

Shigeki Arii and Takayoshi Tobe[1]

1 Introduction

The Liver Cancer Study Group of Japan has been conducting a follow up study of patients with primary liver cancer throughout the country since 1965 [1–7]. Up to December 31, 1987, more than 30,000 patients from 601 hospitals were registered in a computer at Kyoto University. This articel reports the survival rates of patients with hepato-cellular carcinoma and with cholangiocellular carcinoma treated by partial hepatic resection, on the basis of responses received from January 1, 1978, when a prototype of the present question-naire was introduced, to December 31, 1987. Special attention is paid to the survival rates in relation to clinicopathological factors, which provide significant information for estimating the prognosis in patients with primary liver cancer.

2 Results of surgical treatment

The survival rates of patients with primary liver cancer (hepatocellular carcinoma and cholangio-cellular carcinoma) were calculated by the tradit-ional life timetable method of Cutler-Ederer [8]. The date of admission, not the date of diagnosis or initial treatment, is the starting point in the calculation of the survival time. The statistical significancc of differences in the survival pattern was analyzed by the log-rank test.

The abbreviations used here are based on the General Rules for the Clinical and Pathological Study of Primary Liver Cancer [9].

[1] 1st Department of Surgery, Kyoto University Faculty of Medicine, Sakyo-ku, Kyoto, 606 Japan

2.1 Survival rate of hepatocellular carcinoma (HCC) patients treated with curative or non-curative partial hepatic resection

The overall 1-year, 2-year, 3-year, and 5-year survival rates were 71.9%, 56.6%, 45.6%, and 30.9%, respectively (Fig. 1). The survival rates of patients with curative resection were 77.4% at 1 year, 64.8% at 2 years, 55.0% at 3 years and 36.6% at 5 years (Fig. 2), while those of the non-curative group were 66.6%, 47.8%, 34.7% and 23.3%, respectively (Fig. 3).

The difference between the curative and non-curative surgery groups is statistically significant. Curability of surgery was defined by the General Rules for the Clinical and Pathological Study of Primary Liver Cancer.

The survival rates of patients with curative resection in relation to clinical and histo-pathological factors are listed below:

1. *Tumor size* (Fig. 4). In patients with tumors smaller than 2 cm in diameter, the 1-year, 2-year, 3-year, and 5-year survival rates were 86.9%, 81.5%, 74.5%, and 60.5%, respec-tively. Patients with tumors larger than 2 cm in diameter had a poorer prognosis (2.1–5.0 cm: 1 year, 79.3%; 2 years, 67.1%; 3 years, 57.4%; 5 years, 39.3%; 5.1–10.0 cm: 1 year, 74.3%; 2 years, 57.7%; 3 years, 48.0%; 5 years, 26.8%). The differences among these 3 groups were significant.

2. *Tumor number* (Fig. 5). The survival rates of patients with solitary tumors were 80.0% at 1 year, 67.8% at 2 years, 57.2% at 3 years, and 38.2% at 5 years, whereas those of patients with two tumors were 66.8% at 1 year, 48.8% at 2 years, 39.9% at 3 years, and 29.9% at 5 years. There was a significant difference between patients with single tumors and those with two or more tumors, but no significant

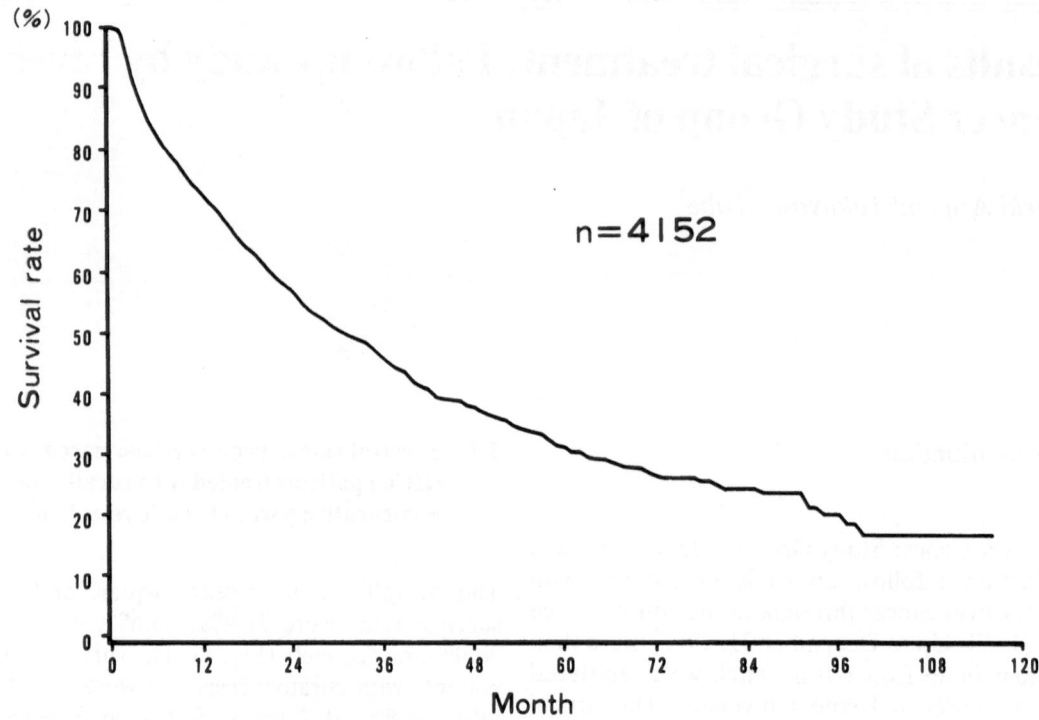

Fig. 1. Cumulative survival rate of HCC patients with partial hepatectomy

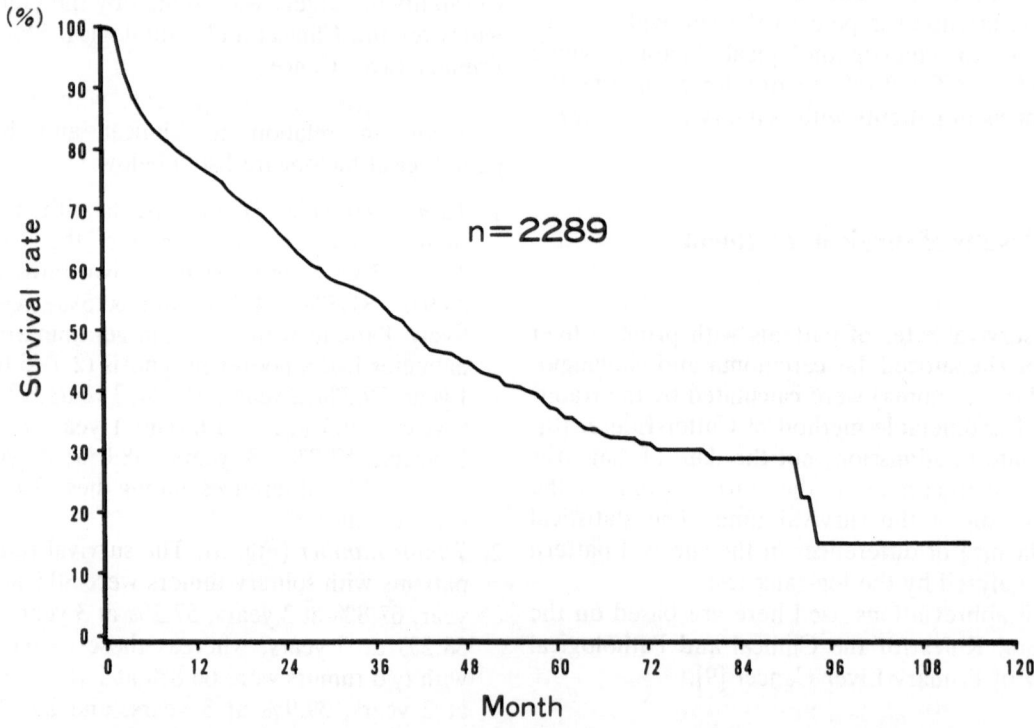

Fig. 2. Cumulative survival rate of HCC patients with curative hepatic resection

Fig. 3. Cumulative survival rate of HCC patients with noncurative hepatic resection

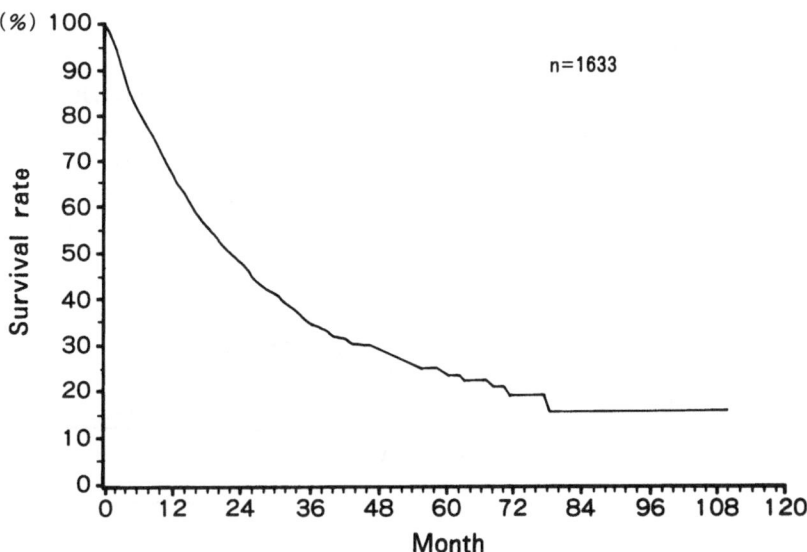

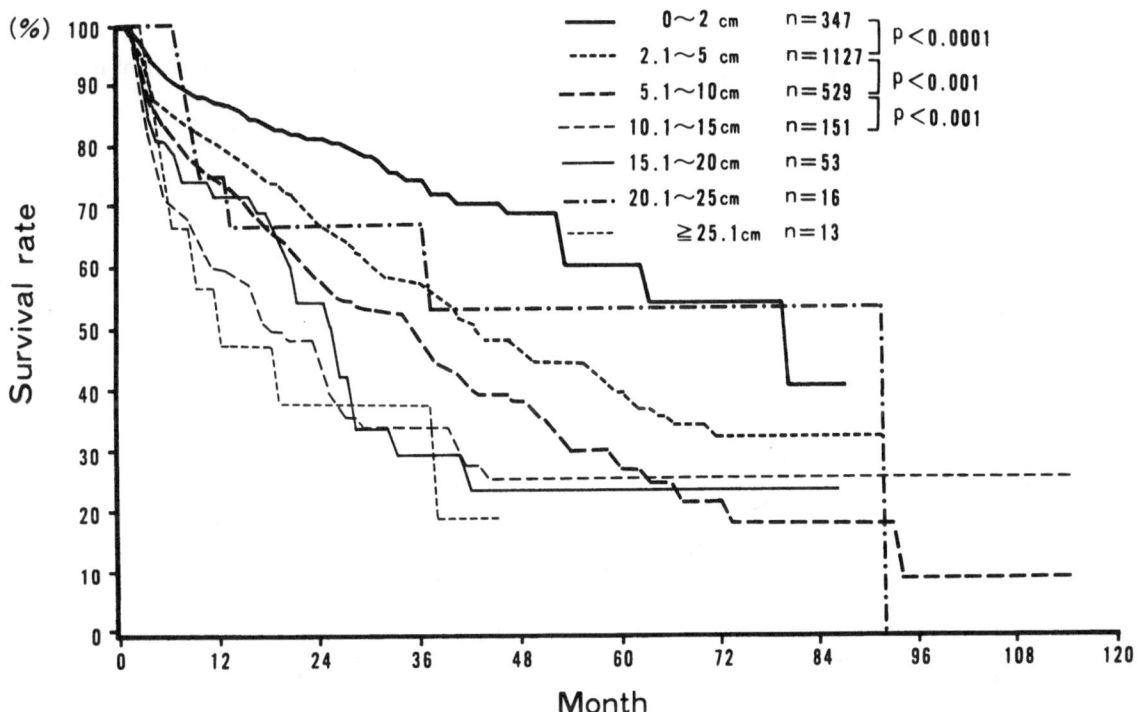

Fig. 4. Cumulative survival rates of HCC patients with curative resection in relation to tumor diameter

difference between those with two tumors and those with three tumors.

3. *Fibrous tumor capsule* (Fc) and *infiltration of cancer cells into tumor capsule* (Fc-inf) (Figs. 6, 7). Capsular formation surrounding the tumor did not significantly influence the survival rate, possibly because a relatively large

proportion of non-encapsulated tumors were small tumors. However, the presence of infiltration of cancer cells into the fibrous capsule of the tumor was related to a low survival rate: in the patients without capsular infiltration, 1-year, 2-year, 3-year, and 5-year survival rates were 81.3%, 71.0%, 61.8%,

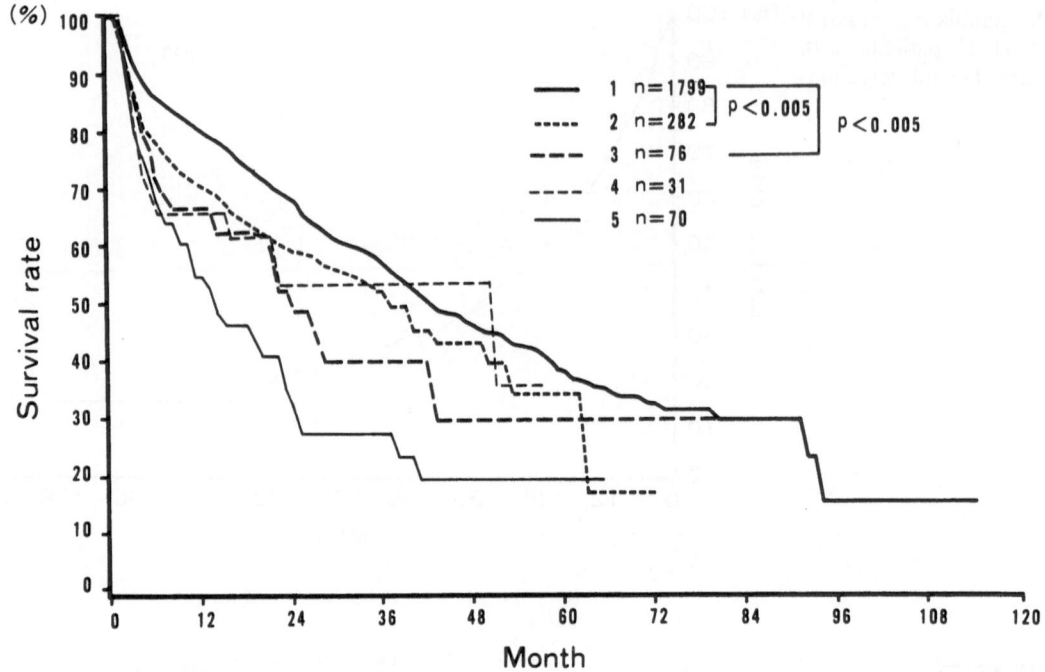

Fig. 5. Cumulative survival rates of HCC patients with curative resection in relation to number of tumors

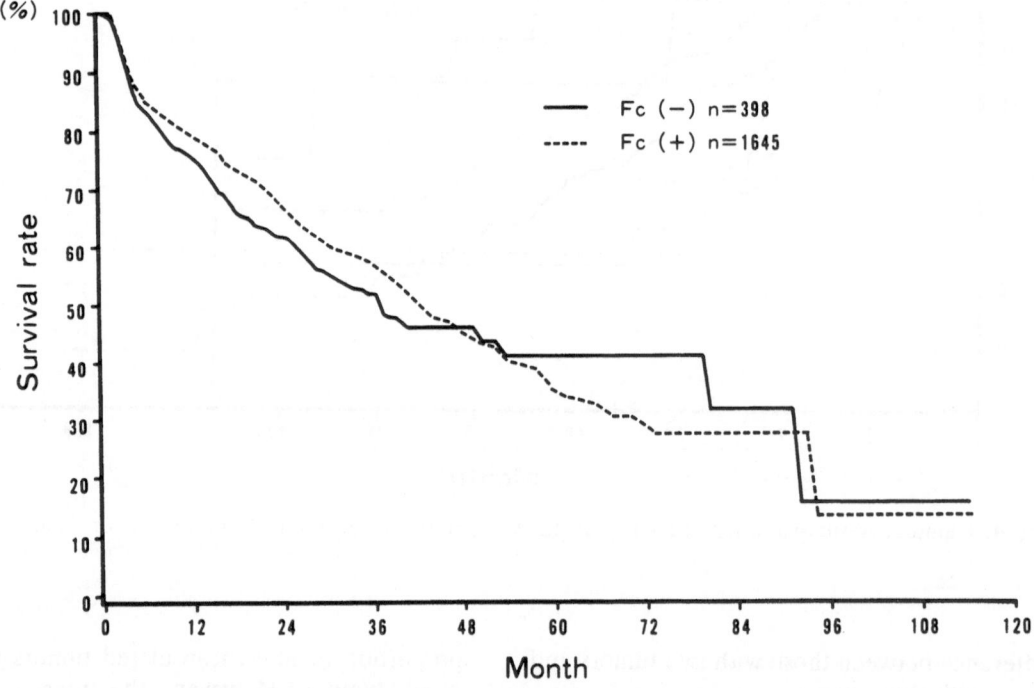

Fig. 6. Cumulative survival rates of HCC patients with curative resection in relation to fibrous tumor capsule. *Fc(−)* and *Fc(+)* represent the absence and presence of tumor capsule, respectively

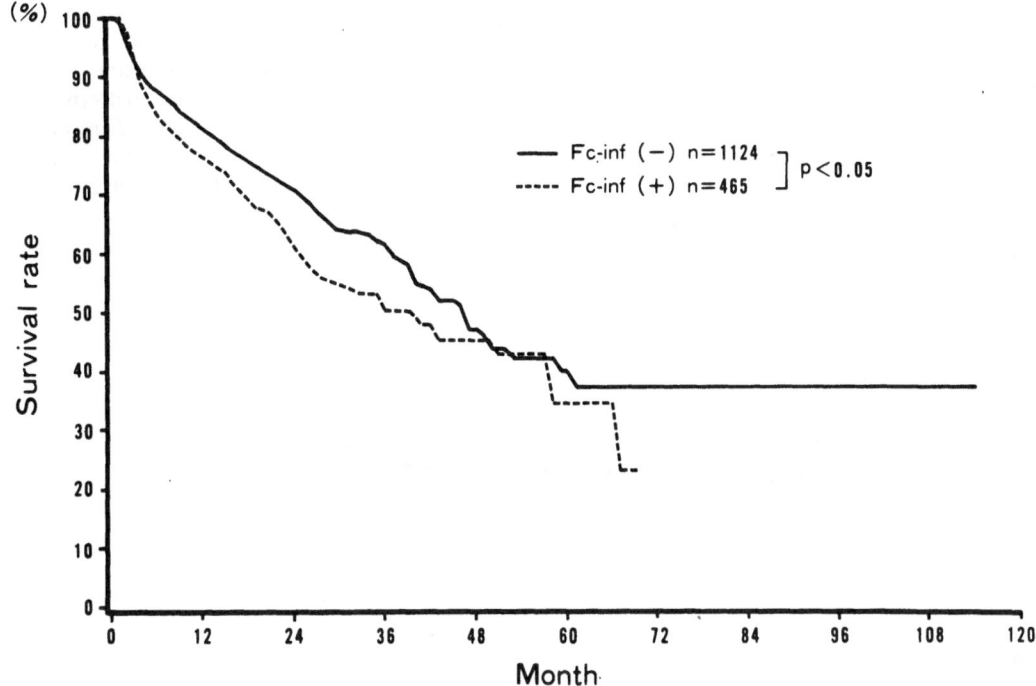

Fig. 7. Cumulative survival rates of HCC patients with curative resection in relation to macroscopic infiltration of tumor capsule. *Fc-inf(−)* and *Fc-inf(+)* represent the absence and presence of macroscopic infiltration, respectively

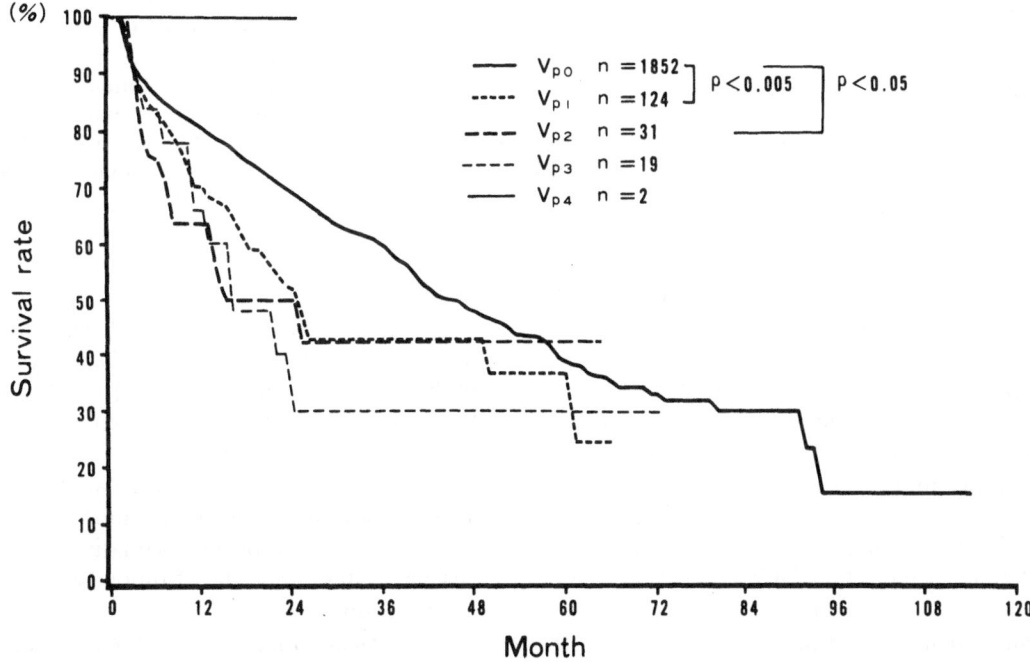

Fig. 8. Cumulative survival rates of HCC patients with curative resection in relation to the degree of macroscopic portal involvement. V_{p0}, no portal involvement; V_{p1}, involvement to more than the 3rd branch of the peripheral tract; V_{p2}, V_{p3}, V_{p4}, involvement to the 2nd branch, 1st branch, and portal trunk, respectively

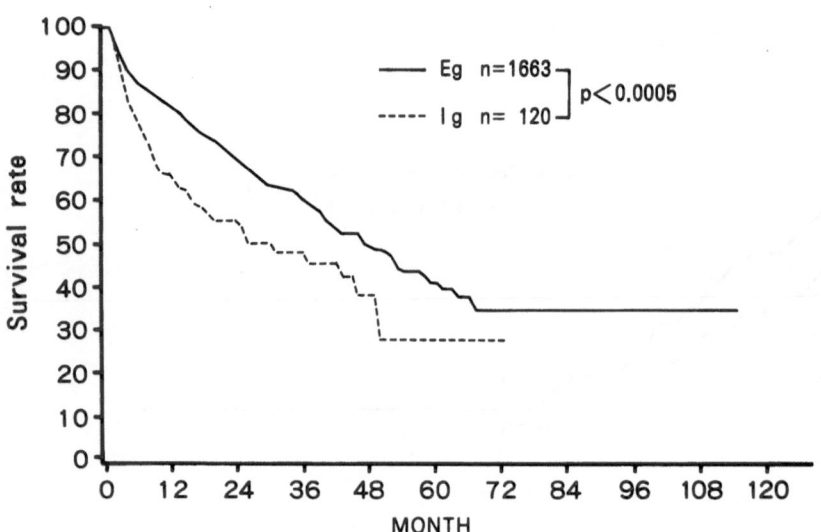

Fig. 9. Cumulative survival rates of HCC patients with curative resection in relation to growth pattern of the tumor. *Eg* and *Ig* represent the expansive and infiltrative growth, respectively

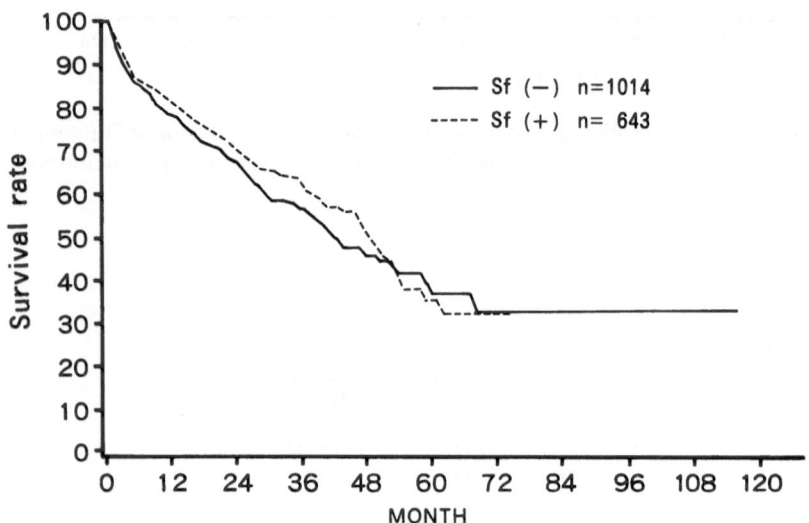

Fig. 10. Cumulative survival rates of HCC patients with curative resection in relation to septum formation in the tumor. *Sf(−)* and *Sf(+)* represent the absence and presence of septum formation, respectively

and 40.1%, respectively, while in those with infiltration, they were 76.6%, 61.2%, 50.3%, and 34.6%, respectively.

4. *Portal vein invasion* of the tumor (Vp) (Fig. 8). There was a significant difference between V_{p0} and V_{p1}, and between V_{p0} and V_{p2}, but no significant difference between V_{p1} and V_{p2} (V_{p0}: 80.4% at 1 year, 69.1% at 2 years, 59.8% at 3 years, 39.0% at 5 years; V_{p1}: 70.4% at 1 year, 52.6% at 2 years, 42.9% at 3 years, 36.8% at 5 years).

5. *Growth pattern* of tumor (Fig. 9). Growth patterns were classified as expansive growth (Eg), in which the tumor had macroscopically clear margins, and infiltrative growth (Ig) with unclear margins. The Eg-group had better survival rates than the Ig-group (Eg: 81.1% at 1 year, 69.1% at 2 years, 59.7% at 3 years, 41.1% at 5 years; Ig: 65.4% at 1 year, 54.9% at 2 years, 47.8% at 3 years, 27.9% at 5 years).

6. *Septum formation* in the tumor (Sf) (Fig. 10). There was no statistical difference between patients with and without Sf.

7. *Grade of anaplasia* of cancer cells (Edmondson-Steiner classification) (Fig. 11). There was no significant correlation between survival rates and the Edmondson-Steiner classification.

8. *Tumor extent* (Fig. 12). The extent of the tumor affected the survival rate significantly. In the H_s group (tumor localized to one Couinaud's segment), the 1-year, 2-year, 3-year, and 5-year survival rates were 85.4%, 78.7%, 69.3%, and 53.3%, respectively.

Fig. 11. Cumulative survival rates of HCC patients with curative resection in relation to the grade of the Edmondson-Steiner classification

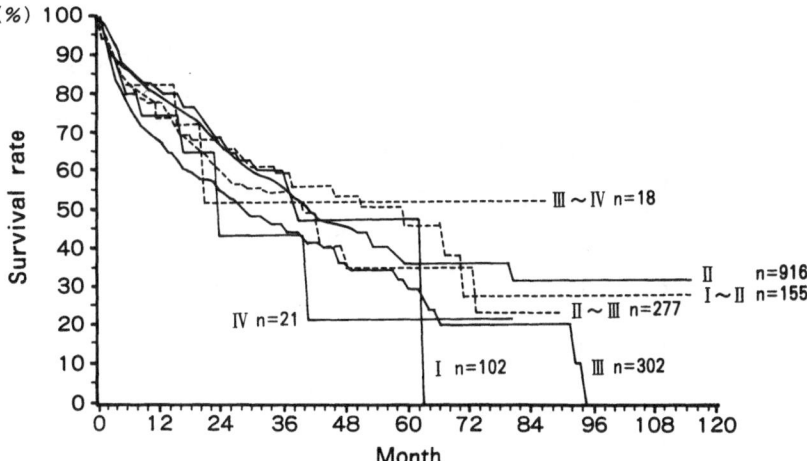

There were statistically significant differences between H_s and H_1, and between H_s and H_2, but not between H_1 and H_2.

2.2 Survival rates of cholangiocarcinoma (CCC) patients treated with curative or non-curative partial hepatic resection

The overall 1-year, 2-year, 3-year, and 5-year survival rates were 54.6%, 38.8%, 31.5%, and 29.8%, respectively (Fig. 13). Patients treated with curative surgery (Fig. 14) had better survival rates than those treated with non-curative surgery (Fig. 15) (curative surgery group: 69.4% at 1 year, 65.5% at 2 years, 43.5% at 3 years, 43.5% at 5 years; non-curative surgery group: 45.5% at 1 year, 22.4% at 2 years, 22.4% at 3 years, 19.6% at 5 years).

Survival rates in relation to clinical and histopathological factors are listed below:

1. *Tumor size* (Fig. 16). All patients with tumors smaller than 2 cm in diameter are alive, but the number of cases (9 patients) is too small to evaluate the significance as a prognostic indicator. In the group with tumors 2.1–5.0 cm in diameter, the survival rates were 62.3% at 1 year, 43.3% at 2 years, 37.9% at 3 years, and 31.6% at 5 years.

2. *Lymph node metastasis* (Fig. 17). In the N_0 group, 1-year, 2-year, 3-year, and 5-year survival rates were 64.2%, 51.4%, 41.9%, and 38.4%, respectively, while in the N_1 group they were 39.7% at 1 year and 29.8% at 2 years—a wide difference.

3. *Type of histology* (Fig. 18). The patients with cystopapillary cholangiocellular carcinoma

have a relatively better survival rate. (microtubular: 51.6% at 1 year, 46.3% at 2 years, 18.4% at 3 years; macrotubular: 56.6% at 1 year, 46.3% at 2 years, 44.7% at 3 years; cystopapillary: 67.9% at 1 year, 58.4% at 2 years, 44.7% at 3 years).

4. *Tumor extent* (Fig. 19). There were no significant difference among the groups, although the H_s group tended to survive longer than the others.

2.3 Survival rate of patients with primary liver cancer treated with transarterial embolization

In this analysis, the patients surveyed were those treated with transarterial embolization (TAE) without surgery. The diagnosis for almost all patients treated with TAE was considered to be HCC even if no histological diagnosis was made, so both histologically proven and unproven patients were listed. Otherwise, the number of patients to be analyzed here would be too small to calculate the survival rate, because most of the patients treated with TAE alone did not have a histological diagnosis. One-year, 2-year, 3-year, and 5-year survival rates in the TAE-group were 58.3%, 34.0%, 20.7%, and 8.3%, respectively (Fig. 20).

3 Discussion

The number of patients with HCC has increased in Japan during the past 10 years, and HCC is now the third cause of cancer death in males. In

S. Arii and T. Tobe

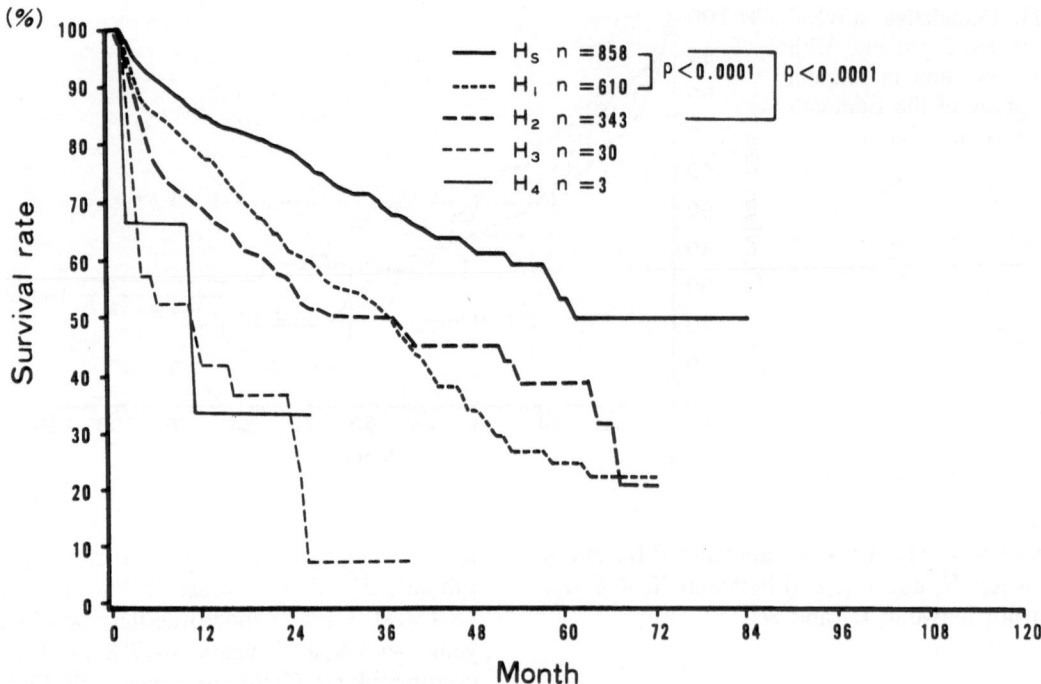

Fig. 12. Cumulative survival rates of HCC patients with curative resection in relation to extent of the tumor. H_s, located in one subsegment (Couinaud's Segment); H_1, located in one segment; H_2, located in two segments; H_3, located in three segments; H_4, located in four segments

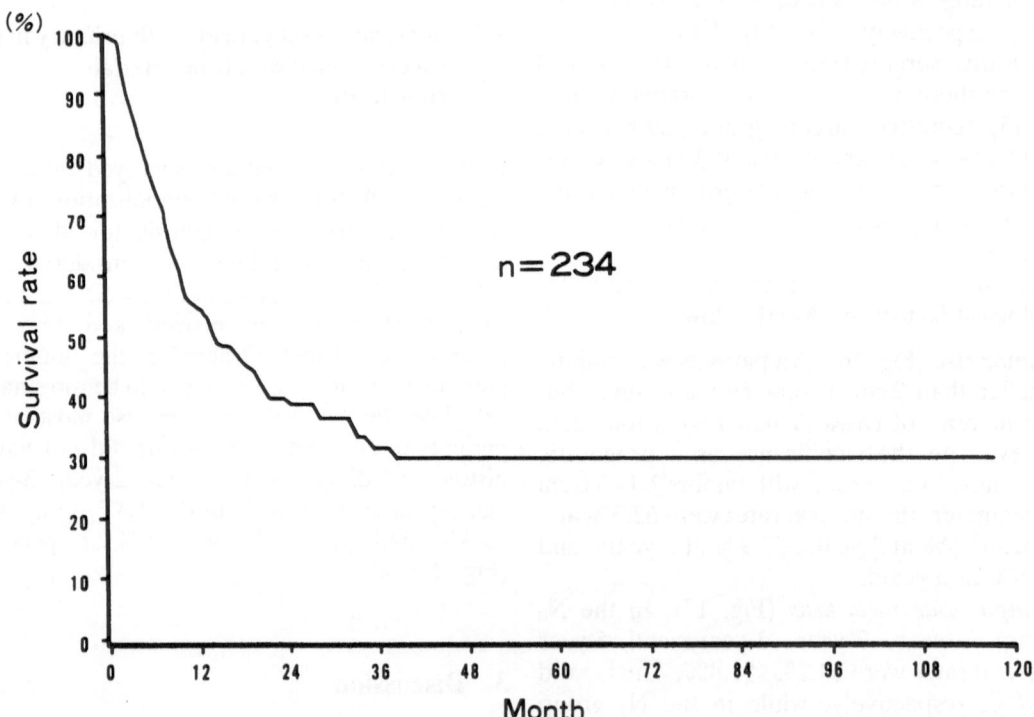

Fig. 13. Cumulative survival rate of CCC patients with partial hepatic resection

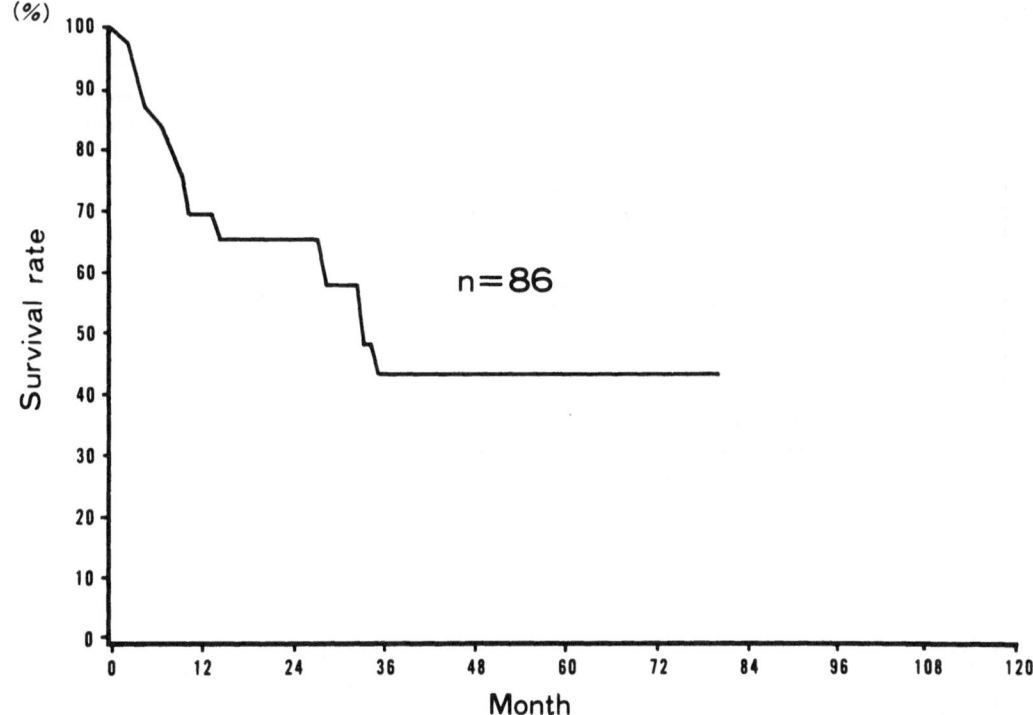

Fig. 14. Cumulative survival rate of CCC patients with curative resection

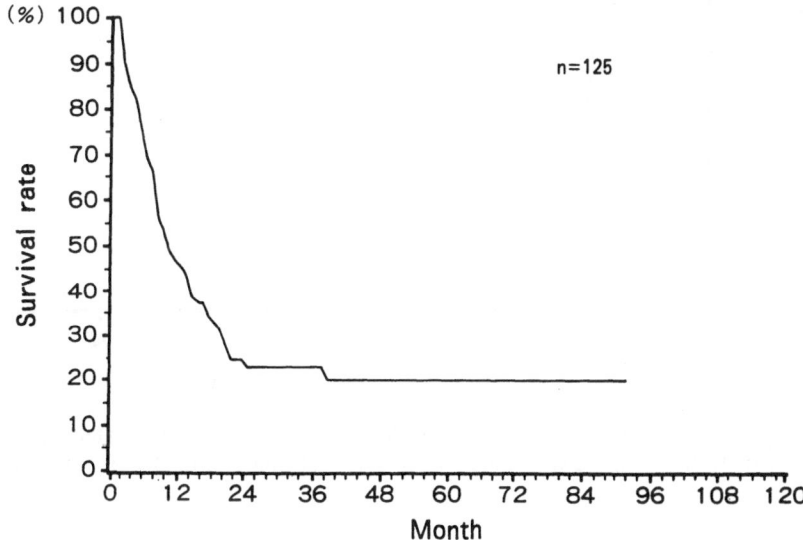

Fig. 15. Cumulative survival rate of CCC patients with noncurative resection

the 1970s, there were very few resectable cases because the tumor was far advanced by the time it was diagnosed and concomitant severe liver cirrhosis was often present. However, the recent development of noninvasive and precise diagnostic modalities, such as computed tomography (CT) and ultrasonography (US), has made it possible to diagnose HCC at an earlier stage, thereby increasing the number of resectable tumors. Furthermore, the operative mortality rate is now lower, because of better pre- and postoperative management, development of surgical

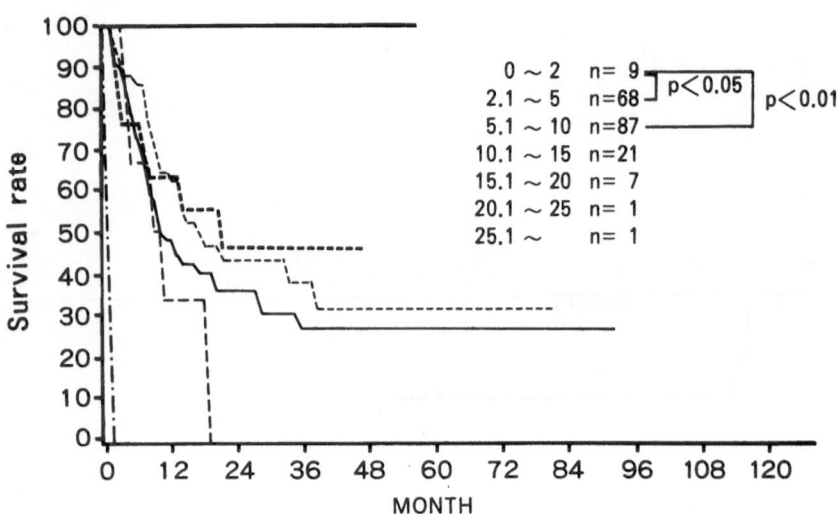

Fig. 16. Cumulative survival rates of CCC patients with partial hepatectomy in relation to tumor diameter (cm)

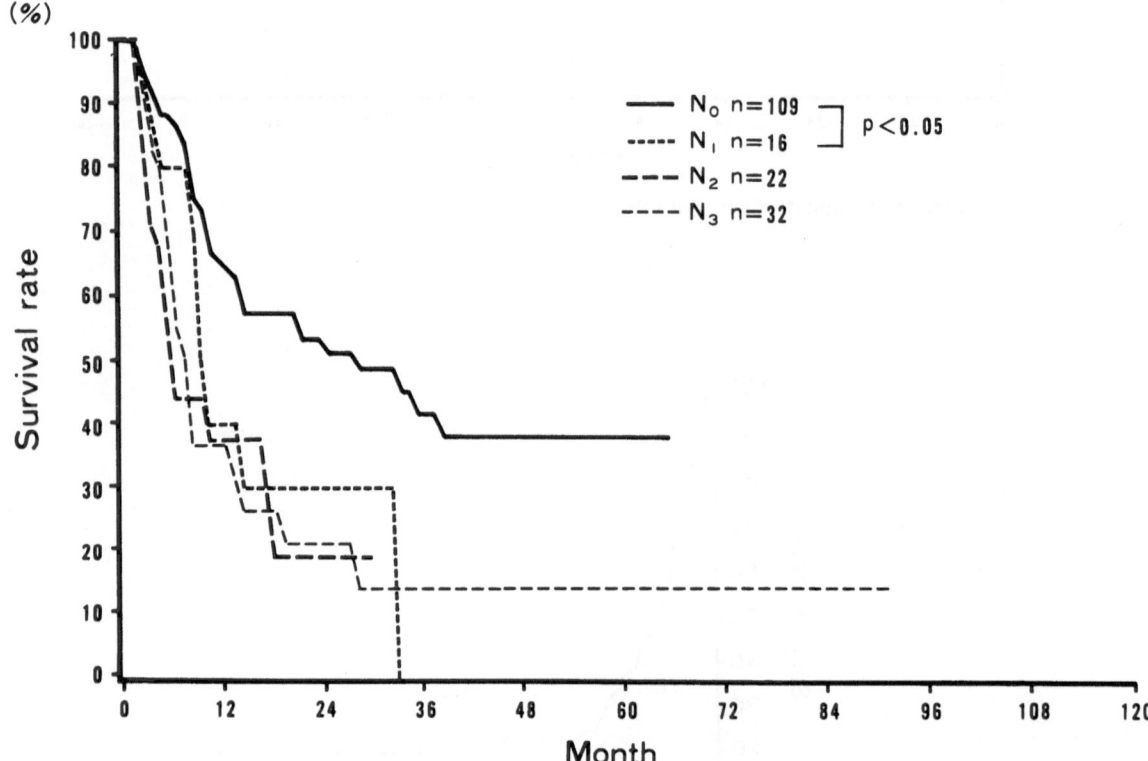

Fig. 17. Cumulative survival rates of CCC patients with partial hepatectomy in relation to the grade of lymph node metastasis. N_0-N_4 are defined by the General Rules for the Clinical and Pathological Study of Primary Liver Cancer

techniques [10] and improved preoperative evaluation of hepatic functional reserve for preventing postoperative liver failure [11–12]. However, despite these great efforts, the results of surgical treatment are still unsatisfactory. Therefore, it is important to investigate the prognostic indicators by analyzing survival rates in relation to clinical and histopathological factors.

In the present study, it was clarified that significant prognostic indicators for HCC are tumor size, number of tumors, tumor extent, growth pattern, capsular infiltration of cancer cells, and portal vein involvement, while those for CCC are tumor size and lymph node metastasis. To our knowledge, this is the first investigation in so many cases throughout the country of prognostic

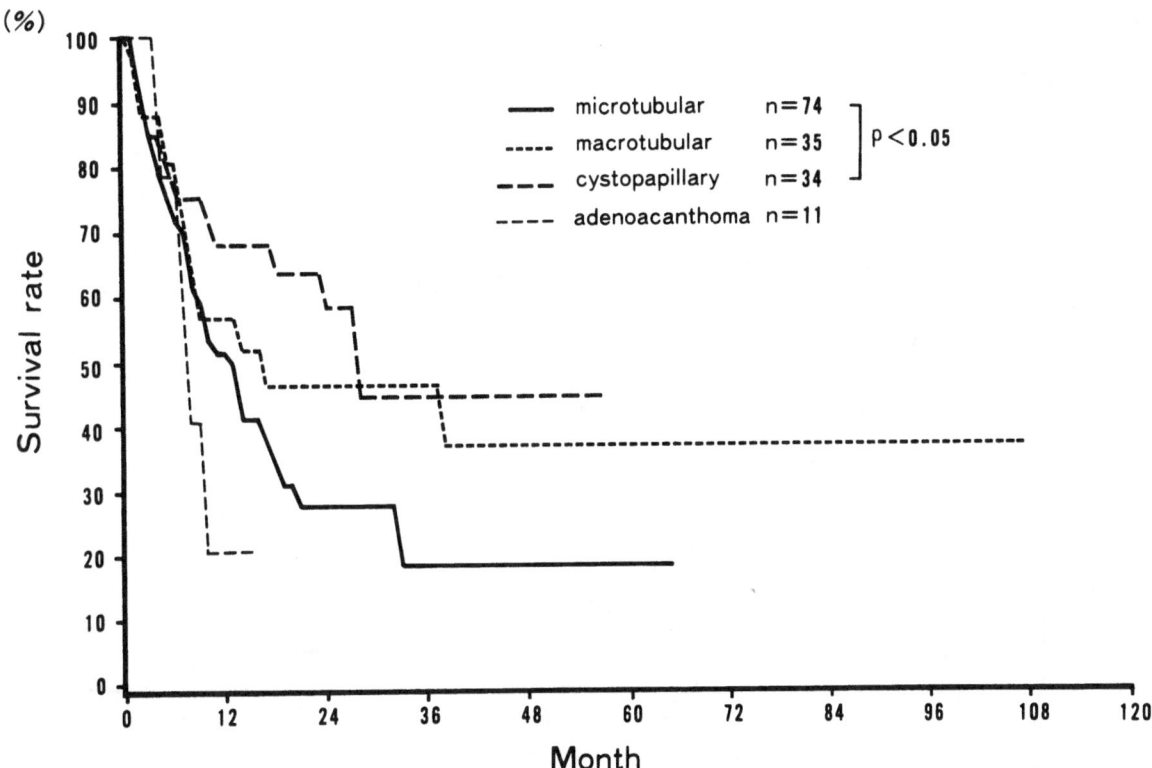

Fig. 18. Cumulative survival rates of CCC patients with partial hepatectomy in relation to the type of histology

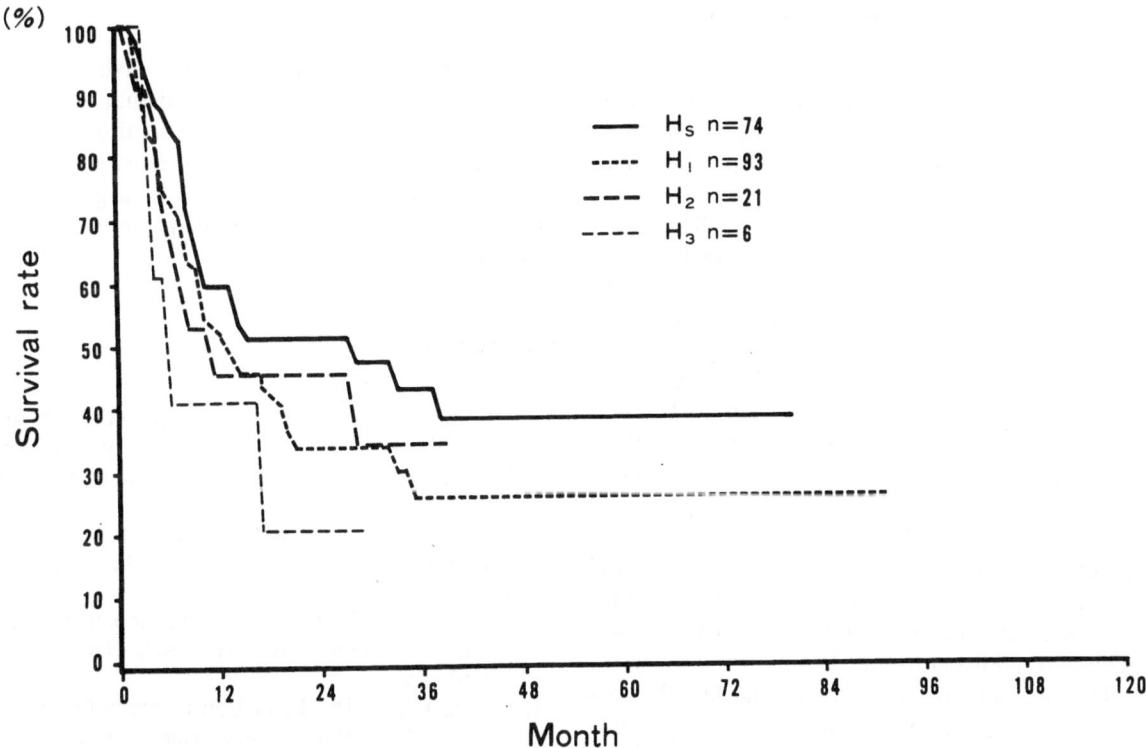

Fig. 19. Cumulative survival rates of CCC patients with partial hepatectomy in relation to extent of the tumor. H_s, located in one subsegment (Couinaud's segment); H_1, located in one segment; H_2, located in two segments; H_3, located in three segments

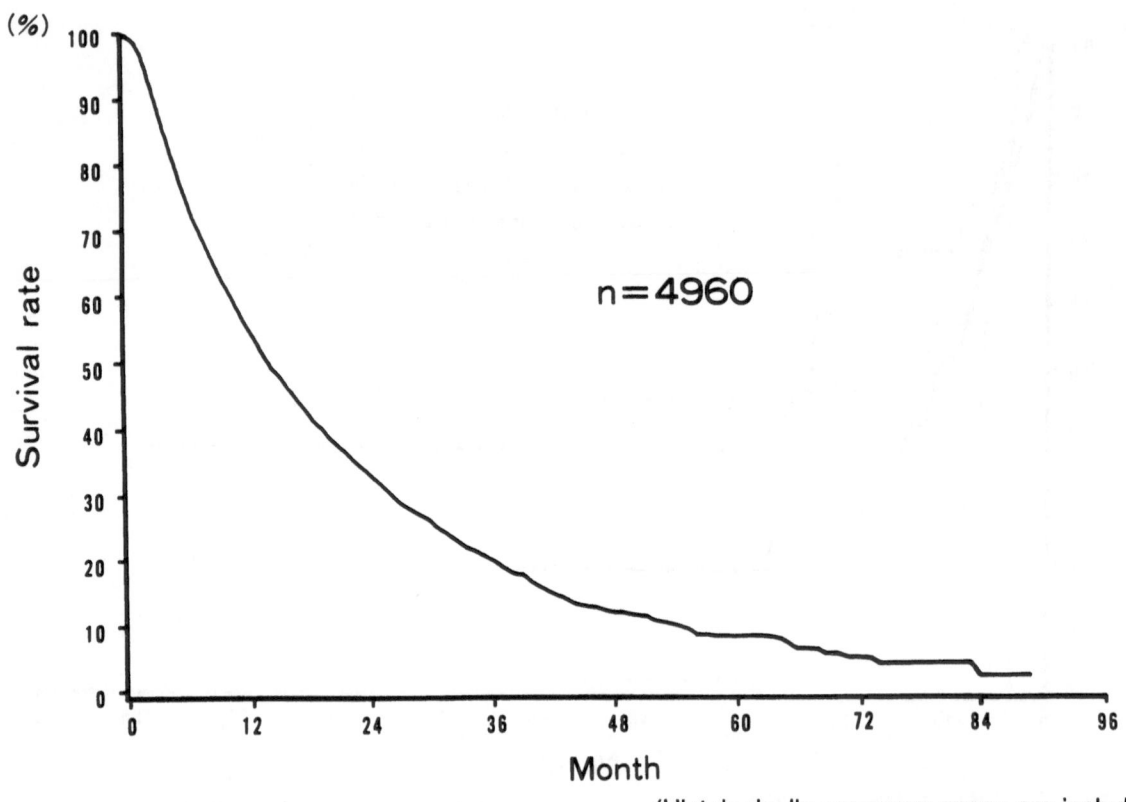

(Histologically unproven cases are included)

Fig. 20. Cumulative survival rates of patients with primary liver cancer treated with transarterial embolization. Histologically unproven cases are included

factors in relation to clinicopathological features. The prognostic factors presented here may correspond closely to the predictive ones for intrahepatic recurrence, because one of the main causes of death after partial hepatectomy is recurrence of the tumor in the remnant liver. Furthermore, intrahepatic recurrence probably plays a role in hepatic failure which is another main cause of death, and in other cases recurrence induces rupture of esophageal varices by involving the portal trunk and causing portal hypertension.

In CCC, the survival curve seems to become almost stable 2 years after surgery. On the other hand, that of HCC patients keeps decreasing even long after operation. This difference implies that in CCC patients, almost all recurrences occur within 2 years after surgery and that in HCC patients the survival rate depends on hepatic failure due to liver cirrhosis and multicentric carcinogenesis in addition to intrahepatic recurrence.

The present survey therefore clarifies the factors affecting the long-term survival of patients with primary liver cancer, especially HCC. However, we should note that only 20% of HCC patients in Japan underwent hepatic resection, mainly because in the remaining patients the

disease and/or associated hepatic cirrhosis was too far advanced for surgery, and that the rate of recurrence in the remnant liver after partial hepatectomy was fairly high. We must therefore investigate ways to improve radical surgery with safety and strive to develop promising new treatments.

References

1. Murakami F, Okamura T, Ohta M, et al. (1970) Liver disease and surgical treatment, particularly hepatic resection and transplantation. Shinryo 23:265–277
2. Ishikawa K, Kosaka K (1973) Results of hepatic resection for primary liver cancer. Acta Hepatol Jpn 14:409–410
3. Ishikawa K (1976) Follow-up Study of patients with primary liver cancer: Report 3. Acta Hepatol Jpn 17:460–465
4. Okuda K and The Liver Cancer Study Group of Japan (1980). Primary liver cancer. Cancer 45: 2663–2669
5. The Liver Cancer Study Group of Japan (1984) Primary liver cancer in Japan. Cancer 54: 1747–1755

6. The Liver Cancer Study Group of Japan (1987) Primary liver cancer in Japan. Cancer 60: 1400–1411

7. The Liver Cancer Study Group of Japan (1990) Primary liver cancer in Japan: Clinicopathologic features and results of surgical treatment. Ann Surg 211:277–287

8. Cutler SJ, Ederer F (1958) Maximum utilization of the life table method in analyzing survival. J Chronic Dis 8:699–712

9. The Liver Cancer Study Group of Japan (1989) The general rules for the clinical and pathological study of primary liver cancer. Jpn J Surg 19:98–129

10. Makuuchi M, Hasegawa H, Yamazaki S (1985) Ultrasonically guided subsegmentectomy. Surg Gynecol Obstet 161:346–350

11. Yamanaka N, Okamoto E, Kuwata K, Tanaka N (1984) A multiple regression equation for prediction of posthepatectomy liver failure. Ann Surg 200:658–663

12. Ozawa K, Aoyama H, Yasuda K, et al. (1983) Metabolic abnormalities associated with postoperative organ failure: A redox theory. Arch Surg 118:1245–1251

Section 2 Conservative and Multidisciplinary Treatment

Transcatheter arterial chemoembolization for unresectable hepatocellular carcinoma

Ryusaku Yamada, Kazushi Kishi, Masaki Terada, Tetsuo Sonomura, and Morio Sato[1]

1 Introduction

Worldwide annual incidence of hepatoma is estimated to be one million cases, with a male to female ratio of 4–5:1. In China, Taiwan, Korea, Japan, and sub-Saharan Africa, the annual incidence is as high as 150 cases per million population [1, 2].

The first choice of treatment is hepatectomy, but hepatomas are often unresectable at the time of diagnosis, because of tumor size, invasion into major vessels, associated liver cirrhosis, or the anatomical singleness of the liver.

According to the 9th report (1986–1987) of the Liver Cancer Study Group of Japan in which 9,564 hepatoma patients were studied, only 1,870 patients underwent tumor resection (20.9%) [2]. The unresectable cases underwent transcatheter arterial chemoembolization or arterial infusion chemotherapy, among other conservative therapies.

In 1977 we developed, and since then have performed, transcatheter arterial chemoembolization (TAE) and related therapies, [3–8]. To date, TAE has been performed on 1,252 patients, 1,061 treated by this means alone. This chapter discusses our experience and approach to TAE for unresectable hepatoma.

2 Alternative therapies

Transcatheter therapies, including hepatic artery embolization and arterial infusion, are currently considered first for treatment of unresectable hepatoma. However, the strategy selected should be based on knowledge of concurrent or traditional therapies; it is essential for clinical transcatheter therapists, who confront every type of difficulty, to have some alternative modalities.

Systemic chemotherapy for the treatment of hepatoma is largely unsuccessful, with a very low response rate ranging from 4%–24% [9–11]. No single agent or combination systemic drug program can be considered standard. The ancillary role of the combination of systemic chemotherapy with regional therapy has not yet been elucidated.

The liver is a radiosensitive organ, and whole liver irradiation at or above 35 Gy in a 3- to 4-week period causes a high incidence of radiation hepatitis [12]. Palliative radiotherapy for pain reduction may be attempted at under 25 Gy. On the other hand, without significant long term morbidity, small portions of the liver can be expressed to 50–60 Gy in 5 or 6 weeks which is the minimum required to control hepatoma [13]. The presence of portal tumor thrombi, hilar lymph node involvement, and localized tumors where TAE or arterial infusion therapy is not applicable or not effective, are indications for radiotherapy.

Hypervascularity of the liver and hepatoma prevent effective local thermo-accumulation in the tumor [14]. However, radiofrequency-induction hyperthermia after TAE may provide an adjuvant effect on ischemic cells, although the net contribution is still to be elucidated [15].

Ultrasound or computed tomography (CT)-guided intratumor ethanol injections [16] may be applicable for small hepatomas when the tumor is not resectable and not treated by TAE or arterial infusion.

[1] Department of Radiology, Wakayama Medical College, Wakayama, 640 Japan

3 Transcatheter approaches for unresectable hepatoma

In principle, the first choice of treatment for unresectable hepatoma is TAE, which has both selective ischemic and chemotherapeutic effects on the tumor. Alternatively, arterial chemoinfusion, with or without temporary vascular occlusion is considered when the main portal vein or the right first-order branch is obstructed by thrombi.

3.1 Catheterization [17, 18]

3.1.1 Sheath
Usually a femoral approach is employed in the Seldinger method. A long sheath is useful for kinky atherosclerotic arteries, while a long, curved sheath is useful for a brachial approach for a precipitous downgoing celiac artery or for continuous infusion.

3.1.2 Catheters
Five French (5 Fr) pre-shaped catheters with soft tips for super selective insertion [19] into the target vessels: These catheters include RH, RC2, RLG, RIM, Mikaelsson, YS-long-tapered, O-LL, and other types.

The 5Fr-RH type can be readily and smoothly inserted into the proper hepatic artery or further distal branches in most cases. The Tracker-18 catheter (Target Therapeutic Inc. California, USA) allows a coaxial approach through a 5.5 Fr catheter, and reaches smaller arteries with less intimal damage. An embolic mixture of Gelfoam particles, degradable starch microspheres (DSM), or Lipiodol can pass through the catheter lumen.

4 Angiographic assessment

In principle, all feeding arteries of the tumor should be identified, and the extent of a tumor, e.g., portal or inferior vena cava thrombi, should be elucidated before treatment is begun. Initially, arterial portography is performed. After infusion of 20–40 mg of prostaglandin E_1 or other vasodilators into the superior mesenteric artery, contrast medium is injected at a dosage of 40–50 ml in 5–7 sec for arterial portography, or of 15 ml in 3 sec for digital subtraction angiography. The entire hepatic arterial blood supply is studied, including the variant anatomy [20]. The cystic artery and the pericholedochal arteries are carefully assessed because these arteries communicate with the proper hepatic, gastroduodenal, or other arteries to some extent [21–23]. The inferior phrenic artery may play an ancillary feeding role.

When portal vein invasion is present, a typical thread and streak sign can be seen on angiography. Slow infusion hepatic arteriography, or balloon occluded angiography, angiographic computed tomography (CT), or digital subtraction angiography may be the most effective way to find a small tumor or detect a hypervascular tumor. Another method for detecting smaller tumors is by infusion of Lipiodol [24, 25]. This is based on the absence of Kupffer cells and the lack of lymphatic drainage in the tumor, both of which are present in normal tissue. When Lipiodol is injected into the hepatic artery, the droplets disperse into smaller particles, reaching the peripheral vessels and lodging there. Then Lipiodol is partially swept away by scavengers while it is retained in the tumor [26, 27].

A study of the acute toxicity of Lipiodol infusion into the hepatic artery of normal beagle dogs found body weight loss and decreased intake of foods [21]. Transient elevation of serum glutamic oxaloacetic transaminase (SGOT), serum glutamic pyruvic transaminase (SGPT) and serum alkaline phosphatase (SALP) were common. All treated animals showed Lipiodol retention in the portal vein and sinusoid. Focal necrosis and inflammatory cell infiltration in the liver parenchyma and interlobular cholangitis were observed in over one-half of the cases. The results of this experimental study led us to conclude that the dosage of Lipiodol should be restricted to less than 0.2 ml per kg [28].

5 Embolization therapies

5.1 Embolic material and method of delivery [19]

For tumor embolization, embolic materials are commonly mixed with anticancer drugs. Injection of embolic material should be carefully monitored under fluoroscopy to avoid unexpected reflux which tends to occur when the blood flow becomes slow. Following embolization, a common hepatic or celiac arteriogram is performed to

Fig. 1. A gelatin sponge block is cut into small pieces of one cubic millimeter, then soaked in a contrast media containing anticancer agents

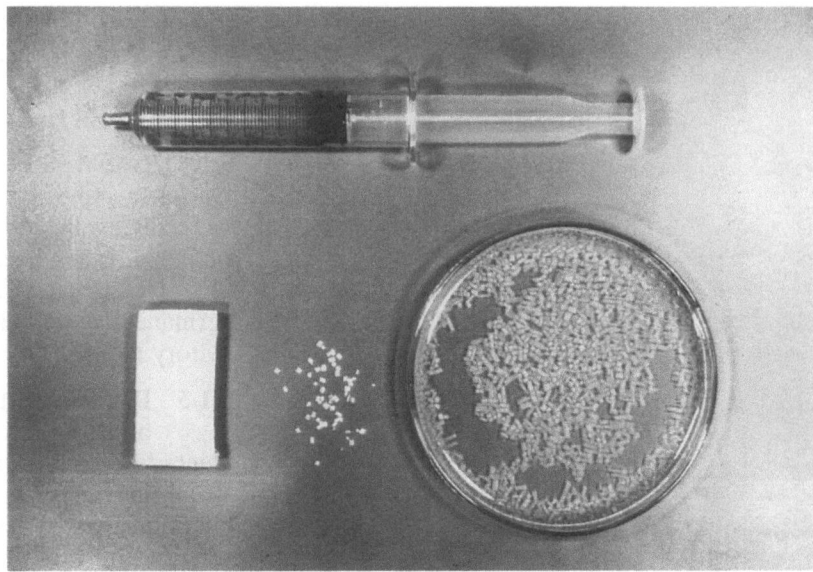

assess the results. Care should be taken not to disperse the embolic materials when contrast media is injected.

5.1.1 Gelatin sponge (Gelfoam) particles
Gelatin sponge particles are a commonly used embolic material which is less flammable and non antigenic. It is available as Gelfoam, Spongel, or Spongostan. A gelatin sponge block is sliced with a blade and cut with scissors into particles 1 mm in size (Fig. 1). The particles are then soaked in a mixed solution of anticancer agents and low osmolarity water-soluble contrast medium. Adriamycin 20 mg and mitomycin C 10 mg are mixed together are mixed together to form an chemoembolic materials.

Pain during and after TEA is reduced by the use of low osmolarity contrast media [29, 30]. Intolerable vascular pain has been associated with the use of high osmolarity contrast media in this setting. The TAE for hepatoma brings about selective coagulation necrosis of a tumor without damage to surrounding liver parenchyma [6].

Toxicity of gelatin sponge embolization was also studied with 25 dogs. Analysis of the results showed that fragments of the gelatin sponge reached neither sinusoids nor hepatic veins, but that almost all of them stayed within small hepatic artery branches with a diameter larger than 50 μm, where secondary thrombosis had occurred. Absorption of a gelatin sponge occurs within 2 weeks. None of the twenty dogs tested died, but two of them showed small foci of infarction and some showed vacuolar degeneration

of hepatocytes, both of which were mild and reversible [6].

5.1.2 Gelatin sponge powder
Gelatin sponge powder is usually used in combination with gelatin sponge particles. The powder causes more peripheral arterial occlusion because it is smaller in size, varying from 30 to 600 μm, with stronger ischemic effect on tumor tissue.

Therefore, inadvertent embolization with gelatin sponge powder can cause infarction of not only peripheral liver but also gallbladder, bile duct, pancreas and small intestine.

5.1.3 Lipiodol (ethiodol) injection therapy
Lipiodol is said to retain selectively in the tumor [24, 25, 27], a fact that has led to its therapeutic use in hepatoma patients, in which it is used as a carrier of anticancer agents. SMANCS/Lipiodol, a mixture of lipiodol and styrene maleic acid neocarzinostatin, has been recently applied with fairly good results for the treatment of unresectable hepatomas (Fig. 2) [31, 32].

Lipiodol infusion followed by gelatin sponge TAE ("Lp-TAE") [33, 34] enhances the effects of TAE; however, it may cause liver infarction. In our animal experiments with Lipiodol infusion followed by gelatin sponge TAE [28], 8 of 19 dogs died within the first week, 9 massive macroscopic liver infarctions were observed in the other 11 dogs tested. The incidence of liver infarction was 100% in those embolized with 0.2 ml per kg of Lipiodol and gelatin sponge particles. Our con-

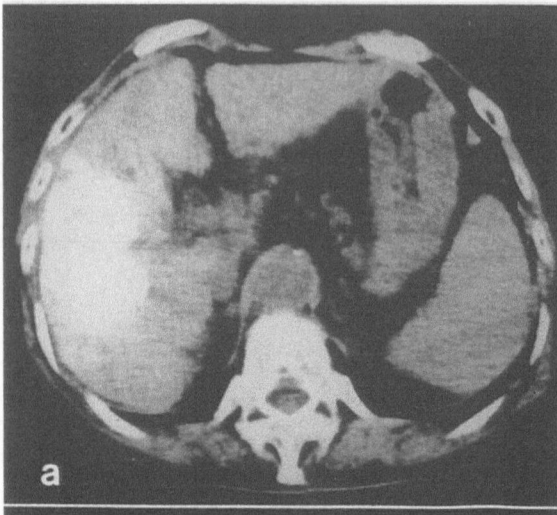

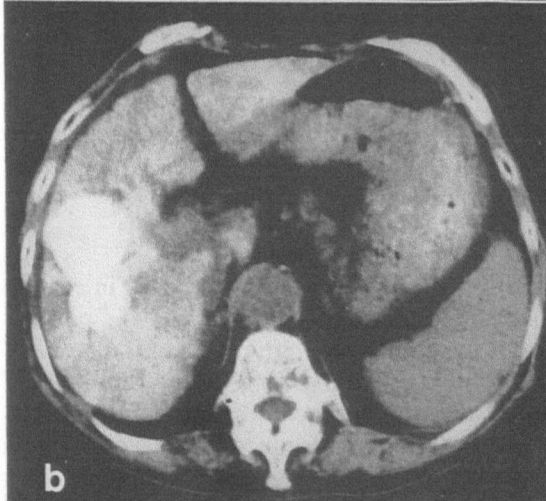

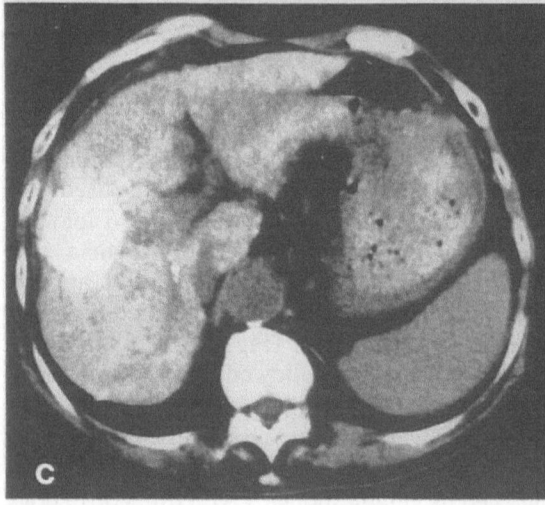

Fig. 2. Lipiodol is selectively retained in the tumor (which was mixed with SMANCS). **a** SMANCS/ Lipiodol accumulates in the tumor. **b** 3 months later, the tumor has decreased in size. **c** 6 months later, the tumor has decreased even further

clusion was that the dosage of Lipiodol infusion followed by gelatin sponge TAE should be limited to below 0.1 ml/kg for the normal part of the liver.

5.1.4 Ivaron particles [35]

Ivaron, a polyvinyl alcohol foam which is commercially available in the United States, reaches smaller arteries because of its smaller diameter (250–600, or 600–1,000 μm), and occludes more permanently due to its nonabsorbable and inflammatory nature.

5.1.5 Degradable starch microsphere infusion [36]

Degradable starch microsphere (Pharmacia) is 40 μm in diameter. Within half an hour, this temporarily occludes blood flow at the precapillary arterioles during degradation by the serum amylase. DSM is used as a mixture with anticancer agents, injected through a catheter into the hepatic artery, and attains a higher local concentration during the quarter or half an hour of the blockade. However, the tumor vessel of the hepatoma is usually more coarse than that of the secondary tumor, and the reported dosage for complete occlusion varies wildly from 150 mg to 2,700 mg [37]. If the tumor vessel is too large to be occluded by the usual administration of DSM, the balloon catheter technique [38] may be helpful.

5.1.6 Steel coil embolization

Similar to arterial ligation therapy, the steel coil usually has a weak ischemic effect on the tumor because the coil occludes only larger arteries and keeps peripheral vascular lumen open. This coil is also used in hepatic blood flow redistribution when the arterial flow needs to be changed prior to embolization or arterial infusion.

5.2 Arterial infusions

5.2.1 Bolus hepatic arterial infusion of anticancer agents

Bolus hepatic arterial infusion (so-called one-shot infusion) of anticancer agents can temporarily attain a higher drug concentration in the tumor. The drug is immediately diluted, however, and washed out by the blood flow. One-shot infusion was earlier thought to produce a higher concentration of anticancer agents in the tumor than systemic chemotherapy, but the result was not satisfactory. Currently, angiotensin-II induced hypertensive chemotherapy is proposed to enhance the effect of drugs on the basis that elevation of blood flow into the tumor increases the

Fig. 3. Changes in serum AFP level of 100 patients after hepatic arterial embolization

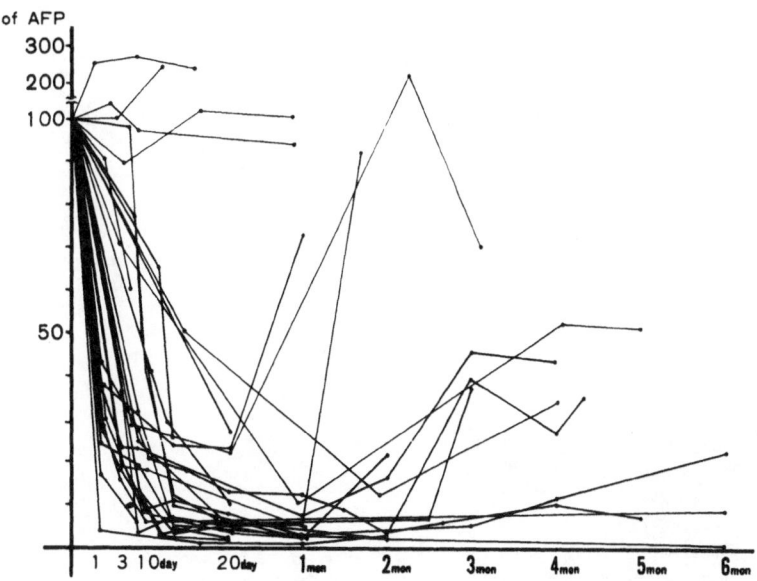

volume of the anticancer agent in the tumor tissue because the tumor vessels lack autoregulation and responsiveness to vasoconstrictors [10].

5.2.2 Balloon-occluded artery infusion [38, 39]

We have developed a balloon occluded artery infusion method (BOAI) using a double-lumen balloon catheter [38]. An anticancer drug solution is infused through the end-hole of the balloon catheter under temporary blockade of blood flow by inflation of a balloon attached to the catheter tip. Adriamycin 20 mg, Mitomycin C 10 mg, Urokinase 24,000 units, and cis-diammine dichloroplatinum 25–50 mg were mixed and diluted with saline to make 300 ml of solution. With the balloon occlusion, the infused drug was hardly diluted by blood flow; it reached the tumor tissue at a high concentration and stayed there much longer than if administered by bolus arterial infusion. In one study [38], Xenon-133 activity ratio of the tumor area to non-tumor area was 7.49:1 in BOAI, and 3.38:1 in one-shot arterial infusion. BOAI may be the therapy of choice when the hepatoma cannot be treated by embolization therapy due to portal obstruction or for some other reasons.

6 Effects of transcatheter arterial chemoembolization

The initial one hundred cases of this series showed a marked decrease of serum alpha-fetoprotein (AFP) immediately after TAE.

Although the value had a tendency to rise again in some cases 1 or 2 months later, re-embolization kept it low (Fig. 3).

Follow-up angiography, which was usually performed one month after TAE, revealed the reduction or disappearance of tumor vessels and stain in all cases with some variety. Tumor stains and tumor vessels were selectively eliminated after TAE despite recanalization of the embolized hepatic artery and recovery of its original blood flow.

The CT findings after TAE agree with the results of angiography [40]. In most cases, before TAE the tumor was identified only as an area of slightly decreased density on CT; 3 to 4 days after TAE it showed a marked decrease in density without any decrease in density of the surrounding liver parenchyma, which indicated selective necrosis of the tumor. Furthermore, sequential CT examinations revealed that the contrast medium containing anticancer agents had remained selectively in the tumor tissue at a high concentration until 48 hours after TAE, although the liver parenchyma surrounding the tumor showed no accumulation of contrast medium. Figure 4 shows an example of selective accumulation of contrast medium in the tumor for more than 24 hours after TAE.

These observations on the dynamics of anticancer agents were also confirmed by measurement of the drug concentration in a surgical specimen of the tumor tissue obtained 48 hours after TAE (Fig. 5) [41]. Figure 5 reveals the correlation between concentration of anticancer agents and that of contrast medium.

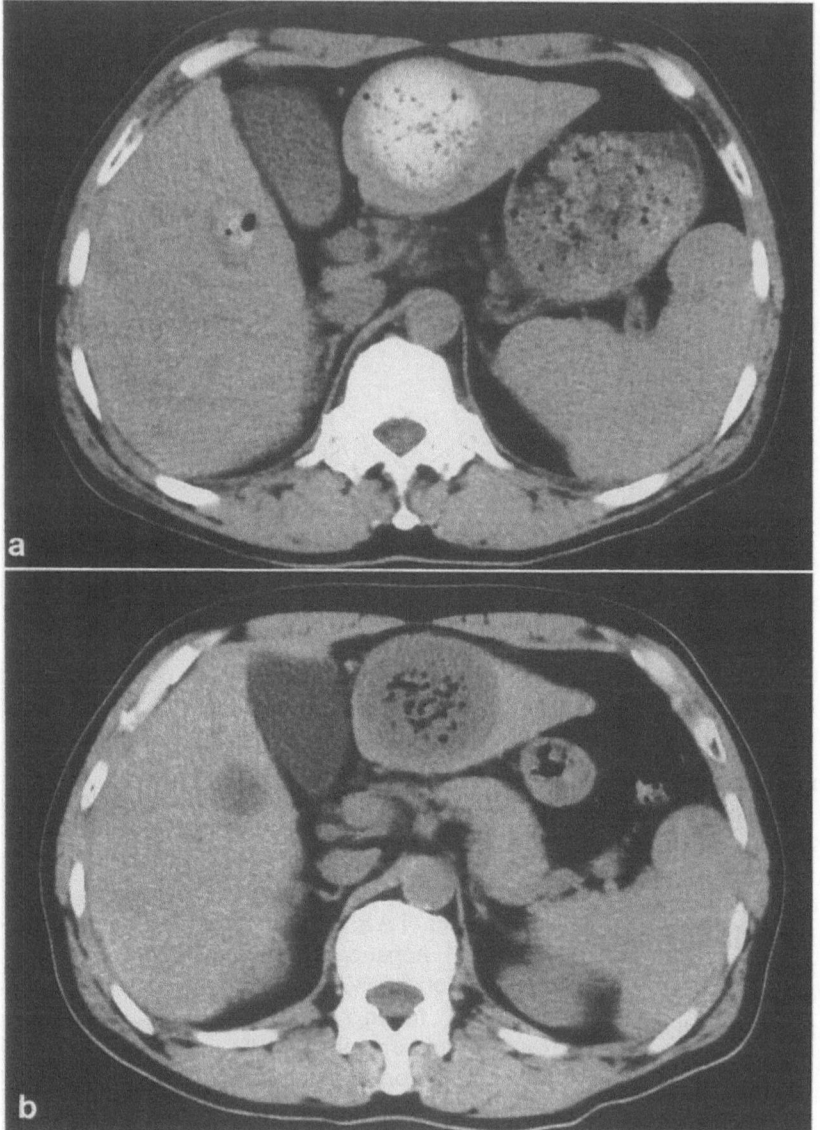

Fig. 4. A 48-year-old male with HCC in the left lobe and small daughter nodule in the right lobe. **a** 24 hours after TAE, contrast media containing Adriamycin and Mitomycin C remained selectively in the tumors at a high concentration. **b** 10 days later, the tumor necrosis was completed

7 Side effects and complications of TAE [6, 42–44]

The primary side effect of TAE, post embolization syndrome, includes daily intermittent fever usually under 39°C, abdominal pain, nausea and vomiting, abdominal fullness, and appetite loss. Those symptoms usually diminish spontaneously within a couple of weeks. Nausea and vomiting fade first, and the fever, usually seen from the first day, and its duration seems to relate to the intensity of tumor necrosis and the size of the tumor. Antifebrile drugs are effective for this fever. The severe abdominal pain may be due to infarction of the gallbladder [42] resulting from cystic artery embolization, pancreatitis resulting from pancreatic artery embolization, or possibly other reasons [43]. Laboratory examinations may reveal leucocytosis, fibrinogen fluctuation, C-reactive protein (CRP) elevation or electrolyte imbalance.

Liver damage appears with elevations of SGOT, SGPT, serum lactate dehydrogenase (LDH), serum glutamate pyruvate transaminase, total bilirubin, alkaline phosphatase (ALP), prolongation of prothrombin time, and decreases in cholineesterase, antithrombin III, fibrinogen, and serum albumin, most cases of which are transient and return later to original levels (Fig.

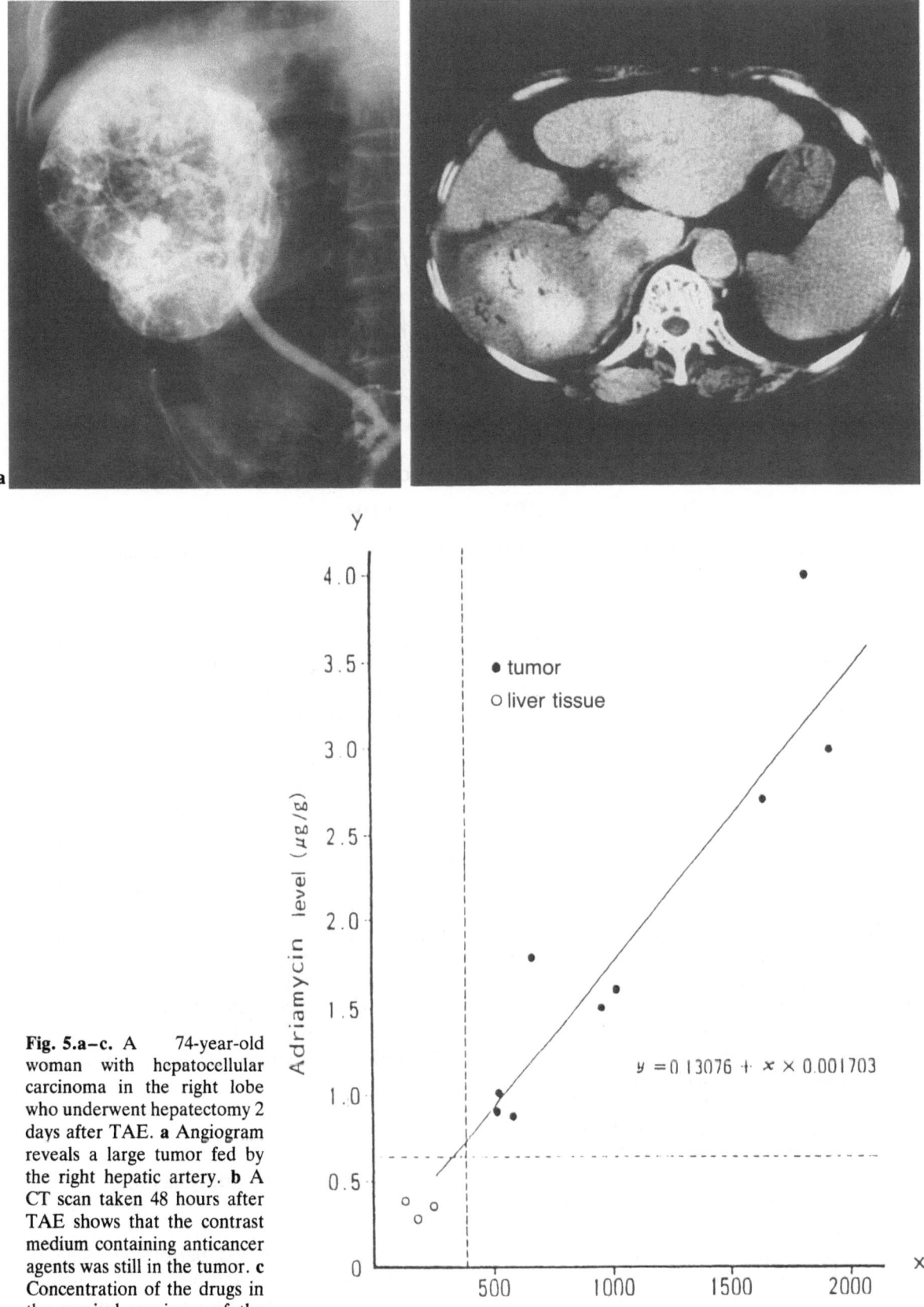

Fig. 5.a–c. A 74-year-old woman with hepatocellular carcinoma in the right lobe who underwent hepatectomy 2 days after TAE. **a** Angiogram reveals a large tumor fed by the right hepatic artery. **b** A CT scan taken 48 hours after TAE shows that the contrast medium containing anticancer agents was still in the tumor. **c** Concentration of the drugs in the surgical specimen of the tumor tissue

$y = 0.13076 + x \times 0.001703$

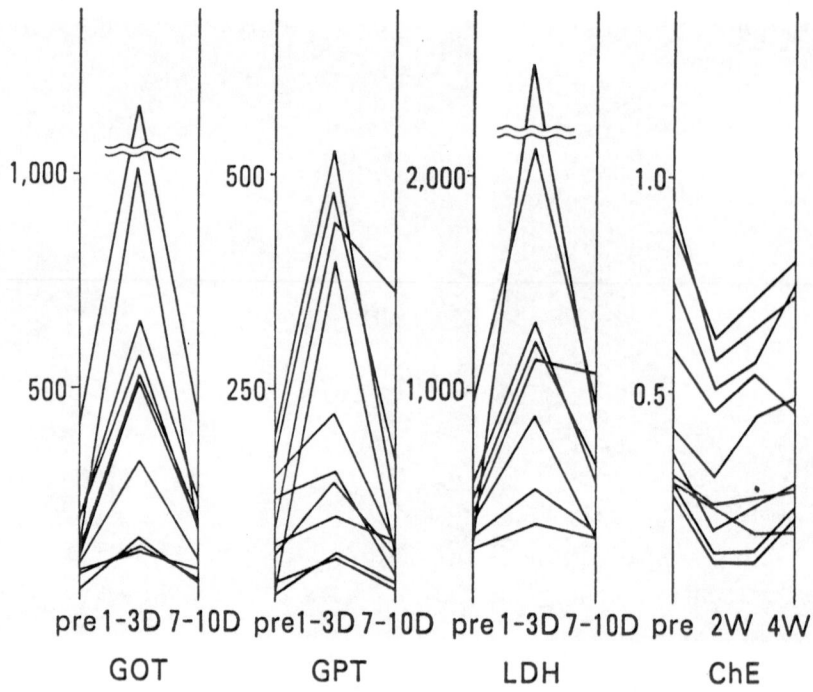

Fig. 6. Changes in SGOT, SGPT, SLDH, and cholinesterase (CLE) after embolization

6). However, severe cases need intensive care for liver function before the onset of acute hepatic failure. Acute gastric mucosal lesions frequently occur and require medication.

8 Results in cumulative survival

From June 1977 to May 1989, 1,252 cases of hepatoma underwent TAE in our Department of Radiology, Wakayama Medical College, or in the Department of Radiology, Osaka City University Hospital. One thousand sixty-one cases were treated by TAE alone, 181 cases underwent hepatectomy after TAE, and 10 had hepatic artery ligation after TAE.

The cumulative survival curve for these 1,061 patients with unresectable hepatoma showed that the 1, 2, 3, 4, and 5-year survival rates were 51, 28, 13, 8, and 6%, respectively (Fig. 7). Among them, 9 cases survived more than 5 years, and the longest survived 10 years and 3 months.

The cumulative survival curve of 66 small hepatomas with a diameter less than 5 cm treated with TAE alone showed that the 1, 2, and 3-year survival rates were 72, 55, and 47%, respectively (Fig. 8). The cumulative survival after resection

of hepatoma (Fig. 9) at 1 year and 3 years is approximately 71.9% and 55.0%, respectively. In comparison with the survival of surgically resected cases, the results of embolization therapy were almost equal to or a little worse than those of hepatectomy.

Hepatomas with main portal vein obstruction due to tumor invasion showed worse results than those without its obstruction in TAE. Of patients with main portal obstruction who were excluded from TAE, 91 were treated by balloon occluded artery infusion or SMANCS/lipiodol infusion therapy. Of those 91, 16 cases showed recanalization of main portal obstruction and marked reduction of tumor size.

During the period of this study we had 40 cases of 3-year survival and 7 of 5-year survival. The longest survivor is still living 8 years after TAE.

9 Prognostic factor analysis [30]

A statistical analysis was performed using the proportional hazard model on the 30 prognostic factors in 134 patients with unresectable hepatoma treated by TAE [30]. Ascites, tumor size,

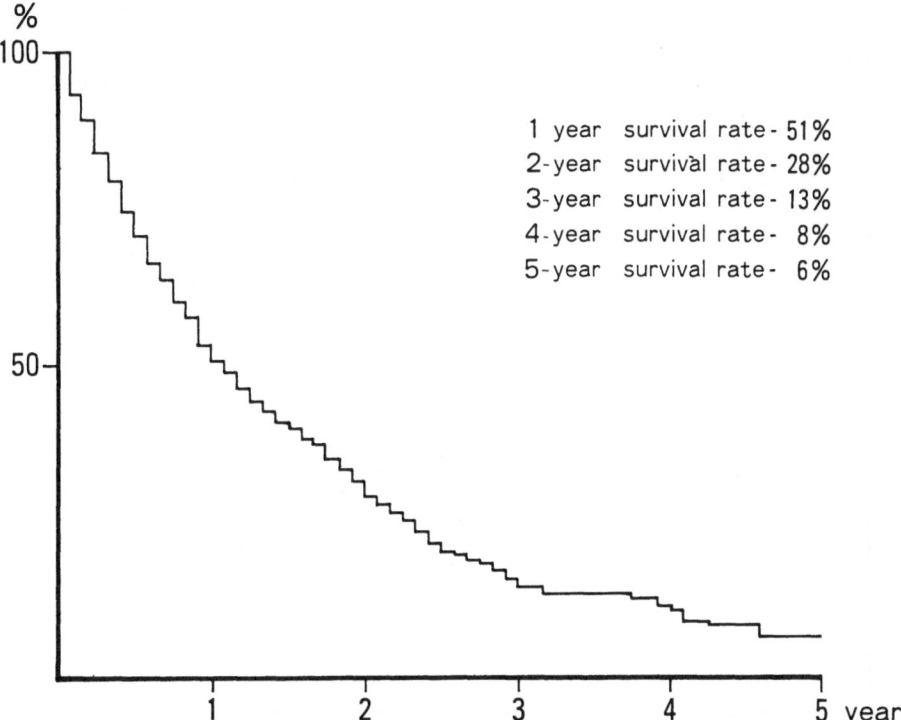

Fig. 7. Cumulative survival rate of hepatoma patients treated by TAE (1,061 cases)

total bilirubin, and extension of the tumor were found to be the factors which influenced the prognosis the most. The proportional hazard model was: λ (t, x) = λ_0 (t) {1.19* ([ascites] − 1.19) + 0.63* ([tumor size] − 1.59) + 0.22* (total bilirubin mg/dl − 1.18) + 0.18* ([extension of tumor] − 1.44)}, where 1.0 was given when the case was free from ascites, tumor size was under 5 cm, and tumor extension was under 20% (E1), respectively, otherwise 2.0 was given for each factor.

10 Discussion

Since 1977, TAE therapy for hepatocellular carcinoma has been widely performed [35, 45–47], not only in Japan, but also in other Asian countries. We have performed TAE therapy in patients with various malignant tumors, including lung cancer, HCC, renal cellular carcinoma, uterine cancer, and urinary bladder cancer. Our best results were obtained in HCC. Seventy five percent of unresectable HCC in our series showed objective tumor reduction or necrosis, classified as complete response or partial re-

sponse. This response rate was far better than reported rates of hepatic artery infusion of anticancer agents in HCC.

The one-year survival rate in this series was 51%. The series consisted only of unresectable cases due to advanced stage of the tumor and/or accompanying liver cirrhosis, which also supports the efficacy of this therapy. A marked decrease in AFP values after TAE was observed in 90% of cases, also supporting efficacy of the therapy.

Angiographic findings were extremely interesting after TAE, all of which indicated a reduction or disappearance of tumor vessels and an increase in the avascular area in the tumor, despite recanalization of the embolized arteries with consequent restoration of original blood flow. This fact can be interpreted as indicating selective necrosis of the tumor, which was corroborated by the findings on CT [48, 49] that indicated that only the necrotized tumor tissue was visualized as a low density area and the surrounding liver tissue was free of any change in density.

Sequential CT examination also disclosed a selective accumulation of contrast medium in the tumor tissue for 48 hours or more after TAE, which means that TAE is a good drug delivery system; this is regarded as a targetting chemo-

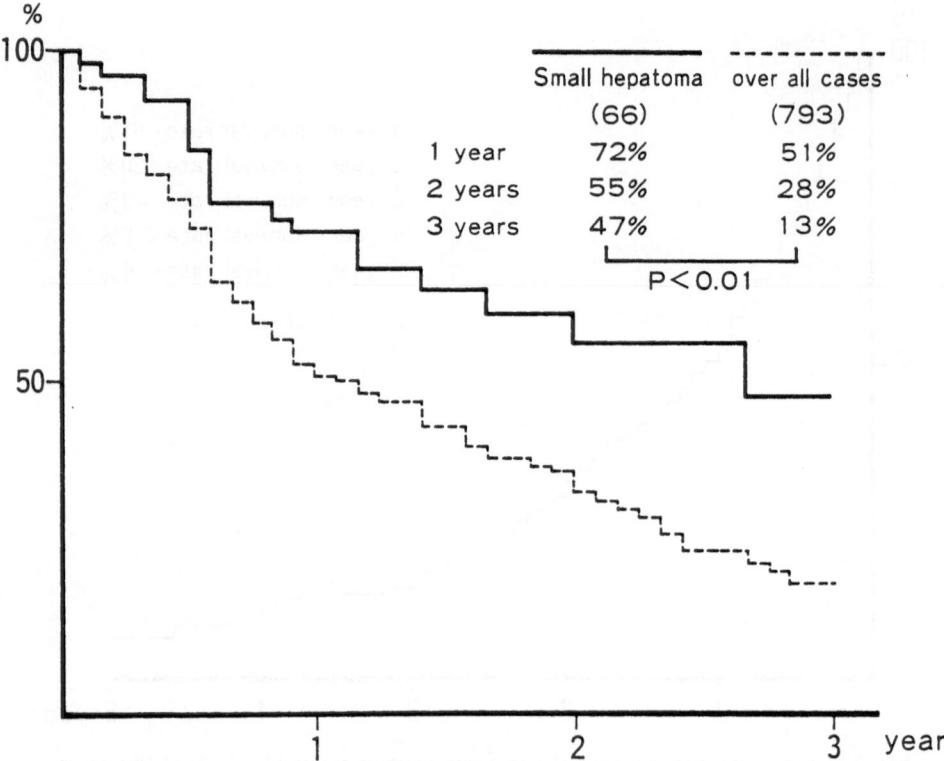

	Small hepatoma (66)	over all cases (793)
1 year	72%	51%
2 years	55%	28%
3 years	47%	13%

P < 0.01

Fig. 8. Cumulative survival rate of small hepatoma treated with TAE ($\phi \leqq 5$ cm)

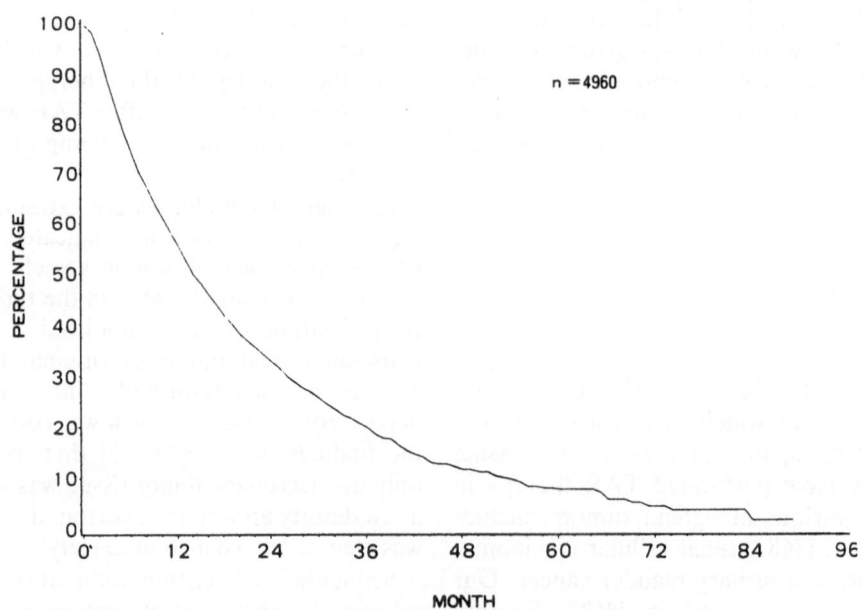

n = 4960

Fig. 9. Cumulative survival rate of hepatoma patients after hepatic resection. From the 9th report of the Liver Cancer Study Group of Japan

therapy known as "chemoembolization." For this reason, TAE for HCC can be expected to produce both ischemic and chemical necrosis of the tumor.

As we reported in 1983 [44], there were 5 patients who died of hepatic insufficiency within 1 month following TAE in whom portal veins were obstructed by tumor thrombi and invasion. In these cases, extensive necrosis was histologically observed, not only in the tumor tissue but also in the liver parenchyma, which seemed to be due to obstruction of both the hepatic artery and the portal vein. Based on these fatalities, it is considered that TAE is contraindicative in cases with main portal vein obstruction.

A prospective randomized clinical trial [50] may settle the question of whether TAE can be an effective therapy for preoperative treatment of hepatoma. However, TAE prolonged the survival of patients with recurring hepatoma after resection [1].

Thus, from long-term results it can be concluded that transcatheter arterial chemoembolization is the most effective conservative therapy for unresectable HCC, and almost the same results can be expected in treatments for metastatic liver cancers [51].

References

1. Liver Cancer Study Group of Japan Survey and follow-up study of primary liver cancer in Japan, Report 6 (in Japanese). (1979) Acta Hepatol Jpn
2. Liver Cancer Study Group of Japan Survey and follow-up study of primary liver cancer in Japan, Report 9 (in Japanese). (1991) Acta Hepatol Jpn, 32:1138–1147
3. Yamada R, Nakatsuka H, Nakamura K, Sato M, Itami M, Kobayashi N, Minakuchi K, Onoyama Y, Kanno T, Monna T, Yamamoto S (1980) Hepatic artery embolization in 32 patients with unresectable hepatoma. Osaka City Med J, 26:81–96
4. Kobayashi N (1987) Experimental and clinical study of a new embolic material for treatment of malignant tumor; Gelatine sponge-containing carboquone. Acta Radiol Jpn, 47:1127–1144
5. Satoh M, Kitayama K, Kishi K, Shioyama Y, Tsuda M, Terada M, Maeda M, Hamachi J, Daimon M, Tanaka H, Sonomura T, Nakatani K, Kawabata M, Yamada R (1988) Usefulness of a 5 Fr sized preshaped balloon catheter: So-called interventional balloon catheter (in Japanese). Acta Radiol Jpn, 48:924–926

6. Satoh M, Yamada R (1983) Experimental and clinical studies on the hepatic artery embolization for treatment of hepatoma (in Japanese). Acta Radiol Jpn, 43:977–1005
7. Yamada R, Kishi K (1991) Embolotherapy for palliative treatment of unresectable hepatoma. ed. S. Kadir, B.C. Decker. In: "Current Practice of Interventional Radiology."
8. Yamada R, Nakatsuka H, Nakamura K, Sato M, Tamaoka K, Takemoto K, Minakuchi K, Yamaguchi S, Tamaki M, Monna T, Onoyama Y, Yamamoto S (1979) Transcatheter arterial embolization therapy in unresectable hepatomas—experience in 15 cases (in Japanese). Acta Hepatol Jpn, 20:595–603
9. Barone C, Astone A (1987) Phase II trial with mitoxantrone in advanced hepatocellular carcinoma (abstract). ECCO-4, p 49
10. Ensminger WD, Gyves JW (1983) Regional chemotherapy of neoplastic diseases. Pharmacol Ther, 21:277–293
11. Okazaki N, Yoshino M, Yoshida T, Hizikata A, Hasegawa H (1986) Systemic chemotherapy of hepatocellular carcinoma (in Japanese). Gan To Kagaku Ryoho, 13:1584–1588
12. Perez CA, Brady CW (1987) Textbook of Radiotherapy. Lippincott, Philadelphia
13. Nagashima T (1989) The study of radiotherapy for hepatocellular carcinoma (in Japanese). Acta Radiol Jpn, 49:1141–1151
14. Yamada R, Tsuji K, Kishi K, Suwa K, Mitsuzane K, Tanaka K, Sato K, Kawabata M, Maeda M (1988) An attempt of hyperthermia with balloon catheter and immunochemotherapeutic agent. Radiat Med, 6:79–84
15. Hasegawa H (1988) Annual report of cancer research, supported by the Ministry of Health and Welfare of Japan National Cancer Center (in Japanese). pp 69–77
16. Suyama Y, Horishi M, Ebisu S (1987) US guided ethanol injection therapy for small liver cancer (in Japanese). J Jpn Soc Cancer Ther, 22:818–826
17. Chuang VP, Soo CS, Carrasco CH, Wallace S (1983) Superselective catheterization technique in hepatic angiography. Am J Roentgenol, 141:803–811
18. Ring EJ, McLean G (1981) Interventional radiology: Principles and techniques. Little, Brown and Company, Boston
19. Rosch J, Potter CT, Brown MJ (1972) Selective arterial embolization: A new method for control of acute gastrointestinal bleeding. Radiology 102:303–306
20. Reuter SR, Redman HC (1988) Gastrointestinal Angiography, (3rd edn) Saunders, Philadelphia
21. Bookstain J, Cho KJ, Davis GB, Dail D (1982) Arterioportal communication: Observations and hypothesis concerning trans-sinusoidal and transversal type. Radiology 142:581–590

22. Cho KJ, Lunderquist A (1983) The peribiliary vascular plexus: The microvascular architecture of the bile duct in the rabbit and in clinical cases. Radiology 147:357–364

23. Lin G, Lunderquist A, Haegerstrand I, Boijsen E (1984) Postmortem examination of the blood supply and vascular pattern of small liver metastasis in man. Surgery, 96:517–526

24. Ohishi H, Uchida H, Yoshimura H, Ohue S, Ueda J, Katsuragi M, Matsumoto N, Hosogi Y (1985) Hepatocellular cartinoma detected by iodized oil: Use of anticancer agents. Radiology, 154:25–29

25. Yumoto Y, Jinno K, Tokuyama K, Araki Y, Ishimizu T, Maeda H, Konno T (1985) Hepatocellular carcinoma detected by iodized oil. Radiology, 154:19–24

26. Kishi K, Satoh M, Sonomura T, Tsuda M, Tanaka H, Shioyama Y, Terada M, Sato M, Yamada R (1989) Experimental study on acute toxicity of hepatic arterial ethiodol infusion (abstract). RSNA '89, Scientific program

27. Matsui O, Takashima T, Kadoya M, Kitagawa K, Hirose J, Kameyama T, Choutou S, Miyata S (1987) Mechanism of Lipiodol accumulation and retention in hepatic tumors. Analysis in cases with simple Lipiodol injection (in Japanese). Acta Radiol Jpn, 47:1395–1404

28. Satoh M, Kishi K, Shioyama Y, Tsuda M, Terada M, Shirai S, Tanaka H, Nakatani K, Sonomura T, Maeda M, Daimon M, Hamati J, Kawabata M, Yamada R (1990) Effects of experimental hepatic artery embolization with Lipiodol and gelatin sponge on liver tissue (in Japanese). Nippon Acta Radiol, 50:107–113

29. Lasser EC, Lang JH, Hamblin (1980) Activation systems in contrast idiosyncrasy. Invest Radiol, 15:S2–S5

30. Shioyama Y (1989) A study on prognostic factors for survival of the patients with hepatocellular carcinoma treated by transcatheter arterial embolization (in Japanese). J Wakayama Med Soc, 40:449–458

31. Konno T, Maeda H, Iwai K (1983) Effect of arterial administration of high molecular weight anticancer agent SMANCS with lipid lymphographic agent on hepatoma: A preliminary report. Eur J Cancer Clin Oncol, 19:1053

32. Miller D, O'Leavy TJ, Girton M (1987) Distribution of iodized oil within the liver after hepatic arterial injection. Radiology, 162:849–851

33. Nakamura H, Hashimoto T, Oi H, Sawada S (1988) Iodized oil in the portal vein after arterial embolization. Radiology, 167:415–417

34. Nakamura H, Tanaka T, Hori S, Yoshioka H, Kuroda C, Okamura J, Sakurai H (1983) Transcatheter embolization of hepatocellular carcinoma: Assessment of efficacy in cases of resection following embolization. Radiology, 147:401–405

35. Chuang VC, Wallace S (1981) Hepatic artery embolization in the treatment of hepatic neoplasms. Radiology, 140:51–58

36. Dakhil S, Ensminger W, Cho K, Niderhuber J, Doan K, Wheeler R (1982) Improved regional selectivity of hepatic arterial BCNU with degradable microspheres. Cancer, 50:631–631

37. Yamada T, Matsuoka T, Manabe T, Takashima S, Kobayashi N, Tamaoka K, Nakajima T, Nakatsuka H, Nakamura K, Minakuchi K, Onoyama Y (1986) Clinical trial of degradable starch microspheres (DSM) in the treatment of hepatic malignancies by intra-arterial infusion of anticancer drugs: Relationship between quantity of DSM and blockade of arterial blood flow (in Japanese). Nippon Acta Radiol, 46:1259–1266

38. Kawabata M (1988) Development of balloon occluded arterial infusion (BOAI) and its clinical application in hepatocellular carcinoma (in Japanese). J Jpn Soc Cancer Ther, 23:118–129

39. Yano S, Tarumi T, Yamamoto T, Tamura K, Nakaya A (1989) The clinical studies of intermittent hepatic arterial occlusion with infusion chemotherapy for unresectable hepatocellular carcinoma associated with arterioportal or arteriovenous shunts (in Japanese). J Jpn Soc Cancer Ther, 24:99–108

40. Takayasu K, Moriyama N, Muramatsu Y, Suzuki H, Yamada T, Hasegawa H, Okazaki N (1984) Hepatic arterial embolization for hepatocellular carcinoma: Comparison of CT scans and resected specimens. Radiology, 150:661–665

41. Tsuda M, Yamada R, Sato M, Tanaka K, Nomura S, Tsuji K, Terada M, Shioyama Y, Maeda M, Kishi K, Nakatani K, Sonomura T, Hiroaki T (1990) The movement of antineoplastic solution in transcatheter hepatic arterial embolization (in Japanese). Acta Radiol Jpn, 50:504–511

42. Kuroda C, Iwasaki M, Tanaka T, Tokunaga K, Hori S, Yoshioka H, Sakurai M, Okamura J (1983) Gallbladder infarction following hepatic transcatheter embolization. Radiology, 149:85–89

43. Makuuchi M, Sukigara M, Mori T, Kobayashi J, Yamazaki S, Hasegawa H, Moriyama N, Takayasu K, Hirohashi S (1985) Bile duct necrosis: Complication of transcatheter hepatic arterial embolization. Radiology, 156:331–334

44. Yamada R, Sato M, Kawabata M, Nakatsuka H, Nakamura K, Takashima S (1983) Hepatic artery embolozation in 120 patients with unresectable hepatoma. Radiology, 148:397–401

45. Kato T, Nemoto R, Mori H (1981) Arterial chemoembolization with microencapsulated anticancer drug: An approach to selective cancer chemotherapy with sustained effects. JAMA, 245:1123–1127

46. Sato Y, Fujiwara K, Ogata I, Ohta Y, Hayashi S, Itai Y, Furui S, Oka H (1985) Transcatheter arterial embolization for unresectable cases with liver cirrhosis evaluated by comparison with other conservative treatments. Cancer, 55:2822–2825

47. Wallace S, Charnsangavej C, Carrasco CH, Bechtel W (1984) Ethanol for hepatic artery embolization. Radiology, 152:821–822

48. Furui S, Otomo K, Itai Y, Iio M (1984) Hepato-cellular carcinoma treated by transcatheter arterial embolization: Progress evaluation by computed tomography. Radiology, 159:773–778

49. Takayasu K, Moriyama N, Muramatsu Y, Suzuki M, Yamada T, Kishi K, Hasegawa H, Okazaki N (1985) Intrahepatic portal vein branches studied by percutaneous transhepatic portography. Radiology, 154:31–36

50. Hase M, Sako M, Fujii M, Ueda E, Nagae T, Shimizu T, Hirota S, Konno M (1989) Experi-mental study of embolo-hyperthermia for treat-ment of liver tumor (in Japanese). Acta Radiol, Jpn, 49:1171–1173

51. Kishi K, Yamada R, Shirai S, Mitsuzane J, Satoh M, Shioyama Y, Tsuda M, Terada M, Sonomura T, Tanaka H, Kawabata M (1989) Transcatheter therapies of metastatic liver tumors (in Japanese). Surgical Therapy, 61:702–710

52. Okuda K (1986) Primary liver cancer: Quadrennial review lecture. Dig Dis Sci, 31:133s–146s

CHAPTER 26

Arterial infusion therapy: Lipiodol-cytostatics with and without embolization

Yoshiyuki Shimamura, Masanori Ishii, Masato Ono, Fujio Makita, Ryuzo Sekiguchi, Masahiro Yoshino, Peter Gunvén, and Kaoru Abe[1]

1 Introduction

The liver has a dual blood supply by the arterial and portal systems. Primary and secondary liver tumors are mainly nourished arterially, as first suggested by Breedis and Young [1]. This knowledge has guided numerous attempts to affect the growth of liver tumors by reduction of the nutritive arterial flow and/or addition to it of anti-tumor agents. In both cases, some selectivity of action is expected because the normal liver is to a great extent also supplied by the portal venous flow. The regional infusion of toxic agents could be expected to give diminished side effects as compared to systemic treatment because the agents may be more or less cleared or modified by passage through the liver.

2 Intra-arterial administration of anti-tumor agents

A number of cytostatic drugs have been used for arterial liver perfusion, one of the most popular being 5-FUDR (5-fluoro-2'-deoxy-β-uridine) infused by means of an implantable pump to aviod repeat arterial catheterizations and to obtain a prolonged infusion that reaches a larger proportion of tumor cells as they go through sensitive phases of the cell cycle. Even though a substantial percentage of treated patients, mostly with colorectal metastases, had objective tumor responses, the few controlled studies that have been done have failed to translate this into a convincing prolongation of survival, as reviewed by Sugarbaker and Kemeny [2]. The regional intra-arterial administration of other anti-tumor agents, e.g. tumor necrosis factor [3], is presently being evaluated.

3 Reduction of arterial blood flow

Ligation of liver arteries affects tumor growth only temporarily, even after extensive devascularization by division of the ligaments of the liver. This is due to the rapid formation of collaterals, that feed the tumor and cannot be employed for further therapeutic measures [4]. A logical development is, therefore, the implantable vascular occluder described by Bengmark and coworkers [5], that is similar to a miniature tourniquet which is placed surgically around the liver arteries. It can be inflated temporarily via a subcutaneous injection port, enabling treatment in the patients' homes. The treatment periods should theoretically be frequent and short to affect tumor growth without stimulation of collateral formation. Periods of 45–90 minutes twice or three times daily have been used but the optimal schedule is not known and the long term results must be awaited before the indications for this treatment modality are defined. The same is true for its combination with intraperitoneal infusions of cytostatic drugs.

Another means to reduce the arterial blood supply to the liver is arterial embolization. A variety of materials have been employed. As with hepatic artery ligation, permanent occlusion by steel coils or other unresorbable materials leads to formation of collaterals that nourish the regrowing tumors and make further similar treatment impossible. Degradable embolizing agents have therefore been used, including gelatin

[1] National Matsudo Hospital 123-1 Takatsuka-shinden Matsudo, Chiba, 271 Japan

sponge or powder, starch microspheres, and iodized oily preparations.

4 Combinations of intra-arterial anti-tumor agents with reduced arterial blood flow

We have used a trans-arterial, repeatable chemoembolization procedure for liver tumors [6]. It first occludes the peripheral, small tumor vessels by a mixture of oily X-ray contrast medium and a cytostatic drug. Immediately after this, larger central afferent vessels are occluded by means of gelatin cubes. We shall here describe a chemoembolization method, Lipiodol-transarterial embolization (L-TAE), and our experiences with it.

4.1 Indications and contraindications for chemoembolization (L-TAE)

We performed L-TAE in all cases of liver tumors, because it serves both diagnostic and therapeutic purposes. According to our experience, computed tomographic (CT) scanning after embolization is a very sensitive method to detect small hepatocellular carcinomas (HCC). The scanning should be delayed for three to four weeks, after which time most of the non-specific staining of the liver has disappeared.

The procedure is sometimes modified by the exclusion of gelatin sponge cubes, in which case we call it Lipiodol-transarterial infusion (L-TAI). This modification is used when there is serious liver dysfunction or when we investigate a patient within the first postoperative month, as is often done after non-radical liver resection. Other indications are if we cannot perfuse only the liver, or during follow-up of resected HCC if we do not find signs of tumor in the preceding arteriography at the same session. The CT scanning is performed about two weeks after L-TAI because the Lipiodol is washed out rapidly when central arteries are not occluded.

With regard to the therapeutic effects of the chemoembolization, direct proof has not been provided by randomized controlled studies. The frequent near-total postembolization tumor necrosis leads us to believe that retardation of tumor growth and prolongation of life can follow. We therefore use the technique as a postoperative adjuvant treatment after curative resections of

multiple HCCs or solitary HCCs larger than 2 cm in diameter, and smaller tumors unless they are very highly differentiated. For similar reasons, we have adopted a policy of debulking resections of large HCCs even in the presence of unresectable disease, if about a 90% reduction of tumor volume can be achieved. Remaining tumors are then controlled by repeated chemoembolizations. With this strategy, we have obtained five year survival rates of about 25% after non-curative resections for HCC in 85 patients, including cases with advanced portal venous tumor thrombi. Another indication for chemoembolization is inoperable HCC.

Newer applications of the procedure are in combination with external beam radiotherapy or with percutaneous ethanol injection into tumors. The addition of radiotherapy seems to be effective in patients with intraportal tumor thrombi of HCC. The ethanol injections seem to create a zone around the tumor that is deprived of portal blood supply. This zone of potential tumor invasion is therefore possibly affected by the reduction of arterial blood flow after embolization.

Contraindications that should be observed are failure to position the catheter so that the embolizing mixture reaches only the liver, in which case we can use Lipiodol-doxorubicin without gelatin sponge as described above (L-TAI). Another theoretical contraindication is extensive arteriovenous shunting, in which case we could expect some pulmonary embolization with Lipiodol, as reported for its use in lymphangiography. Furthermore, occlusion of the main portal trunk without collateral formation, as demonstrated by portography during superior mesentericography in the same angiography session, contraindicates the embolization. We have, however, embolized a few patients with occlusion by intraportal tumor metastases of the right or left lobar portal branch without mortality. We do not embolize with the catheter in a wedge position, or with the use of large injection pressure. Under such circumstances, there is risk for extrahepatic spread of the agents that instead should be carried by the blood stream to the liver.

4.2 Technique for chemoembolization

4.2.1 Vascular access
The treatment modality can be administered percutaneously, e.g. via the femoral artery with the use of a Seldinger technique. The catheter

tip should be positioned in the proper hepatic artery to avoid spilling of the agents into the gastroduodenal artery. If the catheter has a balloon at its tip, with the lumen opening distal to the balloon, the tip can be positioned in the common hepatic artery. Inflation of the balloon before embolization will revert the blood flow in the gastroduodenal artery so that the embolizing mixture is directed exclusively to the liver. Recently, we have used permanent catheters placed percutaneously, via the femoral artery or the subclavian artery under ultrasonic guidance. Two versions of prototype injection ports have been developed but are not presently available commercially. They have small chambers so that the gelatin cubes used can be flushed out completely, and they can be buried subcutaneously under local anesthesia.

Another possibility is that a permanent catheter is operatively inserted into the gastroduodenal artery with its tip at the level of the wall of the liver artery. This catheter has a notched tip to permit its fixation by ligatures, and is connected to a subcutaneous infusion port as described bove.

Due to vascular variations, double catheters, arterial ligation, or placement of an implantable vascular occluder may be necessary to allow treatment of the entire liver. For an example, one patient had a left hepatic artery that originated proximally to the gastroduodenal artery. A vascular occluder on the common hepatic artery proximal to the left hepatic artery after inflation directed part of the infused embolizing mixture into the left hepatic artery by retrograde flow.

4.2.2 The embolizing mixtures

For peripheral embolization of the smaller tumor vessels, 5 ml of an iodinated ethyl ester of the fatty acid of poppyseed oil (Lipiodol Ultra Fluid, André Gelbe Laboratory, France) are mixed with 2.5 ml of 60% meglumine diatrizoate (Urografin, Schering AG, Berlin) and 100 ml of the aminoglycoside antibiotic dibekacin sulfate (Panimycin, Meiji Seika, Tokyo). Doxorubicin (Adriamycin) in a dose of 20–40 mg, or 50 mg of the newer anthracycline 4-epidoxorubicin (Farmorubicin), is added and the mixture is shaken vigorously for ten minutes. The resulting droplets are between 40 and 200 microns in size and remain in suspension for several hours.

For the ensuing central embolization of larger vessels, 10 ml of 75% Urografin are mixed with about 0.6 ml of 1 mm large cubes of Gelfoam gelatin sponge (Ferrosan, Copenhagen, Denmark).

As mentioned above, we observe some contraindications to the administration of this embolizing agent.

4.2.3 The embolization procedure

The first mixture, Lipiodol-doxorubicin with antibiotic and Urografin, is slowly injected without too much pressure under fluoroscopic guidance until it reaches the periphery of the liver and the flow becomes very slow. Usually, the tumors retain contrast to a much greater extent than normal liver tissue. As described under section 4.1, we stop the treatment at this stage in some cases. The second embolizing mixture, Gelfoam and Urografin, is then immediately injected until blood flow almost stops.

4.2.4 The schedule for embolization

The first embolization is done during investigation of a suspected liver tumor. If resection is intended, it can be performed as soon as post-embolization CT scans have been obtained, usually about three weeks after embolization, unless liver function tests have not returned to pre-embolization values. In the latter case, we await their return to the baseline.

Post-resection embolizations can start about one month after hepatectomy but with gelatin sponge cubes excluded from the embolizing mixture. Regular embolizations are then started about three to four months later. In the adjuvant setting, they are repeated at intervals of four months in the first postoperative year, and twice in the second year, followed by yearly embolizations. With non-radical resections or recurrence, we aim at treatments every fourth months for as long as possible.

4.3 Results of chemoembolization (L-TAE)

We have found that Lipiodol is retained in most hepatocellular carcinomas and also incompletely in some secondary liver tumors, as reported for its use in diagnostic radiology [7–10]. We perform the embolization routinely in all cases of suspected liver tumors and have therefore, often after hepatectomy, been able to verify the tumorous nature of contrast-retaining lesions and to assess the degree of postembolization necrosis in such lesions.

4.3.1 Liver function tests

The following describes our initial experience after preoperative embolizations, during which time patients stayed in a hospital and were moni-

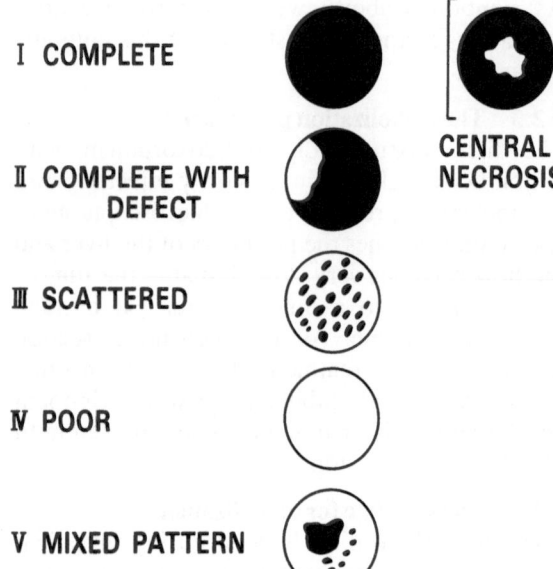

I COMPLETE

II COMPLETE WITH
       DEFECT

CENTRAL
NECROSIS

III SCATTERED

IV POOR

V MIXED PATTERN

Fig. 1. Schematic examples of various Lipiodol staining patterns of HCCs observed on CT scans 3–4 weeks after L-TAE

Table 1. Relationship between tumor size and the pattern of Lipiodol staining in CT scans of HCCs 3–4 weeks after L-TAE

Tumor size (cm)	Staining pattern on Ct scan					Number of tumors
	I	II	III	IV	V	
<2	8	1	0	3	1	13
2~5	16	12	4	4	3	39
5~10	4	4	3	2	2	15
>10	0	1	4	2	1	8
Number of tumors	28	18	11	11	7	75

tored biochemically. In 23 evaluable cirrhotic patients, bilirubin and transaminases (glutamic oxaloacetic [GOT], and glutamic pyruvic transaminase, [GPT]) either did not rise significantly or returned to pre-treatment levels within one month, in most cases within one week. The maximum levels observed before embolization was bilirubin 1.9 mg/dl (upper limit of normal is 1.0), GOT 200 units/l and GPT 80 units/l (upper limits of normal 40 and 35, respectively).

Six patients with chronic active hepatitis were evaluated. All of them returned to pretreatment levels of bilirubin and transaminases within three weeks after embolization. Three of them had one or more parameters elevated before treatment, with a maximum bilirubin value of 4 mg/dl. Patients without histological changes in the resected liver and without signs of portal hypertension all had reversible biochemical changes after embolization.

4.3.2 Tumor necrosis

The extent of necrosis could be evaluated in tumors resected after embolization. The usual interval between embolization and resection was one month, later if bilirubin and/or transaminase elevations after embolization normalized slowly.

The degree of necrosis in the tumors ranged between near-complete and virtually none. We have related it to the size of the tumor and its staining pattern with Lipiodol on post-embolization CT

scans of 75 solitary HCCs. Five types of staining patterns could be distinguished, as shown in Fig. 1. The types were clearly related to the tumor size, as shown in Table 1.

We visually estimated the percentage of tumor areas in the CT slices that were stained by Lipiodol, and compared this figure to the microscopically observed degree of necrosis in the resected tumor. A correlation was observed between the visually estimated and microscopically observed variables, in particular when the staining pattern was massive or patchy. There was also a relationship betwen the other staining patterns so that the summarized results from all patients in Fig. 2 reveal a good correlation. In particular, the two extremes of much or little staining in the CT scans correlated well to a great and small extent of tumor necrosis, respectively.

There was a correlation between the tumor size and extent of necrosis so that tumors larger than 5 cm rarely had massive necrosis after L-TAE and such necrosis was rare after L-TAI of tumors of all sizes (Fig. 3).

Further analysis with regard to capsule formation and the absence or presence of microscopically verified capsular invasion revealed the patterns in Fig. 4, i.e., encapsulated tumors were more often necrotized than non-encapsulated tumors of the same size. Necrosis was always incomplete in tumors larger than 10 cm, as well as in second tumors in the same individuals that were less affected by the treatment than main tumors of comparable sizes. Similarly, very well differentiated or borderline tumors were not hypervascular and were less affected by L-TAE than other tumors of the same size.

The extent of histological necrosis after L-TAI, i.e., with exclusion of the central arterial occlusion by gelatin sponge, was considerably less

Fig. 2. The relationship between visually estimated extent of Lipiodol staining in CT scans of HCCs 3–4 weeks after L-TAE and the extent of histological tumor necrosis in subsequently resected specimens. The overall pattern (main tumors only)

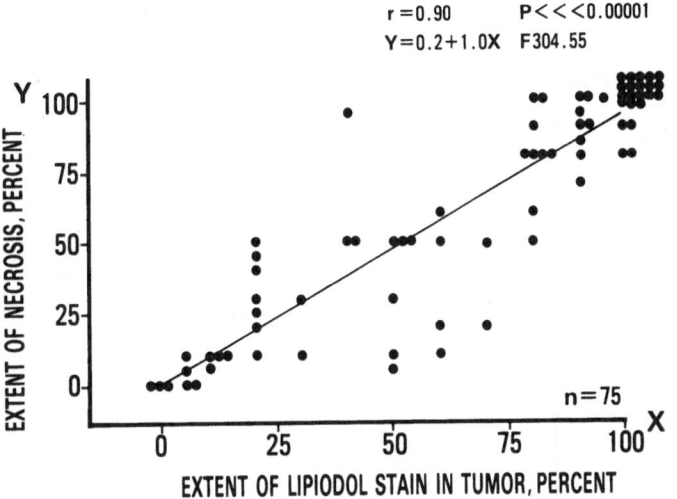

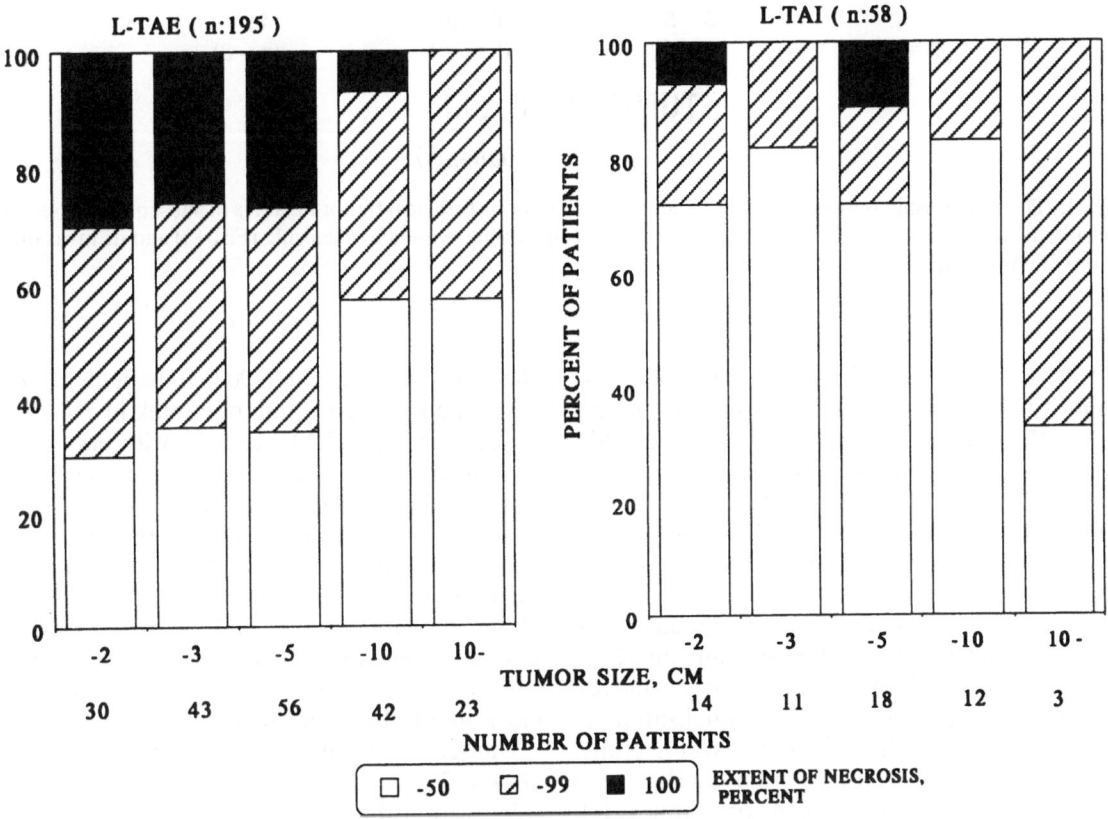

Fig. 3. The relationship between tumor size and the extent of histological tumor necrosis in subsequently resected specimens. Comparison of L-TAE and L-TAI

than after L-TAE and, with few exceptions, less than 60%. In 18 of 26 tumors studied, there was virtually no necrosis even though 15 of them were smaller than 5 cm in diameter (Fig. 4). The interval between embolization and resection seemed to be without importance within the range of 2.5–6 weeks studied, so that regeneration did not seem a very fast phenomenon.

4.3.3 Tumor markers
Serum alpha-fetoprotein levels in HCC usually decreased logarithmically after embolization,

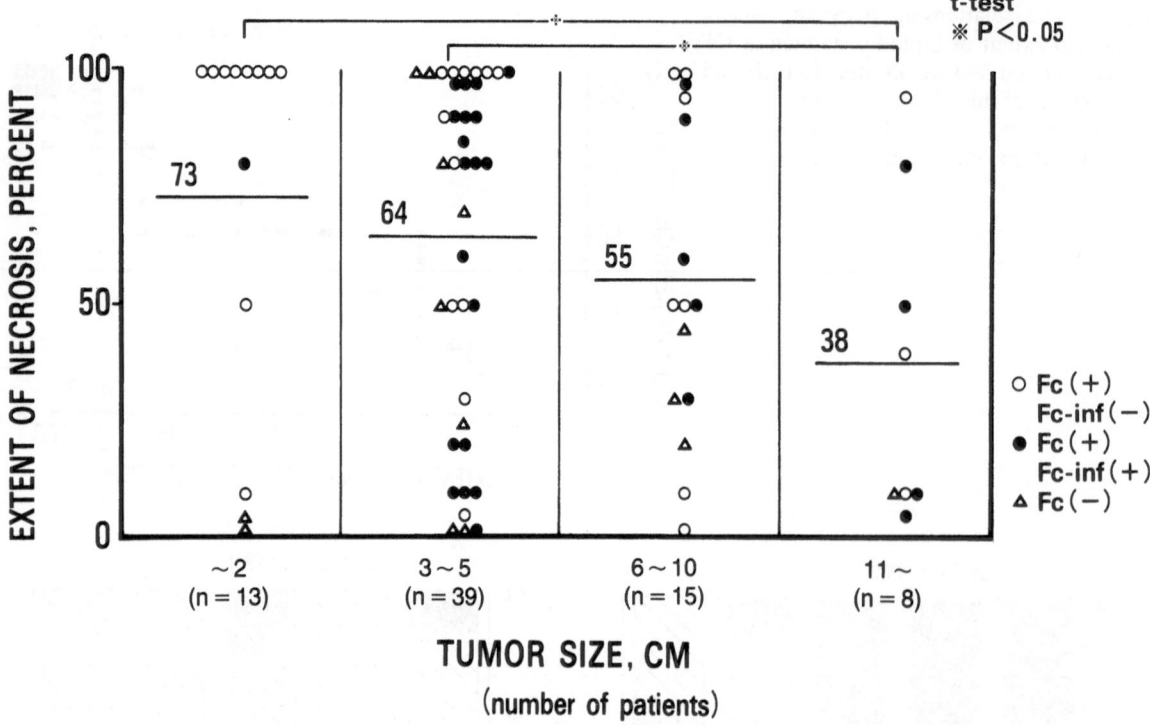

Fig. 4. The relationship between tumor size and the extent of histological tumor necrosis in subsequently resected specimens, with further subdivision of the tumors according to the presence of capsule [Fc (+)] and its invasion by tumor [Fc-inf (+)]

but increased in a small minority of patients. A majority of patients with more than a 50% reduction of the level of the marker had more than 80% necrosis of their tumors. This extent of necrosis was seen in only a minority of patients with either decreased or increased levels of the tumor marker. However, the correlation was not absolute.

One patient with cholangiocellular cancer had a pre-embolization level of 1,100 units/ml of the serum marker CA 19-9, 5,900 after 8 days, and 820 just before surgery 26 days after embolization, at which time about half of the tumor was necrotic.

It therefore seems that serum markers can either decrease, be unchanged, or increase following histologically effective embolizations. The increases can be speculated to result from liberation of the marker from the dying tumor cells, just as vasoactive substances occasionally can give severe symptoms following embolization of liver deposits of carcinoid. They may also result from activation of non-tumorous liver tissue.

4.3.4 Side effects
Regular side effects of minor clinical importance were fever, nausea and pain. Body temperatures

above 37.5°C occurred in 90% of patients after L-TAE and subsided within one week in 55%. The incidence after L-TAI was 85% with only 8% of patients being febrile longer than one week. Usually, the fever did not exceed 39°C.

The pain was mostly located in the upper right abdominal quadrant and subsided within one week. It required analgesic medication in 53% of the patients after L-TAE and in 46% after L-TAI. Sometimes narcotic analgesics were needed, and in a few cases, a thoracal epidural block had to be performed.

Nausea occurred in 37 and 23% of patients after L-TAE and L-TAI, respectively, and subsided within three days. A few patients vomited on the day of treatment, but usually oral intake could be resumed the same day, and there was little or no abdominal distension.

Gall bladder necrosis was not encountered at exploration after L-TAE but seems to constitute a real risk when gelatin powder is used for embolization instead of gelatin sponge cubes. In eleven consecutive routine cholecystectomies for the purpose of hepatectomy, eight specimens showed slight—moderate inflammation. In one of them, however, a gall stone was present. Liver necrosis was sometimes seen in small areas, correlating to areas of Lipidol accumulation on post-embolization CT scans. In such cases, Lipiodol was often seen in portal branches in the same region on plain X-ray films immediately after embolization, suggesting arterio-portal shunting. These small necrotic areas did not give rise to clinical problems.

There was no mortality after embolization alone in our material. A total of 1,362 embolizations have presently been performed with two treatment-related deaths early in our experience, when we gave full L-TAE about one month post-operatively. After this, the immediate postoperative treatment was reduced to L-TAI without gelatin cubes and no fatalities have occurred. When resection was performed after embolization, there were four postoperative deaths among 33 cirrhotic patients and two deaths among nine patients with chronic active hepatitis in our early experience. Better selection of patients for operation has since lowered these figures.

4.4 Theoretical considerations

As discussed previously, a repeatable ischemic treatment is desirable. The agents used in our embolizing mixtures are either soluble or removed by phagocytosis and will, therefore, disappear within the course of time so that collateral formation does not occur and renewed therapy is possible.

Lipiodol and Urografin in the first embolizing mixture are X-ray contrast medias and make it possible to monitor the distribution of the mixture and its effect on the arterial blood flow. Urografin in the second mixture fills the same purpose.

As regards the anti-tumor effect, this can be expected to result from the ischemia caused by vascular occlusion by the Lipiodol droplets and by the gelatin sponge cubes. There may also be a direct effect of the cytostatic drug doxorubicin. It is not known whether doxorubicin affects ischemic tumor cells at low pH so this effect is presently unknown. However, doxorubicin is a potent vascular irritant that frequently gives rise to phlebitis during intravenous administration. It can be expected, that it gives rise to similar changes in some of the tumor vessels where it is retained during embolization and thus adds to the ischemia.

The addition of an antibiotic seems advantageous, because septic complications after liver artery embolization were more frequent in a reported series of embolized patients when no antibiotic was used. The components of the first embolizing mixture are all liquid and can be expected to be washed out from the tumors. Therefore the second embolizing mixture, containing particulate gelatin sponge cubes of $1\,mm^3$ in size, is immediately infused intra-arterially and stops the blood flow in larger, afferent central vessels to prevent this washing out.

The fact that serum alpha-fetoprotein levels decreased only temporarily after embolization, and that very little necrosis was found in a small HCC that was resected three months after embolization, lead us to repeat the treatment when remnant tumor is found or in patients judged to have a high risk for recurrent tumors. The optimal interval between the treatments is not known but practical reasons, including the desired interval of three weeks between embolization and diagnostic CT scans, have made us to repeat the embolizations every three months.

The strategy of non-radical resection of HCC, followed by repeated embolization was developed on the basis of the observations that large tumors were frequently less affected by embolizations than smaller ones, and that second tumors regularly were less necrotized than the main tumors. Probably, the main tumors attracted more of the embolizing agents because of their vascularity. Furthermore, postembolization necrosis of large tumors can give severe toxic reactions, and this also prompts their removal. If thus large tumors are removed, the remaining smaller tumors should be controlled with repeated embolizations without severe side effects. Empirically, we found that a reduction by about 90% of the tumor mass gave the best results. The extent of necrosis could be predicted by the vascularity as seen on X-ray films. This feature was not changed appreciably after repeated embolizations, so that repeated embolizations seemed possible. The favorable outcome of this strategy, except in HCC with spread to large portal venous branches, seems to confirm the reasoning, as well as an observed survival improvement as compared to stage-matched historical controls. As an example of its application, we present the following case report.

Case report. A 56 year old male with chronic active hepatitis developed abdominal pain. Ultrasonography and CT scans revealed a main tumor with a diameter of 16 cm in segments 7–8 with satellites in the entire liver. Liver function

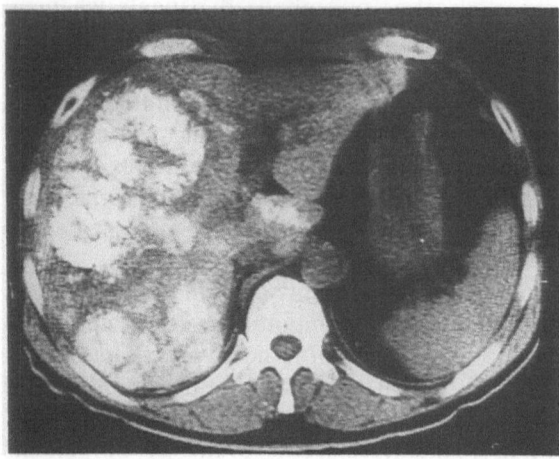

Fig. 5. CT scan of the largest tumor in a patient with multiple HCC 17 days after L-TAE

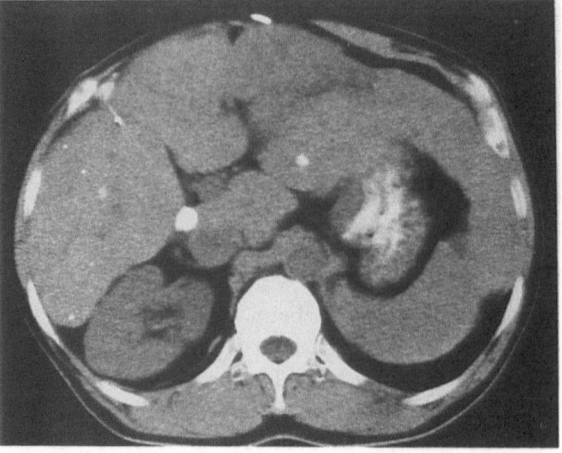

Fig. 7. CT scan of the liver of the patient in Figs. 5–6, 34 months after resection. There is complete staining of scattered small tumors

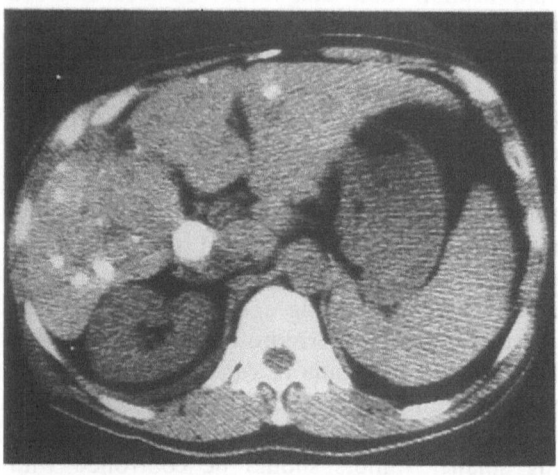

Fig. 6. CT scan of the liver of the patient in Fig. 5 two months after resection, three weeks after the first postoperative L-TAE. There is complete staining of the remaining small tumors

and L-TAE two weeks later, without severe side effects, was followed by CT scanning after three weeks, showing intense staining of the remaining small tumors (Fig. 6). This staining pattern was, in our experience, predictive of a large extent of post-embolization necrosis. Treatment continued and a postembolization CT scan 34 months after resection (Fig. 7) demonstrated multiple small intensely stained foci in the liver. Extrahepatic metastases, including one in the left adrenal gland, developed and the patient died three years after resection.

Acknowledgments. Supported by a grant from the Comprehensive 10-Year Strategy for Cancer Control. Peter Gunvén was a recipient of a fellowship from the Foundation for Promotion of Cancer Research.

tests including ICG[15] were essentially normal. L-TAE was performed followed by CT scans 17 days later (Fig. 5). This embolization was followed by prolonged fever and anorexia with temporary deterioration of the general condition. The main tumor and its adjacent lesions in segments 7, 8 and 4 were resected 6 weeks after L-TAE with the finding of hepatocellular carcinoma, Edmondson grade 2, with invasion of its capsule and intraportal tumor growth (Vp1). Less than half of the tumor was necrotic but the intraportal tumor growth was almost completely viable. A catheter was placed via the gastroduodenal artery into the hepatic artery

References

1. Breedis C, Young G (1954) The blood supply of neoplasms in the liver. Am J Pathol 30:969–985
2. Sugarbaker PH, Kemeny N (1989) Treatment of metastatic cancer to liver. In: DeVita Jr VT, Hellman S, Rosenberg SA (eds) Cancer. Principles and practice of oncology (3rd edn) J B Lippincott, Philadelphia, pp 2275–2298
3. del Giglio A, Zukiwski AA, Ali MK, Mavligit GM (1991) Severe, symptomatic, dose-limiting hypophosphatemia induced by hepatic arterial infusion of recombinant tumor necrosis factor in

patients with liver metastases. Cancer 67: 2459–2461

4. Bengmark S, Rosengren K (1970) Angiographic study of the collateral circulation to the liver after ligation of the hepatic artery in man. Am J Surg 119:620–624

5. Bengmark S, Jeppson B, Lunderquist A, Tranberg KG, Persson B (1988) Tumor calcification following repeated hepatic dearterialization in patients: A preliminary communication. Br J Surg 75: 525–526

6. Shimamura Y, Gunvén P, Takenaka Y, Shimizu H, Shima Y, Akimoto H, Arima K, Takahashi A, Kitaya T, Matsuyama T, Hasegawa H (1988) Combined peripheral and central chemoembolization of liver tumors. Experience with Lipiodol-doxorubicin and gelatin sponge (L-TEA). Cancer 61:238– 242

7. Caron J, Laval-Jeantet M, Lamarque JL, Huguet JF, Caron-Poitreau C (1973) Exploration artériographique des cancers secondaires du foie: Intérêt des iodo-lipides par injection artérielle. Sem Hôp Paris 50:3367–3376

8. Nakakuma K, Tashiro S, Hiraoka T, Ogata K, Ootsuka K (1985) Hepatocellular carcinoma and metastatic cancer detected by iodized oil. Radiology 154:15–17

9. Ohishi H, Uchida H, Yoshimura H, Ohue S, Ueda J, Katsuragi M, Matsuo N, Hosogi Y (1985) Hepatocellular carcinoma detected by iodized oil: Use of anticancer agents. Radiology 154:25–29

10. Yumoto Y, Jinno K, Tokuyama K, Araki Y, Ishimatsu T, Maeda H, Konno T, Iwamoto S, Ohnishi K, Okuda K (1985) Hepatocellular carcinoma detected by iodized oil, Radiology 154: 19–24

CHAPTER 27

Preoperative portal vein embolization for hepatocellular carcinoma

Hiroaki Kinoshita, Kazuhiro Hirohashi, and Shoji Kubo[1]

1 Introduction

Advances in diagnostic imaging and new surgical techniques have improved the outcome for many patients with hepatocellular carcinoma (HCC). However, in Japan, more than 70% of patients with HCC have cirrhosis of the liver [1], and resection of the liver of such patients is often limited by the cirrhosis. Therefore, nonsurgical treatments such as transcatheter arterial embolization (TAE) or percutaneous ethanol injection therapy have been developed and are used widely as adjuvant therapy. TAE was first used to treat HCC patients by Goldstein et al. [2], who reasoned that most of the blood flow to the tumor is supplied by the hepatic artery. However, according to a study by the Liver Cancer Study Group of Japan [3], TAE is effective against the main tumor, but not against small intrahepatic metastases or tumor thrombi; it is particularly ineffective against tumor thrombi.

Honjo et al. [4] tried portal branch ligation as a treatment for liver cancer in 20 patients in whom hepatic resection was not indicated. For the three patients with cirrhosis of the liver as well, the mean survival after this procedure was 4.5 months. They speculated portal branch ligation affected the tumor both directly by decreasing blood flow to the peripheral area of the tumor and indirectly by reducing arterial blood flow to that lobe of the liver, which would affect the central part of the tumor. However, histological effects on the main tumor and tumor thrombi were not evaluated.

We devised a method to embolize the portal vein by percutaneous transhepatic portal cath-

eterization [5], and have tested whether portal vein embolization (PVE) before surgery had an anticancer effect. During that study, we noticed that the volume of the untreated region of the liver seen on computed tomograms (CT) increased after PVE. In 1920, Rous and Larimore [6] tried ligation of a portal branch in rabbits. The affected lobe shrank, and hypertrophy of the nonligated lobe occurred. Ozawa et al. [7] investigated the effect on liver metabolism of ligation of a portal branch. We completely ligated about 70% of the portal branches in the liver of rats, and found that polyamine metabolism and DNA synthesis of the nonligated lobes are accelerated [8]. PVE seems to cause regeneration and hypertrophy of the liver, which may be beneficial as a kind of preparation for resection of the liver even for patients with cirrhosis of the liver.

2 Technique of PVE and clinical course after PVE

2.1 Technique of PVE

First, under sonographic guidance, a 6.5 F catheter introducer is used in selective puncture with a steel needle by the Seldinger method of a portal branch in the noncancerous area, and the introducer is brought to the first branch, either left or right. Then, through the introducer, a catheter is inserted into the portal trunk, and portography is done with vertical and horizontal beams, which serve both to clarify the ramifications of the intrahepatic portal veins [9] and to detect portal invasion, such as portal thrombi. The branch to be embolized is identified. Then, a 6.5 F double-lumen balloon catheter is introduced up to the branch of the portal vein supplying the area to be resected. The balloon is inflated and embolic

[1] Second Department of Surgery, Osaka City University Medical School, 1-5-7 Asahi-machi, Abeno-ku, Osaka 545, Japan

284 H. Kinoshita et al.

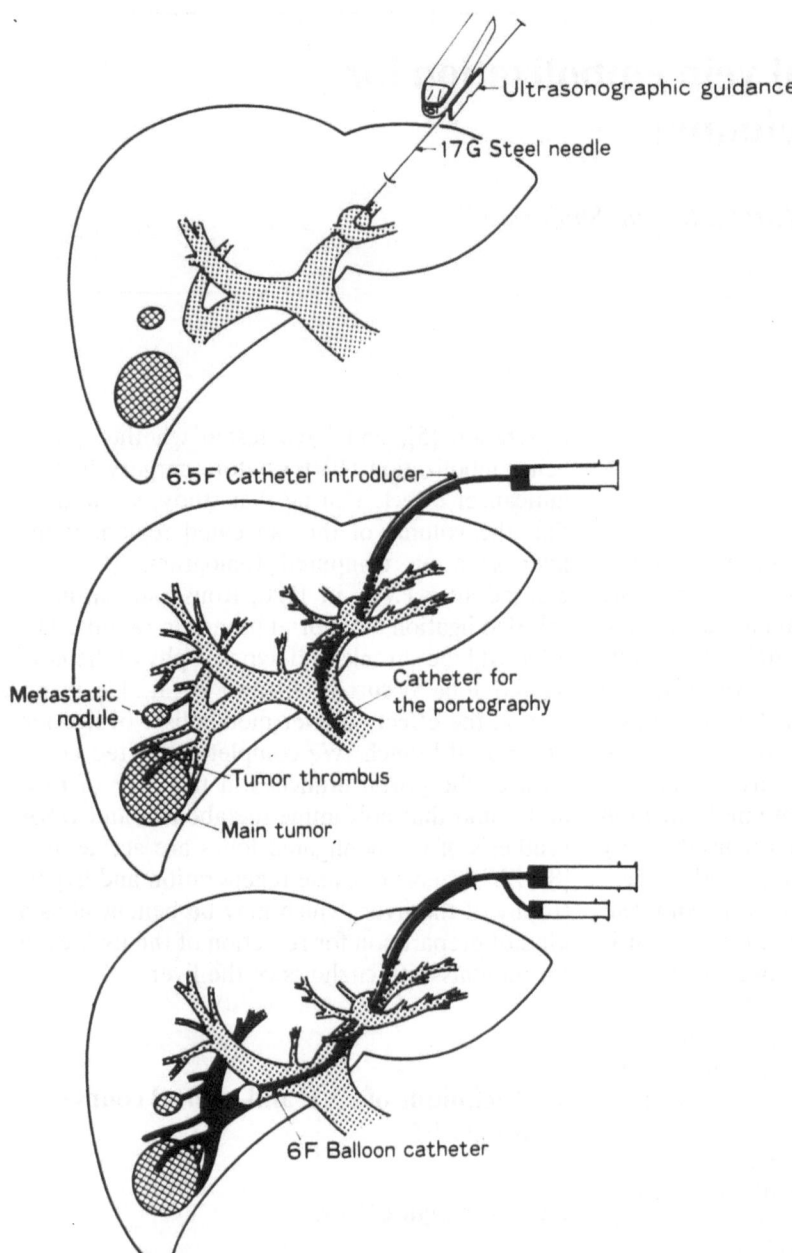

- Ultrasonographic guidance
- 17G Steel needle

6.5F Catheter introducer

Metastatic nodule

Catheter for the portography

Tumor thrombus

Main tumor

6F Balloon catheter

Fig. 1. Procedure for portal vein embolization (PVE). *Top*, the portal vein is punctured under sonographic guidance. *Middle*, percutaneous transhepatic portography (PTP). *Bottom*, a 6.5 F balloon catheter is introduced into the portal branch to be embolized, and the embolic material is injected. (From [10] with permission)

materials such as an adhesive mixture of fibrin (6.4% fibrinogen mixed with an equal volume of 5 units of thrombin per ml of water) with iodized oil (Lipiodol) added to give radiopacity, are injected under fluoroscopic control (Fig. 1) [10]. Abdominal X-ray films are taken after PVE so that the completeness of the embolization can be checked. In our study [10], the portal branch embolized by this procedure was the left first branch (L-1) in 7 patients, the right first branch (R-1) in 37, the right second branch (R-2) in 13, and a more peripheral branch (R-3) in 7 (Fig. 2) [10]. After embolization, the balloon catheter was pulled out and the part of the portal vein punctured was identified. Then, the puncture wound of the liver was blocked with Gelfoam particles through the lumen of the introducer to prevent intraperitoneal bleeding. Usually, TAE was done by the method developed by Yamada et al. [11], PVE was done about 2 weeks later, and hepatic resection was done about 2 weeks after the PVE.

Fig. 2. Pictures taken during PVE. Radiopaque areas show an embolus in the portal vein. The portal branch embolized by this procedure is the left first branch (*L-1*), the right first branch (*R-1*), the right second branch (*R-2*), and a more peripheral branch (*R-3*). (From [10] with permission)

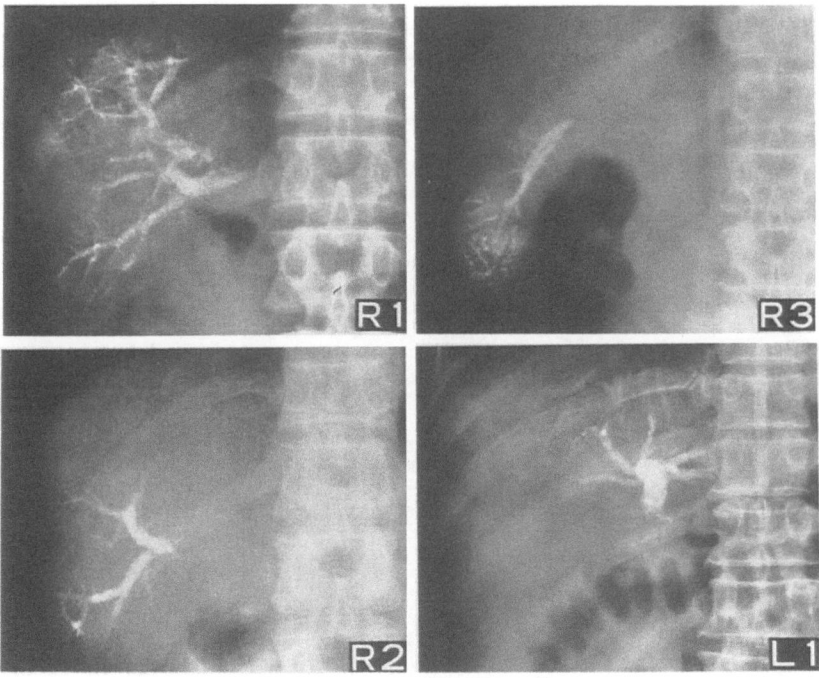

2.2 Clinical course after PVE

Immediately after PVE, portal pressure increased by 20–140 mm H_2O. Most patients had abdominal pain and fever after PVE. These side effects were mild and transitory.

There was often a transitory rise in the leucocyte count compared with the baseline values before PVE. Aspartate aminotransferase (AST) and alanine aminotransferase (ALT) increased in almost all patients, but the increases were transitory. All three values returned to the baseline within 2 weeks after PVE, because canalization of the hepatic artery to the noncancerous area generally occurred within this time. The extent of these measured changes was directly proportional to the embolized area. These changes were similar to those caused by TAE, but their extent was less, so PVE seemed to be safer. CT from before and after PVE were compared. Usually, in patients who underwent embolization of the R-1, the volume of the area not directly affected by this procedure (the left lobe) increased greatly (Fig. 3). The volumes of the lobes of the liver were calculated by computer [12], and changes in different groups of patients classified by the area of the embolization were compared (Fig. 4). After PVE, the embolized lobe tended to become smaller, and the lobe not embolized tended to become larger. The increase in the volume of the nonembolized lobe was largest in the R-1 group.

At laparotomy, the segment affected by PVE was dark red, which made a line demarcation between the embolized and the nonembolized part of the liver. Portal branches were filled with the embolic material. A histological study of the cancerous region affected by PVE is described below. In the noncancerous areas affected by PVE, hepatic cells were atrophied and sinusoids were dilated. The sinusoids were filled with erythrocytes and had been infiltrated by phagocytes. In 4 patients in whom recanalization of the artery had not occurred, there were scattered foci of infarction, in which the hepatic cells were necrotic. In 2 of these 4 patients, there was an abscess in the peripheral part of the segment affected by TAE and PVE. Not only hepatic cells but also mucosa of the bile ducts were necrotic in these 2 patients. The abscess was resected when the liver was resected as scheduled.

3 Anticancer effect of PVE seen by histology and survival rates

3.1 Histological study

A histological study of the cancerous region of the segment occluded by TAE plus PVE was done.

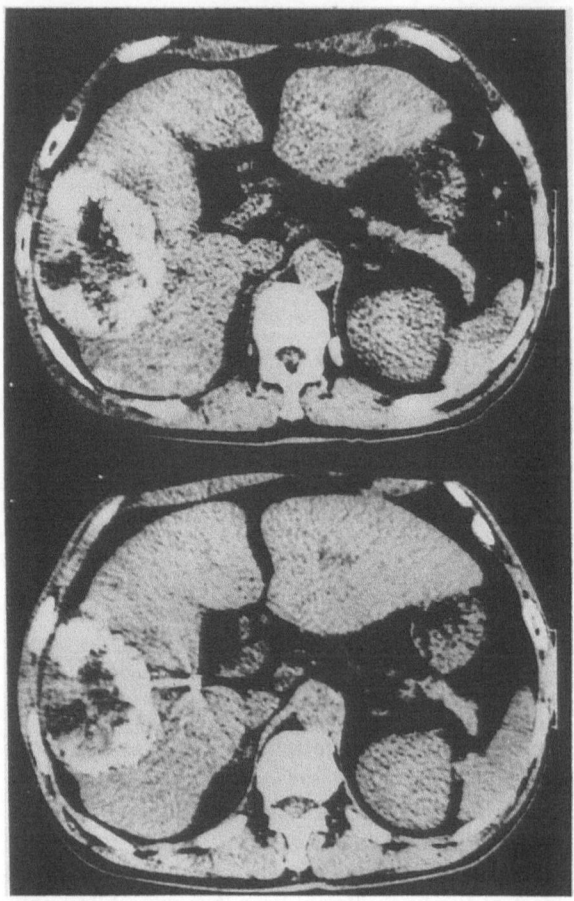

Table 1. Pathohistological changes in cancerous areas after TAE only or after TAE plus PVE

	Procedure	
Pathohistological changes	TAE only	TAE plus PVE
Complete necrosis of		
main tumor	18/60 (30%)	20/33 (61%)
intrahepatic metastases	3/20 (15%)	6/20 (30%)
capsular invasion	2/32 (6%)	3/24 (13%)
portal thrombus	0/13 (0%)	0/9 (0%)
Anticancer effect on		
capsular invasion	13/32 (41%)	12/24 (50%)
portal thrombus	3/13 (23%)	6/9 (67%)

(From [10] with permission)

We also examined these regions after TAE alone in 60 other patients not part of the PVE study. In our 33 subjects who underwent TAE plus PVE before surgery, 20 of the 33 main tumors and 6 of the 20 intrahepatic metastases were completely necrotic. In 12 of the 24 cases of capsular invasion and 6 of 9 portal thrombi found, anticancer effects were seen histologically. The histological findings were better than those for the patients treated by TAE alone (Table 1) [10].

3.2 Comparison of survival rates

The longest follow-up period for a patient who underwent resection after TAE plus PVE has now reached 6.5 years. Survival rates for patients who underwent resection after TAE and PVE tended to be better than those for patients who

Fig. 3. Computed tomograms before and after portal vein embolization (PVE). *Top*, before PVE. *Bottom*, two weeks after PVE. The left lobe is larger than before

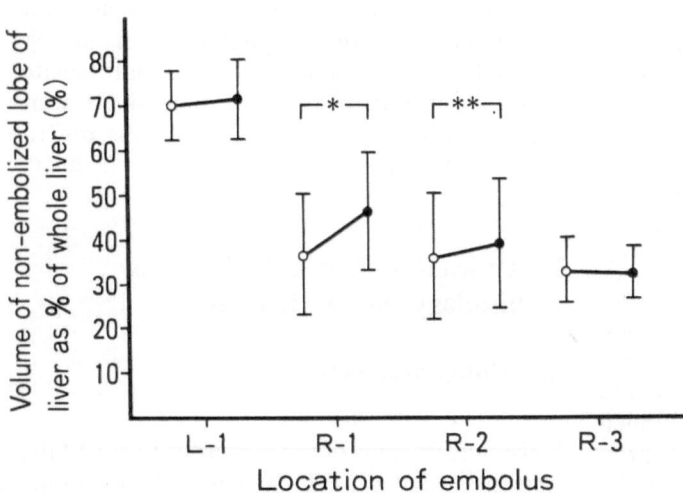

Fig. 4. Comparison of the mean volume of the nonembolized lobe after PVE with the embolus in different positions of portal branches. *Bars*, mean ±SD; *open circles*, before PVE; *Solid circles*, after PVE; *, $P < 0.01$ and **, $P < 0.05$, compared with the values before PVE. *L-1*, left first branch; *R-1*, right first branch; *R-2*, right second branch; *R-3*, more peripheral branch

Fig. 5. Comparison of survival rates for patients with liver cancer given different treatment. *Solid circles*, TAE plus PVE plus resection; *open circles*, TAE plus resection; *crosses*, resection only

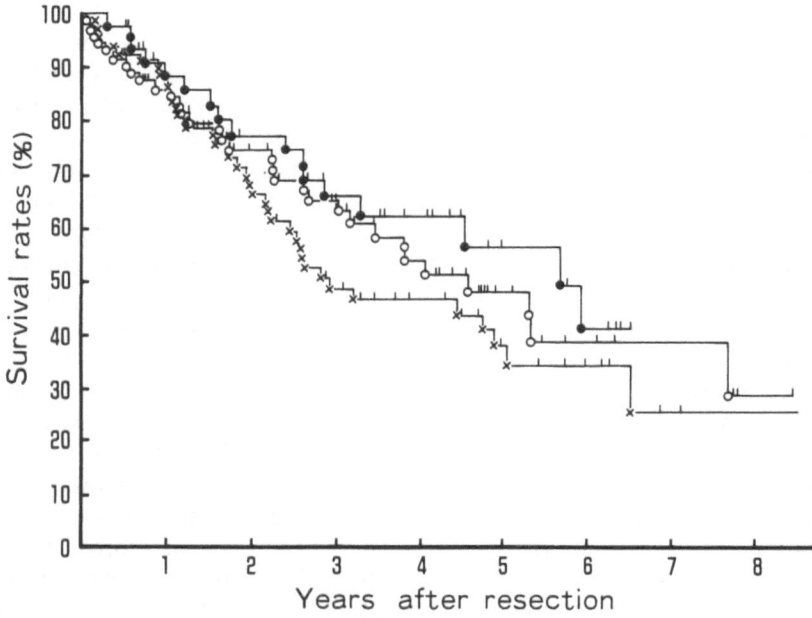

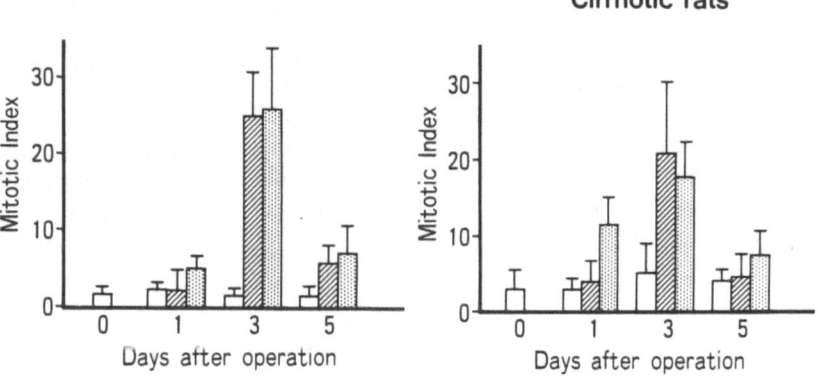

Fig. 6. Mitotic index of the nonembolized part of the liver after PVE in healthy rats and cirrhotic rats. The mitotic index is the number of hepatocytes in mitosis per 1,000 hepatocytes. *Bars*, mean +SE; *no shading*, sham operation; *hatched area*, portal branch embolization; *dotted area*, partial hepatectomy

underwent TAE and resection and those for patients who underwent resection only. The stage of the tumor in the patients treated by resection after TAE and PVE tended to be higher than those in the patients in the other groups (Fig. 5).

4 Extended surgical indications and increased safety of more radical hepatectomy

We investigated in rats whether the increased volume of the nonembolized lobe arose because of regeneration of the liver. In this experiment,

male Wistar rats were used, some healthy and some with cirrhosis caused by CCl_4. The portal branch that supplied 70% of the liver was embolized with isobutyl-2-cyanoacrylate. The weight of the part of the liver that was not embolized increased after PVE, but that of the embolized part decreased. Mitosis of hepatocytes of the nonembolized part of the liver significantly increased after PVE in both the healthy and the cirrhotic rats (Fig. 6). Differences from rats that underwent partial hepatectomy instead were not significant. These results showed that PVE induced cell proliferation in rats, and suggested that the increase in volume of the nonembolized lobe after PVE in humans is caused by regeneration of the liver. Even in rats with cirrhosis, PVE caused cell proliferation, and therefore liver regeneration, although the effects were not as strong as in the healthy rats.

Yamanaka and Okamoto [13] estimated the safe limits of hepatic resection before surgery using a prognosis score. This is calculated from the parenchymal hepatic resection rate, measured on CT, tests of 15-minute indocyanine green retention ($ICGR_{15}$) as an index of the functional impairment of the liver, and age. If the prognosis score is 50 points or more, it is likely that liver resection will cause liver failure after surgery. We calculated the prognosis score before PVE and 2 weeks after. Because the embolized lobe tended to decrease in volume after PVE, the non-embolized lobe tended to increase, the resection rate decreased. Subsequently the prognosis score decreased after PVE. The decrease was significant in the R-1 and the R-2 groups.

We also investigated whether this procedure improved the postoperative course after liver resection. In rats, when endotoxin (2.5 mg/kg) was injected after 70% partial hepatectomy, only 28% (5/18) of the rats survived. When PVE was done 1 week before partial hepatectomy, 65% (11/17) of the rats survived after the injection of the endotoxin. Serum levels of AST, ALT and total bilirubin (T-bil) 6h after the injection of 0.5 mg/kg endotoxin in the partially hepatectomized rats after PVE were all significantly lower than in the partially hepatectomized rats without PVE.

Serum levels of AST, ALT, T-bil, and prothrombin time (PT) were also estimated in patients who underwent right lobectomy with or without PVE. There were no significant differences in ALT or T-bil between these two groups, but the changes in AST and PT in the patients with PVE were significantly smaller than in the patients without. Two of 15 patients (13%) who underwent right lobectomy without PVE died after surgery because of liver failure. One of 21 patients (5%) who underwent right lobectomy after PVE died after surgery. Liver function in the patients who underwent right lobectomy with PVE (14 of these 21 patients had cirrhosis of the liver) was worse than in the patients who underwent liver resection without PVE (4 of 15 patients had cirrhosis).

Therefore, PVE extended the surgical indications for patients with HCC and made surgery safer even if the patients had cirrhosis of the liver.

5 Indications for and limitations of PVE

5.1 Indications for PVE

Portal catheterization was occasionally impossible because the intrahepatic portal vein could not be seen clearly by sonography. Portal catheterization is not indicated for patients with ascites

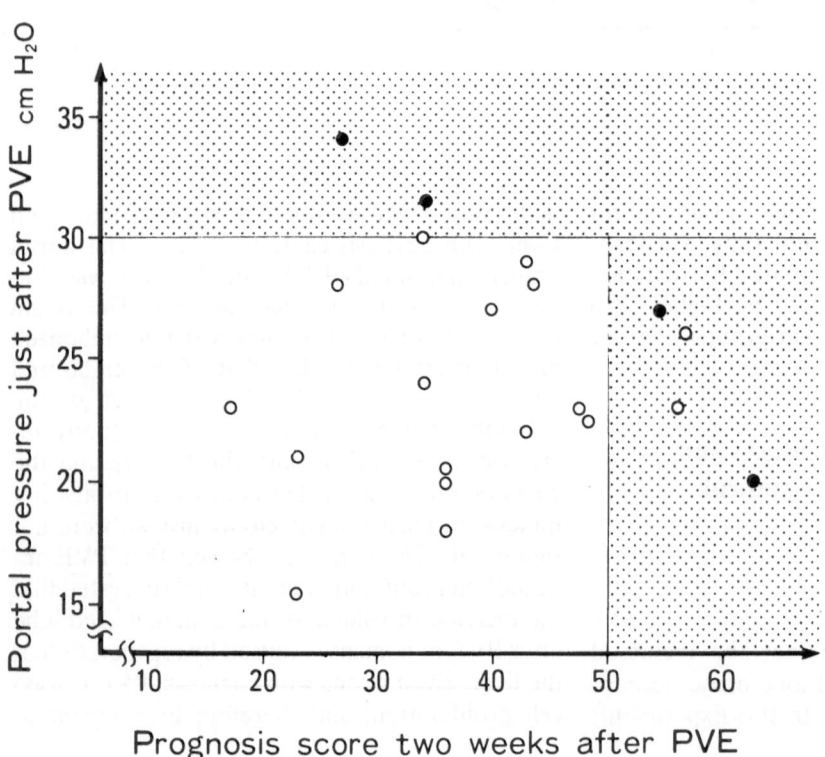

Fig. 7. Postoperative course, prognosis score, and portal pressure after PVE. *Solid circles*, Patients who developed liver failure; *open circles*, patients who did not develop liver failure

or patients who cannot control their breathing during the puncture.

For patients with HCC in both lobes, PVE cannot be carried out.

Other investigators [14] have done TAE and PVE simultaneously to cause infarction of the liver, including the cancer. If this is done, the segment embolized should be limited, because the infarction of the liver may lead to liver abscess and impair liver function.

To extend indications for surgery, PVE at the R-1 is necessary because only PVE there significantly lowers the prognosis score. Patients who need right lobectomy and with a prognosis score of 40 points or more are indicated.

5.2 Limitations of PVE

TAE plus PVE gave fairly satisfactory anticancer effects, but viable areas remained in metastatic or invasive lesions such as portal thrombi. Therefore, if possible, surgery is needed to treat the liver cancer.

To establish the limitations of PVE in extending the indications for surgery, the postoperative course of 21 patients who underwent right lobectomy with preoperative PVE was studied retrospectively. The signs of liver failure were ascites refractory to treatment, gastrointestinal bleeding, hepatic coma, or jaundice (T-bil >5.0 mg/dl). Four of the 21 patients had one or some of these signs of liver failure; 3 of these 4 patients recovered from the liver failure and the other patient died because of liver failure 27 days after surgery. Portal pressure just after PVE in 2 of the 4 patients who later developed liver failure was more than 30 cm H_2O. The prognosis score 2 weeks after PVE in 2 of the 4 patients who later developed liver failure was more than 50 points (Fig. 7). Thus, if portal pressure just after PVE is more than 30 cm H_2O or the prognosis score 2 weeks after PVE is more than 50 points, the amount of liver that is to be resected should probably be limited or another treatment should be selected.

6 PVE as a method for evaluation of remaining liver function

In 16 patients who underwent right lobectomy with PVE, the change in the volume of the liver before any treatment and 4 weeks after liver resection was calculated. This showed the rate of increase in the remaining liver (left lobe). The relationship between the rate of the increase in the remaining liver and the liver resection rate calculated from the volumes before and two weeks after PVE was studied, as was the relationship between the rate of increase in the values of $ICGR_{15}$ before and two weeks after PVE. The rate of the increase in the remaining liver was correlated with the resection rate calculated from the volumes before PVE ($r = 0.84$, $P < 0.001$) and from that after PVE ($r = 0.82$, $P < 0.001$). The rate of the increase in the remaining liver was also correlated with the value of $ICGR_{15}$ before PVE ($r = -0.52$, $P < 0.05$) and that after PVE ($r = -0.73$, $P < 0.001$). Therefore, the rate of the increase in the remaining liver was more strongly correlated with the test results after PVE than those before PVE. These results suggest that the condition after liver resection more closely resembles that after PVE than that before PVE. Evaluation of the clinical course after PVE by portal pressure, resection rate, $ICGR_{15}$, and prognosis score was useful when decisions about the treatment, including surgical treatment, were being made. PVE might give useful information for estimation of the remaining liver function.

7 Conclusions

Patients with HCC often have other liver disorders, such as chronic hepatitis and cirrhosis. Liver resection is the most effective therapy for HCC, but the other disorders prevent its use in some patients. We started to use PVE as adjuvant therapy to improve the outcome of surgical treatment. Our results suggest that PVE strengthened the anticancer effect of TAE. PVE causes regeneration of the nonembolized lobe and atrophy of the embolized lobe, which extends the surgical indication for patients with liver cancer and makes surgery possible even if the patient has cirrhosis of the liver. Evaluation of the clinical course after PVE is useful when decisions about the operative method to be used are being made. PVE is useful as one preparation for liver resection for liver cancer and might be effective as a kind of therapy in the multiplicative therapy for this disease.

Acknowledgment. This study was supported in part by a Grant-in-Aid for Cancer Research from the Ministry of Health and Welfare, Japan.

References

1. Liver Cancer Study Group of Japan (1990) Primary liver cancer in Japan. Clinicopathological features and results of surgical treatment. Ann Surg 211: 227–87
2. Goldstein HM, Wallace S, Anderson JH, Bree RL, Gianturco C (1976) Transcatheter occlusion of abdominal tumors. Radiology 120:539–545
3. Hasegawa H (1983) Recent progress and results of a group study of hepatectomy following the transcatheter arterial embolization using gelatin sponge particles of CO_2 microbubbles (in Japanese). Naika 52:555–559
4. Honjo I, Suzuki T, Ozawa K, Takasan H, Kitamura O, Ishikawa T (1975) Ligation of a branch of the portal vein for carcinoma of the liver. Am J Surg 130:296–302
5. Kinoshita H, Sakai K, Hirohashi K, Igawa S, Yamasaki O, Kubo S (1986) Preoperative portal vein embolization for hepatocellular carcinoma. World J Surg 10:803–808
6. Rous P, Larimore LD (1920) Relation of the portal blood to liver maintenance: A demonstration of liver atrophy conditional on compensation. J Exp Med 31:609–632
7. Ozawa K, Takasan H, Kitamura O, Mizukami T, Kamano T, Takeda H, Ohsawa T, Murata T, Honjo I (1971) Effect of ligation of portal vein on liver mitochondrial metabolism. J Biochem 70: 755–764
8. Kubo S, Matsui-Yuasa I, Otani S, Morisawa S, Kinoshita H, Sakai K (1986) Effect of portal branch ligation on polyamine metabolism in rat liver. Life Sci 38:1835–1840
9. Inoue T, Kinoshita H, Hirohashi K, Sakai K, Uozumi A (1986) Ramification of the intrahepatic portal vein identified by percutaneous transhepatic portography. World J Surg 10:287–293
10. Kinoshita H, Sakai K, Iwasa R, Hirohashi K, Kubo S, Fujio N, Lee KC (1988) Results of preoperative portal vein embolization for hepatocellular carcinoma. Osaka City Med J 34:115–112
11. Yamada R, Sato M, Kawabata M, Nakatsuka H, Nakamura K, Takashima S (1983) Hepatic artery embolization in 120 patients with unresectable hepatoma. Radiology 148:397–401
12. Okamoto E, Kyo A, Yamanaka N, Tanaka N, Kuwata K (1984) Prediction of the safe limits of hepatectomy by combined volumetric and functional measurements in patients with impaired hepatic function. Surgery 95:586–592
13. Yamanaka N, Okamoto E (1983) Multiple regression equation evaluating the resectability for liver tumors (in Japanese). Nippon Geka Gakkai Zasshi 84:126–134
14. Nakao N, Miura K, Takahashi H, Ohnishi M, Miura T, Okamoto E, Ishikawa Y (1986) Hepatocellular carcinoma: Combined hepatic, arterial, and portal venous embolization. Radiology 161: 303–307

CHAPTER 28

Percutaneous ethanol injection for patients with small hepatocellular carcinoma

Masaaki Ebara, Kazuhiko Kita, Masaharu Yoshikawa, Nobuyuki Sugiura, and Masao Ohto[1]

1 Introduction

Hepatocellular carcinoma (HCC) arises in patients with chronic liver diseases, particularly in those with liver cirrhosis, at a rate of more than 80% in Japan [1, 2]. Because of periodic examinations with ultrasonography (US) [3, 4] and serum alpha-fetoprotein (AFP) measurement [5, 6] in high-risk patients with liver cirrhosis or chronic hepatitis, a large number of small HCC, often smaller than 2 cm, have been diagnosed during follow-up of such patients.

Surgical resection is considered to be the most curable treatment for such small HCC. However, poor liver function sometimes precludes surgery [7]. Furthermore, it has also been observed that recurrence of HCC in the remnant liver occurs with a high incidence within a short time after the resection [8]. Therefore, to improve the survival of patients with small HCC, it is imperative to develop a new treatment which is non-invasive and yet as effective as surgical resection. Transcatheter arterial embolization (TAE) is widely performed in Japan as an alternative to resection but it does not necrotize cancer cells infiltrating intra- or extracapsule and hypovascular HCC, and it often causes considerable damage to hepatic parenchyma [9].

Ethanol immediately dehydrates or coagulates tissue in a dose-dependent manner upon contact, and it also causes vascular occlusion. Thus, coagulative necrosis of cancerous nodules and the adjacent hepatic parenchyma can be expected, and the therapeutic effect may be equal to surgical resection if the procedure is performed correctly. The US-guided puncture technique [10] permits experienced sonographers to insert a needle into a target as small as 10 mm with ease. In 1982, we began percutaneous ethanol injection (PEI) for small HCC [11], and so far a dramatic therapeutic effect has been reported not only by us [12, 13] but also by several other investigators [14–16]. It was revealed that tumor size was reduced remarkably following PEI, and HCC that had been treated by PEI appeared almost completely necrotized upon resection. From our long-term observation in a large series of patients with small HCC, the therapeutic effects of PEI on prognosis, the most significant evaluation of the treatment, has also been better than that of untreated patients with small HCC [17] and has been quite comparable to surgery.

2 Indication

PEI is indicated for patients with HCC as follows: Lesions no larger than 3 cm and less than 3 in number; lesions detectable by US; no gross ascites; no bleeding tendency; serum albumin more than 2.8 g/dl; bilirubin less than 3.0 mg/dl; and no other severe disease. Our preliminary study in animals indicates that the distance and breadth through which the injected absolute ethanol spreads is indeed limited [11]. Infiltration of cancer cells around an HCC nodule is much more frequent if its size is greater [18]. For this reason, PEI is not indicated for HCC of more than 3 cm in diameter; the candidate HCC is preferably 2 cm or less in size and the number of lesions should be few, possibly 3 or less.

In case the tumor is situated protrusively at the surface of the liver, possible bleeding from it should be considered. Nevertheless, we performed PEI on 3 patients with such a lesion and as yet no bleeding or seeding of cancer cells has been

[1] First Department of Medicine, School of Medicine, Chiba University, Chiba, 280 Japan

Table 1. Comparison of Patients with Small HCCs between PEI Group and Untreated Group

		PEI	Untreated
No. of patients		112 (89 males, 23 females)	27 (23 males, 4 females)
		134 lesions	29 lesions
Age			
	average	58.1 ± 7.2 yrs.	57.0 ± 7.4 yrs.
	range	41 to 76 yrs.	45 to 71 yrs.
No. of tumors			
	one	93 patients (83.0%)	25 patients (92.5%)
	two	16 (14.3%)	2 (7.4%)
	three	3 (2.7%)	0
Diameter of main tumors			
	≤1 cm	6 tumors (5.4%)	1 tumor (3.7%)
	>1, ≤2 cm	70 (62.5%)	16 (59.3%)
	>2, ≤3 cm	36 (32.1%)	10 (37.0%)
Child's classification			
	"A"	60 patients (53.6%)	11 patients (40.7%)
	"B"	33 (29.5%)	6 (22.2%)
	"C"	19 (17.0%)	10 (37.1%)

experienced. Thus PEI seems to be applicable to any lesion seen by US.

3 Patients

During the 7-year and 5-month period between August 1, 1983 and December 30, 1990, PEI was carried out on 134 lesions in 112 patients with small HCC (Table 1). Patients consisted of 89 males and 23 females aged from 41–76 years, averaging 58.1 ± 7.2 (s.d.). Among these patients, 60 (53.6%) were heavy drinkers (>76 ml of ethanol/day for more than 10 years), 13 (11.6%) were positive for HBsAg antigen, and 24 (21.4%) had received blood transfusions in the past. The final diagnosis of HCC was established with a histological biopsy using a 21 gauge needle under sonographic control [10, 18] in 78.6% (n = 88), and diagnostic imagings including contrast-enhanced computed tomography (CT), angiography and magnetic resonance imaging (MRI). Diagnosis of HCC by the imaging procedures was made when at least two of the following three findings were demonstrated: early enhancement and quick de-enhancement in dynamic CT [19], "ring sign" by MRI [20], and arterial neovasculature by hepatic arteriography.

Out of the 134 tumors in these patients, there was 1 lesion in 93 patients (83.0%), 2 lesions in 16 patients (14.3%) and 3 lesions in 3 patients (2.7%). The size of the main tumor was 1 cm or less in 6 patients (5.4%), 1 to 2 cm in 70 patients (62.5%) and 2 to 3 cm in 36 patients (32.1%). Of these 134 tumors, 109 (81.3%) were located in the right lobe of the liver and the others 25 (18.7%) in the left lobe. All these patients has liver cirrhosis, with the severity of liver dysfunction being classified as Child's A in 53.6% (n = 60), Child's B in 29.5% (n = 33) and Child's C in 17.0% (n = 19) [21]. Serum AFP levels measured by radioimmunoassay ranged from 0 to 2,663 ng/ml at the time of the treatment.

For evaluation of the therapeutic effect of PEI, 27 patients with HCC less than 3 cm in size who did not receive any specific treatment for cancer served as controls. There were no significant differences in age, size of tumor, or liver dysfunction between the two groups (Table 1). Tumor size was measured by US and the largest tumor was adopted for analysis if there was more than one lesion.

4 Procedures

Instruments for PEI consist of a 22 gauge Chiba needle (length 15 cm), a short extension tube and a 5 ml syringe. If a lesion is situated immediately below the diaphragm and is visualized only by a sector scanner, PEI is performed using a sector probe with a specially designed attachment.

The procedures for PEI are as follows: Under local anesthesia a 22-gauge Chiba needle is introduced percutaneously into a tumor or its marginal area through a puncture probe under sonographic control [10]. Absolute (99.5%) ethanol is slowly injected from a 5 ml syringe through the needle while it is being withdrawn little by little in order to produce as much necrosis as possible inside as well as around the mass. The amount of ethanol injected each time is 2–6 ml. The injection is repeated twice a week for up to 4–6 sessions, depending on the tumor size. When ethanol is injected into the target area, high echoic drops are sometimes seen running through a neighboring vessel without spreading over the lesion. On such occasions, the needle is withdrawn and re-inserted. In the first treatment session, the needle is positioned in the center of the lesion; the adjacent areas considered not to have changed by US examination are chosen as the injection site in subsequent sessions. While removing the needle immediately after ethanol injection, 1–2 ml of 1% lidocaine is injected to dilute the ethanol, which would flow back through the needle track into the peritoneal cavity and cause pain.

This procedure is repeated until the original US pattern is completely replaced by one which persists for some time in the tumor as well as in the surrounding area. Although the tumor may become blurred following PEI, it is usually ascertainable and accurate aiming is possible for subsequent injections.

5 Injection of ethanol

In all, 446 sessions of ethanol injection were given, with the total amount of ethanol injected varying from 5–46 ml depending on tumor size: An average 6.0 ± 2.8 ml in 12 HCCs (≤ 1 cm), 11.7 ± 4.7 ml in 60 (>1, ≤ 2 cm) and 18.8 ± 9.2 ml in 29 (>2, ≤ 3 cm). However, additional PEI was necessary for one lesion in each of 5 patients within 6 months after the first PEI because follow-up dynamic CT demonstrated an enhanced area in these lesions at the early phase.

6 Pathological effect and reduction of tumor size

To evaluate the therapeutic effect of PEI on HCC, five surgically resected HCCs on which PEI had been performed earlier were examined histopathologically [12]. Three of the 5 HCCs were completely necrotized, and a direct rela-

tion was observed between the total amount of ethanol injected and the degree of necrosis. According to other reports, solitary lesions smaller than 5 cm in size appeared completely necrotic in 10 of 14 lesions on subsequent surgical resection [14–16]. These results suggest that HCC smaller than 3 cm can be completely necrotized if a suitable amount of ethanol is injected properly.

No tumor against which PEI was performed has shown regrowth or enlargement so far. Reduction of tumor size after PEI was studied in 67 main HCC followed regularly by US for more than 6 months. The percentage reduction was calculated from the equation: $(a \times b - a' \times b')/(a \times b) \times 100$ (%), where a is the longest axis and b the shortest perpendicular axis before PEI, and a' and b' the same after PEI. All 67 HCC decreased in size, and 28 of them (41.8%) became undetectable by US and remain so even now. The reduction rate at 6 months after PEI was 100% (i.e., disappearance of tumor) in 13 of the 67 HCC (19.4%), >50% reduction in 36 (53.7%), and >30% in 59 (88.1%). The disappearance rate for tumors studied by US in relation to the original size was 33.3% of 12 HCC (≤ 1 cm), 26.5% of 34 HCC (>1, ≤ 2 cm) and 9.5% of 21 HCC (>2, ≤ 3 cm).

7 Post-treatment follow-up

Post-treatment follow-up included a US scan every other month, and a dynamic CT scan at 1–2 months after PEI and then every 6 months. Additional injection of ethanol was given if any of these imaging modes showed incomplete tumor necrosis. Observation periods after PEI in these patients were one year or less in 19 patients (17.0%), 1–2 years in 15 patients (13.4%), 2–3 years in 13 patients (11.6%), 3–4 years in 20 patients (17.9%), 4–5 years in 29 patients (25.9%), 5–6 years in 10 patients (8.9%), and more than 6 years in 6 patients (5.4%).

8 Evaluation of therapeutic effect by imaging and serum AFP level

Sonograms of the 67 main HCCs followed for more than 6 months were classified into three patterns before treatment: Hypoechoic (low

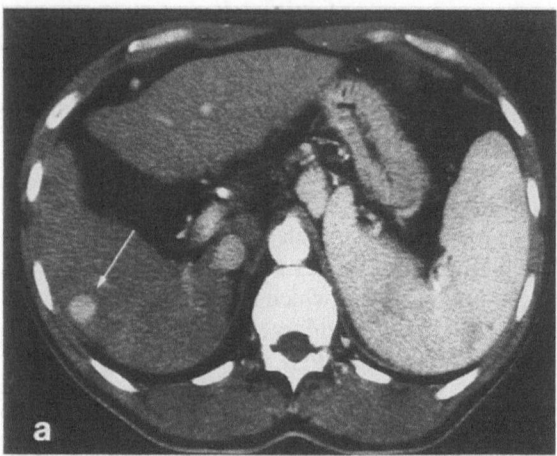

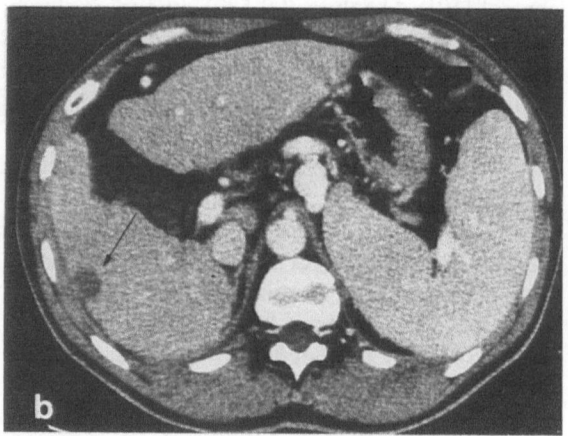

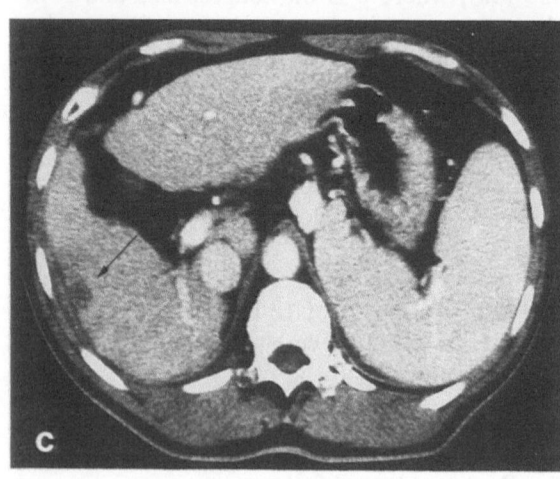

Fig. 1. a Contrast-enhanced CT with bolus injection shows a hypervascular tumor (*arrow*) measuring 25 mm in diameter at the early phase. **b** At 3 weeks after injection of 20 ml of ethanol, the whole tumor including the surrounding liver parenchyma changed to avascular area (*arrow*) at the same phase by dynamic CT. **c** At 18 months after PEI, the lesion decreased in size slightly with low density

echo) in 37 HCC (55.2%), hypoechoic rim (low periphery) in 25 HCC (37.3%) and hyperechoic (high echo) in 5 HCC (7.5%) [17]. About 1 month after PEI, 25 (37.3%) of the lesions had changed to a pattern of hyperechoic rim (high ring), 8 (11.9%) to one of hypoechoic rim surrounding a tumor (low halo) and 20 (29.9%) to one of both high ring and low halo [12]. The clinical diagnosis of complete necrosis of the tumor has not yet been established, although certain sonographic patterns such as high-ring and/or low halo appear to be a sign of the high efficacy of PEI [12].

Dynamic contrast-enhanced CT seems more useful than US for such evaluation (Fig. 1). Contrast-enhanced CT with the intravenous bolus injection technique was carried out for a main lesion in 48 patients before PEI, and 40 of them (83.3%) were visualized. Of these, 30 lesions (62.5%) were enhanced at the early phase and the remaining 10 (20.8%) were only de-enhanced at the late phase. Follow-up dynamic CT by the same technique showed that all 30 lesions and their surrounding liver parenchyma were no longer enhanced, and all 10 lesions and their surrounding liver parenchyma were visualized as low density areas both at the early and late phases. The tumor turned avascular after PEI, as did the region around it. This unenhanced area probably corresponds to the necrosis produced by ethanol.

MRI was performed on 41 patients before treatment and 33 main lesions (80.5%) were detected. Twenty-four (58.5%) showed high intensity on a T2-weighted image (T2WI) before treatment and 16 (39.0%) had changed to low intensity within 1 month after PEI (Fig. 2). T2WI is considered to be useful for therapeutic evaluation of PEI because if a low intensity mass is seen on a T2WI after PEI, which is very uncommon before treatment, it may indicate coagulation necrosis caused by PEI. Such characteristic changes were observed shortly after PEI, mostly within one month.

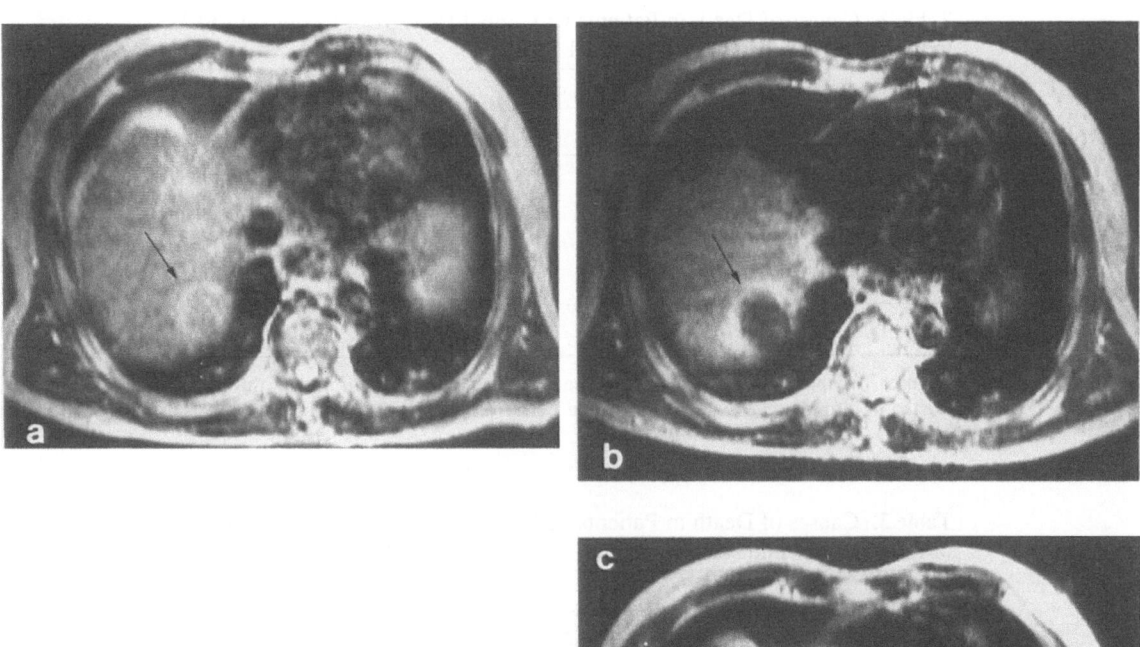

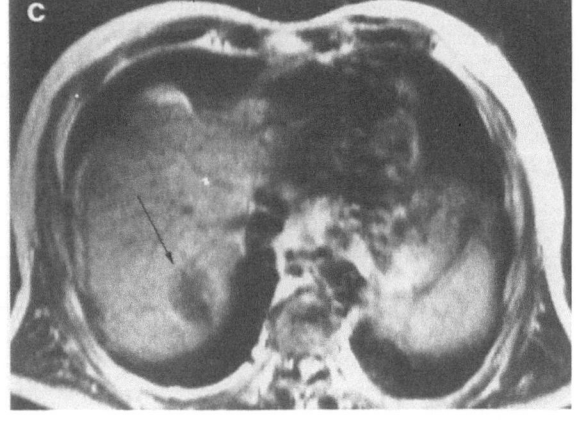

Fig. 2. a MRI with T2-weighted image (TR = 1,500 msec, TE = 80 msec) demonstrates a high intensity mass (*arrow*) measuring 18 mm in diameter at the posterior segment. **b** Two weeks after injection of 13 ml of ethanol into this lesion, it changed to a low intensity one by T2-weighted image. **c** At 18 months after PEI, the lesion was reduced in size but the intensity increased slightly

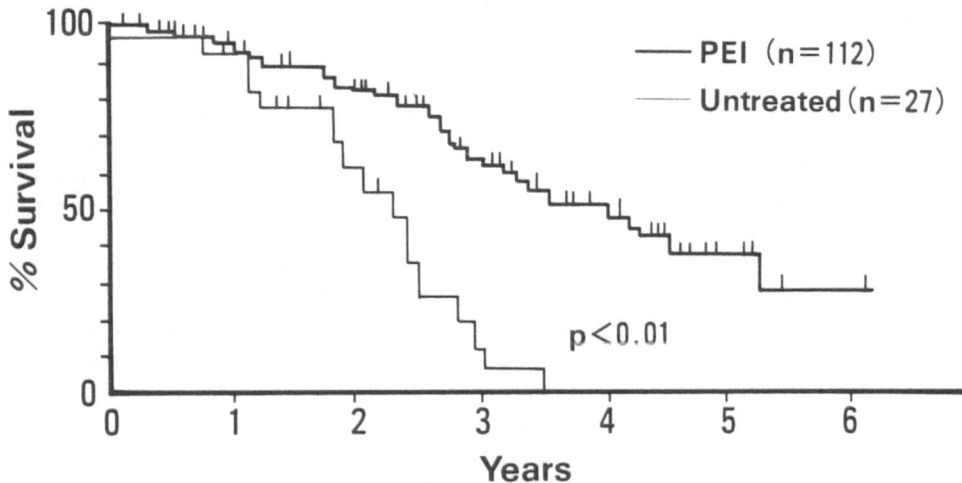

Fig. 3. Survival curves of patients with small HCC (*thick line*) after PEI (n = 112) and (*thin line*) untreated (n = 27) ($P < 0.01$)

Table 2. Causes of Death in Patients with Small HCC Who Underwent PEI in Comparison with Those Untreated

	No. of Patients	
Causes of death	PEI	Untreated
Invasion of cancer[a]	9 (23.1%)	9 (56.3%)
Rapture of tumor	3 (7.7%)	0
Hepatic failure due to liver cirrhosis	16 (41.0%)	4 (25.0%)
Esophageal bleeding	5 (12.8%)	2 (12.5%)
Others	6 (15.4%)	1 (6.3%)
Total	39 (100%)	16 (100%)

[a] Cancer occupied more than 50% of the liver in volume and/or tumor thrombus existed in bifurcation or main trunk of the portal vein at the time of death

Table 3. Causes of Death in Patients with Small HCC Who Underwent PEI in Relation to Child's Classification

	Child's classification		
Causes of death	A (n = 60)	B (n = 33)	C (n = 19)
Invasion of cancer[a]	5	4	2
Rapture of tumor	1	0	2
Hepatic failure due to liver cirrhosis	4	2	10
Esophageal bleeding	2	3	0
Others	3	2	1
Total	15	11	13

[a] Cancer occupied more than 50% of the liver in volume and/or tumor thrombus existed in bifurcation or main trunk of the portal vein at the time of death

Although both CT and MRI often provide distinct information about whether the treatment was effective or not, the detectability of lesions by the two modalities is still limited, especially when HCCs are smaller than 2 cm [18].

Serum AFP levels were measured immediately before PEI and 1 month after in 47 patients. Before PEI, the AFP level was >1,000 ng/ml in 3 patients (6.4%), 100–1,000 ng/ml in 10 (21.3%), 20–99 ng/ml in 19 (40.4%), and <20 ng/ml in 15 patients (31.9%). After completion of PEI, serum AFP levels decreased markedly in all 3 patients having initial levels of >1,000 ng/ml, and to various degrees in 24 of the 29 patients (82.8%) with AFP of 20–1,000 ng/ml, although they increased by up to 78% in the other 5 patients. However, there was little change between before and after the treatment in those of <20 ng/ml before PEI. Thus, measurement of serum AFP level is another way of evaluating the therapeutic effect when it is higher than 200 ng/ml, but it is of limited use since it is less than 200 ng/ml in nearly 80% of patients with HCC smaller than 3 cm in Japan [18].

Unquestionably, the growth of HCC needs to be checked to confirm the therapeutic effect of PEI by various imaging procedures. Definite proof of the effectiveness would be indicated by a lack of viable tumor cells. However, it is impossible to know the histology of the whole HCC treated by PEI even if thin-needle biopsy is repeatedly performed. It seems possible to evaluate the effectiveness by checking changes of size and pattern of tumors with such imaging modalities. In fact, we were able to confirm the incomplete effectiveness of PEI by dynamic CT in 5 patients and additional PEI was successfully given to obtain complete necrosis.

9 Complications

Complications caused by PEI were not serious and did not necessitate intensive care. Local pain, varying from mild to severe, was experienced by most patients and analgesic treatment was necessary for 9 patients (8.0%). A high fever over 38°C developed on the day of injection and continued for up to 3 days in 46 patients (41.1%). A rise of more than 50% in serum transaminase occurred transiently in 13 patients (11.6%). In 2 patients portal thrombus developed as seen by US, but spontaneously disappeared within 1 month. All these side-effects subsided with supportive treatment.

10 Survival and cause of death

Survival curves for the PEI and untreated groups drawn by the Kaplan-Meier method indicated that the median survival time was *4.1* years in the former and *2.4* years in the latter, and that, overall, the former was significantly better than the latter ($P < 0.01$) (Fig. 3). In the PEI group, the 1-year survival rate was 93.9%, 2-year 84.3%, 3-year 63.0%, 4-year 48.5%, 5-year 39.2% and 6-year 29.4%. In contrast, survival time from tumor detection in the untreated group showed a sharp decrease from 2 years to 3 years: 1-year survival rate was 92.1%, 2-year 61.5%, and 3-year 7.0% (Fig. 3).

Causes of death in the PEI and untreated groups were compared (Table 2). In the PEI group, 39 patients died; direct causes of death were hepatic failure without advanced cancer (cancer occupying more than 50% of the liver in volume and/or tumor thrombus in bifurcation or main trunk of the portal vein) in 12 patients, variceal bleeding in five, hepatic failure with advanced cancer in 16, bleeding from the tumor in five and other causes in six. In the untreated group 16 patients died; causes of death were hepatic failure with advanced cancer in six, bleeding from tumor in three, hepatic failure without advanced cancer in four, variceal bleeding in two and cerebral hemorrhage in one. Analysis of these causes in relation to Child's classification is shown in Table 3. Up to now, 15 of 60 Child's A patients (25%), 11 of 33 Child's B patients (33.3%), and 13 of 19 Child's C patients (68.4%) have died. The most common cause of death was hepatic failure due to liver cirrhosis, especially in the patients with Child's C.

Although the survival rates after PEI were correlated significantly with pre-PEI liver function, they were not related to the initial size of the main lesion or to the number of lesions. Survival time in the PEI group in relation to Child's clas-

sification at the time of treatment were as follows: 1-year survival was 96.2% in Child's A, 89.8% in Child's B and 93.8% in Child's C; 2-year survival was 94.1%, 89.8% and 49.2%; 3-year survival was 71.6%, 72.1% and 25.3%; 4-year survival was 58.1%, 55.5% and 16.9%; 5-year survival was 50.9%, 48.5% and 0%, respectively. Survival times in both Child's A and B were significantly longer than in Child's C ($P < .01$) (Fig. 4).

Survival times of the patients with HCC smaller than 2 cm were compared with those of patients with HCC between 2 and 3 cm. Although the survival rate of those with smaller HCC was greater for 1 year ($P < .05$) and 2 years ($P < .01$), there was no significant difference on the whole. There was also no significant difference regarding the number of tumors, although patients with a single nodule tended to survive longer than those with multiple nodules.

11 Recurrence

The major difficulty with PEI is that of recurrence in different areas in the liver, and surgical resection shares the same problem [8]. To evaluate the incidence of recurrence of new lesions after PEI, 40 patients with HCC not larger than 3 cm who underwent surgical resection during our study period were compared with the 112 PEI cases. The recurrence of tumors apart from the original one was seen in 56 PEI patients (50%). The exact site of recurrence was evaluated in 36 patients with 45 recurrent tumors; the recurrent tumor appeared in the same segment as the primary one in 33.3% (15 tumors) and in a different segment in 66.7% (30 tumors).

Cumulative recurrence rates for HCC in the PEI and the operation groups calculated by the Kaplan-Meier method are shown in Fig. 5. The rates were 28.3% in the PEI group and 28.4% in the operation group in one year, 54.0% and 54.8% in 2 years, and 63.0% and 63.8% in 3 years, respectively. There was no significant difference between the two groups by the generalized Wilcoxon test. The average size of the first recurrent tumor detected by US in each patient was 18.9 ± 8.5 mm (n = 56) in the PEI group. The recurrence rate was lower in patients with a single lesion 2 cm or less in size than those with a lesion bigger than 2 cm and those with multiple lesions. The 40 resected patients

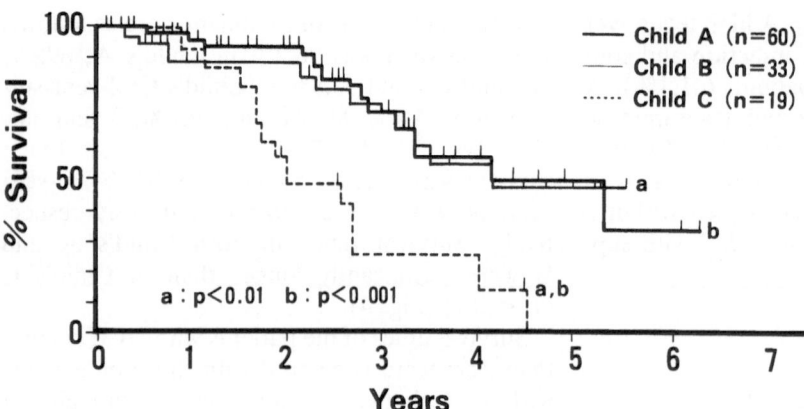

Fig. 4. Survival curves of patients with small HCC after PEI in relation to Child's classification. (*thick line*) grade A (n = 60), (*thin line*) grade B (n = 33), (*dotted line*) grade C (n = 19). **a**: $P < 0.01$, **b**: $P < 0.001$

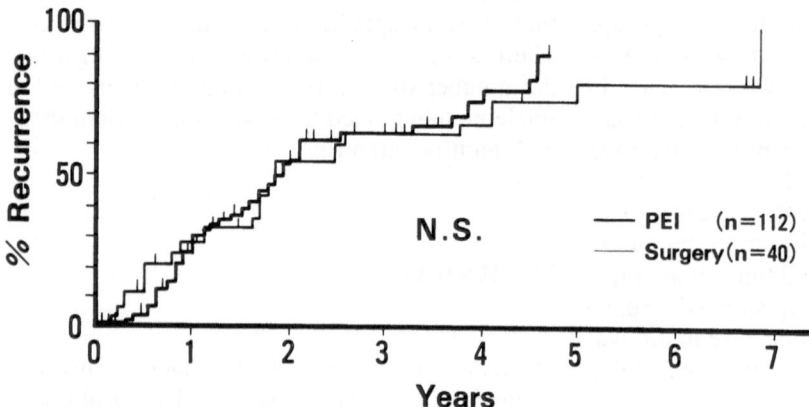

Fig. 5. Recurrence curves of new lesions of HCC after PEI (*thick line*) in comparison with post-surgical resection (*thin line*)

with HCC smaller than 3 cm had a recurrence rate practically the same as that for the patients treated by PEI. According to several recent studies, newly emerging HCC after treatment can be either metastatic from the primary lesion or developing de nouveau [22]. In order to improve the prognosis of patients with such recurrences, it is important to detect them as early as possible so that PEI may be given again. PEI has the advantage of being able to be performed repeatedly as long as tumors consist of not more than 3 lesions and are sized smaller than 3 cm.

The treatments given for recurrence in the PEI group were PEI alone in 51.8% (n = 29), TAE alone in 14.3% (n = 8), TAE and PEI combined in 17.9% (n = 10), arterial chemotherapy alone in 3.6% (n = 2), and no special treatment because of poor liver function in 12.5% (n = 7).

12 Illustrative case

The patient (Fig. 6), a 59-year-old man with liver cirrhosis, was being followed by US and AFP measurement every 3 months. In November,

1986, a mass measuring 21 mm with a low echoic periphery pattern was detected by US, and a histological biopsy showed HCC. A total of 16 ml of ethanol in 6 sessions was injected into the tumor. One month later, the tumor size had decreased. Together with changes of the US pattern, the size was reduced by 69.1% after 6 months, and by 83.5% 28 months later. The patient is alive 4 years and 7 months after PEI, without any sign of recurrence.

13 Conclusion

PEI can be performed in almost any patient with HCC because it causes minimal damage to the liver, the exception being those who have severe liver dysfunction. On the basis of long-term observations of a large series of patients, no tumor has been observed to become bigger than before PEI. Therefore, PEI may be considered to have a therapeutic effect comparable to surgical resection in most cases.

Judging from our results, because of the risk of recurrence of new lesions in the remnant of the

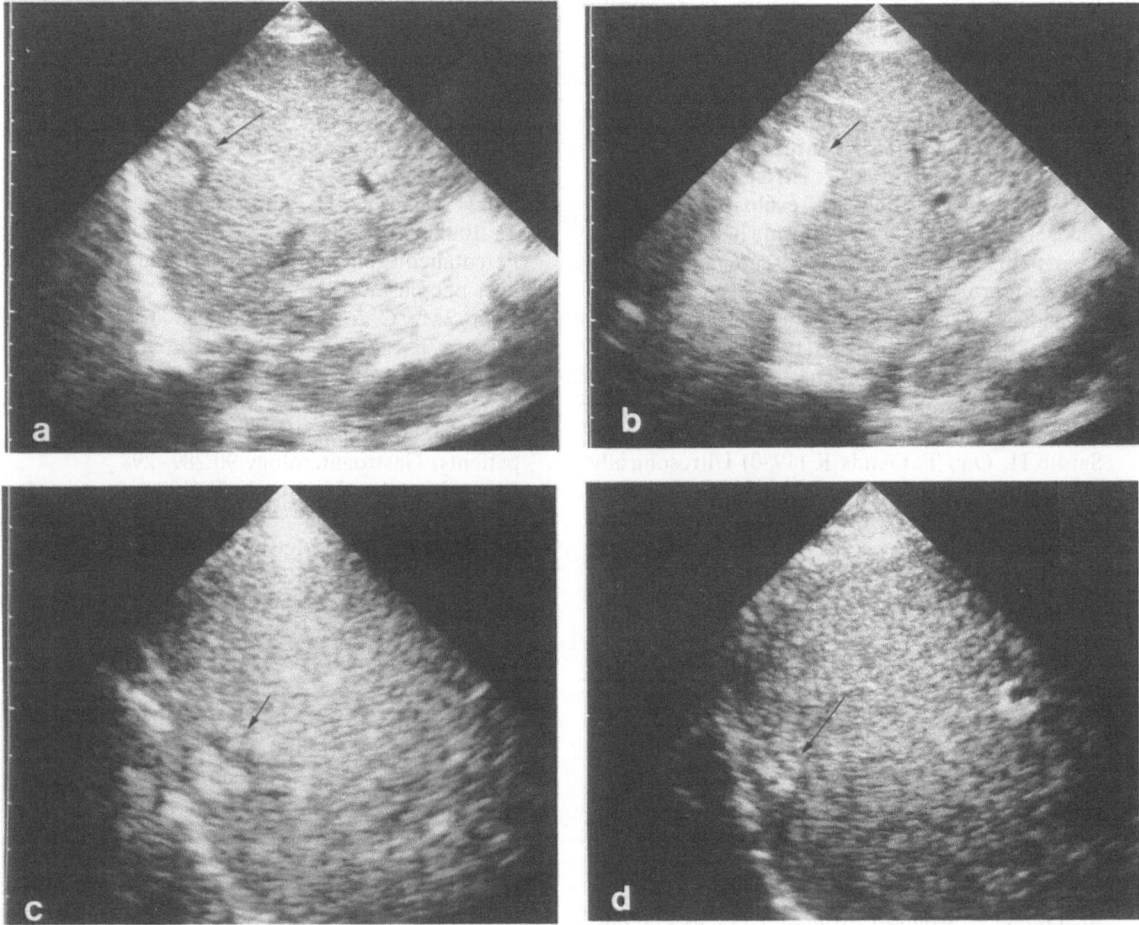

Fig. 6. Sonogram by sector scanner shows a mass measuring 21 mm in diameter with a low periphery pattern (*arrow*) at the 7th segment immediately below the diaphragm of the liver (**a**). For this lesion, a total of 16 ml of ethanol in 6 sessions was injected into the tumor (**b**). After PEI, the lesion was reduced in size and changed in US pattern to high echo (*arrow*) at 3 months (**c**), and to high echo spot (*arrow*) at 24 months (**d**)

liver, the risk of coexisting liver cirrhosis and the operative damage to the liver, PEI might be considered as a viable alternative to surgery for most patients with HCC 3 cm or smaller.

References

1. Okuda K, Fujimoto I, Hanai A, Urano Y (1987) Changing incidence of hepatocellular carcinoma in Japan. Cancer Res 47:4967–4972
2. The Liver Cancer Study Group of Japan (1987) Primary liver cancer in Japan. Cancer 60: 1400–1411
3. Shinagawa T, Ohto M, Kimura K, Tsunetomi S, Morita M, Saisho H, Tsuchiya Y, Saotome N, Karasawa E, Miki M, Ueno T, Okuda K (1984) Diagnosis and clinical features of small hepatocellular carcinoma with emphasis on the utility of real-time ultrasonography: A study in 51 patients. Gastroenterology 86:495–502
4. Sheu JC, Sung JL, Chen DS, Yu JY, Wang TH, Su CT, Tsang YM (1984) Ultrasonography of small hepatic tumors using high-resolution linear-array real-time instruments. Radiology 150:797–802
5. Okuda K, Kotoda K, Obata H, Hayashi N, Hisamitsu T, Tamiya M, Kubo Y, Yakushiji F, Nagata E, Jinnouchi S, Shimokawa Y (1975) Clinical observation during a relatively early stage of hepatocellular carcinoma with special reference to serum alpha-fetoprotein levels. Gastroenterology 69:116–134
6. Kew M (1974) Alpha-fetoprotein in primary liver cancer and other diseases. Gut 15:814–821

7. Kanematsu T, Takenaka K, Matsumata T, Furuta T, Sugimachi K, Inokuchi K (1984) Limited hepatic resection effective for selected cirrhotic patients with primary liver cancer. Ann Surg 199:51–56

8. Takayasu K, Muramatsu Y, Moriyama N, Yamada T, Hasegawa H, Okazaki N, Hirohashi S, Tsugane S (1987) Clinico-radiological evaluation of recurrence in the residual liver following hepatectomy in 97 patients with hepatocellular carcinoma. Jpn J Gastroenterol 84:1424–1432

9. Yamada R, Sato M, Kawabata M, Nakatsuka H, Nakamura K, Takashima S (1983) Hepatic artery embolization in 120 patients with unresectable hepatoma. Radiology 148:397–401

10. Ohto M, Karasawa E, Tsuchiya Y, Kimura K, Saisho H, Ono T, Okuda K (1980) Ultrasonically guided percutaneous contrast medium injection and aspiration biopsy using a real-time puncture transducer. Radiology 136:171–176

11. Sugiura N, Takara K, Ohto M, Okuda K, Hirooka N (1983) Treatment of small hepatocellular carcinoma by percutaneous injection of ethanol into tumor with real-time ultrasound monitoring. Acta Hepatol Jpn 24:920

12. Ohto M, Ebara M, Watanabe Y, Sugiura N, Shinagawa T, Okuda K (1988) Percutaneous ethanol injection (PEI) therapy for small hepatocellular carcinoma: Evaluation of its utility on the basis of tumor-images and survival after therapy. Japanese J of Medical Imag 7:25

13. Ebara M, Ohto M, Sugiura N, Kita K, Yoshikawa M, Okuda K, Kondo F, Kondo Y (1990) Percutaneous ethanol injection for the treatment of small hepatocellular carcinoma: Study of 95 patients. Journal of Gastroenterol and Hepatol 5:616–626

14. Livraghi T, Festi D, Monti F, Salmi A, Vettori C (1986) US-guided percutaneous alcohol injection of small hepatic and abdominal tumors. Radiology 161:309–312

15. Sheu JC, Huang GT, Chen DS, Sung JL, Yan PM, Wei TC, Lai MY, Su CT, Tsang YM (1987) Small hepatocellular carcinoma: Intratumor ethanol treatment using new needle and guidance systems. Radiology 163:43–48

16. Shiina S, Yasuda H, Muto H, Tagawa K, Unuma T, Ibukuro K, Inoue Y, Takahashi R (1987) Percutaneous ethanol injection in the treatment of liver neoplasms. AJR 149:949–952

17. Ebara M, Ohto M, Shinagawa T, Sugiura N, Kimura K, Matsutani S, Morita M, Saisho H, Tsuchiya Y, Okuda K (1986) Natural history of minute hepatocellular carcinoma smaller than three centimeters complicating cirrhosis: A study in 22 patients. Gastroenterology 90:289–298

18. Ebara M, Ohto M, Kondo F (1989) Strategy for early diagnosis of hepatocellular carcinoma (HCC). Ann Acad Med 18:83–89

19. Young SW, Turner RJ, Castellino RA (1980) A strategy for the contrast enhancement of malignant tumors using dynamic computed tomography and intravascular pharmacokinetics. Radiology 137:137–147

20. Ebara M, Ohto M, Watanabe Y, Kimura K, Saisho H, Tsuchiya Y, Okuda K, Arimizu N, Kondo F, Ikehira H, Fukuda N, Tateno Y (1986) Diagnosis of small hepatocellular carcinoma: Correlation of MR imaging and tumor histologic studies. Radiology 159:371–377

21. Child CG, Turcotte JG (1964) Surgery and portal hypertension. In: Child CG (ed) The liver and portal hypertension. WB Saunders, Philadelphia 50

22. Kondo Y, Kondo F, Wada K, Okabayashi A (1986) Pathologic features of small hepatocellular carcinoma. Acta Pathol Jpn 36:1149–1161

CHAPTER 29

Systemic chemotherapy for hepatocellular carcinoma

Nobuo Okazaki, Shuichi Okada, Haruhiko Nose, and Kazunori Aoki[1]

1 Introduction

After a promising preliminary report by Olweny et al. was published in 1975 [1], doxorubicin came into use and was considered the most reliable anticancer agent for hepatocellular carcinoma (HCC). However, in recent well-controlled Phase II trials which included doxorubicin, it was demonstrated that no active anticancer agent for HCC shows more than a 15% response rate reproducibly [2].

Because of the early intrahepatic spread and multicentric carcinogenesis characteristics of HCC, surgical treatment is not always successful. Associated liver cirrhosis is another limiting factor in surgical treatment of patients with HCC [3]. Thus, the median survival of all patients with HCC is less than 6 months, despite recent advances in its diagnosis and treatment [4].

Systemic chemotherapy, the treatment modality for advanced HCC or recurrent HCC after surgery or other treatments, is considered to be a modality which might contribute to improvement of the patient survival rate, as is the case with testicular carcinoma, if a drug active for HCC is developed [5].

2 Indications for chemotherapy

Among the various treatment modalities for HCC, surgical resection [6], percutaneous injection of ethanol into the tumor (PEI) [7], and transcatheter arterial embolization (TAE) [8],

present obvious clinical benefits. In fact, complete cure can be effected only with surgery and PEI. Therefore, patients for whom these treatments are contraindicated, other than those with severe hemorrhagic diathesis or jaundice or at risk of hepatic coma, are considered to be candidates for systemic chemotherapy.

According to the Ninth National Survey of Primary Liver Cancer in Japan, patients who received hepatic resection represent about 20% of total registered primary liver cancer patients, and chemotherapy was performed in about 50% of patients with histologically confirmed HCC [9]. These findings indicate that a large number of patients in Japan are candidates for chemotherapy; thus, development of effective chemotherapy is urgently needed.

Because there is no standard chemotherapeutic regimen for HCC, well-designed phase II studies of new anticancer agents are required for further development of chemotherapy. The following are the minimum eligibility requirements for participation in the phase II trial for HCC which would ensure that valid conclusions are obtained:

1. Unequivocal evidence of HCC
2. Measurable disease
3. Performance status better than 3 by WHO criteria [10] or ECOG criteria [11]
4. Informed consent
5. Disqualification from clinical trials:
   a) Previous chemotherapy within the last month
   b) Previous radiotherapy for the HCC nodule to be evaluated
   c) Previous TAE for the HCC nodule to be evaluated
   d) Leukocyte count less than 3,000, platelet count less than 60,000, total bilirubin greater than 3.0 mg/dl, or serum creatinine greater than 1.5 mg/dl

[1] Department of Internal Medicine, National Cancer Center Hospital, Tsukiji-5-1-1, Chuo-ku, Tokyo, 107 Japan

e) Active infectious process
f) Active heart disease
g) Active double cancer
h) Portal systemic encephalopathy
i) Varices with recent hemorrhage

In HCC nodules treated with radiotherapy or TAE, the mode of tumor response to chemotherapy has been shown to be modified by these treatments [12]. Therefore, any patients with HCC nodules previously treated with radiotherapy or TAE were disqualified from clinical trials to assure precise evaluation of anticancer agents.

3 Response analysis

Chemotherapeutic effects were evaluated by ultrasonography and/or computed tomography, or serial measurement of hepatomegaly. Response was assessed 4 weeks after chemotherapy was started. Complete response (CR) is defined as the complete disappearance of the entire tumor lasting for more than 4 weeks after chemotherapy was started. Partial response (PR) is defined as 50% or greater reduction in the product of the two greatest perpendicular diameters or at least 30% reduction in hepatomegaly without the appearance of new lesions, lasting for more than 4 weeks. Any reduction and/or the duration of response insufficient for classification as PR is classified as minor response (MR). No change (NC) is defined as actually no change or up to 25% progression in tumor size 4 weeks after the beginning of chemotherapy. Progressive disease (PD) is defined as greater than 25% increase in tumor measurements or the appearance of new lesions within 4 weeks after the beginning of treatment. These criteria for response analysis are identical with those of ECOG [11].

Serial determination of serum level of alpha-fetoprotein (AFP) is also helpful in the early recognition of tumor response to chemotherapy [13, 14], although grading of tumor response strictly on the basis of serum levels of AFP seems to be difficult.

There are few studies on the mode of response to chemotherapy in patients with HCC, because of the small number of responders at any given institution. In our experience, the speed of tumor regression varies from case to case, and probably depends on the degree of associated liver cirrhosis, even if complete tumor necrosis is

suspected on the basis of dynamic CT-scan. Modification of criteria for analysis of HCC response to chemotherapy might be necessary after analysis of response in a large number of subjects.

4 Dose schedule

There is no established dose schedule for anticancer agents proven to be effective for HCC. The following are the dose schedules employed in the present clinical phase II trials for HCC:

1. Tegafur [15], 600 mg/m^2, orally twice a day for more than 4 weeks
2. UFT (combination of uracil and tegafur at molar ratio of 1:4) [16], 400 mg/m^2, orally 3 times a day for more than 4 weeks
3. Doxorubicin [15], 30 mg/m^2, intravenously, for 2 consecutive days every 4 weeks
4. Etoposide [17], 80 mg/m^2, intravenously, for 5 consecutive days every 4, weeks
5. Mitoxantrone [18], 10 mg/m^2, intravenously, every 3 weeks
6. Gamma-interferon [19], $16 - 24 \times 10^6$ units, intravenously, for 5 consecutive days, every 2 weeks
7. Cisplatin [20], 80 mg/m^2, intravenously, every 4 weeks, with hydration sufficient to prevent renal failure

5 Results

5.1 Tumor response

Table 1 shows results obtained using systemic chemotherapy with various anticancer agents in

Table 1. Results for clinical trials for systemic chemotherapy for hepatocellular carcinoma

Drug	Number of patients	Number of responders	Response rate (%)
Doxorubicin	17	1	6
Tegafur	15	1	7
UFT	26	1	4
Etoposide	21	1	5
Mitoxantrone	22	2	9
Gamma interferon	14	0	0
Cisplatin	26	4	15
Total	141	10	7

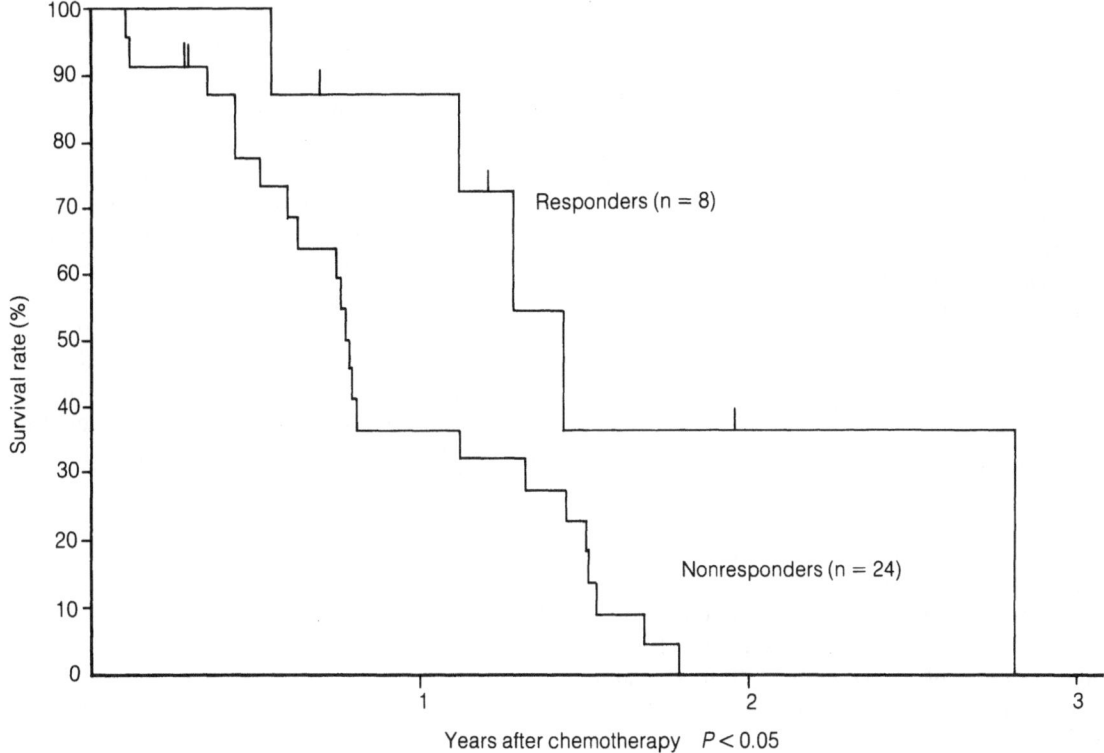

Fig. 1. Survival curves of responders and non-responders of patients with hepatocellular carcinoma to systemic chemotherapy. There was a significant difference ($P < 0.05$) between the two curves

the present phase II clinical trial [15–20]. If regression of tumor size and/or decrease of serum level of AFP was observed 4 weeks after the start of chemotherapy, the chemotherapy was continued until the development of mild toxicities; if no tumor effect was observed, chemotherapy was stopped.

All anticancer agents except cisplatin showed a response rate of less than 10%; the overall response rate was 7%. The response rate for high dose gamma-interferon was 0%. The response rate for cisplatin, which is still under phase II study, was 15% [20]. All responders listed in Table 1 showed PR, and none showed CR.

5.2 Toxicity

Toxicity of tegafur and of UFT, a derivative of 5-fluorouracil, was mostly gastrointestinal in nature, and was mild and tolerable [15, 16]. Gastrointestinal toxicity of cisplatin was more severe than that of tegafur or UFT, even with concomitant use of antiemetica, but was still tolerable [20]. Toxicity of doxorubicin, etoposide

and mitoxanrone was hematological; white blood cell and platelet counts were their lowest 2 weeks after the beginning of treatment, but recovered to their initial levels within the next 2 weeks. Leukocytopenia was usually more severe than thrombocytopenia [15, 17, 18]. Alopecia was observed in doxorubicin and etoposide [15, 17], but not in mitoxantrone [18]. The most common adverse effect of interferon was pyrexia [19].

Table 2. Clinical trials reported in the literature: Systemic chemotherapy for hepatocellular carcinoma

Drug	Response rate (%)	Reference
Doxorubicin	44 (22/50)	[21]
	11 (6/52)	[22]
	12 (5/43)	[23]
	3 (2/60)	[24]
Epirubicin	17 (3/18)	[25]
	9 (3/33)	[26]
Mitoxantrone	6 (2/33)	[27]
	0 (0/34)	[28]
Tegafur	7 (1/15)	[29]
Etoposide	13 (3/24)	[30]
	0 (0/18)	[31]
Cisplatin	5 (1/20)	[32]
	6 (2/35)	[28]

5.3 Survival

Figure 1 shows the survival curves of 8 responders to systemic chemotherapy and that of 24 non-responders. For each responder, 3 nonresponders matched for age, sex, and various prognostic factors were selected from 97 nonresponders. There was a significant difference between the median survival time for the 8 responders (17.5 months) and that for the 24 nonresponders (9.7 months) [13].

6 Discussion

Since 1980, we have used various types and doses of anticancer agents for the treatment of HCC, since no one established dose schedule proven to be effective for HCC has been found. Results for the present phase II clinical trial are summarized in Table 1. The overall response rate was only 7%.

Table 2 shows the results of recent well-controlled phase II studies of treatment for HCC reported in the literature [21–32]. Olweny et al. confirmed their results obtained in a preliminary study on doxorubicin originally conducted in 1980 [1, 21]. However, the high response rate they found has not been duplicated in any subsequent study [22, 23, 24]. The limited clinical benefits of doxorubicin were clearly demonstrated in a well-controlled study by Chlebowski et al. [22]. Fifty-two HCC patients with good performance scores were treated with a 75 mg/m^2 dose of doxorubicin every 3 weeks. A partial response was observed in 6 patients, and the overall response rate was 11%. All recent phase II studies indicated that there is no active drug for HCC (Table 2), and our results confirmed this (Table 1). Patients with HCC may therefore be considered candidates for investigation of protocols.

Results for combination chemotherapy for HCC have also been disappointing. In 1984, Falkson et al. reported results for a randomized clinical trial for HCC [23]. Their treatment regimens were as follows: 1) intravenous doxorubicin, 2) intravenous 5-fluorouracil plus methyl CCNU (N-(2-chloroethyl)-N'-cyclohexyl-N-nitrosourea), 3) intravenous 5-fluorouracil plus streptozotocin, and 4) intravenous 5-fluorouracil plus methyl CCNU, doxorubicin, and streptozotocin. Of these, the four-drug combination regimen showed the best response rate (19%), but 63% of the

patients who received this regimen developed severe toxicity, and the median survival period was only 17 weeks. They concluded that this combination treatment is not acceptable clinically [23].

There is no report showing any clinical advantage in using a multidrug combination for HCC although the synergic effects of cisplatin and the other anticancer agent have not been fully evaluated in HCC patients. However, it is a generally true that no improvement in response is obtained when an anticancer agent that does not have single-agent activity is added. Therefore, the development of a new active anticancer agent is a cardinal necessity for effective chemotherapy in HCC [33].

References

1. Olweny CLM, Toya T, Katongole-Mbidde E, Mugerwa J, Kyalwazi SK, Cohen H (1975) Treatment of hepatocellular carcinoma with adriamycin. Preliminary communication. Cancer 36:1250–1257
2. Falkson G, Coetzer B (1987) Chemotherapy of primary liver cancer. In: Okuda K, Ishak KJ (eds) Neoplasms of the liver. Springer-Verlag, Tokyo, pp 331–326
3. Okamoto E, Yamanaka N, Toyosaka Y, Tanaka N, Yabuki K (1987) Current status of hepatic resection in the treatment of hepatocellular carcinoma. In: Okuda K, Ishak KJ (eds) Neoplasms of the liver. Springer-Verlag, Tokyo, pp 353–363
4. Okuda K, Ohtsuki T, Obata H, Tominatsu M, Okazaki N, Hasegawa H, Nakajima Y, Ohnishi K (1985) Natural history of hepatocellular carcinoma and prognosis in relation to treatment. Study of 850 patients. Cancer 56:918–928
5. Einhorn LH (1981) Testicular cancer as a model for a curable neoplasm: The Richard and Hinda Rosenthal Foundation Award Lecture. Cancer Res 41:3275–3280
6. Yamasaki S, Hasegawa H, Makuuchi M (1981) Clinicopathological observation of minute liver cancer and the new method of hepatectomy. An Analysis of 27 cases. Acta Hepatol Jpn 22: 1714–1724
7. Ebara M, Ohto M, Sugiura N, Kita K, Yoshikawa M, Okuda K, Kondo F, Kondo Y (1990) Percutaneous ethanol injection for the treatment of small hepatocellular carcinoma. Study of 95 patients. J Gastroenterol Hepatol 5:616–626
8. Yamada R, Sato M, Kawabata T, Nakatsuka H, Nakamura K, Takashima S (1983) Hepatic artery embolization in 120 patients with unresectable hepatoma. Radiology 148:397–401

9. The Liver Study Group of Japan (1990) Primary liver cancer in Japan (ninth report)
10. WHO (1979) WHO handbook for reporting results of cancer treatment, WHO Offset Publication, No. 48
11. Oken MM, Greech RH, Horton J, Davis TE, McFadden Carbone PP (1982) Toxicity and response criteria of the Eastern Cooperative Oncology Group. Am J Clin Oncol 5:649–655
12. Okazaki N, Yoshida T, Yoshino M, Okada S, Shimada Y, Moriyama N, Takayasu K (1991) Changes in mode of response to chemotherapy for hepatocellular carcinoma induced by transarterial embolization. A case report. Jpn J Clin Oncol 21:69–67
13. Okada S, Okazaki N, Nose H, Ohkura H, Sugano K, Aoki K (to be published) (1992) Evaluation of chemotherapeutic effects for hepatocellular carcinoma based on survival analysis. Acta Hepatol Jpn
14. Okazaki N, Yoshino M, Yoshida T, Hizikata A, Hasegawa H (1986) Systemic chemotherapy of hepatocellular carcinoma. Jpn J Cancer Chemother 13:584–1588
15. Okazaki N, Yoshino M, Yoshida T, Hijikata A (1985) A controlled study of intravenous doxorubicin versus oral tegafur in patients with hepatocellular carcinoma. J Jpn Soc Cancer Ther 20:556–561
16. Tokyo Liver Cancer Chemotherapy Study Group (1985) Phase II study of co-administration of uracil and tegafur (UFT) in hepatocellular carcinoma. Jpn J Clin Oncol 15:559–562
17. Yoshino M, Okazaki N, Yoshida T, Kanda Y, Miki M, Oda H, Sasagawa Y, Hayashi S, Hoshimoto N (1989) A phase II study of etoposide in patients with hepatocellular carcinoma by Tokyo Liver Cancer Chemotherapy Study group. Jpn J Clin Oncol 19:120–122
18. Yoshida T, Okazaki N, Yoshino M, Ohkura H, Miyamoto K, Shimada Y (1988) Phase II trial of mitoxantrone in patients with hepatocellular carcinoma. Eur J Cancer Clin Oncol 124: 1897–1898
19. Yoshida T, Okazaki N, Yoshino M, Ohkura H, Shimada Y (1990) Phase II trial of high dose recombinant gamma-interferon in advanced hepatocellular carcinoma. Eur J Cancer 26:545–546
20. Okada S, Okazaki N, Nose H, Aoki K, Simada Y (to be published) (1992) Phase II trial of cisplatin for hepatocellular carcinoma. Eur J Cancer
21. Olweny CLM, Katongole-Mbidde E, Bahendeka S, Otim D, Mugerwa J, Kyalwazi SK (1980) Further experiences in treating patients with hepatocellular carcinoma in Uganda. Cancer 46:2717–2722
22. Chlebowski RT, Brzechwa-Adjukiewicz A, Cowden A, Block JB, Tong M, Chan KK (1984) Doxorubicin (75 mg/m^2) for hepatocellular carcinoma: Clinical and pharmacokinetic results. Cancer Treat Rep 68:487–491
23. Falkson G, MacIntyre JM, Moertel CG, Johnson LA, Scherman RC (1984) Primary liver cancer: An Eastan Cooperative Oncology Group Trial. Cancer 54:970–977
24. Lai CL, Wu PC, Chan GCB, Lok ASF, Lin HJ (1988) Doxorubicin verus no antitumor therapy in inoperable hepatocellular carcinoma. A prospective randomized trial. Cancer 62:479–483
25. Hochster HS, Green MD, Speyer J, Fazzini E, Blum R, Muggia FM (1985) 4'Epirubicin (Epirubicin): Activity in hepatocellular carcinoma. J Clin Oncol 3:1535–1540
26. Shiu W, Leung N, Li M, Leug WT, Li AKG (1988) The efficacy of high-dose 4'Epidoxorubicin in hepatocellular carcinoma. Jpn J Clin Oncol 18: 235–237
27. Davis RB, Van Echo DA, Leone LA, Henderson ES (1986) Phase II trial of mitoxantrone in advanced primary liver cancer. A Cancer Leukemia Group B Study. Cancer Treat Rep 70:1125–1126
28. Falkson G, Ryan LM, Johnson LA, Simson IW, Coetzer BJ, Carbone PP, Creech RH, Schutt AJ (1987) A random phase II study of mitoxantrone and cisplatin in patients with hepatocellular carcinoma. An ECOG study. Cancer 60:2141–2145
29. Ohya T, Kikuchi S, Kato K, Takei T, Takeichi M, Nakano S, Watahiki M, Koyama T, Yamamoto M, Komatsu T, Miwa N, Kasugai T, Hisano N, Tuboi Y, Kikuchi S, Tomusa A (1982) Clinical studies of chemotherapy for primary hepatocellular carcinoma. Jpn J Cancer Chemother 9:1623–1627
30. Cavalli F, Rozencweig M, Renard J, Goldhirsch A, Hansen HH (1981) Phase II study of oral VP-16-213 in hepatocellular carcinoma. Eur J Cancer Clin Oncol 17:1079–1082
31. Shiu W, Mok SD, Leung N, Li M, Zacharia A, Li A, Martin C (1987) Phase 2 study of high dose etoposide (VP16-213) in hepatocellular carcinoma. Jpn J Clin Oncol 17:113–115
32. Ravry MJR, Omura GA, Bartolucii AA, Einhorn L, Kramer B, Davila E (1986) Phase II evaluation of cisplatin in advanced hepatocellular carcinoma and cholangiocarcinoma: A Southern Cancer Study Group Trial. Cancer Treat Rep 70:311–312
33. Okazaki N, Yoshino M, Yoshida T (1989) Chemotherapy for hepatocellular carcinoma. Kan Tan Sui 18:239–242

CHAPTER 30

Present status of immunotherapy of hepatocellular carcinoma

Kiwamu Okita[1]

1 Introduction

Systemic treatment of hepatocellular carcinoma (HCC) with conventional chemotherapeutic agents in general seems to be very poor, as well as for other gastrointestinal malignancies. In this sense, trans-arterial embolization (TAE) [1], lipiodolization [2] and percutaneous ethanol injection (PEI) [3] have been expected to be more effective therapy, because those therapies can cause tumor necrosis by direct action. There is no doubt these modalities have brought prolonged the life expectancy of HCC patients.

On the other hand, it has long been recognized that there is a correlation between intact cellular immunity and a favorable prognosis in patients with malignancies. In other words, patients with HCC, whose survival periods are worse among the malignancies, demonstrate decreased natural immunological killer activity in the blood [4, 5]. Therefore, it seems that immune modulation, by enhancing the host's immune response, could provide an avenue for treatment either alone or in combination with other conventional modalities.

Since Sinkovics [6] reviewed immune therapy of human tumors in 1978, several immune modifying agents, which are classified as biological response modifiers (BRM), have become available for human use. This review aims to summarize the present state of immunotherapy of HCC in Japan.

2 Immunological background in patients with HCC

It has been generally accepted that natural killer (NK), cytotoxic T-cells and macrophages are involved in the killing of cancer cells, as shown in Fig. 1, and it is well-known that the function of these cells are depressed in HCC patients. For example, natural killer activity in patients with HCC was lower than that in liver cirrhosis or healthy controls ($P < 0.01$) (Fig. 2).

It has been found that interferon (IFN) and interleukin-2 (IL-2) can augment NK function [7, 8]. In addition, induction of activated killer (AK) cells by IL-2 was reported [9]. The AK cells represent a cytotoxic phenomenon distinct from either the classic cytotoxic T-cells or NK cell system and play a role in the immunosurveillance against malignancies. IL-2 boosted both NK and AK activity of patients, but to a lesser degree in comparison with those of controls when similarly stimulated. NK and AK activity of patients was significantly augmented γ by IFN, but the levels of cytotoxicity were lower in HCC patients than controls. [4] Therefore, they concluded that the relative decrease in NK and AK activity in HCC were due to an altered subpopulation ratio of NK cells and a functional defect of effector cells.

We administered IFN-γ into 2 HCC patients. However, induction of NK activity is minimal and temporary in spite of its continuous administration. This phenomenon was also observed by Dunk et al. [10] who used IFN-α.

Therefore, the evidence mentioned above may indicate not only depressed immunity to HCC, but also difficulty with immunotherapy using BRM.

[1]First Department of Internal Medicine, Yamaguchi University School of Medicine, Ube, Yamaguchi, 755 Japan

recognition of tumor spesific
antigen and / or MHC

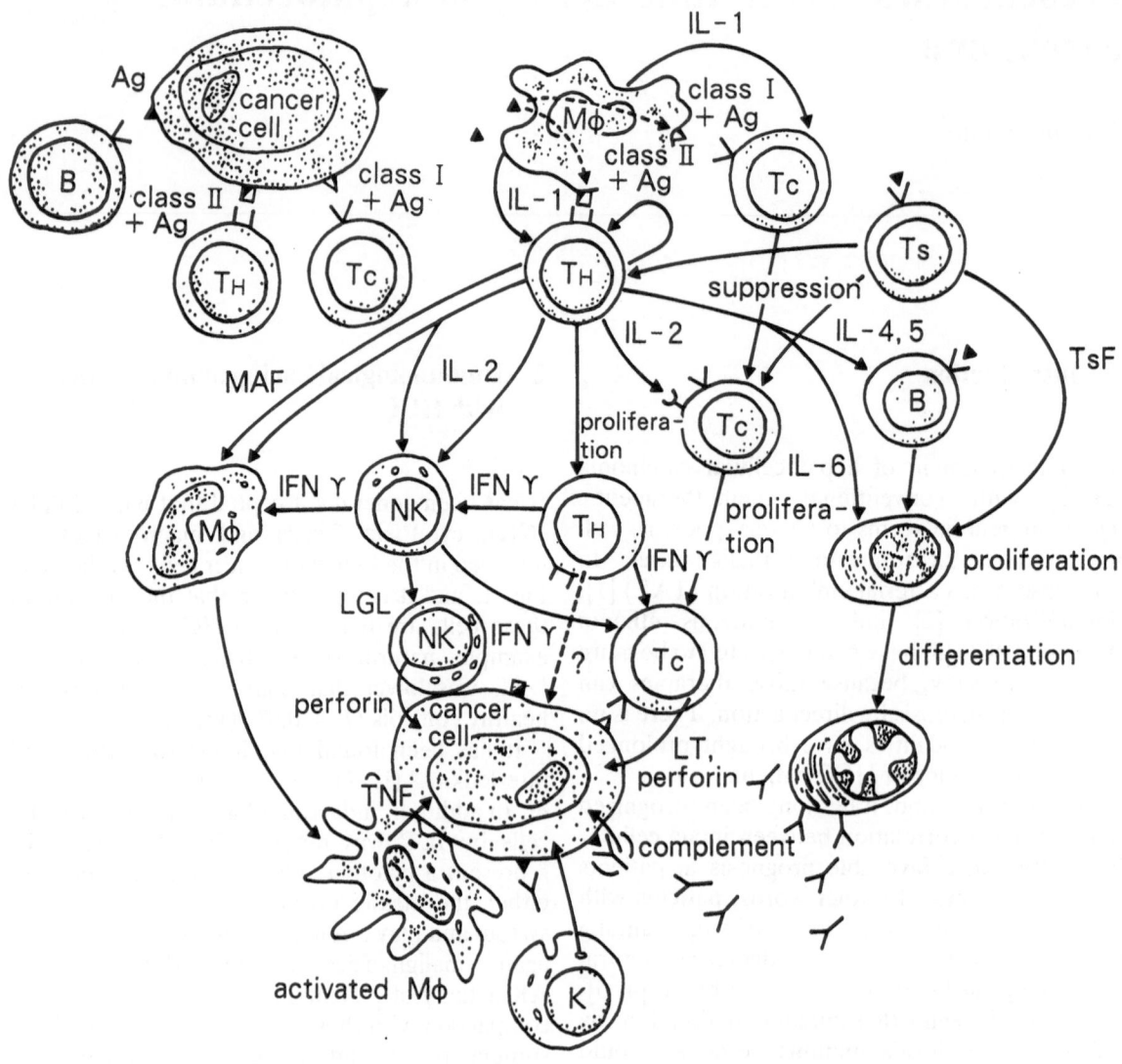

MHC : major histocompatiblity antigen

Fig. 1. Immunological mechanism of recognition of tumor specific antigen and killing of cancer cell. *Tc*, cytotoxic T cell; *Ts*, suppressor T cell; *Tн*, helper T cell; *MAF*, macrophage activating factor; *MHC*, major histocompatibility antigen; *TsF*, suppressor T cell factor; *LGL*, large granular lymphocyte; *Mφ*, macrophage; *LT*, lymphotoxin; *TNF*, tumor necrosis factor; *INFγ*, Gamma-interferon; *IL-1*, interleukin-1; *IL-2*, interleukin-2; *IL-4*, interleukin-4; *IL-5*, interleukin-5; *IL-6*, interleukin-6

3   Interferons (IFNs)

IFN was first discovered by Isaacs and Lindermann [11] in 1957 as an antiviral agent and was subsequently found to have potent anticancer properties. The current nomenclature includes three classifications of IFN such as α which is similar to leuko cyte IFN, β which is similar to fibroblast IFN, and γ which is similar to immune IFN. They each have different properties, however, α and β may share the same cellular receptor. There are several reports describing the therapeutic effect of IFN on HCC. Sachs et al. [12], who admin-

Fig. 2. NK activity in peripheral blood in liver cirrhosis (LC) and hepatocellular carcinoma (HCC). In accordance with progression of chronic liver disesase, NK activity in peripheral blood lymphocytes (PBL) decreased. NK activity was calculated by radioactivity released into the medium from ^{51}Cr labelled K-562 cells destructed by separated PBL

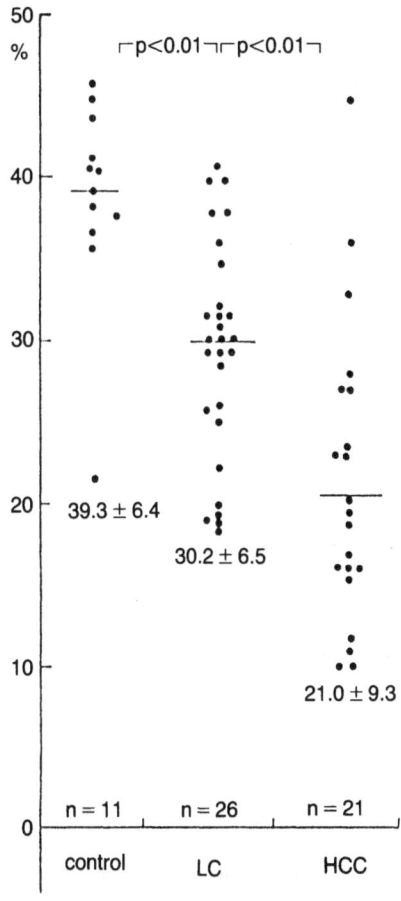

istered 12 MU/m^2 IM injection 3 times per week (low dose) for 12 weeks into 8 HCC patients, and 850 MU/m^2 IM injection 3 times per week (high dose) for the same period into the same number of patients, failed to show the expected effect of IFN. Yoshida et al. [13] treated 15 HCC patients with a high dose of recombinant IFN-γ (16–24 MU, IV injection for 5 consecutive days every 2 weeks) and could not demonstrate favorable effects, at least by the regimen employed. The results [14] of low-dose IFN-γ for HCC were also disappointed.

In conclusion, as this author [15] reviewed "The potential of interferons in malignant disease," and there were no positive reports concerning the usefulness of IFNs in HCC therapy, so far. However, the biological effects of IFNs will be very interesting from the viewpoints of neoplasia therapy as evidenced by us (Fig. 3) and by Dunk et al. [10], and thus the future of IFN therapy should be viewed with some optimism.

4 Adoptive immunotherapy

Adoptive immunotherapy will be one of the more exciting avenues for research of immunotherapy of HCC. Rosenstein et al. [16] demonstrated activation of lymphocytes after incubation with IL-2. In fact, Rosenberg et al. [17] showed that adoptive transfer of lymphokine-activated killer (LAK) cells and recombinant interleukin-2 could mediate regression of colorectal cancer.

In Japan, several institutions [18, 19, 20] have studied the usefulness of adoptive immunotherapy in HCC. Ohnishi et al. [20] treated 10 patients with HCC in very advanced stages, with adoptive immunotherapy using autologus lymphokine-activated killer cells plus recombinant IL-2. In their study, patients received 15 μg per day of recombinant IL-2 consecutively, from day 7 prior to the first leukapheresis, and received 10^9 to 10^{10} lymphokine-activated killer cells once or twice per week intra venously.

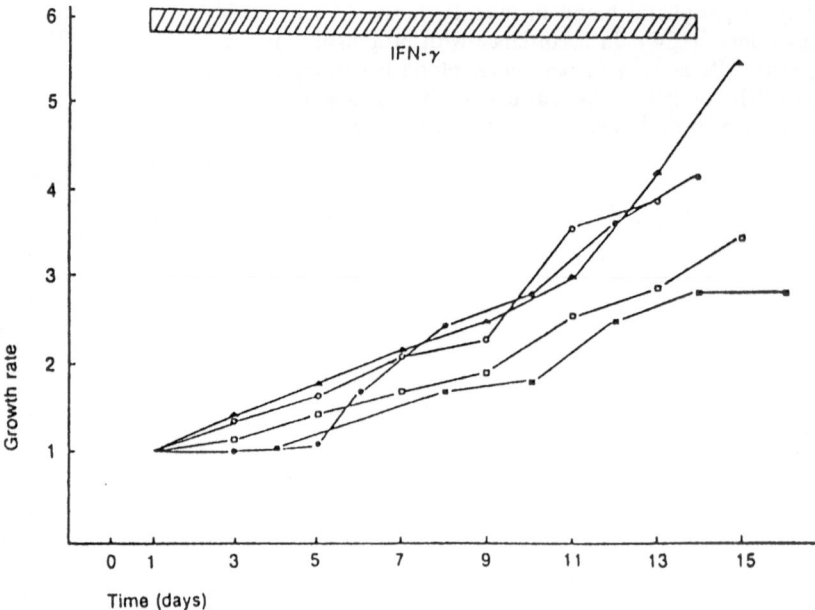

Fig. 3. Antigrowth effect of γ-IFN on human hepatoma cells transplanted into athymic mice. Antigrowth activity with γ-IFN was confirmed dose-dependently. Effect plotted for controls (▲), and mice administered γ-IFN, 1×10^4 IU (□), 1×10^5 IU (■), 2×10^4 IU (○), and 5×10^4 IU (●). Antigrowth activity with γ-IFN was confirmed dose-dependently. [Reproduced with permission from ADIS Press Limited]

By premedication of IL-2 prior to the first leukapheresis, a remarkable increase of lymphokine-activated killer activity was observed in seven out of nine cases in whom lymphokine-activated killer activity had been poorly inducible even at high concentrations of IL-2. However, as a result, they concluded that tumor regression due to adoptive immunotherapy could be expected in small-burden HCC, not in such advanced HCC as entered into their trial. On the other hand, Okuno et al. [18] administered LAK cells generated from autologous spleen cells via selective hepatic arterial infusion into the patients carrying unresectable HCC. Unlike Okuno et al. [18], Ishikawa et al. [19], and Ohnishi et al. [20], Gandolfi et al. [21] performed intratumor echo-guided injection of IL-2 and lymphokine-activated killer cells in HCC in application of echo-guided intralesional injection of ethanol in HCC, so-called percutaneous ethnol injection therapy (PEIT), which has been developed and distributed world wide [22, 23]. According to their experiences with 5 patients, tumor size remained unchanged in 3 of the 4 small HCC, and increased only slightly in the other (over a period of 10 months). As a result, they could not show any effectiveness of adoptive immunotherapy for tumor regression.

So far, there are no reports from Japan which support positively the usefulness of this immunotherapy in HCC, although transient effects such as temporary decrease of serum AFP levels and reduction of ascitic fluid after treatment have been noted.

5 Intratumoral injection of the BRM

5.1 IL-2

Adoptive immunotherapy has been disappointing in the treatment of HCC because of its poor therapeutic effect and the complicated procedures for preparation of LAK cells.

From this point of view, several investigators have treated HCC by means of echo-guided injection of IL-2 in high doses, and they observed an increase of NK and LAK cell activity in peripheral blood. Data reported are still preliminary and do not conclusively determine their efficacy as immunotherapy. However, if intralesional administration of IL-2 can bring expected therapeutic effect, as reported, it has the potential for widespread use because it is simpler than complicated adoptive immunotherapy.

5.2 OK-432

OK-432 is a BRM obtained from Su strain of *Streptococcus pyogenes* (Chugai Co., Tokyo) and composed of dried streptococcal cells containing penicillin G potassium. The mechanisms responsible for the antitumor effect of OK-432 are variable. Direct action on tumor cells and participation of neutrophils, macrophages, NK cells, T-lymphocytes and cytokines have all been reported [24].

The first report of intratumor injection of OK-432 in HCC was performed by Imaoka et al. [25] in 1982. Thereafter, several trials have been performed in the bearers of large HCC or multiple small HCC, but satisfactory results were only obtained occasionally.

Huang et al. [26] selected 7 inoperable patients will small HCC ($\phi < 3$ cm) and achieved total necrosis of the tumors in most cases. They concluded that intra-tumor injection of OK-432 is an alternative treatment for small HCC in operable cases and the effect may be due to the direct tumorcidal mechanism of OK-432.

In any case, a multi-center trial is absolutely necessary for evaluation of this therapy in a scientific manner because the Ministry of Health and Welfare in Japan denied recently the effectiveness of systemic administration of OK-432 in HCC.

6 Tumor necrosis factor

Tumor necrosis factor (TNF) is a macrophage secretory protein with antitumor activity [27]. TNF was first described in the serum of mice treated with BCG and bacterial endotoxin [28]. The serum from such animals contains a factor termed TNF which causes hemorrhagic necrosis of certain tumors growing intradermally in mice [28]. However, there is no reliable information concerning the usefulness of TNF in therapy of the malignant diseases, although severe adverse side effects such as pyrexia, hypotension, hematuria, and so on have been noted after administration of recombinant TNF. For the reasons mentioned above, TNF induction therapy based upon activation of macrophages in vivo has been designed instead of direct administration of TNF. In this therapy, at first, the patients bearing inoperable HCC took intracutaneous injection of a suboptimal dose of OK-432 (2–5KE) for priming, and thereafter were treated via selective hepatic arterial infusion with a large dose of OK-432 (10KE) emulsified with Lipiodol and stearate for elicitation. Fifteen patients were divided into 2 groups: group A is a control group and consists of patients in whom priming was never performed, and group B consists of patients for therapy in whom both priming and elicitation due to OK-432 were employed (Table 1). As shown in

Table 1. Subjects for TNF induction therapy

	Patient	Age	Sex	Tumor size (mm)	Priming	Elicitation
A	E.M.	75	M	45 × 50 (VP 1)[a]	(−)	10KE
	H.T.	68	M	10 × 10, 25 × 10 (VP 0)	(−)	10KE
	T.M.	44	M	180 × 150 (VP 2)	(−)	10KE
	M.H.	49	M	30 × 30 (VP 0)	(−)	10KE
	K.Y.	42	M	180 × 100 (VP 3)	(−)	10KE
	K.H.	62	F	35 × 35 (VP 0)	(−)	10KE
	E.I.	58	M	100 × 50, 15 × 15, 15 × 13 (VP 2)	(−)	10KE
	Z.A.	64	M	105 × 85 (VP 1)	(−)	10KE
	S.N.	68	F	150 × 150 (VP 3)	(−)	10KE
B	M.O.	54	M	23 × 20 (VP 0)	3KE	10KE
	I.O.	66	M	160 × 110 (VP 3)	2KE	10KE
	I.S.	60	M	80 × 80, 60 × 60 (VP 2)	5KE	10KE
	K.H.	56	M	180 × 150, 75 × 60, 65 × 55 (VP 2)	3KE	10KE
	K.Y.	76	M	70 × 68, 33 × 27 (VP 1)	2KE	10KE
	G.T.	58	M	70 × 60, 60 × 60, 35 × 30 (VP 1)	2KE	10KE

[a] Tumor thrombus visualized in portal vein is classified by the general rules accepted by Liver Cancer Study Group of Japan, as follows:
VP 0- no tumor thrombus until visualized 3rd–4th branch of portal vein
VP 1- tumor thrombus in 3rd–4th branch of portal vein
VP 2- tumor thrombus in 2nd branch of portal vein
VP 3- tumor thrombus in main trunk or 1st branch of portal vein

Table 2. Changes of GPT, LDH and AFP after Treatment

Item	Group	Before	1 day after	1 week after	4 weeks after
GPT	A	61.4 ± 40.4	111.7 ± 74.4	104.4 ± 123.7	n.d.[b]
	B	46.2 ± 25.4	232.0 ± 228.5	53.3 ± 18.0	n.d.
LDH	A	354.4 ± 163.2	523.2 ± 170.8	374.4 ± 202.1	n.d.
	B	424.0 ± 213.4	2442.6 ± 3332.3	432.8 ± 237.9	n.d.
AFP[a]	A	100%	n.d.	94 ± 12 (%)	93 ± 83 (%)
	B	100%	n.d.	47 ± 5 (%)	62 ± 72 (%)

[a] [mean value after treatment/mean value before treatment] × 100 (%)
[b] n.d. abbreviation for not determined
values are mean ±S.D.
AFP, alpha fetoprotein; GPT, glutamic pyruvate transaminase; LDH, lactate dehydrogenase

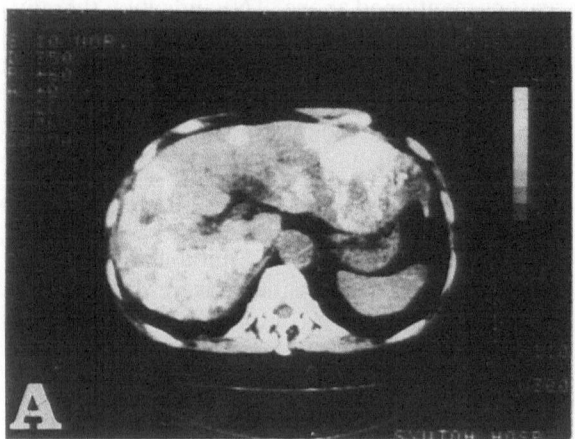
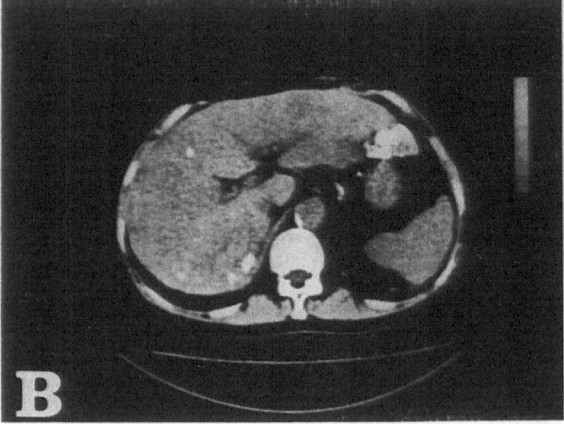

Fig. 4. Tumor regression after TNF induction therapy. Four months after TNF induction therapy, remarkable shrinkage of HCC was confirmed by CT. In parallel with tumor regression, serum AFP level returned to normal. **A** HCC indicated with pooling of Lipiodol occupies almost entire liver. At this time, his serum AFP level was 22,260 ng/ml. **B** CT taken at 4th month after TNF induction therapy reveals remarkable shrinkage of tumor size, as shown by the reduction of Lipiodol accumulated areas. Serum AFP level was reduced to 2.8 ng/ml

Table 2, liver function was impaired much more in group B, and decrease of AFP was also observed in this group as compared with group A. One example in whom a favorable therapeutic effect was observed is shown in Fig. 4. A Lipiodol-CT scan taken immediatly after treatment indicates remarkable accumulation of lipiodol in the entire liver, but the image after 4 months clearly shows reduction of the lesion. In parallel with tumor regression, the serum AFP level decreased from 22,260 ng/ml to 2.8 ng/ml. In this preliminary trial, temporary adverse effects such as pyrexia, hypotension and hematuria were observed, but were tolerable.

On the basis of our preliminary results, it seems that it is worthwhile to establish a dose of OK-432 for priming and elicitation or more suitable agent(s) for induction of TNF in vivo.

Therapy inducing TNF in vivo may be an alternative treatment for inoperable HCC.

7 Radioimmunotherapy

There has been increased interest in radioimmunotherapy using radiolabelled antibodies, polyclonal or monoclonal, for the treatment of human cancer in recent years. However, there are no conclusive reports concerning this therapy in Japan to date.

Liu et al. [29] started radioimmunotherapy for the patients with HCC using ^{131}I-labelled antibody against α-fetoprotein(^{131}I-anti-AFP). They treated 11 patients by perfusion via arterial catheters with ^{131}I-anti-AFP. Tumor regression was observed in 8 patients who received radioimmunotherapy. They concluded that the attack by ^{131}I-anti-AFP induces some change in the biological behavior of the malignant cells so that they became more sensitive to conventional chemotherapeutic agents.

Tang et al. [30] treated 25 patients with surgically proven nonresectable and pathologically proven HCC by radioimmunotherapy using ^{131}I-anti-human HCC isoferritin IgG(^{131}I-isoFtAb) intrahepatic arterial infusion as a part of multimodality treatment. Of the 25 patients, seven (28.0%) received second-look resection after marked shrinkage of the tumor. Of the five patients with 2-year survival in their series, four were in the second-look resection group. Thus, they concluded that radioimmunotherapy using ^{131}I-isoFtAb might be one of the modalities of choice, particularly in the conversion of nonresectable to resectable HCC in a well-designed multimodality treatment regimen.

Radioimmunotherapy investigation to date has focused on tumor regression or life-prolongation based upon a double attack, immunological and radiological, on the cancer. Further investigation regarding immunomodulation in vivo with this therapy should be performed in order to evaluate radioimmunotherapy.

8 Conclusion

In this chapter, the present situation of immunotherapy of HCC was discussed. In general, immunotherapy is very attractive from the aspect of tumor immunology. Unfortunately, there are no conclusive reports indicating a favorable effect of immunotherapy on HCC, however, there were some exceptions where it brought remarkable tumor regression. Therefore, each type of immunotherapy discussed here should be evaluated by a randomized well-controlled trial to obtain more objective results. Otherwise, immunotherapy will not receive support from clinical oncologists interested in HCC therapy.

References

1. Yamada R, Sato M, Kawabata M, Nakatsuka H, Nakamura K, Takashima S (1983) Hepatic artery embolization in 120 patients with unresectable hepatoma. Radiology 148:397–401
2. Kanematsu T, Inokuchi K, Sugimachi K, Furuta T, Sonoda T, Tamura S, Hasuno K (1984) Selective effects of lipiodolized antitumor agents. J Surg Oncol 25:218–226
3. Shinagawa T, Ukaji H, Iino Y, Isomura S, Yamaguchi H, Ishizuka M, Sugiura N, Ohto M (1985) Intratumoral injection of absolute ethanol under ultrasound imaging for treatment of small hepatocellular carcinoma. Attempts in three cases. Acta Hepatol Jpn 26:99–105
4. Hirofuji H, Kakumu S, Fuji A, Ohtani Y, Murase K, Tahara H (1987) Natural killer and activated killer activities in chronic liver diseases and hepatocellular carcinoma: Evidence for a decreased lymphokine-induced activity of effector cells. Clin Exp Immunol 68:348–356
5. Saibara T, Ohnishi S, Sakaeda H, Yamamoto Y (1989) Defective function of lymphokine-activated killer cells and natural killer cells in patients with hepatocellular carcinoma. Hepatology 9:471–476
6. Sinkovics J (1978) Immunotherapy of human tumors. Pathobiol Ann 8:241–273
7. Trinchieri G, Sourtoli D, Kopronski H (1978) Spontaneous cell mediated cytotoxicity in humans: Role of interferon and immunoglobulins. J Immunol 120:1849–1855
8. Henry CS, Karibayashi K, Kern DE, Gillis S (1981) Interleukin-2 augments natural killer cytotoxicity. Nature 291:335–338
9. Grimm EA, Mazumder A, Zhang HZ, Rosenberg SA (1982) Lymphokine-activated killer cell phenomenon. Lysis of natural killer-resistant fresh solid tumor cells by interleukin-2-activated autologous human peripheral blood lymphocytes. J Exp Med 155:1823–1841
10. Dunk AA, Ikeda T, Pignatelli M, Thomas HC (1986) Human lymphoblastoid interferon: In vivo and in vitro studies in hepatocellular carcinoma. J Hepatol 2:419–429
11. Isaacs A, Lindermann J (1957) Virus interference. The interferon. Proc R Soc Lond [Biol] 147:259–267
12. Sachs E, Di Bisceglie AM, Dusheiko GM, Song E, Lyons SF, Schoub BD, Kew MC (1985) Treatment of hepatocellular carcinoma with recombinant leukocyte interferon: A pilot study. Br J Cancer 52:105–109
13. Yoshida T, Okazaki N, Yoshino M, Ohkura H, Shimada Y (1990) Phase II trial of high dose recombinant gamma-interferon in advanced hepatocellular carcinoma. Eur J Cancer 26:545–546

14. Forbes A, Johnson DJ, William R (1985) Recombinant human gamma-interferon in primary hepatocellular carcinoma. J R Soc Med 78: 826–829

15. Okita K, Kaneko T (1990) The potential of interferon in malignant disease. Drugs 39:1–6

16. Rosenstein N, Yron I, Kaufmann Y, Rosenberg SA (1984) Lymphokine-activated killer cell lysis of fresh syngenic natural killer-resistant murine tumor cells by lymphocytes cultured in interleukin-2. Cancer Res 44:1946–1953

17. Rosenberg S, Lotze M, Muul L, Leitman S, Chang AE, Ettinghausen SE, Matory YL, Skibber JM, Shiloni E, Vetto JT, Seipp LA, Simpon C, Reichter LM (1985) Observations on the systemic administration of autologous lymphokine-activated killer cells and recombinant interleukin-2 to patients with metastatic cancer. N Engl J Med 313:1485–1492

18. Okuno K, Takagi H, Nakamura T, Nakamura Y, Iwase Z, Yasutomi M (1986) Treatment for unresectable hepatoma via selective hepatic artery infusion of lymphokine-activated killer cells generated from autologous spleen cells. Cancer 58:1001–1006

19. Ishikawa T, Imawari M, Moriyama T, Ohnishi S, Matsuhashi N, Suzuki G, Takaku F (1988) Immunotherapy of hepatocellular carcinoma with autologous lymphokine-activated killer cells and/or recombinant interleukin-2. J Cancer Res Clin Oncol 114:283–290

20. Ohnishi S, Saibara T, Fujikawa M, Sakaeda H, Matsuura Y, Matsunaga Y, Yamamoto Y (1989) Adoptive immunotherapy with lymphokine-activated killer cells plus recombinant interleukin-2 in patients with unresectable hepatocellular carcinoma. Hepatology 10:349–353

21. Gandolfi L, Solmi L, Pizza GC, Berfoni F, Muratoori R, De Vinci C, Bacchini P, Morelli MC, Corrado G (1989) Intratumoral echo-guided injection of interleukin-2 and lymphokine-activated

killer cells in hepatocellular carcinoma. Hepatogastroenterology 36:352–356

22. Livraghi T, Festi D, Monti F, Salmi A, Vettori C (1986) US-guided percutaneous alcohol injection of small hepatic and abdominal tumors. Radiology 16:309–312

23. Sheu J-C, Huang G-T, Chen D-S, Sung J-L, Yang P-M, Lin T C-T, Chuang C-N (1987) Small hepatocellular carcinoma: Intratumor ethanol treatment using new needle and guidance systems. Radiology 163:43–48

24. Ishida N (1986) Immunopotentiating activities of OK-432. In: Ishida N (ed) OK-432: Recent advances in the understanding of its mechanism of action. Excerpta Medica, Amsterdam, pp 41–84

25. Imaoka S, Sasaki Y, Ishikawa O, Ouhigashi H, Koyama H, Iwanaga T, Terasawa T (1986) Immunochemotherapy in human hepatocellular carcinoma using the streptococcal agent OK-432. J Clin Oncol 4:1645–1651

26. Huang G-T, Yang P-M, Sheu J-C, Hsu J-L, Sung J-L, Wang T-H, Chen D-C (1990) Intratumoral injection of OK-432 for the treatment of small hepatocellular carcinoma. Hepatogastroenterology 37:452–456

27. Old LJ (1985) Tumor necrosis factor. Science 230:630–632

28. Carswell EA, Old LJ, Kassel RL, Green S, Fiore N, Williamson B (1975) An endotoxin-induced serum factor that causes necrosis of tumors. Proc Natl Acad Sci USA 72:3666–3670

29. Liu Y-K, Yang K-Z, Wu Y-D, Gang Y-Q, Zhu D-N (1983) Treatment of advanced primary hepatocellular carcinoma by ^{131}I-anti AFP. Lancet I:531–532

30. Tang Z-Y, Liu K-D, Bao Y-M, Lu J-Z, Yu Y-Q, Chen Z-C, Zhou X-D, Yang R, Gan Y-H, Lin Z-Y, Fan Z, Hou Z (1990) Radioimmunotherapy in the multi-modality treatment of hepatocellular carcinoma with reference to second-look resection. Cancer 65:211–215

CHAPTER 31

Radiofrequency hyperthermia and radiotherapy for hepatocellular carcinoma

Yasushi Nagata, Mitsuyuki Abe, Masahiro Hiraoka, Shinitirou Masunaga, Keizo Akuta, Yasumasa Nishimura, Masaji Takahashi, Shiken Jo, and Mototsugu Koishi[1]

1 Introduction

Malignant liver tumors can be classified into three types: hepatocellular carcinoma (HCC), cholangiocarcinoma, and metastatic tumors. HCC can be further divided into three subtypes: massive, nodular, and diffuse. Most patients with liver tumors are not good candidates for surgical treatment and many chemotherapy regimens do not show good results in these patients. At Kyoto University Hospital, radiofrequency (RF) capacitive heating equipment has been used since 1979 for the treatment of deep-seated tumors [1, 2], and since 1983 we have applied it to liver tumors. Here we report the clinical results of thermotherapy for HCC.

2 Materials

One-hundred and thirty-seven patients with malignant liver tumors treated between 1983 and 1990 were enrolled in this study. The diagnosis was established by computed tomography (CT), angiography, ultrasound, serum tumor markers, and biopsy as was necessary. The 137 tumors consisted of 88 HCCs, 11 cholangiocarcinomas, and 38 metastatic liver tumors. In 78 patients (59%), the intratumor temperature was monitored during hyperthermia and more than 4 sessions of hyperthermia treatment were performed. We evaluated the thermometry data and clinical effects of hyperthermia on these 78 patients. The ages of the patients ranged from 22 to 83. Sixty-five patients (82%) were men and 13 (18%) were

women. The 78 tumors consisted of 44 HCCs, 6 cholangiocarcinomas, and 28 metastatic tumors. Primary lesions were colon carcinoma in 14 cases, gastric cancer in 5, pancreatic and thymic cancer in 2, and tumors of the soft tissue, ureter, gall bladder, lung, parotid, and uterus in one case each. Intratumor temperatures could not be measured in 57 patients because of the following reasons: Poor liver function with a bleeding tendency in 31 cases (54%), inaccessible tumor location in 6 cases (11%), massive ascites in 7 cases (12%), and patient refusal in 13 cases (23%). Twenty-three of the 137 tumors were treated less than 4 times. In 16 of those cases (70%) this was due to the poor general condition of the patient, while severe thermal pain was responsible in 5 cases (22%) and other complications in the remaining 2 cases (9%).

3 Methods

3.1 Hyperthermia technique

Radiofrequency capacitive heating equipment (8 MHz; Thermotron RF-8; Yamamoto Vinyter Co. Ltd., Osaka, Japan) was used for hyperthermia. Two opposing 25-cm electrodes were generally selected for heating liver tumors. The electrodes were covered with a water, pad, and a saline solution maintained at 5°C was perfused through the pads to avoid excessive heating of the skin and subcutaneous fat. Heat was then applied through a pair of electrodes placed on opposite sides of the liver, mostly in the anteroposterior direction and sometimes in the lateral direction. Furthermore, an overlay water bolus was placed under the electrode to eliminate the edge effect. The power which could be endured by the

[1] Department of Radiology, Faculty of Medicine, Kyoto University, Kyoto, 606 Japan

patients was in most cases between 800 W and 1,300 W. Our standard treatment protocol was to administer hyperthermia for at least 40 minutes twice a week for a total of 8 sessions. Some patients received two or three sessions of treatment. Blood pressure and pulse rate were monitored every 5 minutes during hyperthermia, and body temperature was measured before and after treatment.

3.2 Temperature measurement

Temperatures were measured using thin Teflon-coated copper-constantan microthermocouples (Sensortek, Clifton, NJ, USA). The microthermocouple was inserted into the tumor from the skin surface through a 21 G angiocatheter under ultrasonic guidance. Catheters 15 to 20 cm in length were inserted through the normal liver as deeply into the tumor as possible. The position of the catheter was checked by computed tomography after treatment. During and immediately after treatment, the probe was withdrawn in 1-cm increments, and the temperature was measured at each point through the catheter. When the radiofrequency apparatus interfered with the temperature measurement, it was performed after the power was switched off. In this study, we defined the maximum intratumor temperature as the maximum temperature recorded in the tumor during treatment and the average maximum tumor temperature (T_{max}) as the average of the maximum tumor temperatures for each treatment session. Likewise, the minimum tumor temperature was defined as the minimum temperature recorded in the tumor and the average minimum tumor temperature (T_{min}) as the average of the minimum tumor temperatures.

3.3 Combination therapy

Transcatheter arterial embolization (TAE), radiotherapy, and chemotherapy were combined with hyperthermia according to the patient's liver function and tumor location.

When intra-arterial catheterization of the hepatic artery was possible, we performed TAE with gelatin sponge particles or degradable starch microsphere (DSM) before hyperthermia. Continuous intra-arterial infusion therapy was performed through a catheter operatively inserted via the superficial circumflex iliac artery

[3]. We generally commenced hyperthermia 10 to 14 days after TAE or arterial infusion therapy.

For tumors located in the lateral or posterior segment for which TAE was not indicated, we used radiotherapy combined with hyperthermia. Radiotherapy was administered with 10 MV X-rays using a linear accelerator. The dose was 1.8 Gy daily and 5 sessions a week were performed to give a total dose of 50 to 60 Gy. Hyperthermia was administered twice a week immediately after radiotherapy. We minimized the irradiated volume as much as possible to spare the normal liver tissue using a three-dimensional (3-D) treatment planning machine [4].

Patients with poor liver function who were not suitable for TAE or radiotherapy were given intravenous doxorubicin (20 mg) and/or the immunopotentiator OK-432 (2 KE) before each hyperthermia session.

3.4 Therapeutic efficacy

The therapeutic efficacy was evaluated by the change in tumor size assessed by computed tomography three or four months after the completion of treatment. A complete response (CR) was defined as the complete disappearance of a tumor. A partial response (PR) was 50–99% tumor regression; while no response (NR) was between 50% tumor regression and 25% tumor progression. Progression (P) was defined as a more than 25% increase in tumor size. Serum alpha-fetoprotein (AFP) levels were monitored every week during treatment.

4 Results

Thermal parameters were evaluated for all liver tumors, and therapeutic efficacy was evaluated only for HCC.

4.1 Factors affecting tumor thermal profiles.

4.1.1 Tumor type
We compared T_{max} and T_{min} among HCC, cholangiocarcinoma, and metastatic liver tumors as shown in Fig. 1. There was a wide variation of T_{max} between and within the different tumor types. The average T_{max} was over 42°C for diffuse

Fig. 1. The maximum tumor temperature according to the various tumor types. Cholangiocarcinoma and metastatic liver tumors showed higher tumor temperatures than HCC. Among HCC, the diffuse type showed higher temperatures than the other types

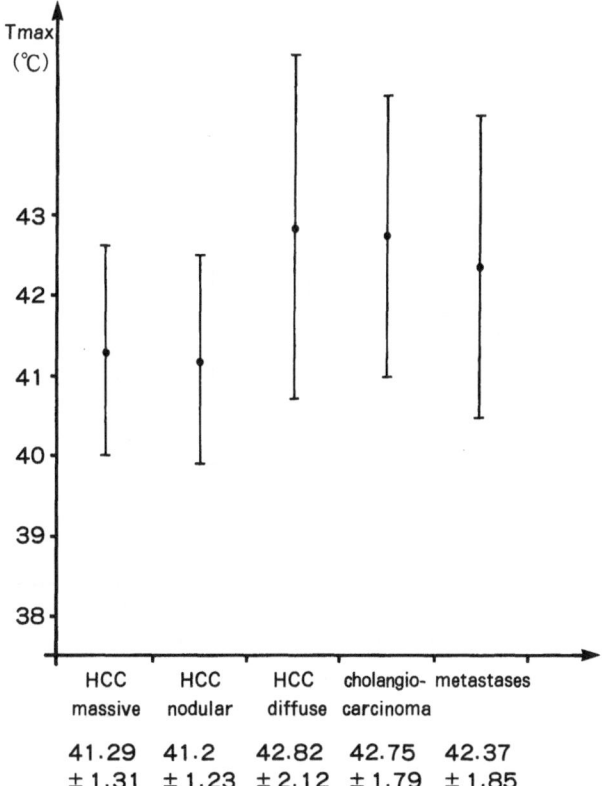

	HCC massive	HCC nodular	HCC diffuse	cholangio-carcinoma	metastases
	41.29 ±1.31	41.2 ±1.23	42.82 ±2.12	42.75 ±1.79	42.37 ±1.85

HCC, cholangiocarcinoma, and metastatic liver tumors, while it was below 41.5°C for massive and nodular HCC. The relationship between T_{min} and tumor type is shown in Fig. 2. We attained a T_{min} above 40.5°C only in metastatic liver tumors.

4.1.2 Tumor volume
The relationship between thermal parameters and tumor volume (assessed from multiple CT slices), was analyzed for 33 HCCs. The maximum tumor temperature did not show any correlation with the tumor volume. Figure 3 shows the relationship of T_{min} to tumor volume. An inverse relationship was noted between the tumor volume and T_{min}.

4.1.3 CT number
The tumor CT number was calculated by averaging multiple CT slices and we then compared the maximum and minimum tumor temperatures with the average CT numbers of 25 tumors. Figure 4 shows the relationship between the maximum tumor temperature and the CT number, with a significant inverse correlation being evident ($P < 0.05/2$). The CT number and the minimum tumor temperature showed a similar relationship but the correlation was not significant.

4.1.4 Temperatures of normal liver (T_{liver}) and subcutaneous fat (T_{fat})
Table 1 summarizes the thermal distributions obtained from 23 HCC patients in whom the temperature data for the normal liver, subcutaneous fat, and tumor (T_{max} and T_{min}) were complete. The T_{liver} was not higher than 41.5°C and the average T_{liver} was 39.8°C. T_{max} was higher than T_{liver} in 20 of the 23 patients, while T_{min} was higher than T_{liver} in 15 cases. The average T_{fat} was 0.3°C higher than the T_{min}. The thickness of the subcutaneous fat was measured by CT scanning at the level of the xiphoid process of the sternum. Most of the patients whose subcutaneous fat thickness exceeded 15 mm could not tolerance more than 4 sessions of hyperthermia and were not enrolled in this study.

4.2 Toxicity

We compared the average blood pressures before and after treatment, with average blood pressure being defined as the lowest blood pressure plus one third of the pressure difference. As seen in Fig. 5, about half the patients showed pressure

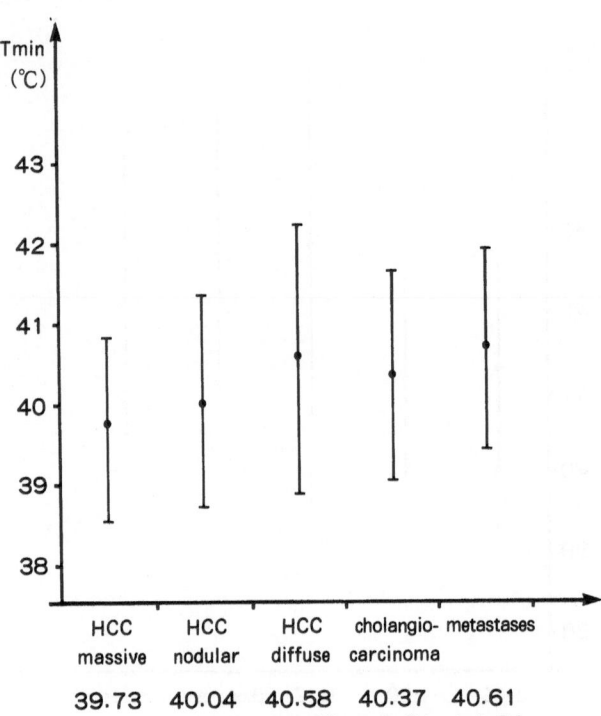

Fig. 2. The minimum tumor temperature according to the various tumor types. Cholangiocarcinoma, metastatic liver tumors, and diffuse HCC showed higher minimum temperatures

HCC massive	HCC nodular	HCC diffuse	cholangio-carcinoma	metastases
39.73 ± 1.13	40.04 ± 1.34	40.58 ± 1.63	40.37 ± 1.21	40.61 ± 1.24

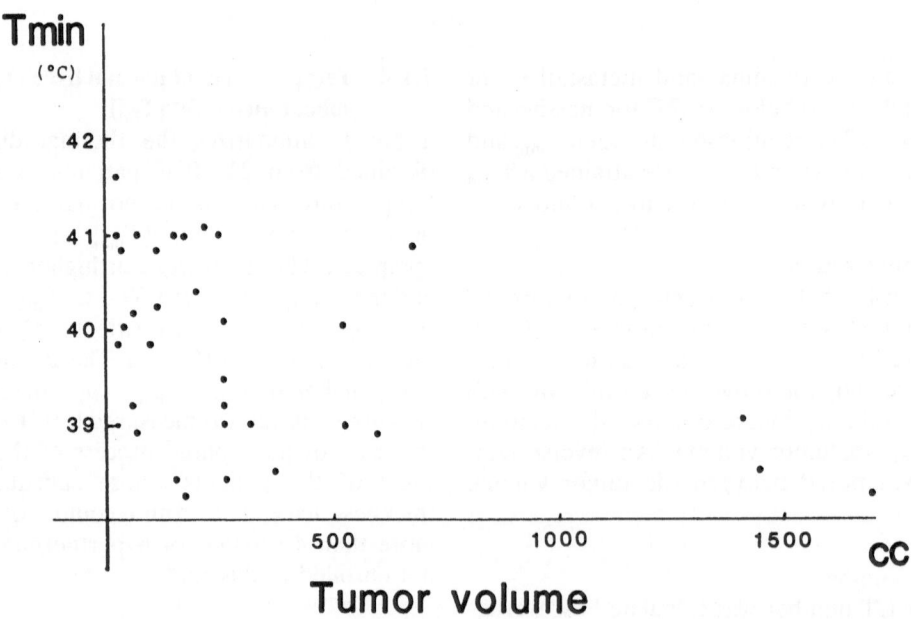

Fig. 3. The relationship between minimum tumor temperature and tumor volume

elevations and half showed decreases. Changes in blood pressure developed quite slowly.

Most patients showed a marked increase in the pulse rate. Figure 6 shows the changes in the pulse rate. The average increase was 15.5 beats/min. A few patients complained of palpitations, which were reduced by lowering the RF power.

Most patients developed sweating during and after hyperthermia. The body temperature eleva-

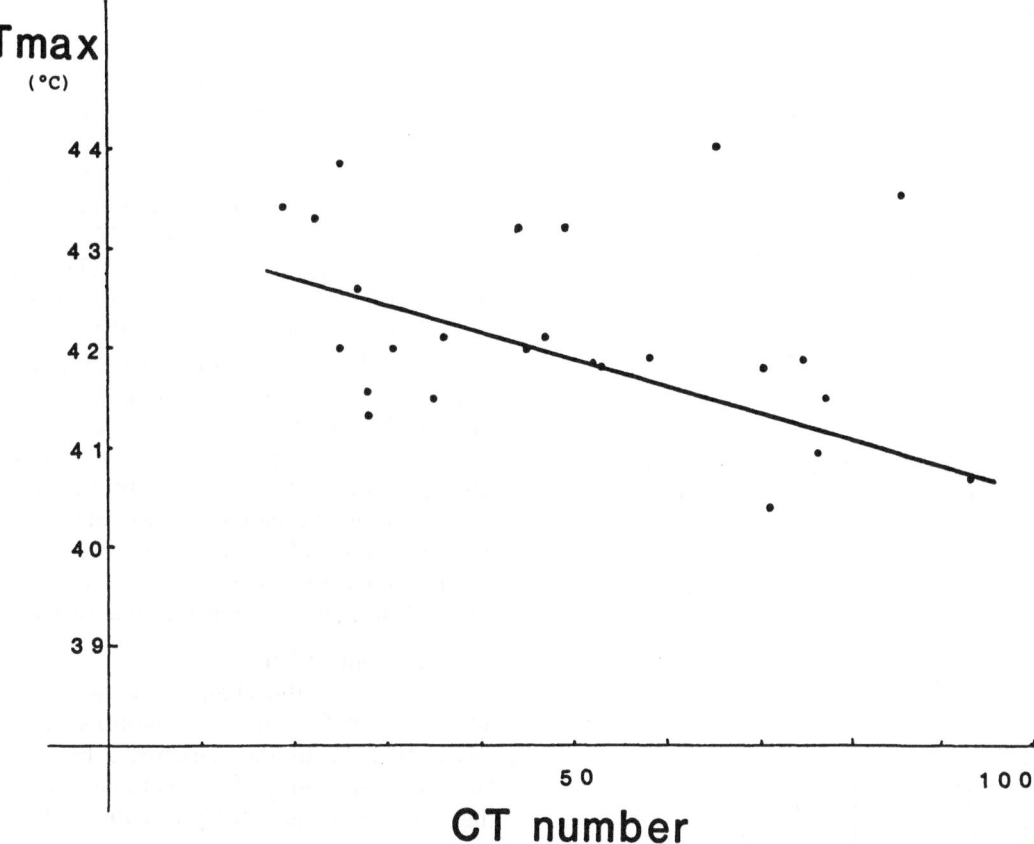

Fig. 4. The relationship between maximum tumor temperature and CT number

Table 1. Thermal distribution of the tumor, normal liver, and subcutaneous fat

Tumor	case no.	T_{max}	T_{min}	Normal liver	Subcutaneous fat	Fat thickness (mm)
H.C.C	1.	43.2°C	41.4°C	40.9°C	41.0°C	3
	2.	39.6	39.4	39.8	41.0	10
	3.	43.4	42.0	41.1	40.2	8
	4.	43.6	41.1	41.4	39.5	3
	5.	41.2	39.8	40.1	41.1	8
	6.	41.5	40.1	38.2	39.3	12
	7.	41.5	40.8	40.1	40.7	5
	8.	42.0	40.4	39.6	38.2	5
	9.	41.0	39.5	39.1	38.4	4
	10.	40.5	39.8	40.1	40.2	12
	11.	41.8	41.0	39.5	41.6	6
	12.	39.9	39.0	40.1	40.6	5
	13.	39.2	38.2	39.5	40.4	10
	14.	39.7	39.2	39.7	40.0	5
	15.	39.4	38.9	38.5	40.3	15
	16.	41.6	40.9	40.5	40.5	7
	17.	40.2	39.0	38.9	41.4	9
	18.	40.8	39.1	38.9	38.7	3
	19.	42.1	41.1	38.6	39.7	7
	20.	42.5	41.0	41.0	40.8	9
	21.	42.0	40.5	40.0	41.0	5
	22.	42.8	41.8	41.0	40.5	5
	23.	39.2	38.9	38.6	41.6	8
Average		41.2	40.1	39.8	40.4	8

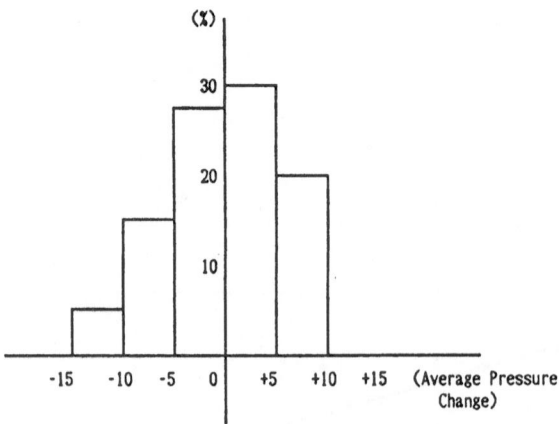

Fig. 5. The average change in blood pressure after treatment (n = 48)

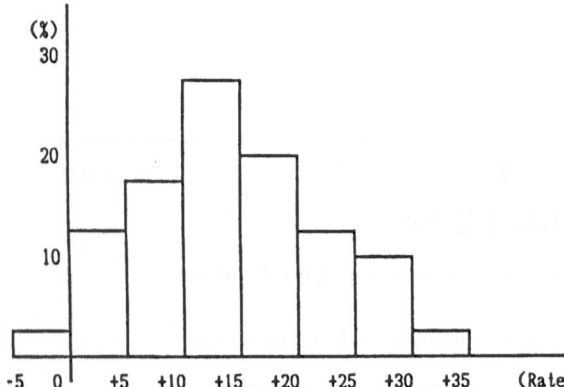

Fig. 6. Changes in pulse rate after treatment (n = 48)

tion was by 0.0 to 3.0°C/(1.1 ± 0.88°C; mean ±SD) immediately after treatment, and decreased again within an hour.

Slight to moderate pain or a mild sensation of heat was noted by every patient. Subacute or chronic complications appeared in 40% of the patients, which limited the number of treatment sessions. Local fat necrosis was the most common side effect to appear during hyperthermia treatment in 15 out of 80 patients (19%), with all cases resolving within 2 months. Transient local pain appeared after treatment in association with the tumor thermometry site in 7 patients (9%), but it resolved within a few hours with analgesics. Intraperitoneal hematoma was detected by CT in 1 patient (1%) and was ameliorated following blood transfusion. Gastric ulcers developed in 4 patients (5%) after treatment.

4.3 Therapeutic efficacy

4.3.1 Local response (Table 2)
Of the 45 HCCs, 11 were treated by hyperthermia in combination with TAE. Two of these showed CR, 3 showed PR, and 6 showed NR. Of the 8 tumors treated by thermoradiotherapy, 6 showed PR and 2 showed NR. Finally, 26 tumors were treated by thermochemotherapy: 6 showed CR, 2 showed PR, 14 showed NR and 4 showed P. Overall, the efficacy rate (CR + PR) was 42% for HCC. Table 3 shows the local response with respect to the minimum tumor temperature. Tumors heated to less than 40°C showed the worst response. Figure 7 shows the cumulative survival rate for HCC treated by hyperthermia. The one-year cumulative survival rate was 49.7%. The median duration of response was 12 months and the longest survival was 92 months, with this patient still being alive at the time of writing.

4.3.2 Serum AFP levels
Figure 8 shows the changes in the serum AFP level from before to three months after treatment. In 83% of the patients, AFP levels decreased immediately after treatment, and in 77% they remained below the pretreatment level after three months.

4.3.3 CT findings
Figure 9 shows the typical CT appearance of HCC before and after thermochemotherapy. The low density area in the tumor before hyperthermia decreased in size at 3 months after treatment, and then disappeared. Atrophic changes appeared in the surrounding normal liver parenchyma after a year. The portal tumor thrombus also disappeared after treatment. Most responders showed findings similar to this case.

5 Discussion

There are several clinical reports on hyperthermia as a treatment for liver tumors [5–7]. Few of them, however, have described any substantial thermometry data. The present study determined the thermal data for liver tumors treated by an 8 MHz RF capacitive heating device.

The average intratumor temperature of HCC was lower than that of cholangiocarcinoma and metastatic tumors. It is generally agreed that blood flow is very influential with regard to temperature elevation. Since HCC has been reported

Table 2. Local response of the tumors according to the type of combination therapy used

	Embolization	Radiotherapy	Chemotherapy	Total
CR	2/11 (18%)	0	6/26 (23%)	8/45 (18%)
PR	3/11 (27%)	6/8 (75%)	2/26 (8%)	11/45 (24%)
NC	6/11 (55%)	2/8 (25%)	14/26 (54%)	22/45 (49%)
P	0	0	4/26 (15%)	4/45 (9%)
	11	8	26	45

Table 3. Local response of the tumors according to the tumor minimum temperature

(°C)

HCC	≧42	≧41	≧40	40>
CR	1	2	3	1
PR	1	2	3	3
NR.P	0	3	6	20

to be more hypervascular than other tumors [8, 9], the cooling effect of its higher blood flow probably explains our results [10, 11]. Also, diffuse HCC is considered to be less vascular than the other types, explaining why diffuse HCCs were better responders to heat than the other types of HCC.

Experimental studies have indicated that the tumor temperature is more readily elevated after TAE [12, 13] due to a decrease in the arterial flow. However, our clinical experience of treating recurrent tumors after TAE (mostly several months after TAE) is that they could not be heated to a high temperature. Recanalization of the tumor vasculature occurring several days after TAE may be responsible for this effect. Thus, hyperthermia should be administered promptly after TAE.

Liver tumors are usually surrounded by normal liver tissue which is abundant in vascularity. The difference between the tumor temperature and the normal liver temperature is not large, as shown in Table 1. Presumably, the tumor temperature, and especially that at the tumor periphery, is greatly affected by the surrounding normal liver temperature. Therefore, a decrease in the vascularity of not only the tumor tissue but also of the normal liver may be necessary to achieve effective heating of the whole tumor.

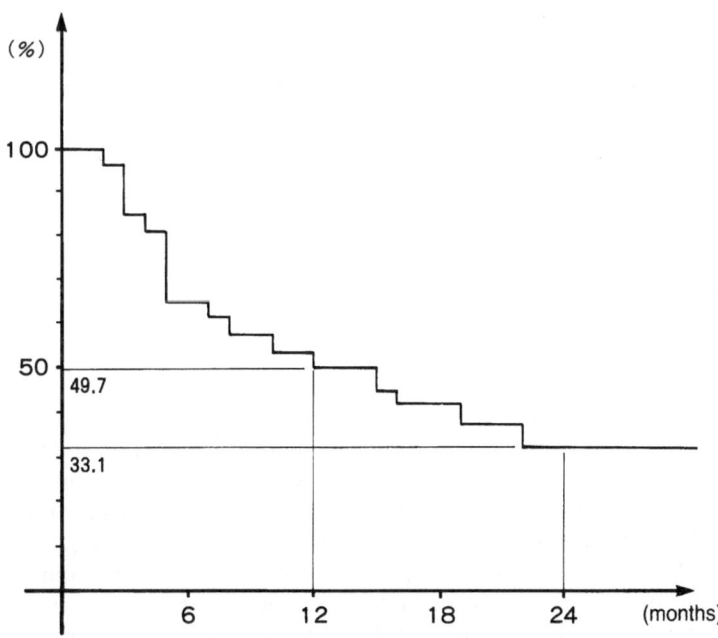

Fig. 7. Cumulative survival rates of hepatocellular carcinoma patients treated by hyperthermia

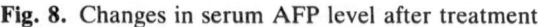

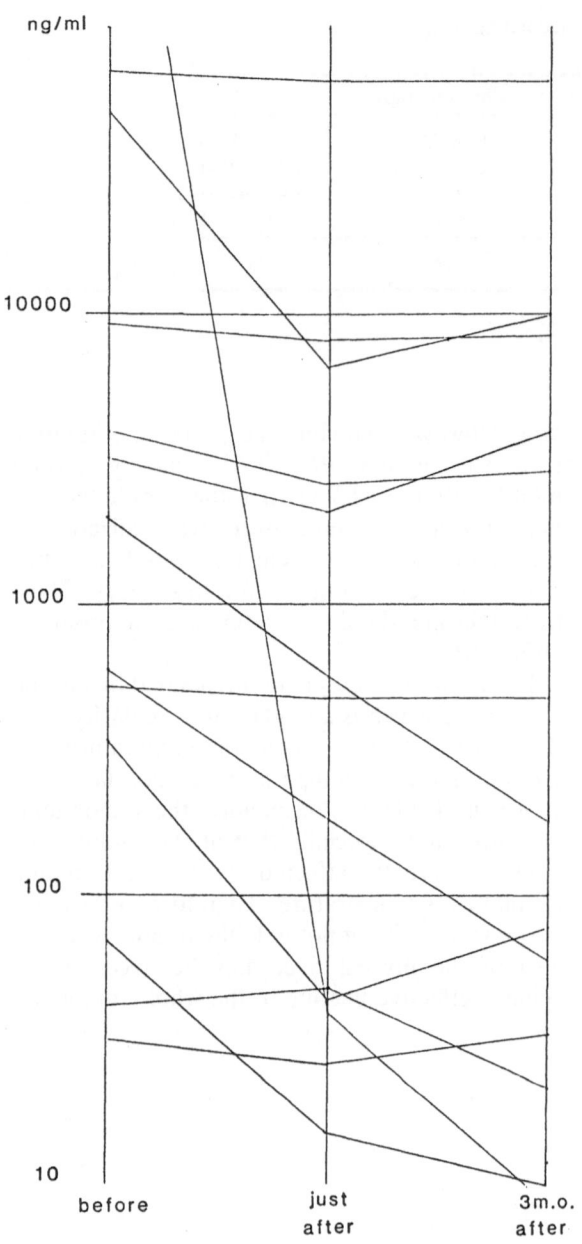

Fig. 8. Changes in serum AFP level after treatment

Tumor size is also an important factor in hyperthermia. The minimum tumor temperature was lower in tumors that were over 500 cm³ in volume when compared to that in smaller lesions. Such large tumors are thought to consist of heterogeneous components, and the tumor periphery adjacent to the normal liver tissue, where therapeutic temperatures are difficult to achieve, also makes up a large portion of such tumors. Accordingly, some form of combination therapy is required to achieve a uniform thermal distribution in these lesions.

The relationship between the CT number and T_{max} was also assessed. Tumors with a low CT

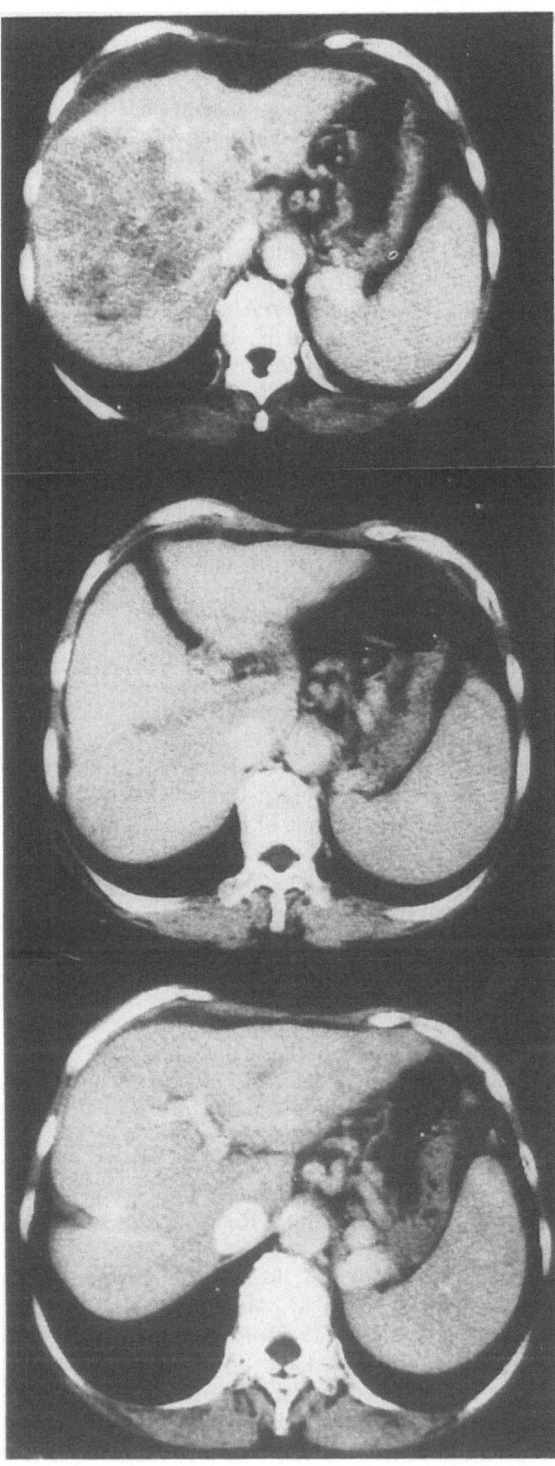

Fig. 9. Typical findings of HCC after hyperthermia by CT. *Upper* Before hyperthermia. Diffuse HCC with a portal thrombus could be seen. *Middle* 3 months after hyperthermia. The low density tumor disappeared and was more enhanced than the surrounding normal liver. *Lower* 36 months after hyperthermia. The area of the previous tumor was atrophic

number were more readily heated, so the CT number seems to be potentially useful as an indicator to predict the degree of temperature elevation of a tumor. Tumors with low CT numbers are considered to be necrotic and to have abundant fatty or fluid-filled compartments. Methods to lower the CT number, such as TAE or direct alcohol injection, might be useful in increasing the heating efficiency of hyperthermia.

It should be mentioned that the method of thermometry used in this study was inadequate, the major reason being the difficulty of achieving the frequent and complete insertion of the thermometers into the tumors. Moreover, the thermal profiles presented did not cover the whole tumor. Non-invasive thermometry methods using CT or ultrasound are definitely needed to improve hyperthermia, but the development of the methods is far from satisfactory.

The general condition of each patient was carefully monitored during hyperthermia. The blood pressure response to hyperthermia differed greatly from one patient to another, although almost all patients showed some similar changes during treatment. In particular, an increase in the pulse rate was usually observed though no significant cardiac complications appeared. Moreover, the increase in body temperature was not dangerous either during or after hyperthermia treatment.

The histopathological effect of hyperthermia on the liver was shown to include damage to the hepatocytes and central veins [14]. Hyperthermia caused bleeding and congestion within the normal liver tissue in the early stage, with fibrosis appearing one month after hyperthermic treatment. The CT changes after hyperthermia can be summarized as follows: The density of the tumor and the normal liver increased immediately after hyperthermia, especially on contrast-enhanced scans. After a few months, the tumor and the surrounding normal liver decreased in size due to fibrosis. These changes coincided very well with the histopathological findings.

On the other hand, radiation also affected the hepatocytes and central veins and evoked congestive changes in the liver. CT findings after radiation were similar to those of venooclusive disease [15]. Therefore, the CT changes of the tumor and surrounding normal liver after hyperthermia were quite similar to those after radiation, suggesting that the effects of hyperthermia and radiation on the liver and the tumor were quite similar.

Radiation therapy can be a useful modality for inoperable liver tumors and for Portal thrombi. However, the tolerance dose of the liver preventing radiation hepatitis is 25–30 Gy. Unfortunately, more than 50 Gy must be administered as a curative dose for liver tumors. Therefore, the radiation field for liver tumors must be limited to a localized small size. Using the 3-D treatment planning system, the treatment volume can be established in an adequate size. The high linear energy transfer (LET) beam, such as a proton beam, is also a good treatment modality for liver tumor. Because of its Bragg peak, the treatment volume or the liver can be small. The treatment result of the proton beam is promising.

Radioisotope can be used for the treatment of HCC. Lipiodol combined with 15–20 mCi of I-131 administered through the hepatic artery is an effective treatment method. About 70–80 Gy can be irradiated within the tumor. Kusumoto et al. [16] reported that 100% of the 20 cases decreased in size.

Radioimmunotherapy proposed by S.E. Order et al. [17] is also an effective method. Forty-eight percent of the 105 tumors decreased in size. However, because the antibody was made from canine and rabbit serum, an allergic reaction was evoked in some cases. To irradiate the tumor with more than 50 Gy, high doses of more than 150–200 mCi of I-131 must be administered.

When CT could not be used for evaluation of therapeutic efficacy, positron emission tomography (PET) with 18F-2-fluorodeoxyglucose (FDG) were sometimes utilized as a functional imaging modality. Of the 17 tumors in which FDG-PET was performed before and after treatment, the change of tumor FDG uptake correlated well with the tumor markers [18].

The number of patients treated was too small to draw a definite conclusion about the therapeutic effects of hyperthermia [19], although some patients did show a dramatic response to this treatment. Furthermore, the response rate of HCC treated by thermoradiotherapy (85%) was quite high. Further clinical trials of hyperthermia for liver tumors definitely appear to be warranted.

References

1. Hiraoka M, Jo S, Dodo Y, Ono K, Takahashi M, Nishida H, Abe M (1984) Clinical results of radiofrequency hyperthermia combined with radiation in the treatment of radioresistant cancers. Cancer 54:2898–2904

2. Abe M, Hiraoka M, Takahashi M, et al. (1986) Multi-institutional studies on hyperthermia using an 8-MHz radiofrequency capacitive heating device (Thermotron RF-8) in combination with radiation for cancer therapy: Cancer 58:1589–1595

3. Nagata Y, Kumada K, Abe M, Ono K, Ozawa K, Hayashido M (1990) Continuous intra-arterial infusion therapy: An alternative approach to the femoral artery. Br J Surg 77:584–585

4. Nagata Y, Nishidai T, Abe M, Takahashi M, Okajima K, Yamaoka N, Ishihara H, Kubo Y, Ohta H, Kazusa C (1990) CT Simulator: A new 3-D planning and simulating system for radiotherapy: Part 2—Clinical Application. Int J Radiat OncolBiol Phys 18:505–513

5. Moffat, FL, Gilas T, Calhoun K, Falk M, Dalfen R, Rostein LE, Makowka L, Hound V, Laing D, Venturi D (1985) Further experience with regional radiofrequency hyperthermia and cytotoxic chemotherapy for unresectable hepatic neoplasia. Cancer 55:1291

6. Storm FK, Kaiser LR, Goodnight JE, Harrison WH, Elliot RS, Gomes AS, Morton DL (1982) Thermochemotherapy for melanoma metastases in liver. Cancer 49:1243–1248

7. Petrovich Z, Langholz B, Kapp DS, Emami B, Oleson JR, Luxton G, Astrahan M (1988) Deep Regional Hyperthermia of Liver. Am J Clin Oncol 12(5):378–383

8. Chuang VP (1983) Hepatic tumor angiography: A subjective review Radiology 148:633–639

9. Reuter SR, Redman HC, Siders DB, et al. (1970) The spectrum of angiographic finding in hepatoma Radiology 94:89–94

10. Samulski TV, Fessenden P, Valdagni R, et al. (1987) Correlation of thermal washout rate, steady state temperatures, and tissue type in deep seated recurrent or metastatic tumors: Int J Radiat Oncol Biol Phys 13:907–916

11. Waterman FM, Nerlinger RE, Moylan DJ, Leeper DB (1987) Response of human tumor blood flow to local hyperthermia: Int J Radiat Oncol Biol Phys 13:75–82

12. Akuta K, Hiraoka M, Jo S, Ma F, Nishimura Y, Takahashi M, Abe M, Marmquist M, Lindbom LO, Lindbom R (1987) Regional hyperthermia combined with blockade of the hepatic arterial blood flow by degradable starch microsperes in pigs: Int J Radiat Oncol Biol Phys 13:239–242

13. Erichsen C, Bolmsjo M, Hugander A, Jonsson PE (1985) Blockade of the hepatic artery blood flow by biodegradable microspheres (Spherex) combined with local hyperthermia in the treatment of experimental liver tumors in rats. Cancer Res Clin Oncol 109:38–41

14. Akuta K, Jo S, Hiraoka M, Nishimura M, Nagata Y, Takahashi M, Abe M (1988) Histological Changes of the normal liver by local hyperthermia.

Part 2—Histopathological Changes of the Rabbit Liver by Local Hyperthermia. Jpn J Hyperther Oncol 4:1–8

15. Fajardo LE, Colby TV (1980) Pathogenesis of Veno-occlusive liver disease after radiation. Arch Pathol Lab Med 104:584–588

16. Order SE, Stillwagon GB, Klein JL, Leichner PK, Siegelman SS, Ettinger DS, Haulk T, Kopher K, Fishman EK (1985) Iodine-131 antiferritin, a new treatment modality in hepatoma: A radiation oncology group study. J Clin Oncol 3:1573–1582

17. Kusumoto Sai S, Shirotani K, Nakada K, Hayashi K, Shoji T (1989) I-131—Lipiodol therapy: Kan Tan Sui. 18:283–288

18. Nagata Y, Yamamoto K, Hiraoka M, Abe M, Takahashi M, Akuta K (1990) Monitoring liver tumor therapy with 18F-FDG Positron Emission Tomography. JCAT 14:370–374

19. Nagata Y, Hiraoka M, Abe M, Akuta K, Takahashi M, Jo S (1990) Radiofrequency thermotherapy for malignant liver tumors. Cancer 65:1730–1736

CHAPTER 32

Multidisciplinary treatment of hepatocellular carcinoma

Kyuichi Tanikawa[1]

1 Characteristic features of hepatocellular carcinoma in Japan

Approximately 90% of hepatocellular carcinoma (HCC) in Japan is associated with chronic liver diseases (mostly liver cirrhosis) and development in the liver is considered to be multicentric. In addition, vascular invasion occurs in the early stages. For these reasons, even small HCC occasionally cannot be removed surgically, and thus, the treatment of HCC is remarkably different from other malignancies. Our studies have indicated that 33.5% of 200 cases of small HCC less than 2 cm in diameter are multinodular [1], and there were recurrent tumors in most cases 5 years after initial successful treatment with surgical resection or percutaneous ethanol injection therapy (PEIT). Autopsy studies have also shown that a high frequency of extrahepatic metastasis is observed in cases with tumors more than 5 cm in diameter. Thus, surgical resection, the preferred treatment of malignancies, is limited. In fact, the Liver Cancer Study Group of Japan reported only about 20% of HCC cases receive surgical resections as the main therapy [2]. Recently, small HCC has been found more frequently due to improved detection methods, and this has resulted in an increase of HCC patients being indicated for surgical resection in our department. Even so, the percentage of HCC patients undergoing surgery is still less than 20% of all HCC cases admitted to our department.

Except for a small number of patients, most of the patients have associated liver cirrhosis and the life span of cirrhotic patients in Japan has, remarkably, been prolonged to over 10 years in 50% of the cases due to recent improvements in medical care. Among the factors determining the prognosis of liver cirrhosis, HCC is the most important and life-threatening complication. The purpose of the treatment of HCC is, generally speaking, to prolong the life of patients with underlying cirrhosis. Rendering a prognosis for HCC patients is very much dependent on cirrhosis.

2 Treatment of small HCC

Small HCC is defined here as a tumor less than 3 cm in diameter. Most small HCC, being found as nodular lesions, are considered to be in an early stage of HCC. Recently, small HCC have been found in quite a large number by a follow-up of patients with chronic liver diseases, especially cirrhosis, using ultrasonography. In fact, about one third of all HCC patients admitted to our department have been found to have small HCC in recent years [1]. In the future, the proportion of therapeutic subjects with small HCC patients is expected to increase when a careful follow-up system for detection of small HCC in chronic liver diseases is established throughout the country.

According to our experience, the criteria for treatment for patients with small HCC less than 3 cm in diameter, patients with good liver function (Child A) and with a single lesion located relatively near the surface of the liver are good surgical candidates. In our experience about one quarter of small HCC cases are indicated for surgery. The patients not indicated for surgery are mostly treated by PEIT [3] in our department. Transcatheter arterial embolization (TAE) is generally not effective for small HCC especially when they are less than 2 cm in diameter because such a small HCC is supplied blood not only from

[1] Second Department of Medicine, Kurume University School of Medicine, Kurume, 830 Japan

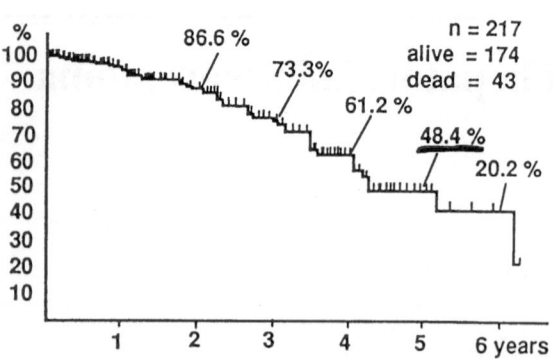

Fig. 1. Survival of patients who received PEIT for small HCC (less than 3 cm in diameter) (Kaplan-Meier method)

the hepatic artery but also from the portal vein. Thus, PEIT is the first treatment of choice for small HCC not indicated for surgery.

The 5-year survival rate for PEIT in 217 cases of small HCC in our department was 48.4% (Fig. 1). A similar survival rate has been reported in another institution [4]. In addition, the 5-year survival rate of PEIT for patients of small HCC with good liver function (Child A) is shown to be 85% in our experience which is superior to the rate for surgical resection [5]. From these results, the prognosis would be not remarkably different in patients with small HCC either treated by surgical resection or by PEIT if the patients have similar clinical backgrounds. However, surgical resection is still the method of choice for complete cure of small HCC in our department.

Our study on the prognostic factors of PEIT has made it clear that cases of small HCC with a high degree of cell atypism have a relatively poor prognosis (Fig. 2). Small HCC generally have a low degree of cell atypism compared to advanced

HCC [6]. From these results, those cases of small HCC with a high degree of cell atypism should be surgically resected relatively widely including the lesion or given extensive chemotherapy after PEIT. In addition, pathologic studies must be carried out on those small HCC with a high degree of cell atypism. The most important method to improve the prognosis after surgical resection or PEIT for small HCC is a careful follow-up every three months and early therapy (mainly PEIT) for a recurrence, because the recurrence of newly developed small lesions occurs in almost all cases 5 years after the initial treatment (Fig. 3).

3 Treatment of advanced HCC

Except for a few cases, most advanced HCC are treated non-surgically. At present, TAE using gel foam mixed with anti-cancer drugs and Lipiodol is used to treat nodular lesions measuring over 3 cm in diameter with relatively good results. TAE is also applied for multiple lesions either simultaneously or at intervals for each respective lesion. As liver failure could occur when TAE is performed in cases with poor liver function, it is necessary to adequately define criteria for performing TAE [1]. At present, we occasionally use Tracker's cathethers, thinner than conventional ones, by which the catheter can be placed at the feeding hepatic artery very close to the tumor lesion. With this method, though, we cannot use gel foam particles because of their large size, and instead, we infuse ethanol through Tracker's catheters for embolization (Ethanol-TAE). Ethanol-TAE can be applied even when

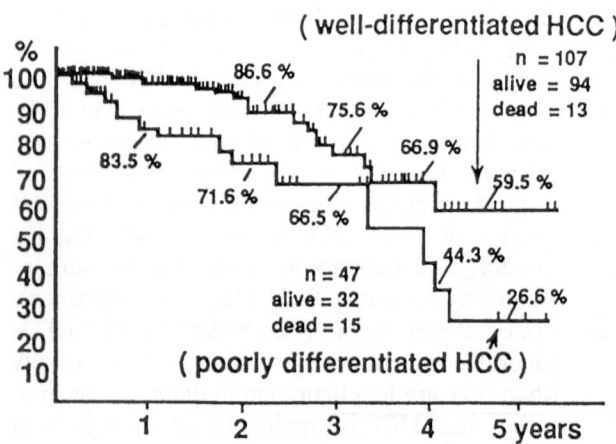

Fig. 2. Survival of patients with well or poorly differentiated small HCC in PEIT

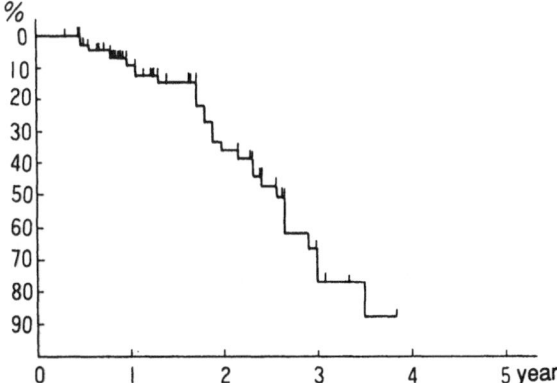

Fig. 3. Recurrence rate of small HCC after PEIT (n = 73)

liver function is relatively poor because embolization is specific for the lesion. Several trials of TAE are desirable as one trial is often not sufficient to necrotize the entire lesion. Our experience indicates that it is necessary to repeat at least twice in a one to two month interval for best results. In Japan, the prognosis of advanced HCC has been remarkably improved by the general use of TAE and the 3-year survival rate of our 374 cases has been around 22.2% (Fig. 4). However, it is, in many cases, impossible to necrotize the malignant tissue completely by TAE alone and a residual malignant tissue often remains in the lesion after TAE. To remedy this problem, TAE has been tried in combination with PEIT [7]. It is still controversial which of the two therapies should be performed first, although our experience suggests performing TAE first. Though we have not yet obtained a long survival time using this combination therapy, there is no doubt that we will have a better result than by TAE alone.

In very advanced HCC in which numerous lesions in both hepatic lobules or diffusely infiltrating lesions are seen, an arterial infusion of anti-cancer drugs is usually indicated. One shot injection of anti-cancer drugs by Seldinger's procedure had formerly been performed. However, at present, arterial infusion therapy has being done using a totally implanted injection port system placed under the skin [8]. By using the

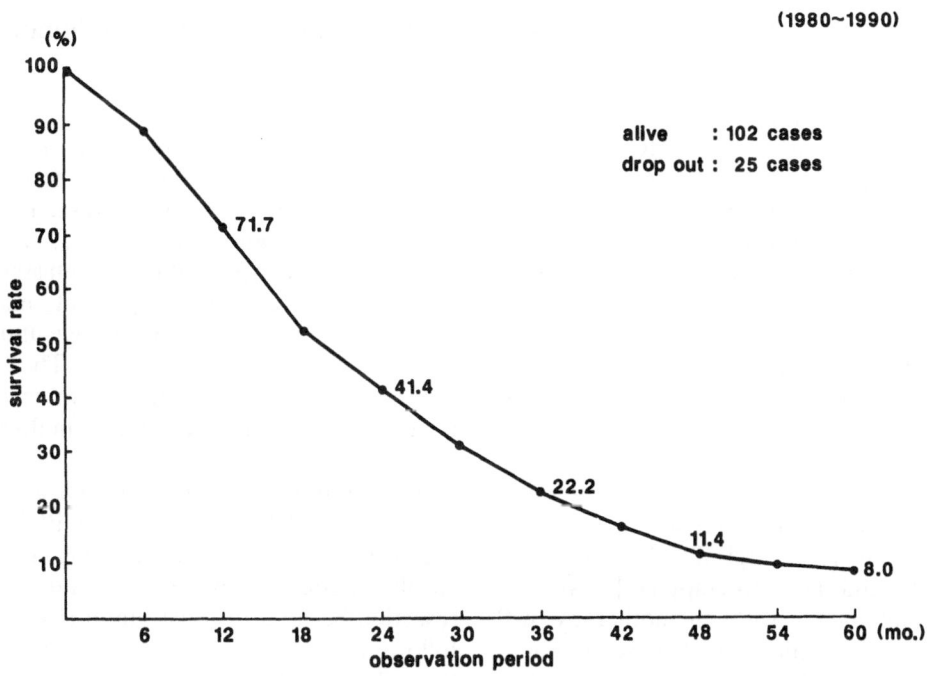

Fig. 4. Cumulative survival rate after TAE treatment in 374 cases

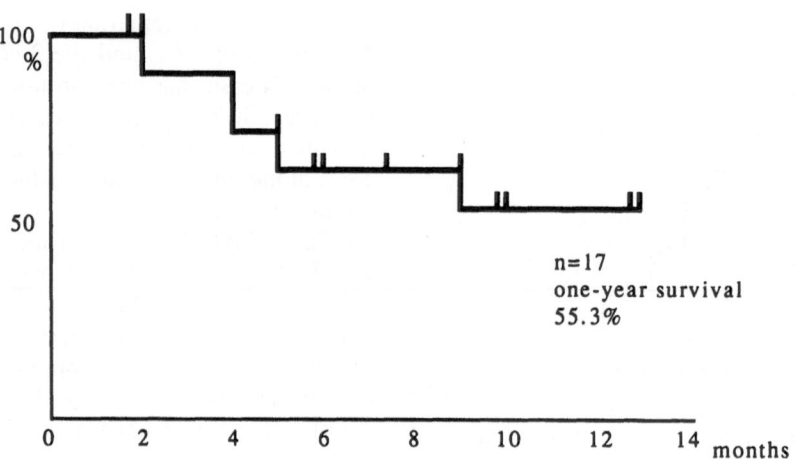

Fig. 5. Effect of arterial chemotherapy using a totally implanted injection port system

tumor stage	No.	Vp factor	No.	Vv factor	No.
II	1	Vp 0	4	Vv 0	11
III	2	1	0	1	0
IV-A	13	2	5	2	5
IV-B	1	3	8	3	1

port it has become possible to perform an arterial infusion of anti-cancer drugs repeatedly with ease and we have recently experienced cases with a remarkably prolonged life (Fig. 5).

The anti-cancer drugs used for HCC at present are adriamycin, mitomycin C and cisplatin. However, no good sensitivity tests of anti-cancer drugs for HCC are known at present. We have used renal subcapsular assay for anti-cancer drugs using liver biopsy specimens obtained by fine needles [9]. Simple and easy sensitivity tests are desired for this purpose.

Extensive vascular invasion often occurs into the portal trunk or hepatic veins in HCC and the prognosis of such cases is very poor and aggressive treatment for those vascular invasions is desired. To prolong the lives of these patients, radiation therapy [10], surgical removal of tumor thrombi [11], and thermotherapy [12] have been tried in combination with chemotherapy with some effect. Indications for these therapies should be established by analysis of their clinical studies.

4 Importance of multidisciplinary treatment

Recurrences occur very frequently in other parts of the liver even after the complete cure of the primary small HCC by surgical resection or PEIT because of its multicentric nature. Most recurrences are not considered to be metastatic lesions from the primary site. At present, many HCC are still found in the advanced stage and they are mostly not cured completely. The evidence indicates that only one treatment is not satisfactory in many HCC cases and multidiscipliary approach is indicated.

In general, cases with recurrence after surgical resection or PEIT are treated by PEIT or TAE except for a few cases again being resected surgically. Patients who receive no satisfactory resection because of large tumor size are usually followed up with extensive chemotherapy through the arterial catheter with a totally implantable injection port system.

Fig. 6. Survival of HCC patients treated by TAE alone or TAE + OK-432

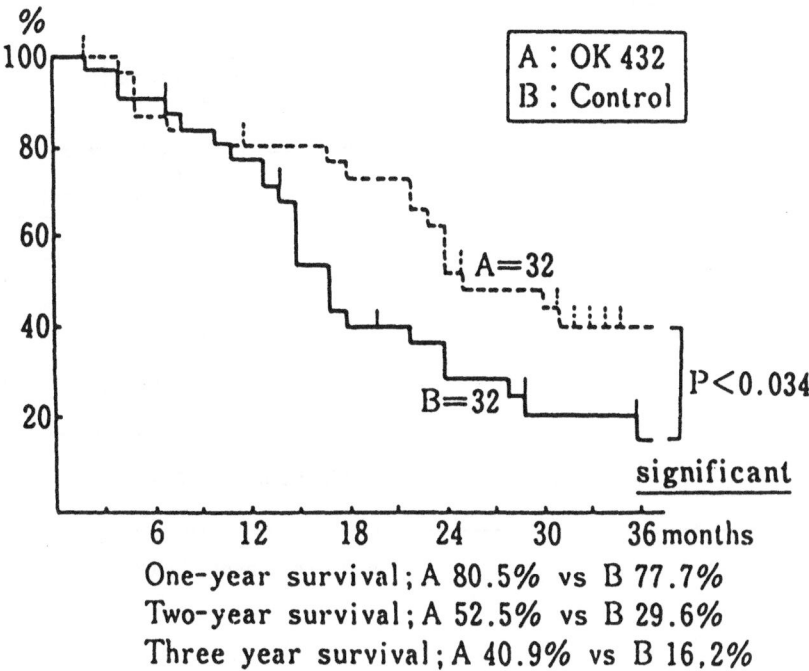

One-year survival; A 80.5% vs B 77.7%
Two-year survival; A 52.5% vs B 29.6%
Three year survival; A 40.9% vs B 16.2%

In Japan, patients who receive surgical resections, PEIT or TAE are usually given anti-cancer drugs orally for a long period of time after those treatments. The drugs used are Tegafur and Carmofur, however, smaller doses of these drugs are generally given compared with other malignancies because most HCC patients tend to have side effects due to associated cirrhosis.

Attention must be paid to hepatic encephalopathy-like symptoms which rarely occur when Carmofur is given in cirrhotic patients and a differential diagnosis is sometimes difficult with true hepatic encephalopathy. A randomized control study on patients receiving successful TAE for an HCC tumor occupying less than 20% of the liver, showed that the 3-year survival rate was significantly longer in ones given an oral administration of an anti-cancer drug with weekly injection of OK-432 (*streptococcus* preparation: Biological response modifier) compared with those given oral anti-cancer drug alone after TAE treatment (Fig. 6) [1]. Experimental studies have shown that OK-432 injection enhances natural killer activity in the liver [13]. In clinical cases, immunological responses against the tumor tissue necrotized by TAE would be enhanced by the injection of potent biological response modifier, OK-432.

Thermotherapy and lymphokine activated killer (LAK) therapy have also been tried in some institutions with some success. Regional hyperthermia, combined with blockade of the hepatic arterial blood flow by degradable starch micropheres, has been proved to be effective in experimental animals and in man [14]. Recently, LAK cells have been given to patients with advanced HCC. Though a decrease in serum tumor markers and tumor size has been seen in some cases, remarkable effects have not been obtained. At present, TAE combined with LAK treatment is tried with better effects [15].

Because of the frequent association of HCC with liver cirrhosis, and because of the multicentric development of lesions, multidisciplinary treatment is important for patients with HCC. Endoscopic sclerotherapy for esophageal varices is occasionally needed in the clinical course of HCC. On the other hand, a small HCC is found often in the follow-up after sclerotherapy. Extensive treatments for HCC occasionally are impossible because of associated bleeding tendency due to hypersplenism in cirrhosis. In such cases, partial splenic embolization by Seldinger's method has been carried out in our department with excellent results [16]. Treatments of HCC are summarized in Fig. 7.

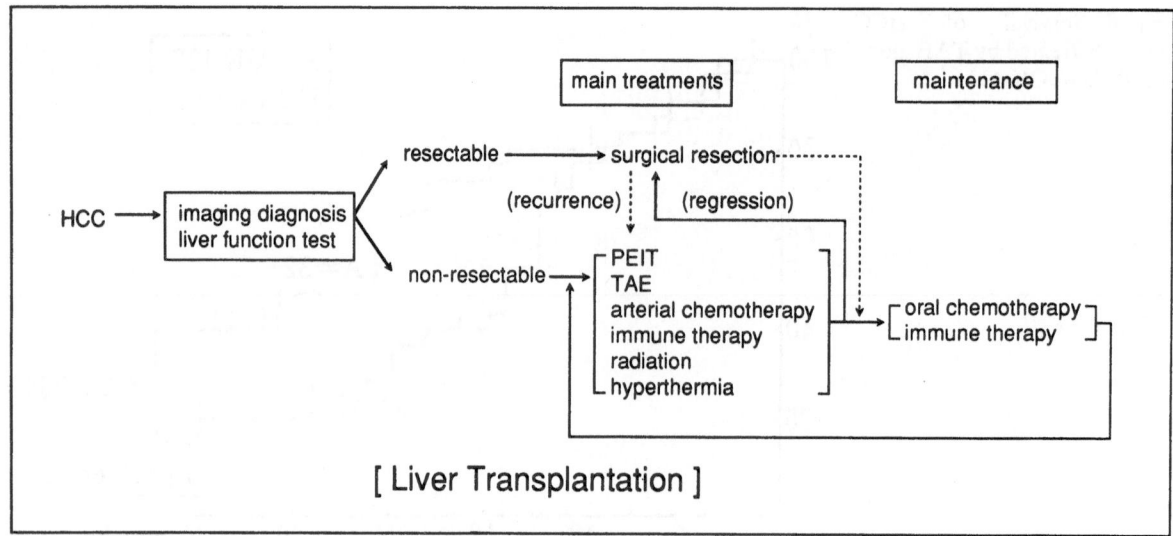

Fig. 7. Treatment of HCC

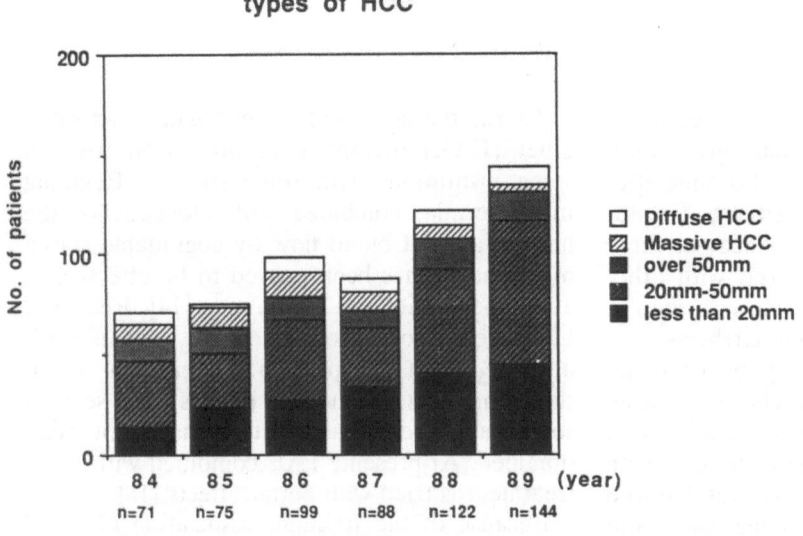

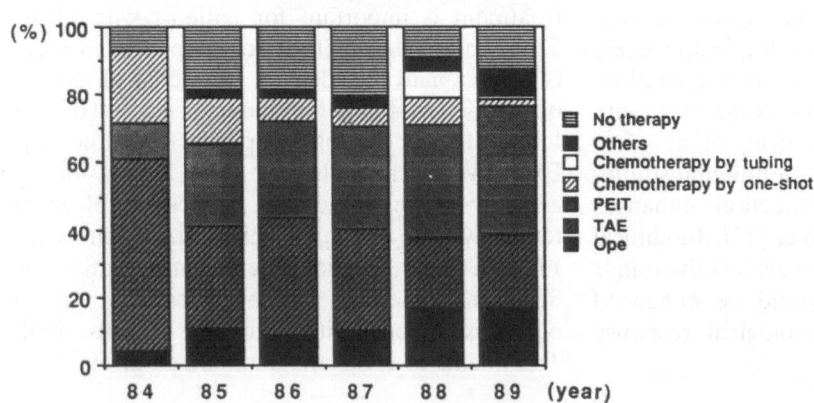

Fig. 8. Changes in type of HCC patients admitted to our department and their treatments

5 Changes of treatment for HCC and future problems

Figure 8 shows the number of admitted HCC patients classified according to their grades of clinical progression and the treatment received for the last 6 years in our department. The treatment for small HCC has become very important as small HCC has been detected more frequently due to careful follow up of patients with chronic liver diseases.

Thus, clinical training of PEIT, the most useful and effective nonsurgical treatment for small HCC, is extremely important to further improve the procedure. In fact, our study indicates that poorly differentiated HCC shows relatively poor prognosis compared with one of well-differentiated small HCC. Thus, special attention must be paid to those small HCC with poor cell differentiation. In those cases, segmental hepatectomy or extensive chemotherapy after PEIT may be indicated for a better prognosis.

The smallest HCC we can find by ultrasound (US) is around 5 to 6mm in size, and it is, at present, impossible to detect lesions smaller than 5mm in diameter by US or by any other imaging diagnostic procedure.

Our previous study has shown that it would take about 4 to 5 years from initiation until the tumor grows to the size of 2 cm by determining the doubling time of tumor volume [17]. It is obvious that the tumor develops a few years before clinical diagnosis of small HCC can be made.

At present, it is important to study methods to diagnose early development of HCC before local detection of HCC by imaging diagnosis can be made. One of the possible approaches is to examine a lectin-reactive alpha-fetoprotein (AFP) [18] by following patients with chronic liver diseases. Liver transplantation has been undertaken for hepatocellular carcinoma in several centers. However, their results are poor in prognosis except for incidental cases and fibrolamellar type. Metastasis is the main cause of death among transplant patients.

In Japan, over 20,000 patients die of HCC and this number seems to be too many for candidates for liver transplantation. In addition, since the prognosis of small HCC patients treated by surgical resection or PEIT is excellent, liver transplantation is not indicated as the first treatment of choice for small HCC. We also have no accurate clinical diagnostic procedures for the

demonstration of extrahepatic metastasis, which is often seen in tumors over 5cm in size on autopsy examination. Thus, at present, liver transplantation for HCC is indicated in cases with no extrahepatic metastasis.

There are many problems to be solved in future for the liver transplantation of HCC. One of them is control of the underlying infection of hepatitis virus because approximately 90% of the HCC we see in Japan are associated with chronic HBV or HCV infection. Prognosis of transplanted patients with chronic infection of HBV has been shown to be poor because of reinfection of the virus in the transplanted liver. Therefore, the means to control associated viral infections, such as the use of interferon, γ-globulin or other treatments, should be established. Good procedures for accurate diagnosis of extrahepatic metastasis are also needed. Improvement of imaging diagnosis and further pathological studies are important areas of study for this purpose.

References

1. Tanikawa K (1991) Recent advance in treatment of hepatocellular carcinoma with reference to the indication. Surg Ther (Geka-Chiryo) 64:172–176
2. The Liver Cancer Study Group of Japan (1990) Primary liver cancer in Japan. Ann of Surg 211:277–287
3. Fujimoto T, Majima Y, Tanaka M, Iwai I, Sakai T, Hirai K, Abe M, Tanikawa K, Kenmochi K (1986) Investigation of percutaneous ultrasono-graphically-guided ethanol injection therapy (PEIT) for treatment of small hepatocellular carcinoma. Acta Hepatologica Japonica 27:1559–1567
4. Ebara M, Kita K, Ohoto M (1990) Therapeutic result of percutaneous ethanol injection (PEI) therapy for small hepatocellular carcinoma—Long-term prognosis and recurrence in non-treated area of the liver. Acta Hepatologica Japonica 31:244–245
5. Tanikawa K (1990) Non-surgical treatment of hepatocellular carcinoma. Jpn J Gastroenterol Surg 23:2492–2496
6. Tanikawa K, Iwai I, Majima Y (1990) Tumor growth rate and cell differentiation in HCC. In: Sung JL, Chen DS (eds) Viral hepatitis and hepatocellular carcinoma. Excerpta Medica, Hong Kong, pp 646–650
7. Tanaka K, Okazaki H, Nakamura S, Hoshino M, Nagase H, Endoh O, Inoue S, Takamura Y (1990)

Evaluation of combination therapy with transcatheter arterial embolization and percutaneous ultrasonographically-guided ethanol injection therapy in patients with advanced hepatocellular carcinoma. Acta Hepatologica Japonica 31: 944–951

8. Gyves JW, Ensminger WD, Miederhuber JE, Dent T, Walker S, Gilbertson S, Cozzi E, Sarran P (1984) A totally implanted injection port system for blood sampling and chemotherapy administration. JAMA 251:2538–2541

9. Fukushima H (to be published) (1991) Subrenal capsule assay using liver cancer specimens obtained by the fine needle biopsy. Kurume Med J

10. Nagashima T, Ryu M, Mukai M, Ariga T, Koh Z, Amano H, Furukawa T, Maruyama T, Yamamoto Y, Odaka M, Isono K, Arimizu N, Uematsu S, Ishikawa T (1987) Therapy of hepatocellular carcinoma complicated with intravascular tumor emboli-Effectiveness of radiotherapy for tumor emboli. Acta Hepatologica Japonica 28:735–744

11. Tsuzuki T, Iida S, Kasajima M, Ueda M, Ozawa I, Ogata Y, Kawada K (1988) Aggressive surgery for patients with hepatocellular carcinoma and hepatoblastoma with tumor thrombi in the portal trunk, hepatic vein, inferior vena cava and right atrium. Acta Hepatologica Japonica 29:1222–1232

12. Nagata Y, Hiraoka M, Akuta K, Abe M, Takahashi M, Jo S, Nishimura Y, Masunaga S, Fukuda M, Imura H (1990) Radiofrequency thermotherapy for malignant liver tumors. Cancer 65:1730–1736

13. Tanaka M, Ogata H, Yoshimoto K, Noguchi K, Sata M, Abe M, Tanikawa K (1989) Harvest of liver sinusoidal large granular lymphocytes (Pit cells) and augmentation of natural killer activity by the administration of OK-432. In: Wisse E, Knook DL, Decker K (eds) Cells of the hepatic sinusoid, Vol 2. The Kupffer Cell Foundation, HV Rijiswijk, The Netherlands, pp 451–455

14. Murata T (1988) Studies on the effectiveness of hyperthermia combined with arterial therapeutic blockage in the treatment of tumors. J Jpn Soc Cancer Ther 23:2709–2731

15. Arakawa K (1989) An immunological and clinical evaluation of combinated TAE-LAK adoptive immunotherapy. Jpn J Gastroenterol 86:1494–1506

16. Hirai K, Kawazoe Y, Yamashita K, Kumagai M, Tanaka T, Sakai T, Inoue R, Eguchi S, Majima Y, Abe M, Toyonaga K, Tanikawa K (1986) Transcatheter partial splenic arterial embolization in patients with hypersplenism: A clinical evaluation as supporting therapy for hepatocellular carcinoma and liver cirrhosis. Hepato gastroenterology 33:105–108

17. Majima Y (1984) Growth rate of hepatocellular carcinoma by ultrasonography and its clinical significance. Acta Hepatologica Japonica 25: 754–765

18. Taketa K, Sekiya C, Namiki M, Akamatsu K, Ohta Y, Endo Y, Kosaka K (1990) lectin-reactive profiles of alpha-fetoprotein characterizing hepatocellular carcinoma and related conditions. Gastroenterology 99:508–518

CHAPTER 33

Multidisciplinary treatment for multiple hepatocellular carcinoma

Ken Takasaki, Atsushi Aruga[1]

1 Introduction

Hepatocellular carcinoma (HCC) is one of the most common malignancies in Japan. However, few HCC patients are candidates for curative surgical resection, due to either associated liver cirrhosis or the presence of multiple tumor nodules in the liver. Several modalities have been used to treat HCC patients including transcatheter arterial embolization (TAE), hepatic arterial infusion, ultrasound (US) guided ethanol injection, radiation, immunotherapy, and hyperthermia, but satisfactory clinical results have not yet been obtained. These non-curative patients can be treated with reduction surgery or hepatic arterial infusion therapy using an implantable injection port (IIP). In this chapter, we will discuss our multidisciplinary treatment of unresectable (non-curative) hepatocellular carcinomas, specially targeting Stage IV-a (IM2,3) multiple HCCs as defined in [1].

2 Methods and patients

2.1 Treated patients with unresectable hepatocellular carcinomas

From April 1, 1987 to August 31, 1990, 254 cases of hepatocellular carcinomas received surgical treatment in our department. Of these, 197 recieved curative resection and 57 were non-curative (Table 1). Among the non-curative cases, 46 patients having multiple tumor nodules

in bilateral lobes of the liver (Stage IV-a due to IM2 or 3) were treated by the following methods: 32 patients received reduction surgery plus hepatic arterial cannulation, and 14 patients received hepatic arterial cannulation only. Tumors were resected whenever possible and cytotoxic T lymphocytes (CTL) induction or carcinostatic agent sensitivity tests were used. For comparison with other non-operative treatments, 30 patients treated by TAE and 10 non-treated patients were studied within the above period of time in our department (Table 2).

2.2 Surgical treatment

Patients who underwent reduction surgery, tumor ennucleation or partial hepatic resection had as much resected as possible within the safety volume judged by their liver function. Implantable injection port, Port-A-Cath (Feither; USA), Infuse-A-port(Infusaid; USA) or Anthron PU catheter (Toray; Japan) were used for hepatic arterial cannulation. The catheter was inserted into the ligated gastroduodenal artery, with the tip set at the common hepatic artery. The other end of the catheter was placed at the site of the injection port subcutaneously (Fig. 1). Cholecystectomy and ligation of the right gastric artery, posterior superior pancreaticoduodenal artery (PSPD), anterior superior pancreaticoduodenal artery (ASPD), and duodenal artery were performed in all patients to minimize the side effects of post-operative infusion therapy.

2.3 Preparation of tumor cells

Hepatocellular carcinoma cells obtained from surgical specimens were used in a sensitivity test

[1] Department of Surgery, Institute of Gastroenterology, Tokyo Women's Medical College, Shinjuku-ku, Tokyo, 162 Japan

Table 1. Operative patients with hepatocellular carcinoma

Total number of operative patients with HCC	254
Curative operation	197
Non-curative operation	57

April 1, 1987–August 31, 1990
Department of Surgery, Institute of Gastroenterology, Tokyo Women's Medical College

Table 2. Patients with stage IV—a (IM2, 3) hepatocellular carcinoma

Reduction surgery plus hepatic arterial cannulation[a]	32
Operative hepatic arterial cannulation[a]	14
Transcatheter arterial embolization (TAE)[b]	30
No treatment[b]	10

April 1, 1987–August 31, 1990
[a] Department of Surgery, Institute of Gastroenterology
Tokyo Women's Medical College
[b] Department of Medicine, Institute of Gastroenterology
Tokyo Women's Medical College

for carcinostatic status and ability to stimulate CTL activity. Tumor tissue was cut into small pieces, around 2–3 mm in diameter, and homogenized in the medium RPMI 1640 with 0.08% collagenase plus 0.01% DNase by a ground glass homogenizer to make a single tumor cell suspensions.

2.4 In vitro sensitivity test for carcinostatic agents

The usual succinic dehydrogenase inhibition (SDI) test using 3-[4,5-dimethyl thiazol-2yl]-2,5- diphenyl-tetrazolium bromide (MTT)[2] as a tetrazolium salt was performed; 1×10^5 tumor cells were put into a 96-well microplate with 100 µl RPMI 1640 plus 10% FCS, and 10 µg/ml of doxorubicin [Adriamycin (ADM)], 10 µg/ml of mitomycin-C (MMC), 20 µg/ml of cisplatin (CDDP), 100 µg/ml of 5-fluorouracil (5-FU), 20 µg/ml of carboquone [Esquinon (ESQ)], 20 µg/ml of epirubicin [Farmorbicine (FARM)] 20 µg/ml of mitoxantrone hydrochloride, and 25 µg/ml of nimustine hydrochloride were added. After 3 days, culture viability of tumor cells was measured by the SDI test. Only those drugs which showed less than 50% SD activity were used for clinical treatment.

2.5 In vitro induction of autologous CTL or lymphokine activated killer (LAK) cell

Autologous peripheral blood mononuclear cells (PBMC) were obtained from HCCs patients by leukocytapheresis using the apheresis system "Hemonetics V-50" (Hemonetic, Mass., USA). After further purification of the PBMC by Ficoll-Hypaque gradient, 2×10^6/ml PBMC were cultivated with 1/50–100 autologous HCC cells, and separated single cells were pretreated with MMC for 5 days in RPMI 1640 supplemented with either 10% autologous serum or pooled human serum, 100 IU/ml of penicillin and streptomycin. On day 5, 1,000 IU/ml of rIL-2 (Shionogi, Osaka, Japan) was added to the culture for further stimulation, and on day 10, the cells were injected via the hepatic arterial catheter. Several doses of rIL-2 were injected after CTL administration for 1 week. Autologous

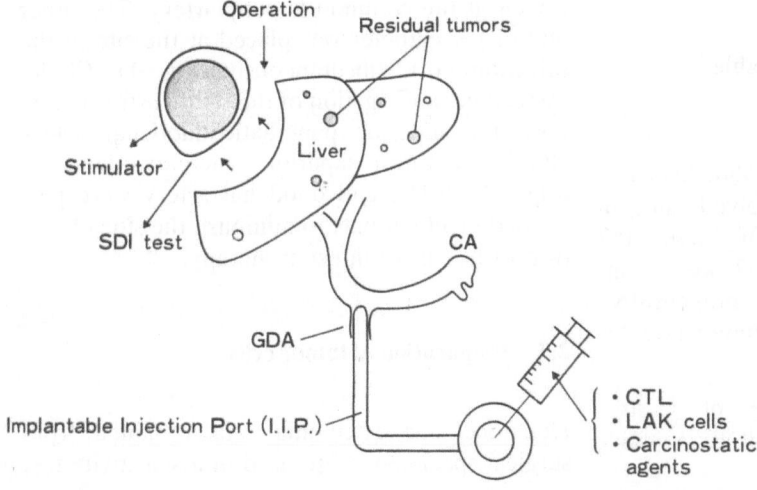

Fig. 1. Our multidisciplinary treatment, reduction surgery plus hepatic arterial cannulation. Tumors are tested for sensitivity to carcinostatic agents or stimulators to induce autologous cytotoxic T lymphocytes (CTLs). *SDI*, succinic dehydrogenase inhibition; *GDA*, gastroduodenal artery; *LAK cells*, lymphokine-activated killer cells

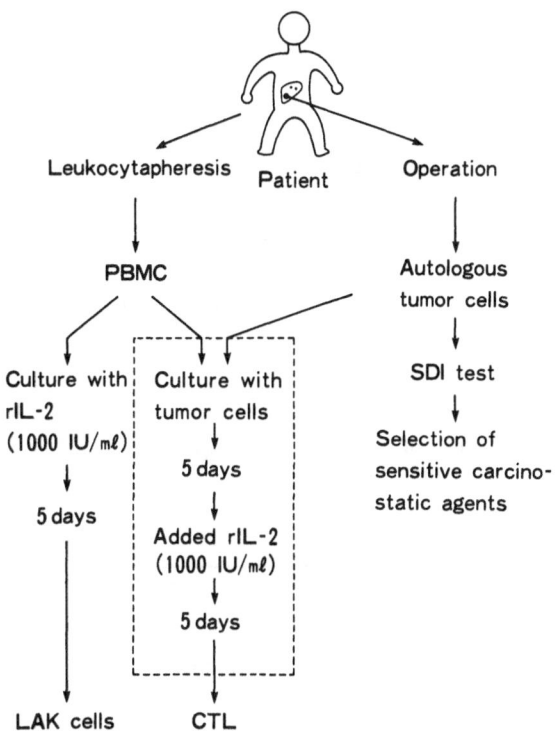

Fig. 2. Treatment scheme for patients with multiple HCCs. *PBMC*, peripheral blood mononuclear cells; *rIL-2*, recombinant interleukin-2

LAK cells were used for patients who could not obtain enough tumor cells by inducement of the CTLs. The patient's PBMC were obtained by leukocytapheresis, and cultivated with 1,000 IU/ml of rIL-2 in RPMI 1640 with the same supplement as the CTL culture. On day 5, the cultured cells were injected via the hepatic arterial catheter and 5×10^5 IU/day of rIL-2 was injected continuously via the SCV catheter for 1 week after LAK cell administration. Three to four killer cell injections were performed in each case.

2.6 Post-operative hepatic arterial infusion to HCC patients

Infusion of autologous killer cells, CTLs or LAK cells are the method of choice over carcinostatic agents. Beginning one week after the operation, leukocytapheresis was performed once or twice a week, and induced autologous killer cells were injected via the hepatic artery. Several doses of rIL-2 were injected during the week following killer cell administration. Three or four injections were given to each patient and they were observed carefully by CT scan or ultrasound. For patients who could not produce autologous killer

cells, or recognize no clinical effects of killer cells, transcatheter hepatic arterial infusion of carcinostatic agents was performed. Within ADM, MMC, CDDP, 5-FU, FARM, and ESQ, the most sensitive agents selected by SDI test were used first for the infusion therapy once every week or two (Fig. 2). Some of them were suspended in Lipiodol ultrafluid (Laboratoire Guerbet, Paris). An infusion of carcinostatic agents was performed as many times as possible on an outpatient basis.

3 Results

3.1 Clinical effects of treated HCC patients

From April 1, 1987 to August 31, 1990, 254 cases of hepatocellular carcinoma were given surgical treatment in our facility. Of these, 197 cases received curative operations, and 57 cases could not be treated curatively. Their survival rates were determined by the Kaplan-Meier method (Fig. 3) and there was significant difference in their survival rate ($P < 0.01$ by generalized Wilcoxon test). There were 46 patients who received non-curative operations, and they had multiple tumors in the bilateral lobes. Some of the remaining patients had either reduction surgery plus hepatic arterial cannulation or hepatic arterial cannulation only (Table 2). Clinical effects were judged by CT scan or ultrasound, 3 CR and 5 PR were obtained (CR + PR = 8/46; 17.4%). The survival rate after operation was estimated by the Kaplan-Meier method and compared with that of other non-operative treatment, TAE, or non-treated patients in our department (Fig. 4). As shown in Fig. 4, patients treated by our multidisciplinary method have obtained a significantly longer survival rate at 1, 2 and 3 years than other patients ($P < 0.001$ by the generalized Wilcoxon test). Patients treated with hepatic arterial cannulation only have not obtained improvement in their survival rate compared with patients treated by TAE.

4 Case report

A 55-year-old man with a 5-year history of chronic hepatitis due to hepatitis-C viral infection was evaluated in October 1989. He had no

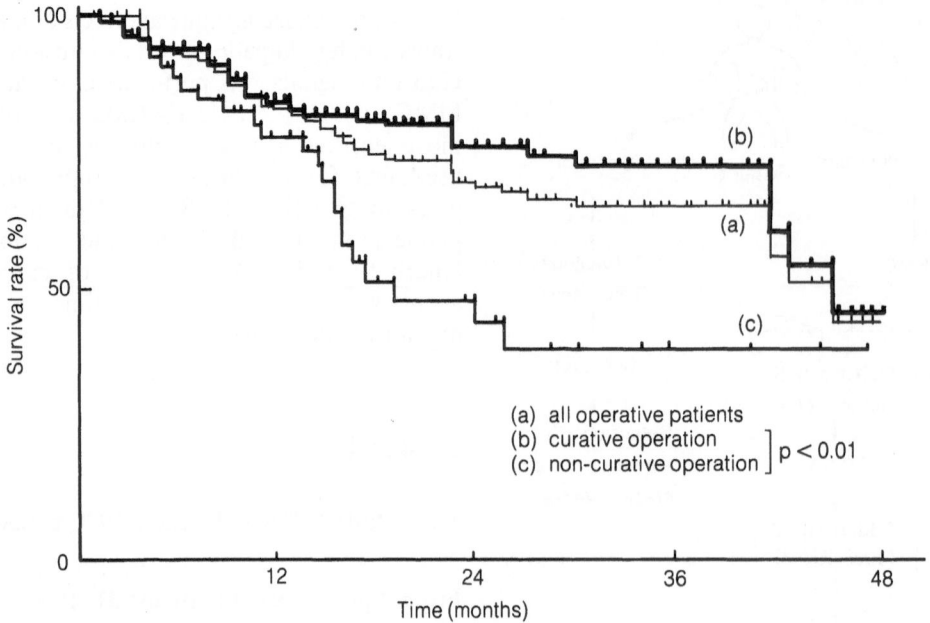

Fig. 3. Survival rate of post-operative patients with hepatocellular carcinoma

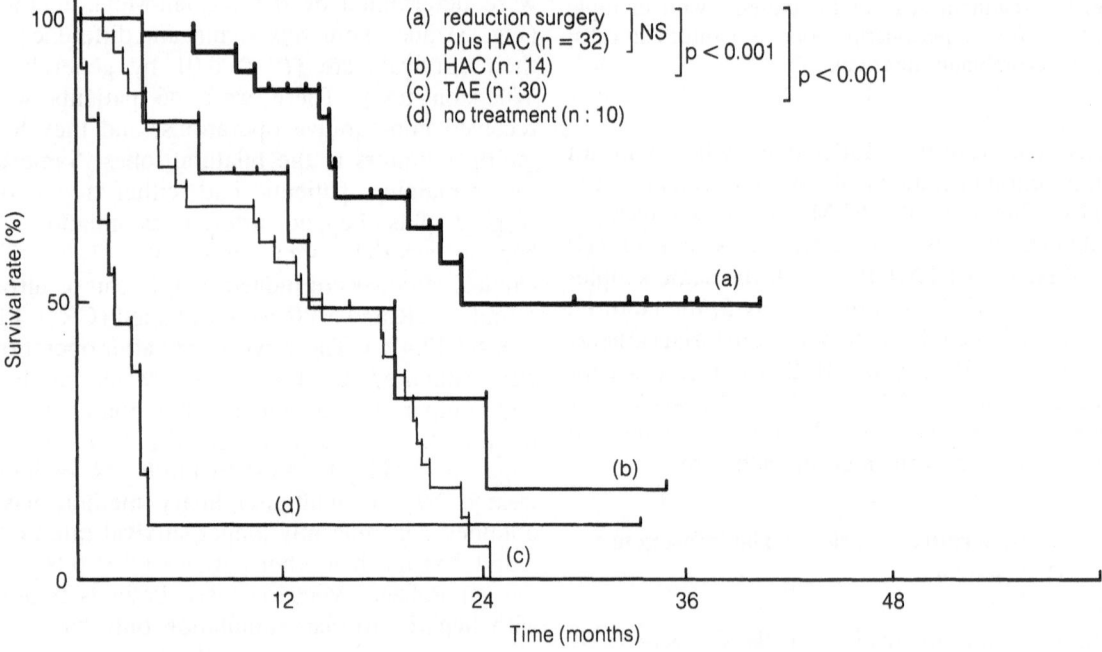

Fig. 4. Survival rate of Stage IV-a HCC patients according to type of treatment. *HAC*, hepaticarterial cannulation; *TAE*, transcatheter arterial embolization

symptoms but the presence of liver tumors was confirmed by routine ultrasound at the other hospital. He was referred to our department on October 27, 1989 and was treated on November 10, 1989. Laboratory data yielded the following results: White blood cell count, 4,010/cc; red blood cell count, 421×10^4/cc; hemoglobin, 13.1 g/dL; platelet count, 8.1×10^4/cc; GOT, 62 KU; GPT, 32 KU; total bilirubin, 2.0 mg/dL; choline esteraze, 0.29 ΣPH; indocyanine green retention test at 15 minutes, 41%; alpha-feto-protein, 90 ng/mL. Ultrasound, CT-scan, and

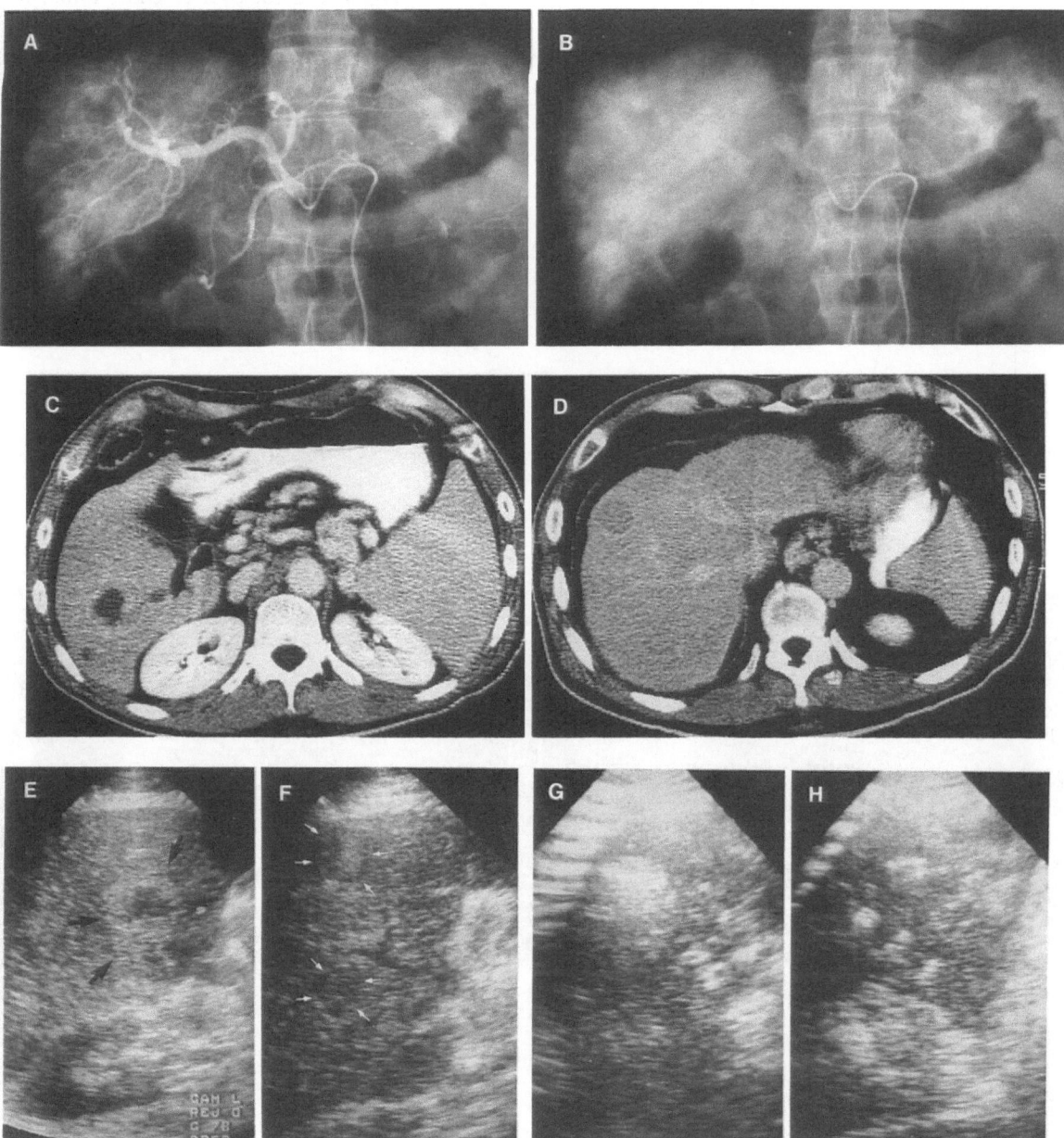

Fig. 5. A–H. Preoperative findings show multiple hepatocellular carcinomas in the bilateral lobes. **A,B** Angiography of the proper hepatic artery. **C,D** Abdominal CT scan. **E,F** Ultrasound. **G,H** CO_2 gas-enhanced ultrasound

celiac angiogram showed multiple tumor nodules in the bilateral lobes of his liver, typical hepatocellular carcinomas (Fig. 5). The largest one was 50×45 mm in diameter at segment S5 in the right lobe. Other tumors were in S6, S7, S8, S3 and S2 segments from 6 mm to 38 mm in diameter. Surgical treatment was performed on November 28, 1989. The tumor existed near the liver surface of S5 segment, and was enucleated, and hepatic

arterial cannulation was performed as described. The ennucleated tumor, about 15 mm in diameter, was separated to 8×10^7 single cells. These cells were used for the carcinostatic agent sensitivity test and in vitro CTL induction. The SDI test showed that the tumor was damaged the most by using adriamycin and mytomicin. Surgical specimens of the tumor showed poorly differentiated hepatocellular carcinoma, Edmondson

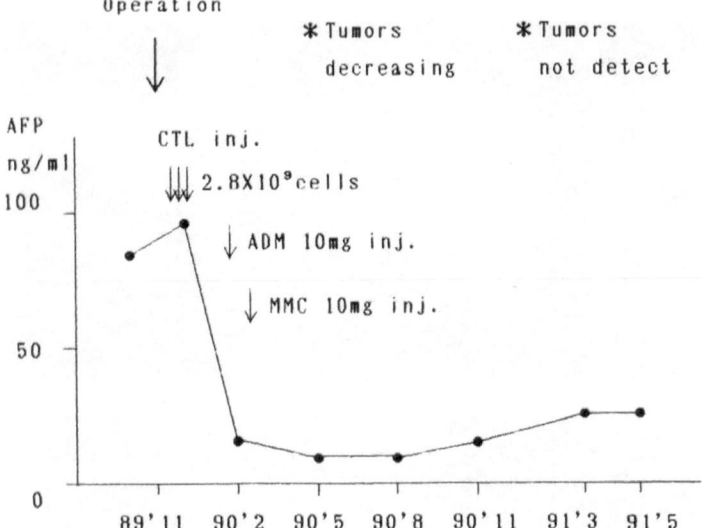

Fig. 6. Clinical course. *CTL*, cytotoxic T lymphocytes; *ADM*, Adriamycin; *MMC*, mitomycin C

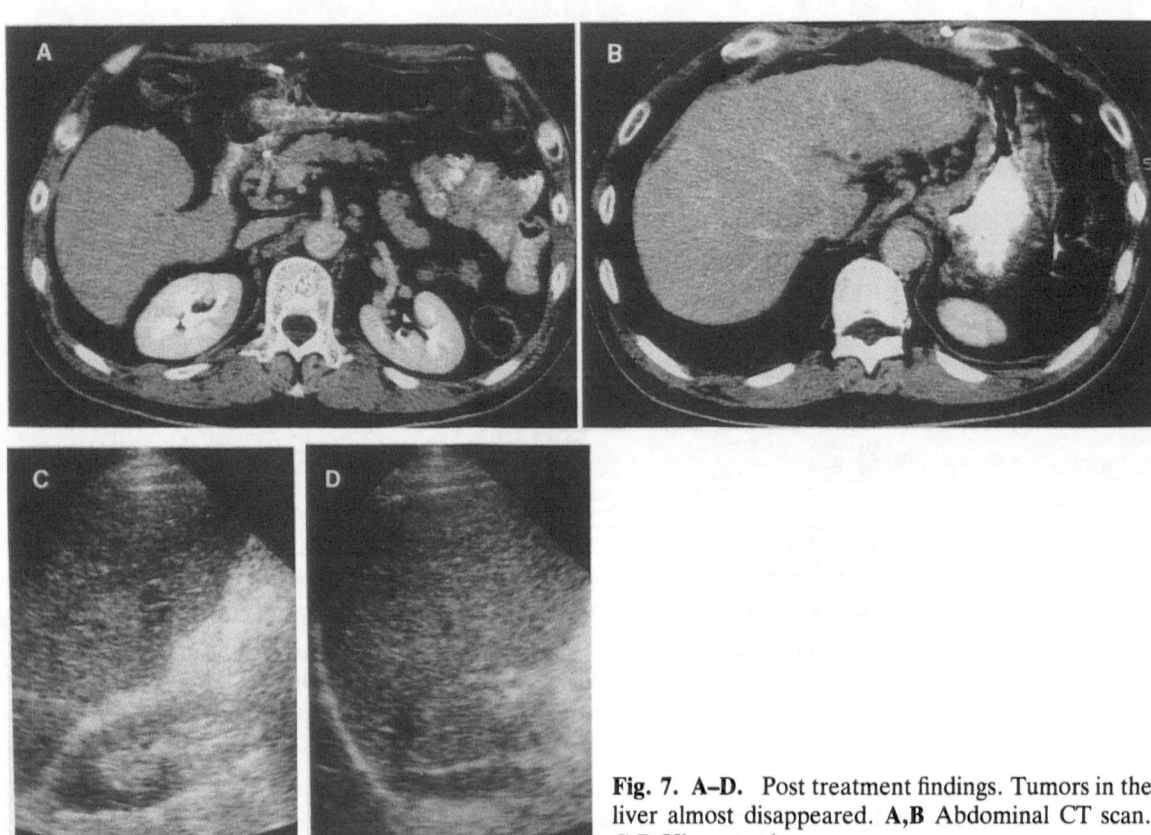

Fig. 7. A–D. Post treatment findings. Tumors in the liver almost disappeared. **A,B** Abdominal CT scan. **C,D** Ultrasound

3. One week after the operation, leukocytapheresis was started once or twice a week, for a total of 4 times in 3 weeks. 4.8×10^9 CTLs and 6.0×10^6 IU rIL-2 (Shionogi; Osaka, Japan) were injected via the hepatic arterial catheter. Two months after the last injection of CTLs, 10 mg of ADM and 10 mg of MMC were injected with 4 ml of Lipiodol (Fig. 6). Four months later, an abdominal CT scan and ultrasound were performed which showed dominant regression and necrosis

of HCCs compared with the pre-treated images. 10 months later, abdominal an CT scan and ultrasound showed no detectable tumor in his liver (Fig. 7) and now, 18 months after the operation, he is living and well.

5 Discussion

Hepatocellular carcinoma is one of the most common malignant neoplasms in Japan. Surgical liver resection, as with the Grisonean sheath core transection we reported [3], has been developed and the number of operations has been increasing every year. However, many HCC patients have difficulties undergoing conventional therapies because of severe liver dysfunction or widespread tumors. HCCs are usually asymptomatic, therefore very few of them are detected in the early stages, although improvement of diagnostic techniques including angio-CT (computed tomography) scan, Lipiodol-CT scan and enhanced ultrasonography by using carbon dioxide gas [4] have been used to detect multiple small tumors. When HCC are non-curable, several therapies, such as TAE, ethanol injection, radiation and immunotherapy, should be performed in combination. However, results such as, regression of the tumor or prolonging survival time have not been satisfactory. In our department, reduction surgery plus hepatic arterial infusion therapy has been successful in terms of improving the prognosis in these advanced HCC patients. One of the most important aspects of our treatment is the implantable drug delivery systems which makes transcatheter hepatic arterial infusion simpler and safer on an outpatient basis [5]. Furthermore, these infusion systems have enabled us to use Lipiodol emulsion with HCC patients. Despite recent advances in the infusion system, many HCC patients have not undergone chemotherapy because of liver dysfunction. Therefore, it is necessary to decrease liver damage which is caused by transcatheter hepatic arterial infusion so that its use can become widespread. Using our methods, effective carcinostatic agents for each case are choosed by sensitivity testing for HCC using the SDI test, thereby preventing the damage caused by non-effective chemotherapy. In our in vitro SDI test, HCCs have been found to have variable sensitivity to MCC, ADM, CDDP, 5-FU, FARM, and

ESQ. We use small doses of the most effective carcinostatic agent as many times as possible in the outpatient clinic.

We have also treated advanced HCCs with in vitro and in vivo studies of adoptive immunotherapy. First we administered LAK cells via the catheter into the hepatic artery. Adoptive immunotherapy using LAK cells was reported by Rosenberg [6] as a treatment for melanoma, colorectal cancer, renal cancer, and others, and was found to be effective. At several institutes in Japan, trans-hepatic arterial LAK cell injections were performed to treat HCC, however very few patients had even partial tumor regression. In our institute, 1 of 9 HCC patients treated by LAK cells obtained 80% tumor regression, but regrowth of the tumor was usually shown within a year [7]. Therefore we attempted to generate more effective killer cells in the form of autologous tumor-specific cytotoxic T lymphocytes. In in vitro culture, autologous tumor-specific CTLs were induced from patient's PBMC plus autologous tumors [8]. CTLs cultured with autologous tumor for 5 days and then added to 1,000 IU/ml rIL-2 for another 5 days have killing activity against autologous tumors, but not allogeneic tumors. These CTLs also inhibit the growth of transplanted autologous tumors in nude mice. Based on these studies, we have effectively used autologous CTLs for clinical treatment of unresectable HCCs. The side effects of CTLs injection are not critical and are easily controlled by medication. These adoptive immunotherapies are suitable for treatment of advanced HCC patients with minimal damage to normal liver tissue and they may become the most important modalities in our treatment.

In the case study reported here, the patient had very poor liver function, 41% ICG-R15, 0.29 cholinesterase (CHE), 2.3 mg/dl of total birirubin and pooling of ascites. Ultrasound showed multiple tumor nodules in bilateral lobes of the liver, and cirrhosis was also present. Most cases judged to be in Stage IV-a are not indicated for resection or TAE and the patients may well die within 6 months. However, our aggressive treatment improved his life expectancy. CTLs induced from autologous PBMC, and selected carcinostatics ADM and MMC were injected. Multiple tumor nodules in the liver have almost disappeared and he is doing well. Three other patients with stage IV-a advanced HCCs treated by our methods have obtained a "complete response" and all of them are healthy and well.

Most HCC patients in Japan have associated liver dysfunction due to cirrhosis and, therefore, excessive injection of carcinostatics may induce liver failure. We carefully selected carcinostatics using SDI testing and treated patients using both carcinostatic agents and autologous killer cells. These multidisciplinary treatments for advanced HCC patients seem to be difficult and time-consuming, but such aggressive trials are necessary to improve advanced cases of HCC.

References

1. Liver cancer study group of Japan (1987) The general rules for the clinical and pathological study of primary liver cancer, (2nd edn), Kanehara, Tokyo
2. Twentyman PR, Luscombe M (1987) A study of some variables in a tetrazolim dye (MTT) based assay for cell growth and chemosensitivity. (1987) Br J Cancer 56:279–285
3. Takasaki K, Kobayashi S, Tanaka S, Saito A, Yamamoto M, Hanyu F (1990) Highly anatomically systematized hepatic resection with glisonean sheath code transection at the hepatic hilus. Int Surgery 75:73–77
4. Takasaki K, Saito A, Nakagawa M, Muto H, Watayo T, Akimoto S, Tanaka S, Yamamoto M, Yamaguchi M, Shimamura Y, Kobayashi S (1986) Enhanced intra-operative ultrasonography. Advanced diagnostic method to determine the tumor bearing area in the liver by intra-arterial and portal injection of carbon dioxide gas. Proc JSUM pp 1061–1062
5. Gyves JW, Ensminger WD, Niederhuber JE (1984) A totally implantable injection port system for blood sampling and chemotherapy administration. JAMA 251:2538–2541
6. Rosenberg SA, Lotze MT, Muul LM (1987) A progress report on the treatment of 157 patients with advanced cancer using lymphokine-activated killer cells and interleukin-2 or high-dose interleukin-2 alone. N Engl J Med 316:889–897
7. Komatsu T, Yamauchi K, Furukawa T, Obata H, (1990) Transcatheter arterial injection of autologous lymphokine-activated killer (LAK) cells into patients with liver cancers. J Clin Immunol 3: 167–174
8. Aruga A, Yamauchi K, Takasaki K, Furukawa T, Hanyu F (1991) Induction of autologous tumor-specific cytotoxic T cells in patients with liver cancer: Characterizations and clinical utilization. Int J Cancer 49:19–24

Part 8   Recurrence

CHAPTER 34

Clinicopathological features of recurrent primary liver cancer in Japan

Susumu Yamasaki, Hiroshi Hasegawa, Tadatoshi Takayama, Tomoo Kosuge, Kazuaki Shimada, and Junji Yamamoto[1]

1 Introduction

In this chapter, the clinicopathological features of recurrent hepatocellular carcinoma (HCC), especially after hepatectomy, are described along with a review of some articles and the author's experiences.

2 Incidence of recurrence after hepatectomy

The recurrence rates after hepatectomy in some Japanese articles ranged from 48.3% to 66.1%, although the periods of observation for follow-up after the hepatectomies were not always given in the reports. The subjects of these reports were HCCs either with a single nodule or with multiple nodules. Matsumata et al. [1] reported a recurrence rate of HCC with a solitary nodule of 36.1% (53/147). Table 1 summarizes the recurrence rates after hepatectomy for HCC from some Japanese articles. The recurrence rates based upon the author's experience at the National Cancer Center Hospital was 57.8% (266/460). The hepatectomies considered here were carried out from October 1974 to September 1990, and the follow-up period continued through the end of 1990. Cases of re-resection, palliative resection and hospital mortality were excluded. Cases in which the date of recurrence detection was not known were also excluded. The cancer-free survival curve is shown in Fig. 1. Two thirds of all recurrences of HCC were detected within

the period from 1.5 years to 2.5 years, as reported by Nagasue et al. [2]. According to the author's case series, one third of the patients operated on had recurrences during the first post-operative year and one fourth of the patients had recurrences during the second post-operative year. In our case series, the latest recurrence was found in the 82nd post-operative month and in the 86th month as reported by Kanematsu et al. [3].

3 Differences between cirrhotic and non-cirrhotic patients

The recurrence rates in cases with normal liver differ from those with diseased liver, chronic active hepatitis (CAH), precirrhosis (pre-LC) and cirrhosis (LC). The cancer-free survival curves of the three case categories: 1) cases with normal liver, 2) cases with CAH or pre-LC, and 3) cases with LC are shown in Fig. 2. The three curves are very similar until the second post-operative year when the curve for normal liver cases thereafter shows lower rates; and after the 52nd month there was no recurrence. The cancer-free survival rate of this group was 36.7% after the 53rd month. That of LC cases, on the other hand, shows a continued sharp decline for another year, declining further to 9% in the 82nd post-operative month. Sasaki et al. [4] reported very similar results in their comparison of cancer-free survival between a cirrhotic-liver group (Group A, n = 121) and a normal-liver group (Group B, n = 37). The cancer-free survival rates of the two groups were almost the same until the third post-operative year and no patients in Group B had recurrences after the 3rd year. Among the Group A patients, recurrences continued until the 5th year.

[1]National Cancer Center Hospital, 5-1-1 Tsukiji, Chuo-ku, Tokyo, 104 Japan

Table 1. The recurrence rates reported in Japanese articles

Author	Recurrence rate	Subject	Period of hepatectomy (year/month)	Period of follow-up
Matsumata et al. [1]	36.1% (53/147)	single nodule	1971/4–1988/3	NK
Nagasue et al. [2]	48.3% (69/143)	overall	1980/1–1988/12	–1989/5
Nagao et al. [5]	66.1% (41/62)	overall	1981/1–1986/12	25–85 months
Author's series	57.8% (266/460)	overall	1974/10–1990/9	–1990/12

NK, not known

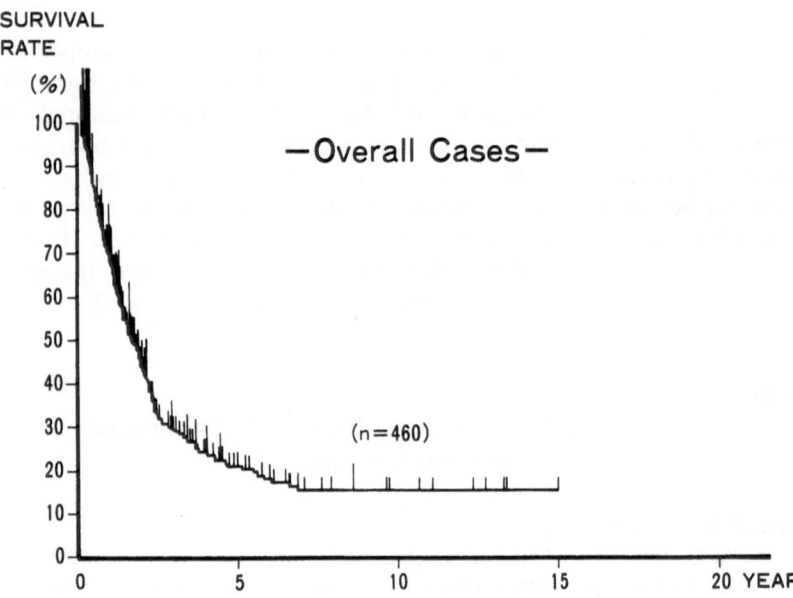

Fig. 1. Cancer-free survival rates of patients operated on at the National Cancer Center Hospital up until September 1990. Operative mortalities and hospital deaths were excluded

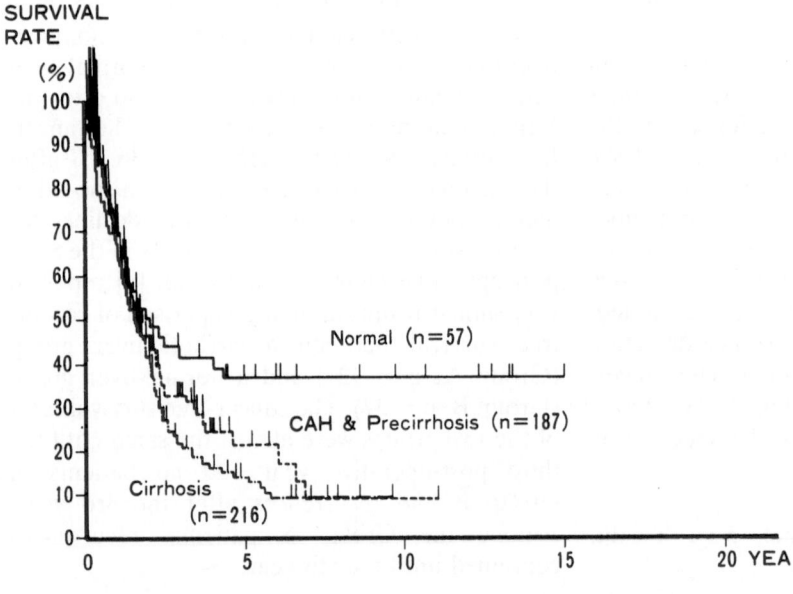

Fig. 2. Cancer-free survival rates of case groups classified by the pathological findings of non-cancerous liver parenchyma on surgical specimens at the National Cancer Center Hospital

Fig. 3. Incidence of recurrence after hepatectomy by site

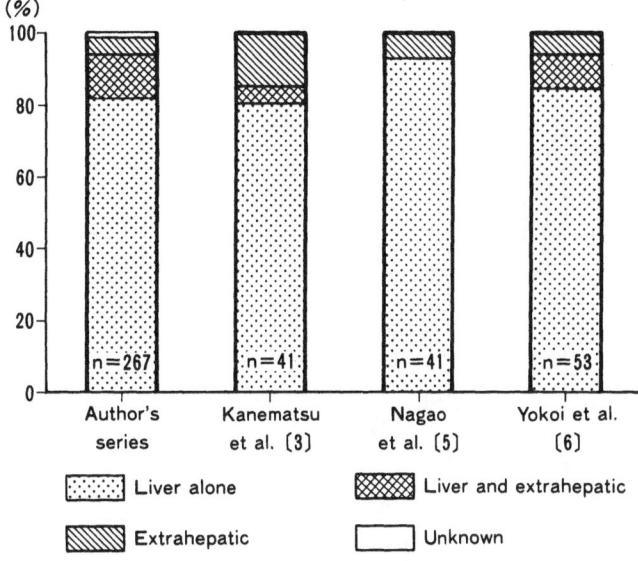

4   **Sites and patterns of recurrence**

Most of the recurrences after hepatectomy occurred in the remnant livers. The lung, bone, lymphnode, adrenal gland, peritoneum and brain were frequent sites of recurrence of HCC, although the incidence of recurrence in those sites was much lower than in the remnant liver. Figure 3 shows the incidence of recurrence in sites which were classified as in the liver alone, in the liver and other viscera simultenously, extrahepatic and unknown, from reported articles [3, 5, 6] and the author's case series. Ninety percent of the recurrences were noted in the liver alone or in the liver along with extrahepatic recurrence.

The patterns of recurrence in the remnant liver are generally classified into three types: A marginal recurrence, B nodular recurrence with a single or a few lesions away from the initially affected area, and C diffuse recurrence over the whole remnant liver. Marginal recurrence is defined as recurring tumor on or within a few centimeters of the surgical margin. Type B recurrences are a single nodule or multiple but few nodules re-developed away from the primary cancer site. Matsumata et al. [1] reported the incidence of these types of recurrence as 21%, 49% and 30% for Types A, B and C, respectively. The same recurrences were 16%, 35% and 49% as reported by Nagasue et al. [2], and 67%, 11% and 22%, as reported by Ezaki et al. [7]. On the whole, this information suggests that these three types of recurrence occur at almost the same frequency.

5   **Prognostic factors for recurrence**

Factors influencing recurrence of HCC were analysed. The clinicopathologic factors were divided into three categories: cancer-related, host-related and surgery-related. To clarify the value of the influence of each factor upon recurrence, the cancer-free survival rates of the groups defined by each factor were compared among the author's cases. The cancer-free survival rate is expressed as a percentage ±SD.

5.1   **Cancer-related factors**

5.1.1   **Solitary or multiple nodules**
The cancer-free survival curves of cases with a solitary HCC (n = 244) and those with multiple HCCs (n = 216) are shown in Fig. 4. There was a significant difference ($P < 0.001$) between the two groups by the generalized Wilcoxon test. Thus, solitary or multiple nodule HCC is a significant prognostic factor in recurrence.

5.1.2   **Size of HCC nodule**
To exclude the influence of other factors, the cancer-free survival rates of cases with a solitary HCC of 5 cm or less in diameter were analysed. The caner-free survival rates in the third year

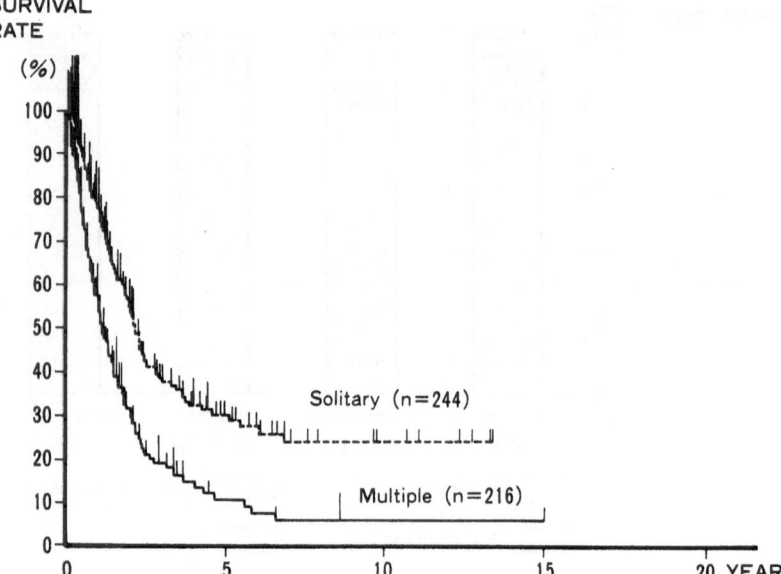

Fig. 4. Comparison of the cancer-free survival rates between patients with a solitary *HCC* and multiple *HCCs*, at the National Cancer Center Hospital

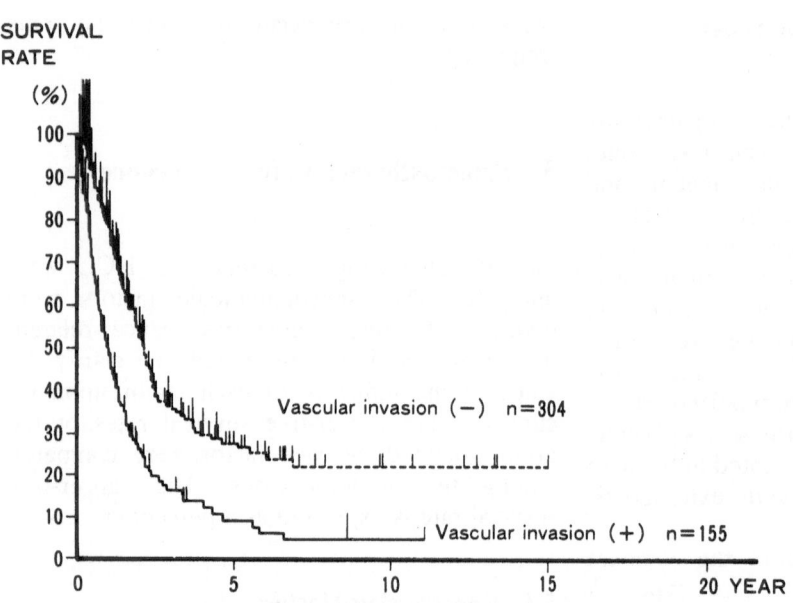

Fig. 5. Comparison of the cancer-free survival rates between patients with vascular invasion of the *HCC* in the surgical specimen and those without at the National Cancer Center Hospital

after hepatectomy for the case groups with a solitary HCC of 2 cm or less (n = 49), 2~3 cm (n = 63), 3~4 cm (n = 49) and 4~5 cm (n = 24) were 48.0 ± 8.8%, 30.2 ± 7.8%, 38.8 ± 8.6% and 37.7 ± 12.3%, respectively. There was no differece between any two groups. That suggests the size of the HCC nodule is not a prognostic factor in recurrence.

5.1.3 Vascular invasion

The most common manner of HCC extension is intrahepatic metastasis through the portal vein branch and tumor thrombi in the portal vein. In some surgical specimens of HCC, macroscopic tumor thrombi are seen in the vascular structures including the portal and hepatic veins as well as in the bile duct. The cancer-free survival rates were compared between cases with and without macroscopic vascular invasion. Intrahepatic metastases are thought to be a product of vascular invasion. Here, the case group with vascular invasion includes cases not only with vascular invasion but also with intrahepatic metastatic nodules. The 5-year cancer-free survival rate of the vascular invasion positive-group (n = 155) was 9.1 ± 3.1% and that of the vascular invasion

Fig. 6. Cancer-free survival rates of patients categorized by the *TNM* stage of the *HCC*

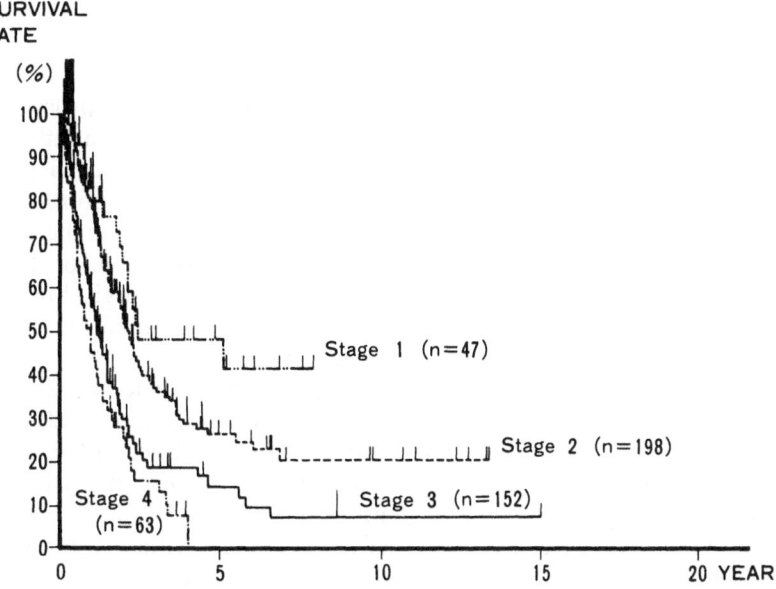

negative-group (n = 304) was 27.6 ± 3.5% (Fig. 5). The difference was significant by the generalized Wilcoxon test ($P < 0.001$). Thus, vascular invasion is one of the strongest prognostic factors.

5.1.4 Differentiation of cancer tissue

In the 200 cases with solitary HCC of 5 cm or less in diameter, the influence of cancer differentiation for recurrence was examined. In 40 of the 200 cases, the degree of cancer differentiation could not be determined because of complete necrosis, mainly due to preoperative hepatic arterial embolization. Edmondson-Steiner's classification [8] was adopted for HCC differentiation. There are four grades in the Edmondson-Steiner classification system, Grade 1 ~ Grade 4. However, cancer differentiation is not always homogeneous in one HCC nodule and we found that four grades were not adequate to distinguish the degree of differentiation observed. So here, the cases were classified into six grades: A, B, C, D, E and F. Grade A (n = 6) is identical to Grade 1 of Edmondson-Steiner's classification; Grade B (n = 27) is a cross-over of Grades 1 and 2; Grade C (n = 47) is identical to Grades 2 Grade D (n = 62) is a cross-over of Grades 2 and 3; Grade E (n = 14) is identical to Grade 3; Grade F (n = 4) is a cross-over of Grades 3 and 4. Grades A and F were ommitted in the analysis of survival rates because the number of cases in these two grades were too small (4 and 6) to yield stastically significant results. The 5-year cancer-free survival rates were 35.6 ± 12.0%, 27.7 ±

8.7%, 22.7 ± 7.1% and 28.6 ± 12.1% for Grades B, C, D, and E, respectively. Thus, cancer differentiation is not a significant prognostic factor in recurrence.

5.1.5 Alpha-fetoprotein

The influence of alpha-fetoprotein (AFP) in recurrence was examined in cases with a solitary HCC of 5 cm or less in diameter. The cases were categorized into 4 groups according to the serum AFP value per unit of cancer volume. Cubic centimeter (cm^3) was used as the unit of cancer volume. Group A was a case group with negative (less than 20 ng/ml) AFP in sera. Groups B, C and D were those with AFP of 1,000 ng/cm^3, or less, AFP between 100 and 100 ng/cm^3 and more than 1,000 ng/cm^3, respectively. The 3-year cancer-free survival rates were 44.7 ± 8.7%, 30.8 ± 8.1%, 36.5 ± 8.0% and 42.7 ± 13.8 for Group A (n = 65), Group B (n = 53), Group C (n = 53) and Group D (n = 14), respectively. Thus, AFP does not seem to be a prognostic factor in HCC recurrence.

5.1.6 TNM stage

The TNM (tumor, node, metastasis) staging system of HCC by UICC (Union Internationale contre le Cancer) uses mainly the tumor size break off at 2 cm, the number of HCC nodules (solitary or multiple) and the presence or absence of vascular invasion [9]. The cancer-free survival rates of the author's case series broken down by TNM stage are shown in Fig. 6. The number of cases in the 4 stages of TNM stages 1, 2, 3 and 4, were 47, 198, 152 and 63, respectively. The 5-year cancer-free survival rates were $48.0 \pm 9.1\%$, $26.1 \pm 4.2\%$, $14.4 \pm 4.3\%$ and 0%, respectively. The 4-year cancer-free survival rate of stage 4 was $7.8 \pm 4.2\%$. The differences among all the stages were significant. Thus, the TNM staging system of HCC is a good indicator in recurrence.

5.2 Host-related factors

As host-related factors, the pathological finding of non-cancerous liver parenchyma, hepatitis B surface antigen (HBs-ag) and liver function were analysed. There were 216 cases with cirrhosis, and 57 with normal liver parenchyma. The remaining 187 cases had intermediate changes in liver parenchyma such as chronic active hepatitis, liver fibrosis and precirrhosis. The 5-year survival rates were $14.1 \pm 3.2\%$, $36.7 \pm 6.9\%$ and $21.7 \pm 5.0\%$ for the cirrhotic, normal and intermediate groups, respectively, as shown in Fig. 2. Between the normal and the other two groups, a significant difference ($P < 0.01$) was observed.

The 5-year cancer-free survival rate of cases positive for HBs-ag (n = 97, $27.1 \pm 5.4\%$) was better ($P < 0.05$) than that of cases negative for HBs-ag (n = 359, $18.7 \pm 3.0\%$). The results were the same whether all cases were analyzed or whether analysis was confined to cases with a solitary HCC of 5 cm or less in diameter. These results seem rather surprising, however, as many cases negative for HBs-ag may also have hepatitis C virus infection. Therefore, no conclusion on the influence of hepatitis virus infection in recurrence should be made until data regarding hepatitis C antibody in hepatectomized cases have been accumulated.

The indocyanin green 15-minute retention rate (ICG R15) was used as an indicator of liver function in the hepatectomized cases. The cases with a solitary HCC were divided into 4 groups according to the values of ICG R15: A) ICG R15 of 10% or less, B) 10–20%, C) 20–30%, D) more than 30%. The 5-year survival rates for A (n = 27), B (n = 86), C (n = 64) and D (n = 67) were $41.3 \pm 11.1\%$, $53.1 \pm 6.8\%$, $11.0 \pm 5.7\%$ and $15.1 \pm 6.1\%$, respectively. A significant difference can be seen between the first two groups and the second two ($P < 0.05$), but not between A and B, or between C and D. This means that recurrences are significantly more frequent in cases with ICG R15 of more than 20%.

5.3 Surgery-related factors

Surgical procedures for patients with HCC, most of whom are cirrhotic, are restricted by the degree of liver dysfunction, though it is clear that a more extensive resection is likely to produce a higher survival rate. Here we discuss the questions of the distance from the tumor edge to the surgical margin (TW), and whether or not an anatomic resection is better than non-anatomic one.

The abbreviation TW is defined by the Liver Cancer Study Group of Japan in The General Rule for the Clinical and Pathological Study of Primary Liver Cancer [10] as follows: Positive TW means macroscopic cancerous infiltration within 10 mm from the cut liver surface in freshly excised specimens. Negative TW means no macroscopic cancerous infiltration within 10 mm from the cut liver surface in freshly excised specimens. The 3-year cancer-free survival rate for negative TW (n = 69) was $33.1 \pm 6.7\%$ with no change at 5-years. The rates for positive TW (n = 337) were $28.6 \pm 3.2\%$ and $15.7 \pm 3.1\%$ at 3 and 5 years, respectively. The difference between the two was not significant.

The influence of the surgical procedure, i.e. anatomic or non-anatomic, in recurrence was examined. The subjects were the cases with a solitary HCC of 5 cm or less in diameter. The surgical procedures compared here were the anatomic subsegmentectomy (Group A, n = 64) and the non-anatomic small range resection (Group B, n = 103) [11]. The 3- and 5-year cancer-free survival rates for Group A were $36.2 \pm 7.7\%$ and $29.9 \pm 7.6\%$, respectively. Those for Group B were $36.6 \pm 6.1\%$ and $25.5 \pm 5.9\%$. The differences were not significant. Thus, no positive prognostic factors were found in the surgical procedure.

As discussed above, the number of HCC nodules (solitary or multiple) and the presence or absence of vascular invasion are definite prognostic factors in recurrence. Pathological change of the non-cancerous liver parenchyma and liver function are weak prognostic factors. The TNM staging system by UICC is a good indicator in recurrence. Tumor size, degree of cancer differentiation, serum AFP level, positive or negative TW, surgical procedure (anatomic or non-anatomic) do not seem to be significant prognostic factors. The influence of hepatitis virus infection remains obscure.

References

1. Matsumata T, Kanematsu T, Takenaka K et al. (1989) Patterns of intrahepatic recurrence after curative resection of hepatocellular carcinoma. Hepatology 9:457–460
2. Nagasue N, Yuyaya H, Chang YC et al. (1990) Assessment of pattern and treatment of intrahepatic recurrence after resection of hepatocellular carcinoma. Surgery 171:217–222
3. Kanematsu T, Matsumata T, Takenaka K et al. (1988) Clinical management of recurrent hepatocellular carcinoma after primary resection. Br J Surg 75:203–206
4. Sasaki H, Imaoka S, Masutani S et al. (1990) Long-term postoperative courses of hepatocellular carcinoma with and without cirrhosis. Jpn J Cancer Chemother 17:435–439
5. Nagao T, Inoue S, Yoshimi F et al. (1990) Postoperative recurrence of hepatocellular carcinoma. Ann Surg 211:28–33
6. Yokoi H, Noguchi T, Kawarada Y et al. (1990) Clinical features and counter-measures against recurrent hepatocellular carcinoma. Jpn J Gastroenterol Surg 23:1331
7. Ezaki T, Yukaya H, Ogawa Y et al. (1989) Recurrent form of hepatocellular carcinoma after partial hepatic resection. Hepato gastroenterology 36:164–167
8. Edmondson HA, Steiner PE (1954) Primary carcinoma of the liver: A study of 100 cases among 48,900 necropsies. Cancer 7:462–503
9. Hermanek P, Sobin LH (eds) (1987) Digestive system tumours: TNM classification of malignant tumours. International Union Against Cancer, 4th edn. Springer-Verlag, Berlin pp 53–55
10. Liver Cancer Study Group of Japan (1989) The General Rule for the Clinical and Pathological Study of Primary Liver Cancer. Jpn J Surgery 19:98–129
11. Yamasaki S, Hasegawa H, Makuuchi M et al. (1990) Significance of systematic subsegmentectomy of the liver for hepatocellular carcinoma from the view point of the long-term result. Acta hepatol Jpn 31:558–564

References

CHAPTER 35

Treatment of recurrent primary liver cancer

Junichi Uchino, Yoshie Une, Yasuaki Nakajima, Naoki Sato, Shinichi Matsuoka, Toshiya Kamiyama, Kazuhito Misawa, Hiroyuki Ishizu, and Kazuhiro Ogasawara[1]

1 Introduction

Resection of the liver offers the most favorable prognosis for primary liver cancer (PLC) [1]. Recently, an increasing number of patients with hepatocellular carcinoma (HCC) have been treated with resection, and the survival periods have been prolonged. However, the rate of recurrence after resection is still high, and there is much room for improvement. [2–5].

Since prevention of recurrent tumors is vital, various modalities of treatment for recurrence have been employed, and prognoses have gradually improved. The methods of treatment may be varied according to the mode of recurrence and should take into account the quality of life of the patients.

2 Mode of recurrence and selection of treatment

Recurrence occurs in approximately 50% of patients after hepatectomy within 3 years. The most frequent site of recurrence is the remnant liver. Extrahepatic metastasis is not common but may occur in the lung, bones, and lymph nodes. About 85% of the recurrences occur within 1 year, so close follow-up examination should be carried out in the first one year after operation.

According to Matsumata's report [6], among 33 patients with intrahepatic recurrences, 7 had recurrence near the resected margin, 5 had nodular recurrence, and 8 had widespread multinodular recurrence within one year after hepatectomy. Hsu et al. [7] described that only 2.4% of HCC were regarded as having true multicentric origin, because recurrence results mostly from intrahepatic dissemination of the portal invasive tumor.

In our series, 186 patients with HCC were followed after hepatic resection between 1978 and 1989. Tumor markers were estimated every month, and a computed tomography (CT) scan and hepatic ultrasonography were done every two or three months. One hundred forty-two patients had satisfactory clinical data for evaluation. Recurrence of HCC were confirmed by postoperative investigation in 75 patients (52.8%). Recurrences were detected within one year in 87% of the patients. The most frequent site of recurrence was the remnant liver (88.5%). This was followed in order by the lung, bone and lymph nodes (Table 1).

Our previous reports on nuclear DNA contents of HCC showed that patients with HCC of diploid pattern had a more favorable prognosis than those with an aneuploid pattern: 3 years survival in 91.6%, and 5 years survival in 61.3% (Fig. 1). Although the recurrence rates do not correlate with the nuclear DNA ploidy pattern, multiple intrahepatic recurrences were somewhat more frequent in patients with the aneuploid pattern than those with the diploid one. This result was not related to the operative procedures for the primary lesion. The most favorable survival rate was obtained in patients with recurrence limited to the liver.

According to the Liver Cancer Study Group of Japan [1], 417 out of 1,374 patients (30.3%) had lymph node metastasis in autopsy. Recurrence in the regional lymph nodes was noted in 2.8% (4/142) in our series. When regional lymph nodes swelling are detected by abdominal CT scan or ultrasound, they can occasionally be resectable. Therefore, strict follow-up of not only the rem-

---

[1] Department of Surgery, Hokkaido University School of Medicine, Kita-ku, Sapporo, Hokkaido, 060 Japan

Table 1. Sites of recurrence of HCC (1978–1989)

Sites	No. patients (%)
Liver	61 (43.0)
Lung	6 (4.2)
Bone	4 (2.8)
Lymph nodes	4 (2.8)
None	67 (47.2)
	142 (100%)
	(Total 186)

nant liver but also the regional lymph nodes increases the chance of re-resection of metastatic lymph nodes as well as recurrence in the remnant liver.

3 Reserve liver function in patients with recurrence

3.1 Overview of patients with re-resected HCC

Re-resection of the liver was carried out in 20 patients over the past 12 years in our department. Fifteen patients had enough clinical data to be analyzed and were investigated. Twelve were male and three were female. The average age was 59.1 years (from 32–76 years) at the initial operation, and 61.0 years at the second operation. The period between the first and second operations ranged from 5 months to 5.6 years, with an average of 22.7 months. The method of the first and second operations were somewhat different. In the first operation, partial resections

were performed in 6 cases, subsegmentectomy in 2, segmentectomy in 3, lobectomy in 3, and trisegmentectomy in 1. The second operation mostly consisted of partial resection, and major hepatectomy was not performed. The postoperative complications after the second operation were liver failure in three, pleural effusion in one and biloma in one.

3.2 Estimation of preoperative reserved liver function

3.2.1 Indicative criteria for hepatic resection
Livers with HCC are often accompanied by hepatic cirrhosis. HCC with liver cirrhosis accounted for 67.7% of total cases of hepatectomy registered with the Japanese Primary Liver Cancer Society [1]. HCC patients with impaired hepatic function require precise resection and accurate estimation of liver resectability. The indicative criteria for hepatic resection has been applied since 1985 using several liver function tests at our institution. This criteria includes serum cholinesterase (CHE), serum albumin (ALB), serum bilirubin (BIL), prothrombin time (PT), and ICG retention rate at 15 min ($ICGR_{15}$). Ninety-one hepatic resections were performed from 1988 to 1990. In four patients, more than two values were abnormal, and two of these patients (50%) suffered from postoperative hepatic failure. In the remaining 87 patients who had one or no abnormal values, liver failure was occurred in four patients (4.6%). From these retrospective view, the criteria is considered to be useful for evaluating the preoperative reserved hepatic functions and resectability for the second hepatectomy as well.

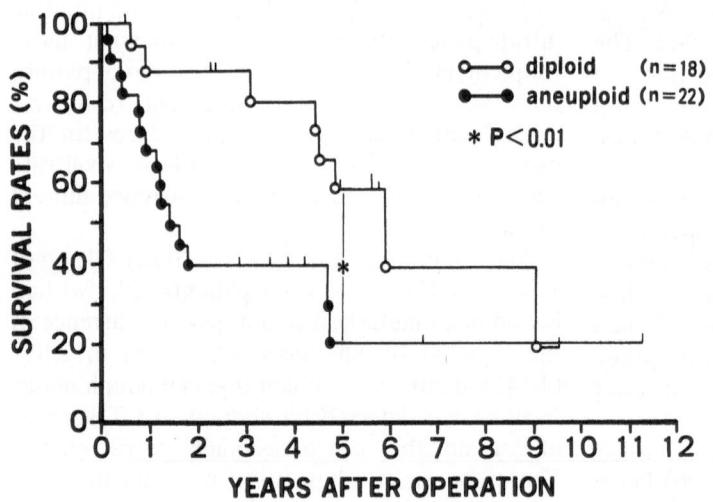

Fig. 1. DNA ploidy pattern and survival rates in recurrent HCC (Kaplan-Meier method)

3.2.2 Reserved liver function in re-resected patients

In the liver function tests, the preoperative serum CHE level was 212 ± 67 IU/l (mean $\pm$SD) before the first operation, and significantly decreased to 179 ± 57 IU/l before the second operation. The $ICGR_{15}$ level was $12.7 \pm 4.9\%$ before the first the operation, and it significantly declined to $17.1 \pm 9.7\%$ before the second operation. Among re-resected patients, one had abnormal CHE and ALB values before the first operation, but he underwent emergent liver resection of the lateral and caudate lobes because of rupture of the hepatoma. Although the postoperative hepatic failure occurred on day 3, he recovered from this complication following treatments that included plasma exchange.

Before the second resection, one patient showed abnormal levels of CHE and $ICGR_{15}$, and two had abnormal values of ALB and $ICGR_{15}$. These three patients had postoperative hepatic failures and died on day 3, 5, and 59. In terms of hepatic reserve function, there is no definite indicative criteria for re-resection of recurrent hepatic cancer. From our experience with re-resection, we found that the hepatic functional reserve had apparently deteriorated before the second operation and postoperative liver failure occurred more frequently than after the first operation. Therefore, the second resection should be carefully selected and undesirable postoperative complications should be minimized by optimal treatment.

4 Repeat hepatectomy for recurrent HCC

Recurrence after liver resection frequently occurs in the remnant liver, so a repeat hepatectomy must be considered for improvement of the prognosis. There have been very few reports comparing the practicability and results of repeat hepatectomy and other therapy (Table 2).

4.1 Clinicopathological study on re-resected HCC

From January 1979 to December 1990, 15 patients with recurrent HCC were treated by re-resection including two patients treated with dissection of metastatic regional lymph nodes. Twelve patients were male and three were female, and the average age was 59.1 years old with a range of 32–76. The tumor sizes at the

Table 2. The 2-year survival rates after treatment for recurrent HCC (%)

	TAE	Re-resection
Uchino 1991	30.0	92.0
Yamazaki 1991 [4]	51.3	92.3
Ozawa 1989 [28]	41.9	62.5
Oka 1990 [3]	64.9	34.3
Mizumoto 1990 [2]	42.0	50.0

TAE, Transcatheter arterial embolization

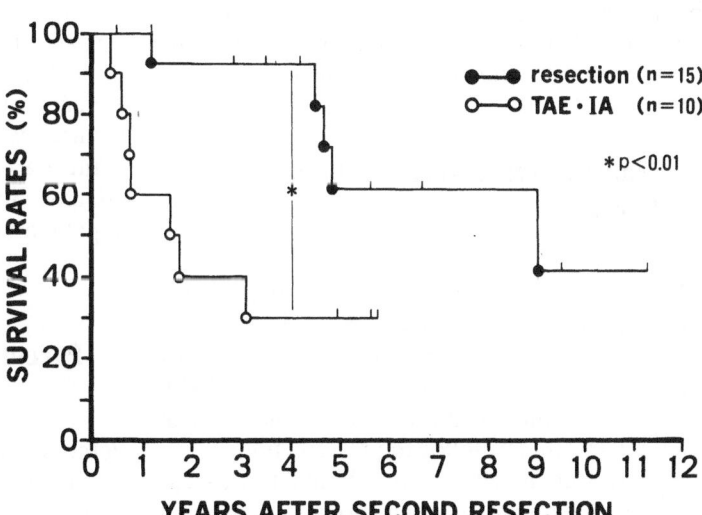

Fig. 2. Treatment for the recurrence in the remnant liver

first resection were 2.5–22 cm in diameter, with an average of 6.0 ± 5.2 cm. At the second resection, the tumors were smaller than those at the first resection with an average of 3.4 ± 1.6 cm, and 1.6–7.2 cm in diameter. Compared with other treatments for recurrence, re-resection showed significantly better results. The five-year survival rates by the Kaplan-Meier method in the re-resected group showed the most favorable results of 66.3% (Fig. 2). This was followed by patients treated with transcatheter arterial embolization (TAE) and intra-arterial chemotherapy.

The DNA ploidy pattern was analyzed in 15 re-resected cases using flow cytometry. Seven were diploid and 8 were aneuploid. The time interval between the initial and the second hepatectomies was 27.6 months and 22.9 months, respectively. The five-year survival rate in the diploid group was significantly higher than that of the aneuploid group, however there were two patients in each group who survived more than 5 years. Kanematsu [8] reported that the second resection was effective in four patients: Three survived for over 2 years, and the longest survival time was 9 years after the second resection. Lange et al. [9] reviewed 11 patients with re-resection on recurrence of HCC. The interval between hepatectomies ranged from 5–132 months. Seven patients died of recurrence of the liver tumor after 11 to 48 months. Four patients have been living without recurrence for 4–54 months with a mean of 33 months.

Repeat hepatectomies for recurrent tumors are technically quite feasible. Low operative mortality rates and prolongation of the survival time also encouraged us to perform second resections of recurrent primary liver cancer. However, the reserve liver function worsens after the first resection in patients with associated liver cirrhosis, therefore, these patients should be carefully selected for repeat hepatectomy.

5 Transcatheter arterial embolization therapy

TAE was reported to improve the prognosis for non-resectable recurrent HCC cases [4, 9]. In our institution, 30 cases were treated by TAE for recurrent hepatic lesions between 1980 and 1989. They showed the second most favorable survival rates for treatment, following re-resection.

Nagasue et al. [10] reported that the 5-year survival rate obtained by chemoembolization of the hepatic artery after the second resection was 26.8%. Takayasu et al. [11] reported on 97 cases with a reference to recurrence in the remnant liver following hepatectomy. TAE for the recurrence was proven to prolong the survival of patients after hepatectomy, and to improve the results of surgery.

Sasaki et al. [12] showed the post-recurrence survival of a group which was treated with regional therapy including chemoembolization of the hepatic artery. The group was significantly better than the non-treated group in the analysis of his 101 hepatectomized patients.

6 Intra-arterial chemotherapy

Intra-hepatic arterial infusion of anticancer agents has proven to be effective for unresectable recurrent HCC. A percutaneons reservoir was recently developed which connects with the intra-arterial catheter enabling us to perform repeated infusion of chemotherapeutic agents.

The intra-arterial chemotherapy under occlusion of hepatic arterial flow may increase the concentration of intra-hepatic drugs in the liver. We created a new reservoir system, which used a balloon to occlude hepatic arterial flow temporarily. Twenty patients with unresectable hepatocellular carcinoma have been treated by this method in the past four years. Twenty-one repeated infusions were possible without any severe side effects. The overall response rate was 65%. Compared with conventional intra-arterial infusion chemotherapy, the 2-year survival rate was significantly improved by this method. A fifty-seven year-old male patient had a recurrence 2 years after resection for HCC, and he underwent this treatment. He is now in good condition 2 years and 8 months after detection of the recurrence.

Intra-arterial chemotherapy is particularly effective when combined with occlusion of the hepatic arterial flow.

7 Percutaneous ethanol injection therapy

Percutaneous ethanol injection therapy (PEI) is a less invasive, and it is an effective therapy for small liver cancer. Recently, PEI has become widespread. It can be used repeatedly and effectively, even on recurrent lesions. The recurrence rate after PEI is almost the same as after hepatic resection in the cases studied: 1 year, 28.9%; 2 years, 59.8%; and 3 years, 73.0% [13]. Ehara et al. [13] reported the usefulness of repeat PEI which they performed on 60.6% of their recurrent cases.

8 Treatment of recurrence in the other organs and lymph nodes

Frequent sites of distant metastases of HCC are the lung, bone, lymph nodes, and adrenal gland. Similar to other malignant tumors with distant metastases, the treatment of HCC with distant metastases is quite difficult. No confirmed treatment has been established yet. The modality of treatment is varied according to the site, the number and the size of the metastatic lesions, the general condition of the patients, the condition of the primary tumor, and status of liver function, and so on. The modalities include surgical resection, chemotherapy, immunotherapy, and radiotherapy. It is also important to consider the quality of life of the patients.

8.1 Surgical resection of the metastatic lesions

Surgical resection of the metastatic lesions can be tried if the metastasis is solitary and resectable, though the presence of the distant metastasis may indicate that the tumor cells have already spread to some other parts of the body as well.

In our department, 42 cases of pulmonary metastasis were seen among all HCC patients. We recently performed lung resection in 3 patients with metastatic lung tumor after resection of HCC. Two of the 3 were solitary lesions. One patient is still alive 18 months after the lung resection with recurrent tumors in the liver, and another patient died of another disease one month after the operation. The remaining 1 patient, a 32-year-old male, had two lesions in the bilateral lungs after right trisegmentectomy of the liver for large advanced HCC. The pulmonary lesions were initially controlled with bronchial artery chemoembolization. However, the tumors showed no response to this therapy, so partial resection of the left lower lobe was performed.

Then right upper and middle lobectomy was performed one month after the first pulmonary resection. He survived and continued his career as a school teacher one year after the last operation without any recurrence (Fig. 3).

One patient, a 56-year-old male, had a solitary lesion in the right lung 6 months after hepatectomy for HCC, and the lesion was resected as a metastasis. However, it was primary lung cancer.

The indications for resection of pulmonary metastasis of HCC are as follows: a) the primary hepatic lesions should be well controlled, b) there should be no other metastatic lesions except lungs, c) all pulmonary lesions should be resected, and d) the respiratory function after pulmonary resection should be conserved.

We performed simultaneous hepatic and bone resection in three patients with solitary bone metastasis. The site of the resected bones were the rib in 2 cases, and the sternum in one. However, all these patients died within a year with recurrent liver disease. Even if the metastatic lesion is solitary and resectable, it is difficult to obtain long-term survival by resection of the lesion. There is, however, a case report of 5-year-survival after hepatic and sternal resection in a patient with HCC with sternal metastasis [14].

The swelled metastatic lymph nodes are detectable by elevation of serum alpha fetoprotein (AFP), and imaging studies such as computed tomography (CT) and magnetic resonance imaging (MRI), so they may be surgically resectable. Recurrence in the lymph nodes were most commonly detected in the hepatoduodenal ligament and the retropancreatic region in our patients. One of the patients died of hepatic recurrence 4 years 10 months after the initial operation. A 59-year-old male has survived and is doing well 3 years after dissection of recurrent lymph nodes, 6 years after the initial hepatectomy. (Fig. 4).

8.2 Chemotherapy

Most distant metastases were multiple, thus making them non-resectable. Chemotherapy will be the first choice of treatment in such patients. There is a case report of bone metastasis of HCC which was reduced completely after steroid therapy [15], and tegafur derivatives were reported to be effective in a case of bone metastasis from HCC [16]. We have experienced a case of lung metastasis which was reduced after intra-

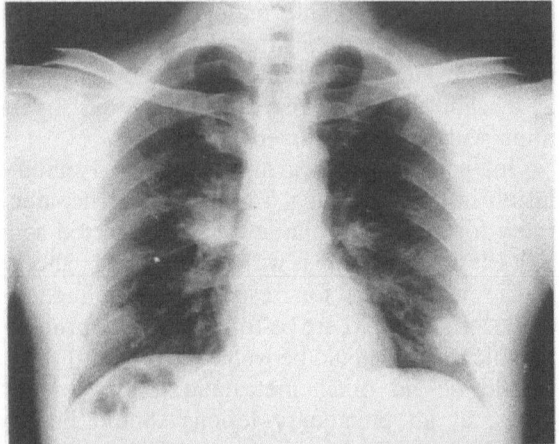

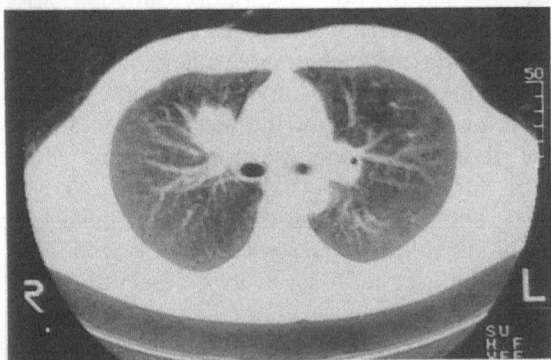

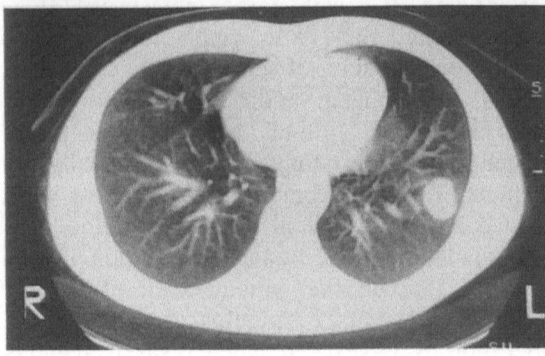

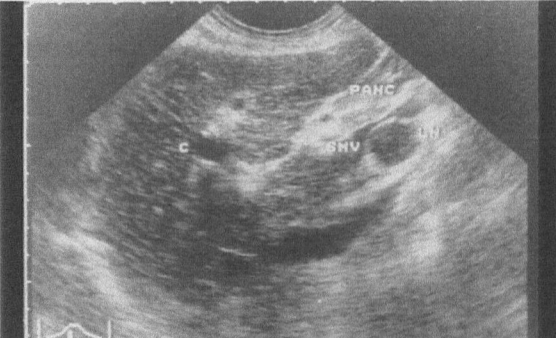

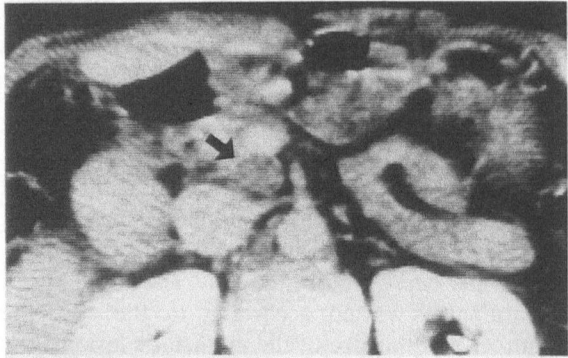

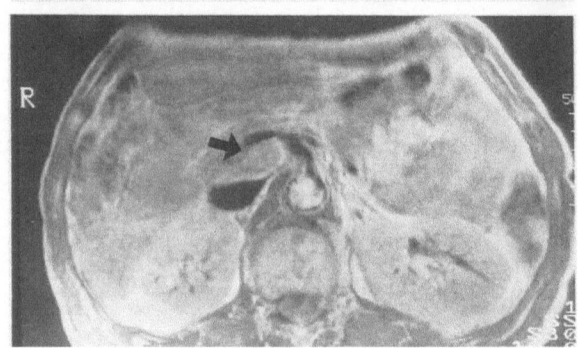

Fig. 4. Recurrence of regional lymph node metastasis in a 59-year-old man. HCC of 3 cm in diameter at segment 5 had been resected 2 years 5 months previously

Fig. 3. Lung metastasis of HCC in a 32-year-old male. Two tumors were demonstrated in right upper lobe (S^3) and left lower lobe (S^9)

venous administration of adriamycin. However, these cases are rather exceptional. In most patients, intravenous or oral chemotherapy has little or no effect on the metastatic lesions.

Intra-arterial chemotherapy or TAE to the feeding artery of the lesions may be more effective. This is because metastatic HCC lesions are usually hypervascular which is similar to the primary lesion. We treated a 32-year-old female patient who developed metastasis to the left iliac bone 15 months after hepatic resection. TAE and

intra-arterial chemotherapy to the feeding artery were carried out in combination with irradiation, and she is alive at present, 45 months after detection of the bone metastasis, though the iliac bone tumor is still present. When the feeding artery to the metastatic lesion is clearly detected, long term palliation can be obtained with such therapies.

We performed bronchial artery infusion chemotherapy and TAE in 2 patients with lung metastases. The size of the tumors was not significantly reduced, but on the follow-up CTs, the density of the lesions became lower which suggested necrotic changes. A 44-year-old male complained of bloody sputum due to invasion of a metastatic lung lesion to the bronchus. TAE was performed to the bronchial artery, which was effective in improving his symptom.

Arterial infusion therapy to the lung metastasis is less effective compared with the other lesions such as bone because the lung tumors are supplied not only by the bronchial artery but also the intercostal artery, and others. Nevertheless, some palliation, including improvement of the symptoms, can be obtained.

8.3 Radiotherapy

Radiotherapy is often performed for bone metastases of HCC, but it is difficult to reduce the tumor size with the usual clinical dose. We treated 6 patients with bone metastasis by radiotherapy, and a partial response was seen in only one patient. Symptoms such as pain, however, were considerably relieved by the radiotherapy in most of the patients.

Though there is a case report of rib metastasis which was effectively treated with ^{60}Co therapy [17], radiotherapy alone has only limited value. Combining radiotherapy and intra-arterial chemotherapy may increase the antitumor effect.

9 Treatment of recurrent cholangiocellular carcinoma

Cholangiocellular carcinoma (CCC) is a relatively rare primary hepatic cancer originating from the intrahepatic bile duct. According to the 8th report from the Japanese Cancer Association [18], the frequency of CCC is 5.5% of all hepatic primary cancer. The tumor is not associated with hepatic disorder, and early detection of lesion is so difficult that resectable tumors are few. Furthermore, the recurrence rate after resection is higher than HCC.

We experienced 36 cases of CCC over the past 30 years. Ten patients were resected (27.0%). The average survival time after hepatectomy was 1.5 years, and the longest survivor lived for 4 years. Causes of death were peritoneal dissemination in 3 cases, tumor recurrence in the remnant liver in 3 cases and unknown in 1.

There are very few reports evaluating modalities to treat recurrence of CCC after resection. There are some differences between those of CCC and HCC. In the analysis of autopsied cases, the recurrent sites were found in the lung, regional lymph nodes, and peritoneal dissemination [19]. Fujita [20] reported that in his 7 radically resected cases, peritoneal dissemination were found in 5, and regional lymph node metastasis in 2. Peritoneal dissemination seems to be common in CCC although it is rare in HCC. Tanaka et al. [21] and Yamamoto et al. [22] reported re-resection of hepatic recurrent lesions which occurred at 8 years and 9 months, and at 1 year and 3 months after hepatectomy, respectively. They have survived for 9 years, and 6 years 2 months since the initial operation, respectively.

Recently, we have been performing intra-arterial infusion chemotherapy at the early period of postoperatively using an implantable reservoir which is expected to help prevent intrahepatic recurrence.

10 Liver transplantation

Liver transplantation is now being tried clinically to treat primary liver cancer. Klompmaker et al. [23] reported, HCC and CCC had the poorest survival and highest recurrence rates. Olthoff et al. [24] indicated that patient selection is extremely important in predicting outcome after transplantation. Hart et al. [25] reported that 6 out of 13 patients (46%) who underwent transplants for HCC developed recurrent tumors, and chemotherapy to treat this is currently undefined. Liver transplantation for recurrent primary liver cancer is unlikely to be successful in the near future unless an effective anticancer therapy is developed for use in combined therapy.

11 Future prospects

Prevention of recurrence after the initial operation is essential. However, at the present time, the recurrence rate is so high that prognosis of patients with HCC depends on how the recurrent disease is successfully treated.

Several clinical trials to prevent intra-operative dissemination have been investigated. Nagao et al. [26] advocates larger hepatic resection for the primary tumors to prevent recurrence. This is because intrahepatic recurrences are considered to be the result of dissemination of the tumor cells during operation by manipulation of the liver via the portal vein.

Matsumata et al. [27] performed ultrasonically guided intra-operative portal embolization with starch microspheres in eight patients with HCC which resulted in no recurrence in the remnant liver to date.

Because the rate of recurrence in the remnant liver after hepatectomy is significantly high, we are now striving to develop promising treatment. We had done highly sophisticated chemoimmunotherapy using splenic lymphokine activated killer (LAK) cells which were induced from the spleen cells obtained from resected spleen at the time of the initial hepatectomy. The spleen LAK cells were injected into the hepatic artery via a subcutaneously implanted reservoir following single administration of adriamycin. Interleukin-2 (Il-2) was infused simultaneously during the first three weeks. A clinical randomized study was performed during January 1989 to July 1990. Patients who were received radical resection were divided into 2 groups: With adriamycin, LAK and Il-2 therapy, and with adriamycin only. At the present time, 2 years from the beginning of the protocol, significantly lower recurrence rates and prolonged survival were obtained in the group with chemoimmunotherapy.

This chemoimmunotherapy may promise to improve the survival rates of patients with resected HCC by suppression of recurrence of the tumor after hepatectomy.

References

1. The Liver Cancer Study Group of Japan (1990) Primary liver cancer in Japan: Clinicopathological features and results of surgical treatment. Ann Surg 211:277–287
2. Imai T, Higashiguchi T, Yokoi H, Noguchi T, Kawarada Y, Mizumoto R (1990) Significance of multidisciplinary therapy for hepatocellular carcinoma. J Jpn Surg Soc 91:1378–1381
3. Kohnosu H, Hironaka T, Tsukamoto T, Horii A, Kan K, Shimode Y, Kubo H, Ohmori K, Makino H, Hamagashira K, Itoi H, Sonoyama T, Naitoh K, Yamagishi H, Oka T (1990) Therapeutic effects for recurrence after resection of hepatocellular carcinoma. Jpn J Gastroenterol Surg 23:2343–2349
4. Yamazaki S, Hasegawa N, Makuuchi M, Takayama T, Kosuge T, Shimada K, Moriyama N, Takayasu K, Muramatsu Y (1991) Preoperative transcatheter arterial embolization (TAE) and TAE for recurrence: A role of TAE from the view point of hepatectomy. Jpn J of Clin Radiol 36:553–557
5. Fujihara S, Okamoto E, Yamaoka N, Katou T, Manabe Y, Furukawa K, Kawamura E (1990) Importance of multidisciplinary treatment for hepatocellular carcinoma. J Jpn Surg Soc 91:1375–1377
6. Matsumata T, Kanematsu T, Takanaka K, Yoshida Y, Nishizaki T, Sugimachi K (1989) Patterns of intrahepatic recurrence after curative resection of hepatocellular carcinoma. Hepatology 9:457–460
7. Hsu HC, Wu TT, Wu MZ Sheu JC, Lee CS, Chen DS (1988) Tumor invasiveness and prognosis in resected hepatocellular carcinoma: Clinical and pathogenetic implications. Cancer 61:2095–2099
8. Kanematsu T, Matsumata T, Takenaka K, Yoshida Y, Higashi H, Sugimachi K (1988) Clinical management of recurrent hepatocellular carcinoma after primary resection. Br J Surg 75:203–206
9. Lange JF, Leese T, Castaing D, Bismuth H (1989) Repeat hepatectomy for recurrent malignant tumors of the liver. Surg Gynecol Obstet 169:119–126
10. Nagasue N, Yutaka H, Chang YC, Yamanoi A, Kohno H, Hayashi T, Nakamura T (1990) Assessment of patterns and treatment of intrahepatic recurrence after resection of hepatocellular carcinoma. Surg Gynecol Obstet 171:217–222
11. Takayasu K, Muramatsu Y, Moriyama N, Yamada T, Hasegawa H, Okazaki N, Hirohashi S, Tsugane S (1987) Clinicoradiological evaluation of recurrence in the residual liver following hepatectomy in 97 patients with hepatocellular carcinoma. Jpn J Gastroenterol 84:1424–1432
12. Sasaki Y, Imaoka S, Fujita M, Miyoshi Y, Ohigashi H, Ishikawa O, Furukawa H, Koyama H, Iwanaga T, Kasugai H, Kojima J (1987) Regional therapy in the management of intrahepatic recurrence after surgery for hepatoma. Ann Surg 206:40–47
13. Ehara M, Kita K, Yoshikawa M, Outoh M (1989) Percutaneous ethanol injection (PEI) therapy for small hepatocellular carcinoma. Geka Shinryou 31:827–834
14. Ogino N, Nakao K, Miyata M, Sakaki S, Takenaka H, Tumori T, Kamiike W, Kawashima Y, Kitagawa A (1985) A case report of primary liver cancer diagnosed by solitary sternal metastasis, surviving 5 years after hepatic resection. Jpn J Gastroenterol Surg 18:1884–1887
15. Ikeda K, Kumada H, Yamamoto A, Murashima N, Yoshida A, Irimoto M, Unakami M, Endo Y (1986) A case of hepatocellular carcinoma presenting regression of bone metastasis in the course of transcatheter arterial embolization therapy. Acta Hepatol Jpn 27:359–365
16. Inada M, Minami Y, Kawata S, Miyoshi S, Imai Y,

Satio R, Noda S, Tamura S, Inui Y, Matsuda Y, Uchida A, Tarui S (1987) A case of hepatocellular carcinoma with bone metastasis which responded to oral administration of UFT. Jpn J Cancer Chemother 14:531–535

17. Egawa H, Horiuchi T, Kashiwagi H, Shimozuma N, Yamane H, Mori K, Kobayashi Y, Nagai Y, Noguchi H, Tabuse Y, Katumi M (1986) Successful ^{60}Co radiation therapy for rib metastasis from hepatocellular carcinoma: A case report. J Jpn Soc Clin Surg 47:393–397

18. Liver Cancer Study Group of Japan (1988) Survey and follow-up study of primary cancer in Japan. Report 8. Acta Hepatol Jpn 29:1619–1626

19. Nakano M, Noguchi T, Ide G (1975) Histopathological study of cholangiocellular carcinoma: A comparison with hepatocellular carcinoma in 61 autopsy cases. In: Hirai H, Tsukada Y (eds) Carcinoembryonic protein and hepatoma, Nankodo, Tokyo, pp 203–210

20. Fujita T (1990) Clinicopathological studies of the resected intrahepatic bile duct carcinoma. Jpn J Gastroenterol Surg 23:36–46

21. Tanaka N, Okamoto E, Toyosaka A, Hida T, Suzuki E, Nose K, Kanno H, Nakamura K (1988) A case of cholangiocellular carcinoma recurred 8 years and 9 months after left hepatic lobectomy. Jpn J Gastroenterol Surg 21:1343–1346

22. Yamamoto T, Ryu M, Ozaki M, Isono K (1989) The management of recurrent hepatocellular carcinoma in residual liver. Asian J Surg 12(2): 88–91

23. Klompmaker IJ, De Bruijn KM, Gouw ASH, Bams JL Sloof MJH (1988) Recurrence of hepatocellular carcinoma after liver retransplantation. Br Med J 296(6634):1445

24. Olthoff KM, Millis M, Rosore MH, Goldstein LI, Ramming KP, Busuttil RW (1990) Is liver transplantation justified for the treatment of hepatic malignancies? Arch Surg 125:1261–1268

25. Hart J, Busuttil RW, Lewin KJ (1990) Disease recurrence following liver transplantaion. Am J Surg Pathol 14:79–91

26. Nagao T, Isono S, Yoshimi F, Sodeyama M, Omori Y, Mizuta T, Kawano N, Morioka Y (1990) Postoperative recurrence of hepatocellular carcinoma. Ann Surg 211:28–33

27. Matsumata T, Kanematsu T, Takenaka K, Sugimachi K (1989) Lack of intrahepatic recurrence of hepatocellular carcinoma by temporary portal venous embolization with starch microspheres. Surgery 105(2):GT188–191

28. Takayasu T, Maki A, Shimahara Y, Mori K, Yamaoka Y, Ozawa K (1989) A study on recurrent hepatocellular carcinoma patients. J Jpn Gastroenterol Surg (Suppl.) 22(6):1471

CHAPTER 36

Pathology, diagnosis, and treatment for small liver cancer

Masao Ohto, Fukuo Kondo, and Masaaki Ebara[1]

1 Introduction

Since the introduction of modern imaging modalities into the diagnosis of liver diseases, the detection of small mass lesions in the liver has become possible and the early diagnosis of hepatocellular carcinoma (HCC) has been established. Regular check-ups with examinations of tumor markers, serum alpha-fetoprotein and ultrasonography (US) for chronic hepatitis and liver cirrhosis are indispensable for making an early diagnosis of HCC. Although conventional diagnostic imaging and radiographic modalities, such as ultrasound, X-ray computed tomography (CT), magnetic resonance (MR), and angiography, are effectively used in detecting small mass lesions of the liver, they cannot discriminate small HCC from benign mass lesions such as large regenerative nodules (LRNs) of cirrhosis. Thus, histological examinations of small mass lesions by percutaneous biopsy under ultrasound image control have become imperative for reaching a final diagnosis of HCC and designing an appropriate treatment regimen. The histological features of small HCCs and standard histological criteria for their biopsy diagnosis are essential, and now they have been established owing to cooperative work by clinicians and pathologists.

In the treatment of small HCC, various therapeutic methods, such as surgical intervention, transcatheter arterial embolization (TAE), irradiation, and anticancer chemotherapy, are generally used. There are, however, some limitations on their performance, depending on the degree of coexisting liver injuries and the extension of the carcinoma in the liver. Further-

more, a few years after treatment, a new HCC often arises if there is a background of liver cirrhosis, which has potential to develop carcinoma. Considering this scenario, the treatment of small HCC should not only be effective against the cancer, but also needs to be such that it will not cause additional damage to the liver. Recent advances in diagnosis and treatment towards this goal have indeed greatly altered the clinical features of HCC.

2 Pathology

2.1 Tumor invasion

To evaluate the clinical significance of HCC tumor size, we histologically examined the relation of tumor invasion to the surrounding liver tissue and tumor size in 47 resected and 8 autopsied HCCs (Table 1) [1]. Intracapsular invasion was seen in almost the same incidence among various tumor sizes. The incidence of invasion into peripheral branches of the hepatic portal veins became higher in parallel with the elevation of tumor size. The incidence of cancer invasion in microvessels and the area surrounding the tumor was much lower in HCCs of less than 2 cm, in comparison with invasion in those larger than 2 cm.

On the basis of these histological findings, HCCs of less than 2 cm should be considered as in the early stage in which cancer invasion is limited in a small area in the liver.

2.2 Cell differentiation and histological features

Table 2 shows the cell differentiation and histological types of HCCs smaller than 2 cm in com-

[1] Department of Medicine and Department of Pathology, Chiba University School of Medicine, Chiba, 280 Japan

Table 1. Microscopic invasion of HCC to surrounding liver tissue

Tumor size (cm)	Invasion			
	Microvessels	Portal branch	Capsule	Extracapsule
<1	1/5　(20)	0/5　(0)	3/3　(100)	1/3　(33)
>1<2	5/15 (33)	2/15 (13)	8/9　(89)	3/9　(33)
>2<3	16/20 (80)	6/20 (30)	11/12 (92)	8/12 (67)
>3<5	11/15 (73)	6/15 (40)	14/14 (100)	10/14 (71)

( ), %

Table 2. Cellular differentiation and histological type of hepatocellular carcinoma

Tumor size (cm)	No. of cases	Cellular differentiation				Histological type			
		well	moderate	poor	anaplastic	Nor	Mid	Macro	others
<2	15	7	8	0	0	9	5	0	1[a]
>2<3	19	3	13	2	1	3	13	2	1[b]
>3<4	10	0	7	3	0	0	7	3	0

[a] scirrhous
[b] anaplastic
Nor, normotrabecular; Mid, midtrabecular; Macro, macrotrabecular

parison with HCCs larger than 2 cm [2]. The incidence of well-differentiated HCC was the highest in HCCs of less than 2 cm and much lower in HCCs of 2–3 cm. No well-differentiated HCCs were present in those larger than 3 cm. We divided the trabecular type of HCC, which is the most commonly seen, into three subtypes: normotrabecular (1–2 cells thick), midtrabecular (3–7 cells thick), and macrotrabecular (more than 8 cells thick).

In HCCs of less than 2 cm, the normotrabecular subtype was seen in 9 of the 15 tumors (60%), while the midtrabecular and macrotrabecular subtypes were common in tumors of a larger size. Well-differentiated normotrabecular HCCs are considered as characteristic histological features of small HCCs. Figure 1 shows the typical histological features of well-differentiated normotrabecular HCC: (1) distinctive nuclear crowding, (2) increased cytoplasmic basophilia, (3) scattered microacinar formation, (4) tumor cell reduction with almost no change of nuclear size, resulting in elevation of nucleo-cytoplasmic (N/C) ratio [3], and (5) overt atypia, such as irregular nuclear shape, prominent nucleoli, or anisokaryosis.

Thus, we consider that HCCs in the early stage showing these histological features gradually transform from normotrabecular subtype into midtrabecular, macrotrabecular, or pseudoglandular subtypes following tumor growth, and then present an increased cellular atypia, a characteristic feature of advanced HCC nodules.

3　Diagnosis

3.1　Current trends

Modern imaging modalities such as US and X-ray CT serve to identify a greater number of patients with HCC and permit an earlier diagnosis by detecting HCC less than 2 cm in diameter (small HCC).

In our hospital, patients with small HCC amount to about one-third of all those with HCC. The clinical symptoms in patients with small HCC are similar to those in patients with chronic hepatitis or liver cirrhosis, because small HCC is so diminutive as not to produce any specific symptoms. The majority of patients with HCC are related to hepatitis virus infection of HCV and/or HBV. The positive anti-HCV (Chiron-antibody, ELISA) of 254 patients with HCC was 60.2%, and the positive HBs-antigen was 18.1%. Those carrying both positive anti-HCV and positive HBs-antigen were 2.4%, and both negative anti-HCV and negative HBs-antigen were 24.0%. Compared to large HCC, small

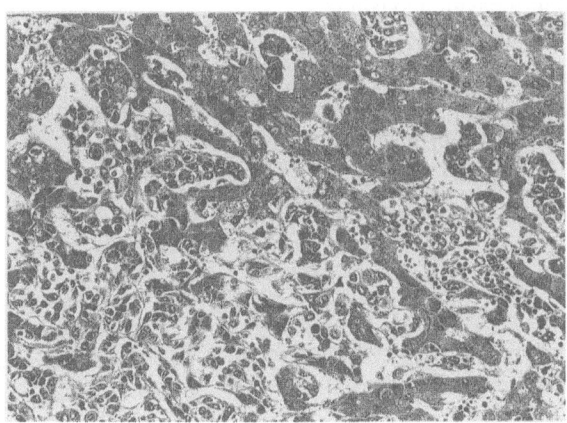

Fig. 1. Resected specimen of a HCC sized 15 mm in diameter. Tumor cells are arranged in normo trabecular manner, 1 to 2 cells thick. When compared with a pseudolobule (*PL*), tumor (*HCC*) cells show distinctive cytoplasmic basophilia and nuclear crowding. Scattered microacinar formation is observed (*arrows*). HCC tissue involves adjacent pseudolobule (*PL*) showing replacing growth pattern. Fibrous tissue (*) is also involved (interstitial invasion). H and E × 80

HCC was more frequently related with positive anti-HCV and less frequently with positive HBs-antigen (Table 3). The relation of small HCC with liver cirrhosis was closer than that of large HCC.

Generally, serum alpha-fetoprotein (AFP) is thought to be useful for screening HCC. However, it showed a level of <20 ng/ml in 39.8% of all 83 patients with small HCC, 20–200 ng/ml in 44.6% and >200 ng/ml in 14.4%, indicating that it is quite limited in terms of reaching an early diagnosis. Recently developed diagnostic ultrasound apparatus, on the other hand, quite readily allows us to detect a tumor of 1–2 cm in diameter [4]. Accordingly, not only clinical symptoms and the level of AFP but also the use of ultrasound

examinations combine to form crucial diagnostic tools for the detection of various types of HCCs.

In order to clinically make early diagnosis possible, regular check-ups with US for HCC should be carried out in patients with chronic hepatitis or liver cirrhosis. According to our study on the growth of HCC, the doubling time (DT) of tumor volume in small HCCs varied considerably [5]. Rapid growth with a DT of less than 3 months was seen in 5 of 27 small HCCs with no specific cancer treatment, intermediate growth with a DT of 3–6 months in 10, and slow growth with a DT of more than 6 months in the other 12. For tumors with a diameter of 1.5–2.0 cm as detected by routine US, the DT was from 3.4–45.6 months (average 14.0 ± 11.3 months). Therefore, in order to make an early diagnosis of such minute HCC with reliability, patients with chronic hepatitis and cirrhosis, considered high-risk in terms of HCC development potential, should undergo regular US examinations every 3 or 4 months.

In the past few years, we have adopted this strategy for early diagnosis and have succeeded in detecting many patients with small HCC. Among 254 patients with HCC treated in the last five years, 29.1% had HCCs of less than 2 cm, 49.2% HCCs of 2–5 cm, and 21.7% HCCs of larger than 5 cm.

3.2 Imaging diagnosis

The detectability of HCC varies according to the kind of imaging modalities and the size of tumors [6]. Our retrospective study revealed that when the tumors were less than 2 cm, the detection rates of tumors by US, CT, MRI, and angiography were 97.8%, 54.0%, 61.1%, and 75.4%, respectively (Table 4). Therefore, among the

Table 3. Clinical features of hepatocellular carcinoma with reference to tumor size

Tumor size	No. of patients	Age	Sex M:F	Anti-HCV	HBs-antigen	Anti-HBC	Associated liver cirrhosis	ICG-15minute clearance	AFP (100 ng ≦/ml)
<2	74	57.6 ±7.3	62:12	50[c] (67.6)	10[b] (13.5)	44 (63.8)	70[b1,2] (94.6)	29.8 ±17.6	9[a1,2] (12.2)
2–5	125	59.4 ±7.3	98:27	74 (59.2)	20 (16.0)	82 (69.5)	102[b2] (81.6)	27.7 ±16.3	50[a1] (40)
5≦	55	58.7 ±6.8	50:5	29[c] (52.7)	16[b] (29.1)	40 (78.4)	45[b1] (81.8)	25.9 ±16.1	29[a2] (52.7)

[a1,2], $P < 0.01$; [b1,2], $P < 0.05$; [c], $P < 0.1$
( ), %

Table 4. Detection of small HCC by various imaging modalities

Tumor size (cm)	Ultrasound (%)	X-ray CT (%)	MRI (%)	Angiography (%)
<1	92.9	11.1		50.0
	(13/14)	(1/9)		(5/10)
1–2	98.7	61.1	61.1	80.0
	(74/75)	(33/54)	(11/18)	(44/55)
2–3	99.0	92.2	92.0	86.1
	(97/98)	(71/77)	(23/25)	(68/79)
3–4	100	97.5	100	97.7
	(48/48)	(39/40)	(14/14)	(42/43)
4–5	100	95.2	100	97.7
	(47/47)	(38/40)	(15/15)	(43/44)

various imaging modalities, US is the most useful for early diagnosis, although it did fail to detect small tumors located below the diaphragm in a few patients.

Echographic patterns of the tumors differ in relation to tumor size. Characteristic echo patterns of HCC, such as ring signs, nodule in nodule, and lateral acoustic shadowing, were not observed in HCCs of less than 2 cm. A low echo pattern appeared in 92.3% of HCCs of 1.0 cm or less, in 59.5% of 1.0–2.0 cm, in 35.8% of 2.0–3.0 cm, and in 11.2% of 3–5 cm. Incidentally, LRNs of cirrhosis are also seen as a tiny tumor with a low echo pattern. A high echo pattern characteristic of small hemangioma was also seen in 5.7% of HCCs of less than 2 cm. Thus, on echograms, it is difficult to discriminate between small HCCs, particularly those less than 2 cm in diameter, and small lesions like hemangioma and LRNs of cirrhosis.

X-ray CT is usually selected to follow US for a detailed examination. In 63 small HCCs, CT revealed 54% of them. However, characteristic findings of HCC, such as ring signs and septum formation, were observed in only 14.3%. By dynamic scan, early enhancement and quick de-enhancement, characteristic findings of HCC, were observed in 47.6% of small HCCs. The CT scan, a modern diagnostic procedure, still has some limitations with regard to early diagnosis, particularly when differential diagnosis is needed [7].

Lipiodol CT, in which several ml of Lipiodol oil contrast medium are injected into the hepatic artery and a CT scan is done 10–14 days later, is useful for detecting small HCCs, particularly minute satellite nodules around the main tumor [8]. This procedure, however, sometimes leads to false-positive and false-negative results, and has the additional disadvantage of leaving a persistent deposition of Lipiodol in the tumor, which there-

after makes the assessment of tumor vascularity difficult.

MRI is similar to CT in terms of detection of small HCCs, and has the advantage of being able to discriminate small HCC from small hemangioma. Both small HCC and hemangioma display low T1 values, but the T2 value of small hemangioma is distinctly higher than that of small HCC.

Hepatic angiography is a most useful procedure for detecting small satellite nodules scattered around the main tumor and also for finding minute HCCs sporadically distributed throughout the liver. It is well documented that both neo-vasculature (tumor vessels) and hypervascularity (tumor stain) are characteristic findings of HCC. Small HCCs showing tumor vessels, however, are less in number when they are smaller in size, and only a discrete tumor stain becomes a characteristic of such small HCCs. When small nodules show an equivocal stain, differential diagnosis between small HCCs and other small mass lesions like LRNs of cirrhosis become almost impossible with angiography [9].

3.3 Percutaneous biopsy

Although various imaging modalities are highly capable of detecting small HCCs, it is difficult to make a final diagnosis of HCC based on this evidence alone. Consequently, percutaneous biopsy under ultrasound image control is performed to allow a final diagnosis on the basis of histological findings in addition to the image findings.

3.4 Histological criteria for biopsy diagnosis

Most small HCCs show histologically well-differentiated normotrabecular HCC in which

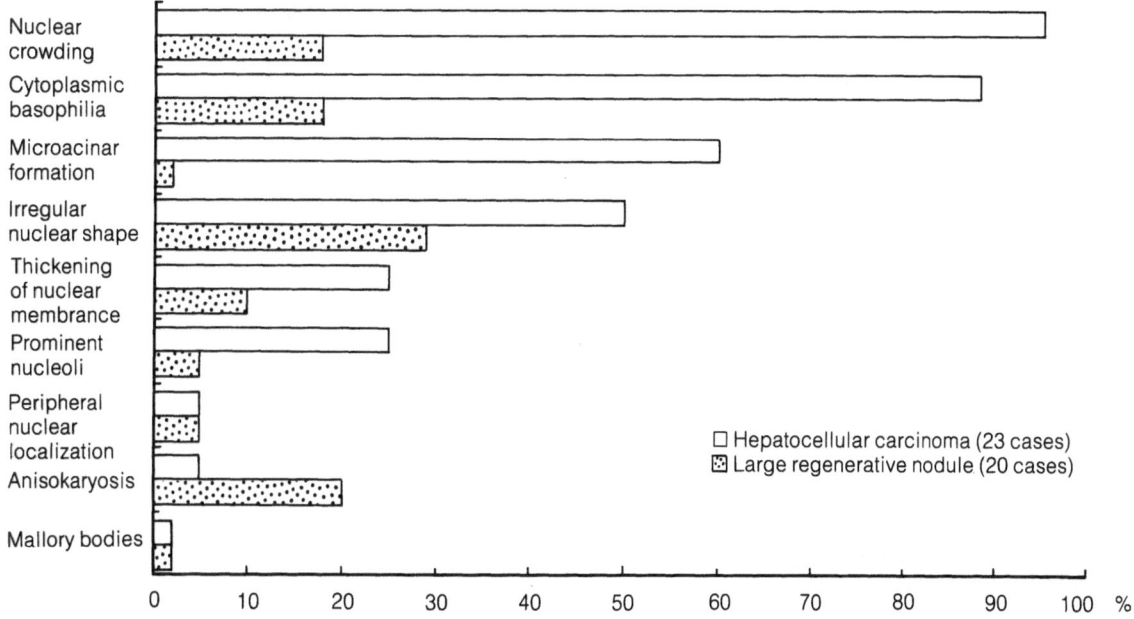

Fig. 2. Cytological and structural atypia found in small hepatocellular carcinoma and large regenerative nodules

overt atypia, such as distortion of liver cell cords, nuclear pleomorphism, and anisokaryosis, are not seen. The classical histological criteria of HCC are therefore not always applicable for small HCCs.

Various cytological and histological criteria have been proposed for histological diagnosis of small HCCs, but there has been no unanimous agreement of their validity. The three cardinal findings (nuclear crowding, increased cytoplasmic basophilia, and microacinar formation) are found in high incidence in HCCs of less than 2 cm and in low incidence in LRNs [2, 10, 11] (Fig. 2). Furthermore, nuclear crowding of double that in the noncancerous tissue is sufficient to make a diagnosis of HCC. Therefore, they are useful in differentiating between small HCC and LRNs. In addition, results showed that all nodules positive for two or more of the three cardinal findings, and/or remarkable nuclear crowding (double that in control tissue) proved to be malignant from clinical evidence during a long follow-up [12].

3.5 Process of percutaneous biopsy

In order to prevent misjudgements in the biopsy diagnosis, the process of biopsy is important, particularly for small HCCs and nodular lesions of the liver (Fig. 3). The biopsy should be carried out in combination with ultrasound image control, thereby allowing the histological specimen to be removed without complications such as bleeding and seeding of cancer cells. In the procedure, two punctures are made for each lesion to avoid sampling errors. Extranodular liver tissue is also obtained for comparison.

Specimens are prepared for microscopic examination following the routine procedure. Before microscopic examination, pathologists should obtain detailed clinical information, especially about the association of liver cirrhosis, because various tumor-like lesions, such as adenoma, nodular regenerative hyperplasia, and focal nodular hyperplasia, often arise in noncirrhotic livers. During microscopic examination, moderately- or poorly-differentiated HCCs can be easily diagnosed from overt cytological or structural atypia.

For differentiation between well-differentiated HCCs and LRNs, the three cardinal histological findings are essential. When nodular lesions show two or more of these cardinal findings and/or nuclear crowding of double that in the control, they can be reliably diagnosed as well-differentiated normotrabecular HCC [2, 12].

When the lesions show the same histological features as the control tissue, the diagnosis is "benign liver tissue" and the possibility of sampling error should be considered as one of

Sampling
1. Two punctures are made for one lesion
2. Extranodular liver tissue is also obtained as control tissue for comparison (change needles to prevent seeding of tumor cells)

Fig. 3. Total process of biopsy diagnosis of nodular lesions in the liver

Microscopic examination
1. Obtain clinical information about association of liver cirrhosis
   a. Associated → Differentiate only large regenerative nodule

   b. Not associated → Differentiate other tumor-like lesions

2. Examine whether overt atypia is present or not in the specimen (① ②)

   a. Present → "moderately or poorly differentiated HCC"

   b. Absent → Evaluate three cardinal findings, (compare with the control tissue (③))

3. Evaluate three cardinal findings ────→ "Well differentiated
   a. Distinctly positive in   normotrabecular HCC"
   two or more items,   (definitive diagnosis)
   and/or remarkable nuclear crowding
   (double that of control tissue (③))

   b. Same histologic feature ────→ "Benign liver tissue"
   as in control tissue   (tentative diagnosis)

   c. Intermediate histologic feature ────→ "Borderline lesion (= adenomatous hyperplasia)"
   between well differentiated HCC
   and benign liver tissue

Re-biopsy
1. In case of "benign liver tissue" or "borderline lesion"

Table 5. Nodule size and histological diagnosis

Tumor size (cm)	No. of cases	Histologic diagnosis			
		LRN	borderline lesion	wd-HCC	cl-HCC
<2	144	28	24	37	55
>2<3	84	0	2	12	70
3≦	151	0	0	6	145

LRN, large regenerative nodule; wd, well differentiated; cl, classical (moderately or poorly differentiated)

the causes for the negative results. When they show histological features lying between well-differentiated HCC and benign liver tissue, the diagnosis is "borderline lesion" or "adenomatous hyperplasia" (AH). At present in Japan, there is a controversy over the histological entity of AH. Highly well-differentiated HCC, LRN with high cellularity, HCC with fatty or clear cell transformation, and tissues from marginal areas of small HCC may be categorized as AH because histological differentiation among them is quite difficult.

Rebiopsy is recommended to confirm the diagnosis when the first biopsy diagnosis is benign liver tissue or borderline lesion (AH). Lesions that are consistent with benign liver tissue both at the first and the second biopsy (a total of four punctures) should be regarded as LRN because the possibility of sampling error has been much reduced by rebiopsy.

Using the biopsy technique under ultrasound image control [13, 14] and the three cardinal histological criteria, we carried out histological examination of 437 nodular lesions of the liver during a period between 1982 and 1990. The results were as follows: 270 HCCs of moderately- or poorly-differentiated type of classical histological features, 55 HCCs of well-differentiated normotrabecular type, 28 LRNs, 26 borderline lesions, and 3 hemangiomas. The incidence of these lesions in relation to nodule size is presented in Table 5. Nodules of smaller than 2 cm consisted of LRNs, borderline lesions, and HCCs, whereas all nodules of 2–3 cm were HCC except for 2 borderline lesions. All nodules of larger than 3 cm were HCC consisting mostly of the moderately- or poorly-differentiated type. These results suggest that nodules of larger than 2 cm arising in cirrhotic liver are probably malignant, while nodules of smaller than 2 cm consisted of well-differentiated HCCs, moderately- or poorly-differentiated HCCs, borderline lesions, and LRNs.

4 Treatment

4.1 Current trends

The treatment for small HCC is decided according to the degree of extension of the malignancy and the severity of coexisting liver injuries. Recently, modern imaging modalities have been able to detect small mass lesions easily, and even small HCCs are seen not only in a single tumor but also in multiple tumors independently distributed throughout the liver. Our data from image findings during the last five years indicated that 34.2% of 20 patients with HCC of less than 2.0 cm, 40.9% of 88 patients with HCC of 2.0–3.0 cm, and 61.0% of 83 patients with 3.0–5.0 cm had multiple tumors.

Whether small HCCs appearing in multiple tumors are due to multicentric development or intrahepatic metastasis is still a major clinical problem, and decisions regarding therapeutic approaches will depend on its resolution.

According to the histopathological findings, cancer invasion is often observed in the pericapsular area and the small portal branches around the tumor even in small HCCs. Considering these clinical and pathological features of small HCCs, treatment needs to be carried out on the basis of a precise diagnosis.

4.2 Surgery

The resectability of the liver is assessed generally on the basis of the levels of serum bilirubin (less than 2.0 mg/dl), serum albumin (more than 3.0 mg/dl), and the ICG 15-minute clearance rate (less than 20%). Furthermore, the tumors must be located in a limited area in the liver, and the severity of the accompanying liver injuries must be taken into consideration. In spite of the increase in the number of patients with small HCC, those with a good indication for resection have not increased as much as could be expected, and therefore no surgical treatments have been preferred for small HCCs.

4.3 Chemotherapy

So far, improvement in the survival of patients with small HCC has not been achieved clinically in treatment with chemotherapeutic agents.

4.4 TAE, chemoembolization

TAE, in which small gel-particles are injected into the hepatic artery through an arteriographic catheter, is commonly adopted in unresectable HCCs as long as the liver functional reserve is Child A and B in severity [15]. This procedure carries the risk of exacerbating coexisting liver damage by blocking the blood supply to the non-cancerous parenchyma of the liver. TAE as a rule causes necrosis in the central part of the tumor in small HCCs, but cancer cells also reside in the peripheral part and in the capsular and pericapsular areas. The complete disappearance of cancer cells after TAE was seen in a few patients with an encapsulated HCC [16]. In a follow-up study on patients with HCCs of 3–10 cm, the survival in those who had TAE treatment was significantly superior to that in those who had no special cancer treatment. However, in those with small HCCs of 2–3 cm, the survival was not improved in comparison to those with no cancer therapy. TAE does not always have satisfactory results, and has some limitations in the treatment of small HCCs.

Recently, chemoembolization has been used as a new therapeutic modality. Here, Lipiodol, an oily contrast medium, works as carrier delivering chemotherapy agents, such as neocarzinostatin,

Table 6. Relationship between small hepatocellular carcinoma treatment and carcinoma extention and coexisting liver injuries

Treatment	Number of tumors	Tumor thrombus within liver	Liver injuries Child's classification
PEI	no more than 3	no	A, B, (C)
TAE	single, multiple	possible	A, B
Chemotherapy	multiple	yes	A, B (C)

( ), possible
PEI, percutaneous ethanol injection; TAE, transcatheter arterial embolization; Chemotherapy, anticancer chemotherapy

mytomycin C, Adriamycin, or cysplatin, to the tumor, where it is then slowly released. TAE using small gel-particles as the embolus is sometimes carried out following chemoembolization in the same session [17]. In this combination therapy, both a long lasting effect on the tumor by the remaining chemotherapy agents and a necrotizing effect on the tumor by blocking the blood supply can be expected to bring good therapeutic results. The liver, however, must have good reserve function to be tolerate such a heavy burden.

4.5 Percutaneous ethanol injection

In HCC patients associated with advanced cirrhosis, treatment should not cause further damage to the liver because they succumb often to hepatic failure soon after. Percutaneous ethanol injection (PEI) under ultrasound image control was developed in order to prevent patients with small HCCs from further damage to the liver after treatment. In Japan as well as in some other countries, PEI has now been accepted as a useful modality in the treatment of small HCCs. (see Chap. 28).

After PEI, all tumors decrease in size and nearly half become undetectable on images. Neither regrowth nor enlargement of the treated tumors are seen. The technique is simple and does not raise complications which might require intensive care. The patient's overall condition is generally unchanged by the treatment, and survival is significantly improved in comparison with that of patients with no specific anticancer treatment [18].

The major problem with PEI is occurrence of new HCC in different areas within the liver after treatment. This seems to be unavoidable because of coexisting liver cirrhosis. Unlike surgical in-

tervention, PEI can be carried out repeatedly for recurring HCCs without damaging the patient's quality of life. So, PEI is an alternative to laparotomy in treatment of small HCCs in a few tumors, particularly when accompanied by liver cirrhosis.

4.6 Indication of treatment

HCC treatment is limited due to the extension of the malingancy and the severity of coexisting liver injuries. In small HCCs, when the patient's liver function is good enough to undergo a combination of therapies, we should consider carrying out multidisciplinary treatment.

In small HCCs with a single tumor, PEI is the first treatment indicated. With multiple tumors, TAE is indicated first, in combination with anticancer chemotherapy (Table 6). Following that, PEI is performed for the main tumors, because in small HCCs, TAE does not always produce complete necrosis.

References

1. Ebara M, Ohto M, Kondo F (1989) Strategy for early diagnosis of hepatocellular carcinoma (HCC). Ann Acad Med Singapore 18:83–89
2. Kondo F, Hirooka N, Wada K, Kondo Y (1987) Morphological clues for the diagnosis of small hepatocellular carcinomas. Virchows Arch [A] 411:15–21
3. Kondo F, Wada K, Kondo Y (1988) Morphometric analysis of hepatocellular carcinoma. Virchows Arch [A] 413:425–430
4. Shinagawa T, Ohto M, Kimura K, Tsunetomi S, Morita M, Saisho H, Tsuchiya Y, Saotome N, Karasawa E, Miki M, Ueno T, Okuda K (1984)

Diagnosis and clinical features of small hepatocellular carcinoma with emphasis on the utility of real-time ultrasonography. A study in 51 patients. Gastroenterology 86:495–502

5. Ebara M, Ohto M, Shinagawa T, Sugiura N, Kimura K, Matsutani S, Morita M, Saisho H, Tsuchiya Y, Okuda K (1986) Natural history of minute hepatocellular carcinoma smaller than three centimeters complicating cirrhosis. A study in 22 patients. Gastroenterology 90:289–298

6. Ebara M, Ohto M, Watanabe Y, Kimura K, Saisho H, Tsuchiya Y, Okuda K, Arimizu N, Kondo F, Ikesira H, Fukuda N, Tateno Y (1986) Diagnosis of small hepatocellular carcinoma: Correlation of MR imaging and tumor histologic studies. Radiology 159:371–377

7. Tsunetomi S (1987) Study of computed tomography in diagnosis of small hepatocellular carcinoma (in Japanese). Chiba Igaku 63:185–195

8. Ohishi H, Uchida H, Yoshimura H, Ohue S, Ueda J, Katsuragi M, Matsuo M, Hosogi Y (1985) Hepatocellular carcinoma detected by iodized oil. Use of anticancer agents. Radiology 154:25–29

9. Sumida M, Ohto M, Ebara M, Kimura K, Okuda K, Hirooka N (1986) Accuracy of angiography in the diagnosis of small hepatocellular carcinoma. AJR 147:531–536

10. Wada K, Kondo F, Kondo Y (1988) Large regenerative nodules and dysplastic nodules in cirrhotic livers: A histopathologic study. Hepatology 8:1684–1688

11. Kondo F, Ebara M, Sugiura N, Wada K, Kita K, Hirooka N, Nagato Y, Kondo Y, Ohto M, Okuda K (1990) Histological features and clinical course of large regenerative nodules: Evaluation of their precancerous potentiality. Hepatology 12:592–598

12. Kondo F, Wada K, Nagato Y, Nakajima T, Kondo Y, Hirooka N, Ebara M, Ohto M, Okuda K (1989) Biopsy diagnosis of well-differentiated hepatocellular carcinoma based on new morphologic criteria. Hepatology 9:751–755

13. Ohto M, Kimura K, Tsuchiya Y, Ebara M (1987) Sonographic guided procedures in the liver and biliary tract. In: van Sonnenberg E (ed) interventional ultrasound. Churchill Livingstone, New York, pp 77–101

14. Ohto M, Karasawa E, Tsuchiya Y, Kimura K, Saisho H, Ono T, Okuda K (1980) Ultrasonically guided percutaneous contrast medium injection and aspiration biopsy using a real-time puncture transducer. Radiology 136:171–176

15. Yamada R, Sato M, Kawabata M, Nakatsuka H, Nakamura K, Takashima S (1983) Hepatic artery embolization in 120 patients with unresectable hepatoma. Radiology 148:397–401

16. Nakamura H, Tanaka T, Hori S, Yoshioka H, Kuroda C, Okamura J, Sakurai M (1983) Transcatheter embolization of hepatocellular carcinoma: Assessment of efficacy in cases of resection following embolization. Radiology 147:401–405

17. Sasaki Y, Imaoka S, Iwanaga T, Miyoshi Y, Ishikawa O, Ohigashi H, Kasugai H, Kojima J, Tanaka S, Fujita M, Kawamoto S, Ishiguro S (1986) New approach of chemoembolization for hepatocellular carcinoma: Lipiodol, cisplatin sandwich therapy (in Japanese). J Jpn Soc Cancer Ther 21:647–654

18. Ohto M, Ebara M, Watanabe Y, Sugiura N, Shinagawa T, Okuda K (1988) Percutaneous ethanol injection (PEI) therapy for small hepatocellular carcinoma: Evaluation of its utility on the basis of tumor-images and survival after therapy. Jpn J Med Imaging 7:25–33

CHAPTER 37

Transplantation for liver cancer

Michio Mito, Hidetaka Ebata, and Masayuki Sawa[1]

1 Introduction

Primary liver cancer patients usually have a poor prognosis due to the expandable nature of the disease, however, considerable progress has been achieved in the treatment of lesions in the last ten years. Recent advances in screening for tumor markers, imaging techniques, and better understanding of the disease have enabled more frequent and earlier detection of tumors as small as 2 cm in diameter even though they are usually asymptomatic. Therefore, a higher resectability rate has been achieved. Furthermore, refined patient selection, perioperative patient care, and surgical techniques have also contributed to a lower mortality and better long-term survival [1].

Extensive surgical excision is the only way to cure patients with primary liver cancer. In a recent Japanese study, partial hepatic resection was performed for hepatocellular carcinoma (HCC) with reasonable patient survival for more than a year [2]. On the other hand, in most large series from the West [3], segmental hepatic resections for patients with HCC revealed early local recurrence and lethal hepatic failure, and only 10–20% of all patients with primary liver malignancies are resectable due to concomitant advanced liver cirrhosis and multifocal liver malignancy [3].

The first clinical liver transplantation was done by Dr. Starzl and his colleagues in 1963 [4]. In the early days of clinical liver transplantation, extensive liver malignancy which could not be treated with conventional surgical procedures was considered to be an ideal indication for this newly developed therapeutic method [5, 6]. Unfort-

unately, long-term follow-up of liver grafting for tumor patients revealed that many cases were lost due to a high incidence of tumor recurrence [7].

The results of liver transplantation have since improved dramatically following remarkable developments in patient care, surgical and organ preserving techniques (Fig. 1) [8], and especially after the introduction of cyclosporin-A (CyA). Thus, orthotopic liver transplantation has become a practical alternative in the treatment of various end-stage hepatic diseases. Overall survival rates of the 1,000 liver graftings treated with cyclosporin steroids at institutes in Denver, Dallas, and Pittsburgh were three times higher than those of 170 recipients treated with azathioprine steroids before 1980. One- and 5-year survival rates were 74% and 64%, respectively. While transplantation was initially met with skepticism at the major transplant centers throughout Europe and the United States due to the initial disappointing results [9, 10], there has been a shift in this attitude towards liver grafting as a treatment of primary liver malignancy.

In this article, we will summarize the present and future status of liver grafting for liver malignancy.

2 Indications

The main indications for liver transplantation are end-stage liver cirrhosis, metabolic and cholestatic diseases, and malignancies and acute hepatic failure (Table 1) [8]. In the early days of clinical liver transplantation, 9 out of 20 liver transplantations were performed at the University of Pittsburgh for patients with liver malignancies [5], and over 70% of the patients treated with liver transplantation at Cambridge/ Kings' College Hospital had liver malignancies

[1] The Second Department of Surgery, Asahikawa Medical College, Nishikagura 4-5, Asahikawa, Hokkaido, 078 Japan

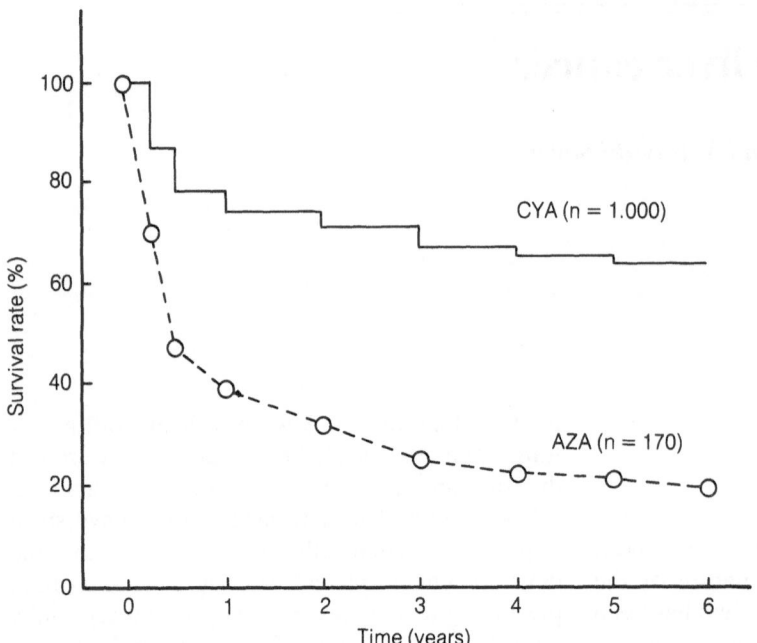

Fig. 1. Overall actuarial survival rates of 1,000 patients treated with cyclosporin steroid therapy (*CyA*) in comparison with overall actual survival rates of 170 patients treated with azathioprine steroid therapy (*AZA*). (From [8] with permission)

Table 1. Liver diseases of adult recipients

Disease	No. patients
Cirrhosis (postnecrotic, cryptogenic, alcoholic)	278
Postnecrotic and cryptogenic	237
HB_sAg positive	36
Alcoholic	41
Primary biliary cirrhosis	165
Primary sclerosing cholangitis	74
Liver-based inborn metabolic errors (Alpha-1-antitrypsin deficiency, Wilson's etc)	35
Primary hepatic malignancy	33
Fulminant hepatic failure	27
Secondary biliary cirrhosis	13
Budd-Chiari syndrome	13
Bile duct cancer	10
Secondary hepatic malignancy	7
Others[a]	11

[a] Cystic fibrosis (3), adenomatosis (2), biliary atresia, cryptococcal cholangitis, congenital hepatic fibrosis, polycystic disease, trauma, lymphoangiomatosis.
(From [8])

[6]. This initial success encouraged the use of liver grafting for more patients with liver malignancy in many transplant centers. However, the number of liver malignancies indicated for liver grafting has now decreased due to the high incidence of tumor recurrence.

At the University of Pittsburgh, primary liver malignancy occupied 13.5% of the cases for which liver transplantation was indicated before the introduction of CyA, and recently only a few percent of liver transplantation have been performed for patients with liver malignancy after the introduction of CyA [11].

In contrast, liver malignancy occupied 33.8% of the cases indicated for liver transplantation at Hanover Medical School between 1972 and 1987 (Fig. 2) [10]. Until now, approximately 30% of the cases indicated for liver grafting were malignant liver diseases at the main European transplant centers [12, 13]. As shown in Fig. 3, there is also a shift similar to that at Hanover at European centers regarding the different types of cases indicated for liver transplantation for benign diseases. Liver grafting for malignant diseases has gone down from 40% to 29.14%, and grafting for acute hepatic failure has risen since 1984 [14]. In 1989, only 20.2% of patients with liver malignancy were recorded in the European Liver Transplant Registry 1989, although a significant number of liver transplantations are still performed for liver cancer [15]. In spite of Starzl's results, the European centers still have a positive attitude towards liver transplantation for primary liver malignancy. At Hanover Medical School, primary liver malignancy is still considered to be one of the indications for liver transplantation on

Fig. 2. Distribution of indications for liver transplantation in Hanover, Germany from 1972–1987. (From [10] with permission)

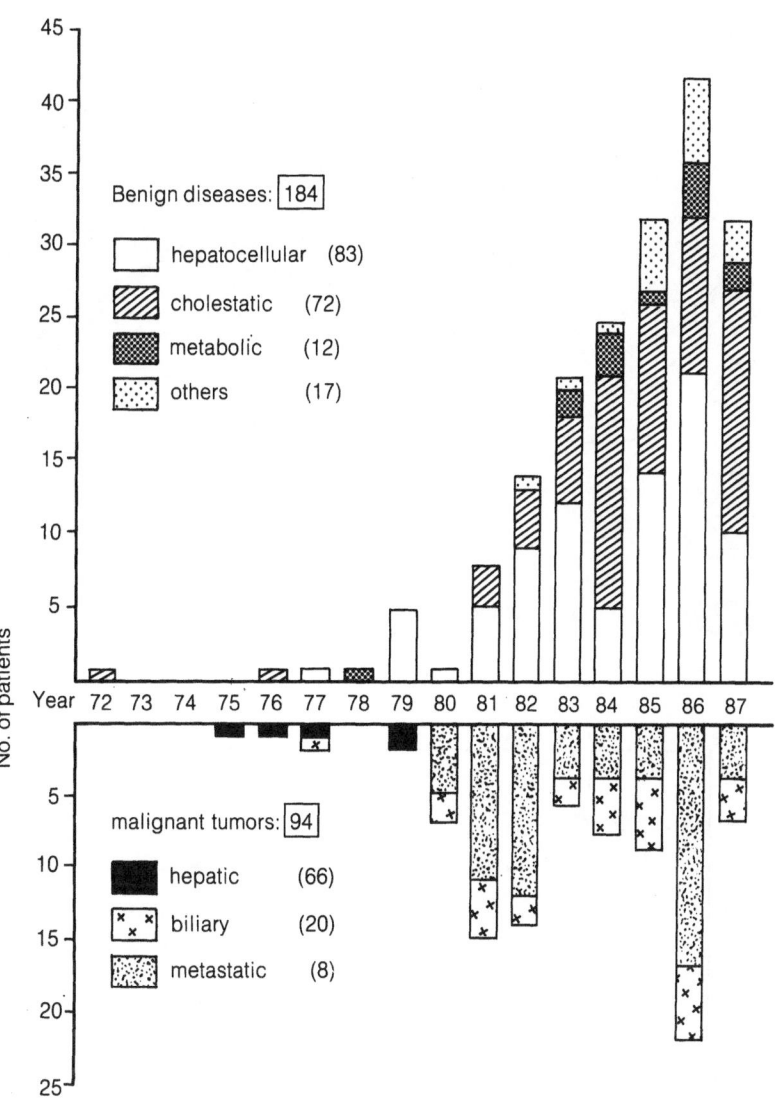

3 Results

According to the report by Iwatsuki et al. [8] on liver transplants for primary liver cancer under cyclosporin steroid therapy, 53 of the 1,000 patients received liver transplantation in the presence of primary liver cancer. Transplantation for 36 of these 53 patients was primarily to treat advanced liver cancer that could not be resected by conventional subtotal hepatectomy due to highly advanced tumor. Eighteen of 36 patients had HCC, 8 had fibrolamellar type HCC, 8 had

the premises of careful patient selection by adequate tumor staging [13].

epitheloid hemangio-endothelioma, 1 had cholangiosarcoma, and another had angiosarcoma. For 17 of 53 patients, total liver replacement was primarily to treat an end-stage non-neoplastic liver disease, but were found to have coincidental primary liver cancer either before transplantation or after examination of the removed whole liver. Fifteen of 17 patients had HCC, 1 had fibrolamellar type HCC, and another had mixed cholangiohepatoma. One- and 5-year survival rates of the 36 patients who received liver replacement for primary liver cancer were 65% and 29%, respectively. The cause of death was tumor recurrence in approximately 90% of the cases. Conversely, 16 of 17 patients who received liver replacement primarily for hepatic failure and whose liver had incidental primary liver cancer were all alive, free of the disease between 3

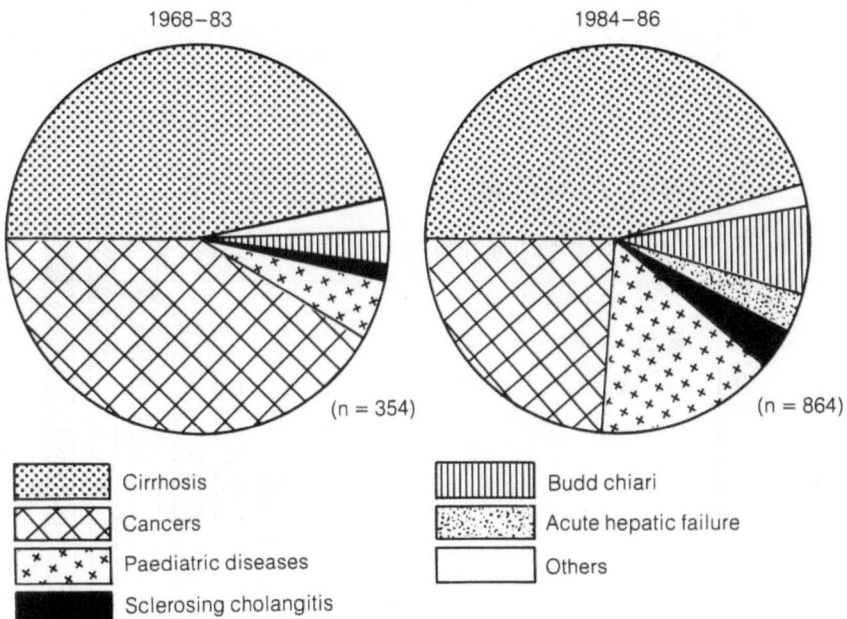

Fig. 3. Changing patterns of primary indications for liver transplantation. (From [14] with permission)

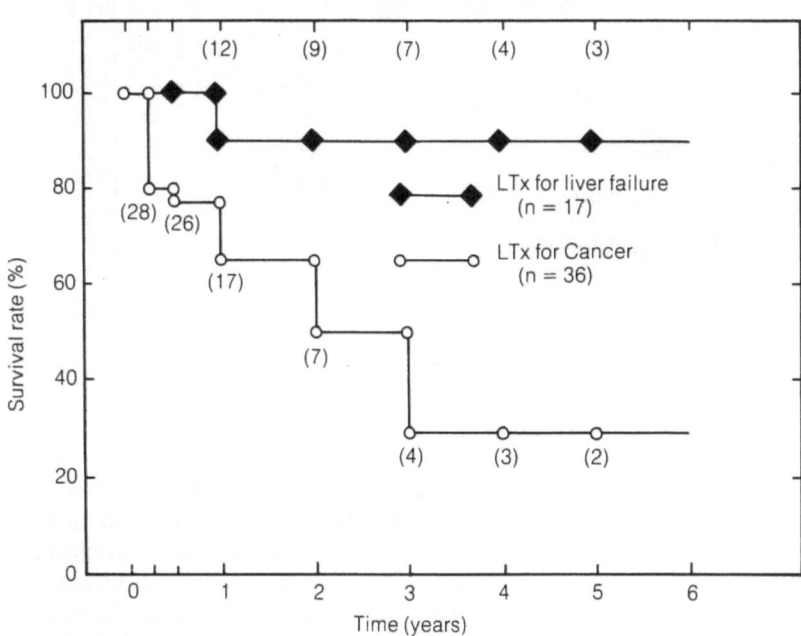

Fig. 4. Survival rates of patients who received transplantation for primary liver malignancy and for liver failure with incidental small malignancies. (From [8] with permission)

months and 6 years (Fig. 4). Only one case with HCC was lost due to tumor recurrence. However, the mere presence of incidental small primary liver cancer did not influence the total survival rates. For the last few years, adjuvant chemotherapy with adriamycin has been applied for patients with primary liver cancer at the University of Pittsburgh, and no significant adverse effects were noted in short trials. In conclusion, Iwatsuki et al. demonstrated that safer and more effective adjuvant chemotherapy and/or immunotherapy are necessary to prevent tumor recurrence.

Between May 1968 and April 1987, 93 patients with liver cancer underwent liver transplantation at Cambridge/King's College Hospital [16]. The 93 patients consisted of 50 with HCC, 26 with cholangiocarcinoma, 5 with angiosarcoma, 1 with epitheloid hemangioendothelioma, 2 with

Table 2. Survey of long-term survival after hepatic transplantation for malignant liver tumors in seven European centers (September 1, 1987)

Histological diagnosis	No. transplant recipients	Survival (n)			Longest survival	Currently alive (n)
		>1 yr	>2 yr	>5 yr		
Hepatocellular carcinoma	73	29	18	7	11 yr 9 mo	21
Hepatocellular carcinoma in cirrhosis	84	19	9	2	12 yr	16
Cholangiocellular carcinoma with/ without cirrhosis	42	11	4	1	6 yr 6 mo	7
Other primary liver tumors[a]	16	4	4	1	5 yr 9 mo	4
Bile duct carcinoma	38	15	6	—	3 yr 11 mo	8
Metastases[b]	43	12	6	—	4 yr 10 mo	12
Total	296	90	47	11		68

Data were compiled from the following contributing centers: Berlin, Birmingham, Cambridge, Hamburg, Hanover, Innsbruck, and Vienna. We would like to thank these European centers for contributing to this collection of data.
[a] Angiosarcoma (seven), hemangioendothelioma (four), hepatoblastoma (three), sarcoma (two).
[b] Colorectal carcinoma (30), mamma carcinoma (four), carcinoid (four), melanoma (two), pheochromocytoma (one), sarcoma (one), teratoma (one).
(From [10])

apudoma, 1 with bile-duct cystadenocarcinoma, and 8 with secondary liver malignancy. Thirty seven of 50 patients with HCC (19 with cirrhosis, and 31 without cirrhosis including 7 with fibro-lamellar type) survived for more than 3 months, and tumor recurrence was observed in 24 patients of the 37. The longest survival time was 11.8 years, and 3 patients survived for more than 5 years. They found no difference in survival rates and tumor recurrence between cirrhotic and non-cirrhotic patients. For patients with metastatic liver cancers, survival times were shorter with little palliation except two patients with carcinoid syndrome. O'Grady et al. [16] suggested that liver transplantation achieved favorable survival as well as considerable palliation of symptoms for a number of patients with primary liver cancer in spite of high incidence in tumor recurrence, but was of little use for patients with secondary liver cancers. According to the statistics from 7 main European transplant centers, a few long-surviving cases were registered after liver transplantation for primary liver cancer, although the 1-year survival rate was at most 30% (Table 2). In order to avoid frequent tumor recurrence, more precise patient selection has been adopted at Hanover Medical School since 1985 after retrospective analysis of their own series [10, 13]. It has become apparent that extrahepatic tumor growth resulted in a lower survival rate. Therefore, Pichlmayr et al. [10] has transplanted liver grafts to patients with HCC only in the hepatic hilar lymph node negative stage. The survival rate in lymph node-positive stages is found to be far worse than that in lymph node-negative stages. The 6-month, 1-

year, and 2-year survival rates for lymph node negative HCC without cirrhosis are 83%, 75%, and 75%; respectively. The same rates for lymph node positive are 33%, 11%, and 11%, respectively. HCC with cirrhosis up to now has revealed less worthwhile results. Moreover, prolonged survival without tumor recurrence was not obtained in patients with cholangiocellular carcinoma or secondary liver cancers. They concluded that hepatic transplantation for selected tumor patients seems justified, and a detailed analysis of the chance of different tumor types for success with this method of treatment is essential.

4 Tumor recurrence

Tumor recurrence after liver transplantation is unavoidable due to the nature of malignant liver diseases. Iwatsuki et al. [8] reported that recurrence of primary liver cancer after liver transplantation was observed in 13 of the 27 patients who survived 6 months. Seven of 11 patients with HCC had tumor recurrence, 3 of which developed within 1 year. Three of 7 patients with fibrolamellar HCC had recurrence. Similarly, 2 of 8 patients with epitheloid hemangioendothelioma had recurrences more than one year after liver grafting. One patient with cholangio-carcinoma had tumor recurrence 23 months after transplantation and died from metastases 31 months after transplantation. They had also 7 patients who received liver graft for secondary liver cancer, and two of them died from recurrence of bile duct carcinoma and adenocarcinoma of unknown origin. One patient with leiomyosarcoma of the small intestine is alive with recurrent tumor 15 months after liver grafting.

According to the report from Cambridge/King's College Hospital [16], tumor recurrence was detected in 24 (64.9%) of 37 patients with HCC who survived at least 3 months after transplantation. This recurrence rate is as high as that reported from the University of Pittsburgh [8]. Among the 7 patients with fibrolamellar HCC, tumor recurred in 3 patients at 6, 9 and 18 months after transplantation. Twelve of 14 patients with cholangiocarcinoma developed tumor recurrence (abdomen, lung, bone, liver, and cervical lymph node). Only 3 of 6 patients with secondary liver cancer survived for 3 months after transplantation, but died between 22 and 41 weeks from tumor recurrence. From Hanover Medical School, the overall incidence of tumor recurrence was reported to be 28 of 95 patients with hepatobiliary malignancy [13]. Clinical observation of patients after transplantation at Pittsburgh and Cambridge confirmed that the dominant sites of detected or documented tumor recurrence were liver, lung, adrenal gland, bone, abdominal cavity, cervical lymph node, and skin [8, 16].

Tumor recurrence in grafted livers is a very interesting phenomenon, but the mechanism remains equivocal.

5 Factors influencing recurrence and prognosis

Recurrence and prognosis of malignant liver tumors depends mainly on the individual nature of each tumor. Tumor size, capsule formation, vascular invasion, and differentiation of a tumor have been suggested as important factors to determine the prognosis of tumors [1, 17, 18]. Incidental HCC showed better prognosis and lower tumor recurrence because incidental HCC was small in size, and only one patient with incidental HCC died from tumor recurrence [8]. On the other hand, O'Grady et al. [16] found no correlation between tumor size and frequency or rapidity of tumor recurrence.

Fibrolamellar HCC is very rare in Asian countries like Japan, but is relatively common in the West and approximately 7% of HCC is of the fibrolamellar variant. This type of HCC is observed solitary in relatively young adults or adolescents with rare concomitant cirrhosis. Their prognosis is better than those of other types of HCC due to slow-growing characteristics, and the 5-year survival rate was reported to be 63% [19]. The characteristic morphological feature of this tumor is polygonal cells with an abundant eosinophilic cytoplasm and uniformly large oval and vesicular nuclei [19]. Nine patients with this type of tumor have been given a transplanted liver graft using CyA [11]. Four of 8 patients with fibrolamellar HCC had tumor recurrence, but survival rates of patient with this type of HCC and epitheloid hemangioendothelioma were significantly higher than those with other types of HCC. The median interval between transplantation and death from recurrence was longer in patients with a well-differentiated tumor on histological examination than in moderate/poorly differentiated tumor. All 3 patients free of detectable malignancy at 2 years after transplantation had well-differentiated tumors [16].

Since 1985, Pichlmayr et al. [10] started a new liver transplant program which emphasized precise patient selection by lymph node metastasis. Median survival then improved significantly within the next 4 years as compared to the preceding era (18.06 vs. 4.0 months) [13]. Alphafetoprotein (AFP) is an internationally accepted tumor marker for HCC. In the majority of patients with HCC, serum AFP dropped immediately after transplantation and rose in relation to tumor recurrence [13, 16]. Ringe et al. observed that tumor-free long-term survivors tended to be those with normal or only slightly elevated AFP levels before transplantation [13].

6 Immunosuppression and liver malignancy

Under immunosuppressive therapy using azathioprine steroid therapy, 1-year survival was only 30% as compared with 65% in patients under CyA steroid therapy. Tumor recurrence after transplantation for primary liver cancer was approximately 70% in both azathioprine and CyA treated patients in the series of the University of Pittsburgh [20]. The Cambridge/King's College Hospital group reviewed the outcome in liver graftings for HCC with specific regard to the frequency and rate of tumor recurrence in those surviving for at least 3 months after the operation

[21]. Tumor recurrence was observed in 12 (66.7%) of 18 patients treated with azathioprine steroid therapy (Group 1) and 13 (68.4%) of 19 patients treated with CyA steroid therapy (Group 2). The average tumor-free interval after transplantation was 0.5 ± 0.3 years (± 1 SD) in Group 1 as compared with 1.1 ± 0.8 years in Group 2 ($P < 0.01$). The interval between the detection of tumor recurrence and the development of associated symptoms has improved from 0.3 ± 0.1 years to 0.9 ± 0.4 years after the introduction of CyA, and the 1-year survival rate has also improved from 25% to 92.3%. While all patients in Group 1 died within 2.1 years following transplantation, 2 patients in Group 2 were alive and asymptomatic at 2.5 and 4.9 years.

Immunosuppressive agents can not avoid promoting tumor growth due to their simultaneous suppression of the recipient's tumor immunity. The introduction of CyA with immunosuppressive therapy did not reduce the incidence of tumor recurrences after liver grafting, but CyA has shown considerable improvement in the palliative effect of liver grafting for liver cancers. It is therefore urgent for those performing liver grafting in hepatic malignancies to develop more selective and safe immunosuppressive agents which do not promote tumor growth after liver grafting.

7 HCC in Japan as an indication for liver transplantation

Tanaka and Tanigawa [22] reported that Japan had a large number of cases with HCC and approximately 19,000 patients have died annually from primary liver cancer in Japan, 95% of which were patients with HCC. The application of liver transplantation for unresectable HCC will be thus a very important matter of discussion in the near future in Japan. In recent years, small HCC (<2 cm in diameter) are being detected and diagnosed by ultrasound-guided biopsy of liver tumors more frequently due to remarkable developments in imaging techniques, and the prognosis of small HCC then improved with conventional hepatic resection and percutaneous ethanol injection therapy (PEIT). The 5-year survival rate for small HCC was elevated to 50%. Small liver cancer (<2 cm in diameter) should not considered to be an indication for liver transplantation except with concomitant end-stage

liver cirrhosis. On the other hand, large HCC (>5 cm in diameter) has shown a high incidence of extrahepatic involvement of tumors and micrometastasis in the lung in spite of palliative therapies, mainly transarterial embolization (TAE). Therefore, liver transplantation plays a small role in the treatment these large HCC because of the high incidence of vascular invasion and extrahepatic tumor involvement soon after liver grafting. Consequently, medium sized HCC (between 2 and 5 cm in diameter) appears to be a possible indication either for conventional hepatic resection or liver transplantation, but it should be noted that even small HCC may have a multicentric nature [22].

At present, Tanigawa et al. have concluded that application of liver transplantation in Japan would be limited only to medium sized HCC which are unresectable due to underlying cirrhosis or multifocal tumor growth.

In recent years, great effort have been made to evaluate the malignant potential of tumors by DNA and/or gene analyses of tumor cells, and small liver cancers can be evaluated in terms of their multifocal characteristics prior to liver transplantation. Small HCC less than 2 cm in diameter would also appear to be an ideal indication for liver grafting provided that it would be diagnosed to be multifocal in an early stage.

8 Future aspect of liver transplantation for liver cancer

8.1 Abdominal organ cluster transplantation for liver cancer

From the results of large series liver transplantation at the University of Pittsburgh, Starzl et al. have a negative attitude towards liver transplantation for liver cancer other than the fibrolamellar type HCC and incidental liver cancer, since liver transplantation for primary liver cancer did not achieve sufficient long-term survival, nor is effective perioperative chemotherapy available after liver transplantation for liver cancer [8].

In the development of human fetus, the liver and pancreas begin as ventral and dorsal diverticula from the portion of the foregut that later diffentiates into the duodenum, and malignant tumors that originate from one of these three organs metastasize to the others. Therefore, Starzl et al. considered that radical excision of most of the foregut could be available for complete removal of tumors in the liver, bile duct, duodenum, stomach, and pancreas [23].

Twenty one patients underwent upper abdominal exenteration (liver, stomach, spleen, pancreas, duodenum, proximal jejunum, terminal ileum, and ascending and transverse colon) for unresectable tumors in the foregut with liver involvement, followed by abdominal organ cluster transplantation (pancreatic-duodenal-hepatic grafts) between July 1988 and January 1990. Seven of them had carcinoma of the bile duct, and four patients had carcinoid. As a result, 8 of 21 patients who underwent transplanted abdominal organ cluster survived and were discharged from the hospital. Of the two patients with HCC and two with cholangiocellular carcinoma who were treated with this original cluster procedure, only one case with cholangiocellular carcinoma survived. Following this, 18 patients were treated with modified cluster (hepatic graft only) between April 1989 and December 1989. Four out of 9 patients with cholangiocellular carcinoma survived, but none of the 4 cases with HCC survived. From January to April 1990, 9 patients had liver replacement and pancreatic islet transplantation under FK 506 and steroids. The patients had either CCC, pancreatic cancer, or HCC. Five of the six survivors are not dependent on insulin treatment following the operation. (Iwatsuki S, Starzl TE, et al. (1991) Cluster transplantation and its variants. Personal communication). In spite of a 20% technically related perioperative mortality, Iwatsuki et al. suggested that a selected group of patients could benefit from this radical surgical approach and that postoperative adjuvant chemotherapy and irradiation should be considered.

8.2 Combined intensive therapy

The miserable prognosis for patients with secondary liver cancers has not been improved by intensive chemotherapy, nor has liver transplantation succeeded in improving the survival rate of the patients. In Innsbruck, combined treatment of metastatic liver disease consisting of total liver replacement and ultra-high-dose cytotoxic chemotherapy (cyclophosphamide 60 mg/kg body weight for 2 days) as well as total body irradiation at 1,000 rad followed by autologous bone marrow reconstitution was tried. There was no associated mortality and relatively low morbidity, and it was surprisingly well tolerated by the liver grafts. They were also able to achieve one long-lasting remission, but rapid tumor recurrence developed in the other two patients. Therefore, Margreiter et al. are of the opinion that, in light of the shortage of organs and the great pains taken, liver transplantation for metastatic disease is not justified at the present time [24].

In contrast, liver grafting for primary liver malignancy has resulted in a better prognosis in selected patients than that for secondary tumors in the liver, and thus the new idea of this combined intensive therapy might be tried and applied in the treatment of primary liver cancer.

9 Conclusion

Liver transplantation is now the treatment of choice for various liver diseases which lead to irreversible hepatic failure in children and adults, but the supply of donor livers is less than the demand. Therefore, prioritization of candidates for liver transplantation should be based on the probability of success or on the urgency of need. It is, however, difficult to predict the probability of success for the majority of patients based on perioperative evaluation of risk, and many patients who might be considered highly risky have an excellent opportunity for survival in the hands of a well experienced transplant team.

We believe that liver transplantation in liver cancer should be indicated in non-resectable tumors without extrahepatic tumor growth or in patients with cirrhosis which excludes major surgery due for functional reasons. More precise patient selection, new immunosuppressors, and refined perioperative therapy are important to achieve better results in liver transplantation for liver cancer.

References

1. Okuda K, Ishak KG (1987) Neoplasms of the Liver. Springer Verlag, Tokyo
2. Nagasue N, Yukaya H, Ogawa Y, Sasaki Y (1986) Clinical experience with 118 hepatic resections for hepatocellular carcinoma. Surgery 99:694–701
3. Bismuth H, Houssin D, Ornowsky J, Meriggi F (1986) Liver resection in cirrhotic patients. A western experience. World J Surg 10:311–317

4. Starzl TE, Marchioro TL, Von Kaulla KN, et al. (1963) Homotransplantation of the liver in humans. Surg Gyn Obstet 117:659–676

5. Iwatsuki S, Klintmalm GBG, Starzl TE (1982) Total hepatectomy and liver replacement (orthotopic liver transplantation) for primary hepatic malignancy. World J Surg 6:81–86

6. Calne RY (1983) Liver transplantation: The Cambridge and King's College Hospital Experience. Grune and Stratton London, pp 306–311

7. Starzl TE, Porter KA, Putnam CW, et al. (1976) Orthotopic liver transplantation in 93 patients. Surg Gynecol Obstet 142:487–505

8. Iwatsuki S, Starzl TE, Todo S, et al. (1988) Experience in 1,000 liver transplants under cyclosporine steroid therapy: A survival report. Transplant Proc 20:498–504

9. Starzl TE, Todo S, Iwatsuki S, et al. (1989) Liver transplantation: An unfinished product. Transplant Proc 21:2197–2200

10. Pichlmayr R (1988) Is there a place for liver grafting for malignancy? Transplant Proc 20:487–492

11. Koneru B, Iwatsuki S, Starzl TE et al. (1988) Liver transplantation for malignant tumors. Gastroenterol Clin N Am 17:177–193

12. Neuberger J, Williams R (1987) Indications and assessment for liver grafting. In: Calne RY (ed) Liver transplantation, 2nd edn. Grune and Stratton, Tokyo, pp 63–75

13. Ringe B, Wittekind C, Pichlmayr R et al. (1989) The role of liver transplantation in hepatobiliary malignancy. Ann Surg 209:88–98

14. Bismuth H, Ericzon BG, Rolles K et al. (1987) Hepatic transplantation in Europe. First report of the European liver transplant registry. Lancet 2:674–676

15. European Liver Transplant Registry (June 1989) Bismuth H. Villejuif, Paris

16. O'Grady JG, Polson RJ, Rolles K, Calne RY, Williams R (1988) Liver transplantation for malignant disease. Ann Surg 207:373–379

17. Okuda K, Nakashima T, Obata H (1977) Clinicopathological studies of minute hepatocellular carcinoma. Gastroenterology 73:109–115

18. Hsu H, Wu T, Wu M, et al. (1988) Tumor invasiveness and prognosis in resected hepatocellular carcinoma. Cancer 61:2095–2099

19. Bermann MM, Libbey NP, Foster JH (1980) Hepatocellular carcinoma: Polygonal cell type with fibrous stroma—an atypical variant with a favorable prognosis. Cancer 46:1448–1455

20. Iwatsuki S, Gordon RD, Shaw BW, Starzl TE (1985) Role of liver transplantation in cancer therapy. Ann Surg 202:401–407

21. O'Grady JG, Johnson PJ, Zaman S, Calne RY, Williams R (1988) Decreased rate of growth of hepatocellular carcinoma recurrance after liver transplantation in patients maintained on cyclosporin immunosuppression. Transplant Proc 20:394–396

22. Tanaka M, Tanigawa K (1990) Prognosis of hepatocellular carcinoma and indication for liver transplantation (in Japanese). Kan Tan Sui 20:821–825

23. Starzl TE, Todo S, Tzakis A, Iwatsuki S et al. (1989) Abdominal organ cluster transplantation for the treatment of upper abdominal malignancies. Ann Surg 210:374–386

24. Margreiter R, Niederwiser D, Frommhold H et al. (1987) Tumor recurrence after liver transplantation followed by high-dose cyclophosphamide, total body irradiation, and autologous bone marrow transplantation for treatment of metastatic liver disease. Transplant Proc 19:2403

Overview of the general rules for the clinical and pathological study of primary liver cancer in Japan

Masayuki Yamamoto and Katsuhiko Sugahara[1]

1 Introduction

The General Rules for the Clinical and Pathological Study of Primary Liver Cancer provides guidelines for case management and research in Japan. These rules were initially published by an individual Cancer Study Group in Japan and some of them were translated into English. In general, most of the information on malignant diseases has come from North America and Europe, but few studies have been forthcoming from Asia. Since primary liver cancer is the third most common malignant disease in Japan and its clinical features are different from those in occidental society, clinical classifications have been established to aide research and treatment.

2 History of the general rules

The number of cases of primary liver cancer, mostly hepatocellular carcinoma (HCC), in Japan have rapidly increased since around 1980. According to the Liver Cancer Study Group of Japan, there were a total of 4,031 cases in the 10 years between 1968 and 1977, and there were 4,652 cases in only two years between 1980 and 1981. This increase is a direct result of improved imaging techniques, such as CT (computed tomography) and US (ultrasonography). As a result of the need to collect and analyze the increasing number of diagnosed cases according to a standardized criterion, the first Japanese edition of The General Rules for the Clinical and

Pathological Study of Primary Liver Cancer was published by the Liver Cancer Study Group of Japan in 1983 [1]. Soon after the first edition was published, data was analyzed from more than 500 institutes belonging to the Liver Cancer Study Group of Japan. This additional data necessitated revision of the Rule and a second edition was published in 1987 in Japanese and in 1989 in English [2].

For comparison with data from other parts of the world, the features unique to HCC in Japan, mostly arising from accompanying liver cirrhosis, had to be defined in the Rule. At the Second International Symposium of the Japanese Society of Gastroenterology in Tokyo in 1987, the theme of "Regional characteristics of hepatocellular carcinoma" [3] was proposed.

In the second edition, the Clinical Stage was defined according to the accompanying liver cirrhosis and liver function in addition to the macroscopic staging of the tumor itself. In cases of severe liver cirrhosis, it was decided that decisions regarding surgical intervention should be made on the basis of liver function as well as extention of the liver tumor. The macroscopic stage was also changed to emphasize the size of tumor, vascular invasion, and the number of tumors. The revised macroscopic stage conforms to the UICC [4] classification for tumor, node, metastasis (TNM).

3 Outline of the third edition of the general rule

Soon after the second edition was published, a new committee was organized to prepare a third edition [5] to keep up with results collected according to the standardized criteria. The

[1]First Department of Surgery, Yamanashi Medical College, Shimakato 1110, Tamaho-cho, Nakakoma, Yamanashi, 409-38 Japan

new criteria that were to be developed were descriptive methods to describe the state of the liver tumor by imaging diagnosis, macroscopic classification of liver cancer including cholangiocarcinoma, and definition of the relative curative resection.

Due to the increasing number of diagnosed cases of liver cancer, several modalities for their treatment, such as transcatheter arterial embolization (TAE), ethanol injection, and immunochemotherapy have been developed and their direct effects on tumors have to be noted according to the standardized methods. Imaging is the only way to diagnose the direct effects of these treatment modalities in non-operative cases. It is also necessary for postoperative follow-up studies to be performed to detect recurrent tumors or tumors not resected at the time of surgery.

The macroscopic classification of liver cancer was divided to three basic types in conformity with Eggel's classifications. Because small tumors are found and operated on more frequently these days, a new classification for small tumors is required. As shown in Fig. 2, subtypes of the nodular type of tumor are re-classified in the third edition. In addition, small tumors located within one segment but with an unclear and irregular border were termed as infiltrative form. On the other hand, big tumors occupying more than one segment with the characteristic of an unclear and irregular border were termed as the massive type.

For small liver cancer that consists of single tumors whose maximum diameter is 2 cm or less, one subtype, "small liver cancer-well differentiated type", was defined. This type should be differentiated from small nodular-type tumors, since well differentiated HCC maintains the preexisting internal structures with unclear borders even though it has often a hyperechoic image on US.

Definition of the curative resection was made in the second edition, but the results revealed that, even after resection, sometimes recurrent tumors appeared in the remnant liver postoperatively. It is possible that minute tumors in the remnant liver were present prior to resection and were simply not detected by the existing imaging techniques before the operation. There remains several problems to be solved to establish a new definition of the curative resection, whether the tumor be synchronous, metachronous multicentric, or metastatic. The curative resection described here is still a provisonal one.

The present rule is more applicable to HCC,

but reports of cholangiocarcinoma have been increasing. Clinical staging and macroscopic staging are also required but were not concluded in the third edition.

4 General rules for the clinical and pathological study of primary liver cancer

4.1 Anatomy

4.1.1 Liver lobes and segments
The right and left lobes, which are divided by Cantlie's line, are each divided into two segments, and together with the caudate lobe, there are five segments. Each segment is divided into upper and lower subsegments except for the caudate lobe.

4.1.2 Lymph node
Lymph node metastasis in liver cancer awaits further study, but for the time being, descriptions should be made in accordance with the general rules for cancer in other organs.

1. Group 1 lymph nodes
   a) Subdiaphragmatic lymph nodes of the upper region of the liver
   b) Lymph nodes in the hepatic porta
2. Group 2 lymph nodes
   a) Lymph nodes in the hepatoduodenal ligament
3. Group 3 lymph nodes
   a) Lymph nodes around the vena cava above the diaphragm
   b) Lymph nodes at the posterior aspect of the pancreas
   c) Lymph nodes along the common hepatic artery
   d) Lymph nodes around the celiac artery
   e) Low thoracic paraesophageal lymph nodes

4.2 Descriptive methods of state of tumor by imaging diagnosis

4.2.1 Location of tumor
The site of a liver tumor should be indicated, according to (4.4) Descriptive methods of operative findings and resected specimens of liver cancer, using the abbreviation for the liver segments (P,A,M,L,C) as described in Fig. 1, and

Fig. 1. Segments of the liver

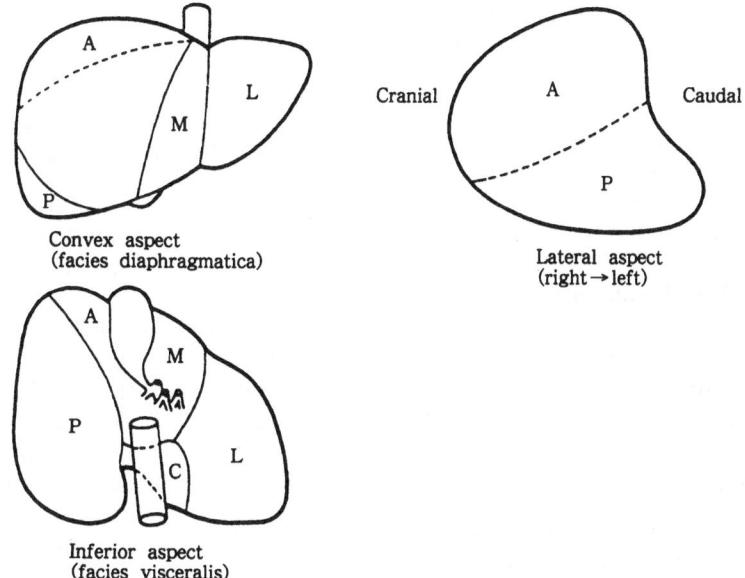

Convex aspect
(facies diaphragmatica)

Lateral aspect
(right → left)

Cranial   Caudal

Inferior aspect
(facies visceralis)

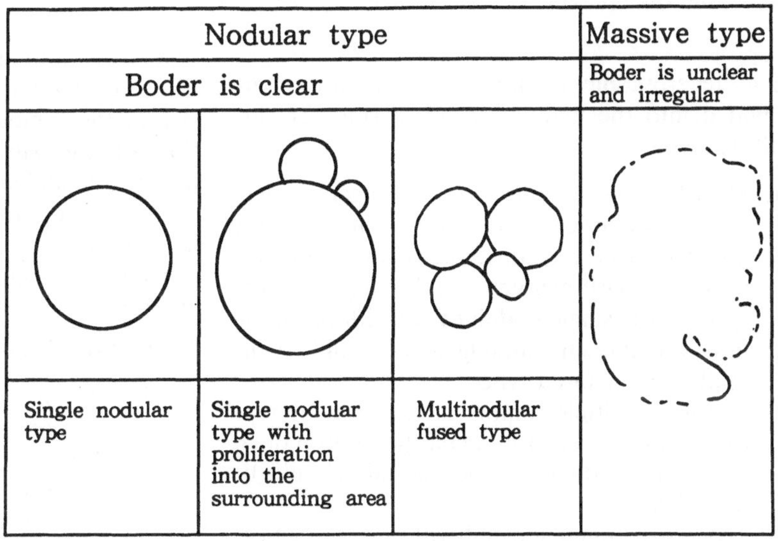

Nodular type			Massive type
Boder is clear			Boder is unclear and irregular
Single nodular type	Single nodular type with proliferation into the surrounding area	Multinodular fused type	

Fig. 2. Types of tumors

adding St for single, Mt for multiple, or Dt for not-countable diffuse tumors.

4.2.2 Size
The size of a tumor should be measured as long diameter (cm) × short diameter (cm). If this is not possible, the longest diameter should be entered.

4.2.3 State of tumor border

1. PD. Poorly demarcated
2. WD. Well demarcated
   a) Fc(+). Clear capsule formation
   b) Fc(−). No clear capsule formation

If a macroscopic type of tumor can be determined by imaging diagnosis according to (4.3) Macroscopic classification of liver cancer, it should be so indicated.

4.2.4 State of internal tumor structure

1. solid
   a) Nc(+). Necrotized in some parts; the Nc% (necrotized percent) should be calculated
   b) Nc(−). No necrosis
2. cystic

Practices of transcatheter arterial embolization (TAE) or ethanol injection should be indicated.

If lipiodol or an anti-cancer drug was used at the same time as TAE, it should be so indicated.

4.2.5   Vascular invasion

Vascular invasion should be examined by imaging techniques, and it should be described according to (4.4) Descriptive methods of operative findings and resected specimens of liver cancer.

4.2.6   Distant organ metastasis (DM)

Metastasis of liver cancer to distant organ is expressed as DM. The metastasized organ as identified from X-rays, scintigraphy, ultra-sonography, computed tomography, magnetic resonance imaging or clinical findings, should be indicated in parentheses.

1. DM_0. No metastasis to distant organs
2. DM_1. Metastasis to distant organs

4.3   Macroscopic classification of liver cancer

The macroscopic findings of liver cancer are divided into the nodular, massive (Fig. 2), and diffuse type.

1. *Nodular type*. In this type of cancer, a clear border can be seen between the cancerous and non-cancerous portions, and it can be divided into three basic subtypes: 1) the single nodular type, 2) the single nodular type with proliferation into the surrounding tissues, and 3) the multinodular fused type.

    When multiple tumors of the nodular type exists in the liver, it is called the multinodular form, and subtype of each nodule should be described.

    A small tumor located within one segment with an unclear and irregular border between the cancerous and non-cancerous portions is treated provisionally as a subdivision of the nodular type, the infiltrative form, and this is indicated in parentheses.
2. *Massive type*. Big liver cancers occupy more than one segment of the liver, and the borders between the cancerous and non-cancerous portions are unclear and irregular. This definition conforms with Eggel's classification of the massive type.
3. *Diffuse type*. The liver as a whole is replaced by a great number of small, disseminated tumor nodules. It is often difficult, when examining the liver surface macroscopically, to distinguish between this type of cancer and cirrhosis of the liver.

4.3.1   Additional factors

In cholangiocarcinoma, in addition to the macroscopic findings described above, examinations should include confirmation of the presence or absence of the following factors.

1. Proliferation of tumors along the intrahepatic bile duct
2. Accompanied by intrahepatic calculi

3. Cholangiocarcinoma, which is primarily found in the liver, is treated as primary liver cancer under this Rule. Those tumors whose predominat location is not clearly either inside the liver or at the porta hepatis are not treated under this Rule. They are regarded as bile duct cancer and treated under The General Rule of the Bile Duct Cancer.

4.4   Descriptive methods of operative findings and resected specimens of liver cancer

Operative findings should be recorded for all cases having undergone laparotomy. When the size of the tumor, macroscopic findings, infiltration of the surrounding tissues, lymph node metastasis, and so on, are unconfirmed because a case was inoperable, the entry should be made in parentheses. When an item is unclear or unknown, "unclear" or "unknown" should be entered.

4.4.1   Location of cancer

1. The *site* of liver cancer should be indicated using the abbreviations for the liver segments (P,A,M,L,C) as described previously and adding St for single or Mt for multiple tumors.
2. When liver cancer is present in *two segments*, the segment containing most cancer should be entered first.
3. When the liver cancer is present in *more than two segments*, the segments should be entered in the order of the amount of cancer present in each segment. For example, single liver cancer in which the majority of the neoplasm is located in the posterior segment, but part of it is also located in the anterior segment should be indicated as St-PA. Moreover if the liver cancer has spread from the medial segment to the lateral segment, and there are also two tumors in the anterior segment, the entry should be indicated as Mt-MLA.

4.4.2   Size and surroundings (H)

The size of the cancer in each segment should be measured, and the length (long diameter), width (short diameter) and thickness (height) entered in cm. The following symbols should also be employed:

1. H_0. Liver cancer is T1 (p. 109) and is present only in one subsegment
2. H_s. Liver cancer is present only in one subsegment
3. H_1. Liver cancer is present in only one segment
4. H_2. Liver cancer is present in two segments
5. H_3. Liver cancer is present in three segments
6. H_4. Liver cancer is present in more than three segments

4.4.3 Macroscopic findings of liver cancer

The macroscopic findings of liver cancer at resection or autopsy are classified into three main types (nodular, massive and diffuse) and then into the subtypes as specified in (4.3). Since it is often difficult to distinguish between the nodular and massive types in inoperable cases, however, entries should be based on local findings, imaging findings, and so on, and should be made in parentheses.

The macroscopic conditions, such as the border between the cancerous and non-cancerous portions, are expressed as follows:

1. Growth type
   a) Expansive growth (Eg). The border between cancerous and non-cancerous tissue is clear.
   b) Infiltrative growth (Ig). The border between cancerous and non-cancerous tissue is not clear.
2. Capsule formation (Fc)
   a) Fc(−). No clear connective tissue capsule is formed around the cancer.
   b) Fc(+). A clear connective tissue capsule is formed around the cancer.
3. Capsule infiltration (Fc-Inf)
   b) Fc-Inf(−). There is no apparent cancer infiltration into the cancer capsule.
   c) Fc-Inf(+). There is cancer infiltration into the cancer capsule and/or outside the capsule.
4. Septal formation (Sf)
   a) Sf(−). No formation of fibrous septa can be seen within the cancer.
   b) Sf(+). Formation of fibrous septa can be seen within the cancer and there is clear lobe formation.
5. Serosal infiltration (Si)
   Serosal infiltration should be classified under

the following four headings on the basis of macroscopic expansion:
   a) S_0. No cancer tissue in the serosa.
   b) S_1. Cancer tissue in the serosa.
   c) S_2. Cancer tissue infiltration to other organs. The name of the infiltrated organ should be noted.
   d) S_3. Ruptured cancer tissue, accompanied by intraperitoneal hemorrhage.

4.4.4 Lymph node metastasis (N)

1. $N_0(-)$. No apparent lymph node metastasis
2. $N_1(+)$. Metastasis to Group 1 lymph nodes
3. $N_2(+)$. Metastasis to Group 2 lymph nodes
4. $N_3(+)$. Metastasis to Group 3 or more distant lymph nodes

5. $N_1(-)$. No metastasis to Group 1 lymph nodes
6. $N_2(-)$. No metastasis to Group 2 lymph nodes
7. $N_3(-)$. No metastasis to Group 3 or more distant lymph nodes

Determination of N_3 metastasis is often difficult in operative cases, $N_2(+)$, $N_3(+)$ are treated as M1 (4.6).

4.4.5 Vascular invasion (V)

1. Vp_0. No tumor embolus in the portal vein
2. Vp_1. Tumor embolus distal to the second branch of the left or right portal veins (not including second branches)
3. Vp_2. Tumor embolus in the second branch of the portal vein
4. Vp_3. Tumor embolus in the first branch, or trunk of the portal vein, or in a branch on the opposite side

5. Vv_0. No tumor embolus in the hepatic vein
6. Vv_1. Tumor embolus in a branch of the hepatic vein
7. Vv_2. Tumor embolus in the right, middle or left hepatic vein trunk, posterior inferior hepatic venous trunk or short hepatic vein
8. Vv_3. Tumor embolus in the inferior vena cava

The first branch of the portal vein consists of a common trunk on the right side and the transverse portion on the left side. The second branch consists of the segment branch trunk on the right side and the umbilical portion on the left side.

4.4.6 Bile duct invasion (B)

1. B_0. No expansion into the intrahepatic bile ducts
2. B_1. Expansion into the intrahepatic bile ducts

3. B_2. Expansion into the intrahepatic bile ducts and further into the extrahepatic bile ducts

4.4.7 Intrahepatic metastasis (IM)

1. IM_0. No intrahepatic metastasis
2. IM_1. Intrahepatic metastasis only in the same segment as the main tumor
3. IM_2. Intrahepatic metastasis in two segments
4. IM_3. Intrahepatic metastasis in three or more segments

The liver segment containing the intrahepatic metastasis should be indicated in parentheses. For example, when the main tumor is present in the posterior segment and another tumor, considered to be metastatic, is found in the posterior segment, the entry should be IM_1 (P). When metastasis is also found in the lateral segment, it should be then IM_2 (PL).

4.4.8 Peritoneal dissemination (Pd)

The degrees of peritoneal disseminating metastasis fall into the following three categories:

1. P_0. No disseminating metastasis in the serosal surface of the entire peritoneal cavity
2. P_1. Disseminating metastasis in the adjacent peritoneum (cranial to the transverse colon, but including the greater omentum), but no metastasis in the distant peritoneum
3. P_2. Disseminating metastasis in the distant peritoneum

Findings from histological examinations of (4.4.3) to (4.4.8) should be written in small letters, such as eg, ig, fc(+), fc-inf(+), sf(+), s_2, n_1, vp_1, b_1, im_2, or p_1.

4.4.9 Evaluation of the cancer infiltration of the resected liver surface

Cancerous infiltration of the resected liver specimens should be evaluated macroscopically and histologically.

1. Macroscopic classification (TW)
   a) TW(−). No macroscopic cancerous infiltration within 10 mm from the cut liver surface in freshly excised specimens
   b) TW(+). Macroscopic cancerous infiltration within 10 mm from the cut liver surface in freshly excised specimens
2. Histological classification (tw)
   a) tw(−). No cancer cells observed histologically within 5 mm from the cut liver surface in fixed specimens
   b) tw(+). Cancer cells observed histologically within 5 mm from the cut liver surface in fixed specimens

Table 1. Clinical stage for hepatocellular carcinoma

Findings \ Stage	I	II	III
Ascites	None	Treatment effective	Treatment ineffective
Serum bilirubin (mg/dl)	below 2.0	2.0–3.0	over 3.0
Serum albumin (g/dl)	over 3.5	3.0–3.5	below 3.0
ICG R_{15} (%)	below 15	15–40	over 40
Prothrombin activity value (%)	over 80	50–80	below 50

The clinical stages for hepatocellular carcinoma should be used as an index for the selection of treatment, but they do not necessarily correspond degree of advancement of the hepatocellular carcinoma.

When clinical stages correspond to two or more items occur in two sites, the higher clinical stage should be used. For example, when the clinical stage is II for three items and III for two items, the case should be classified as Clinical Stage III.

Leukocytopenia, 3,000/mm^3 or less; and thrombocytopenia, 50,000/mm^3 or less, should be noted.

The Clinical Stage for cholangiocarcinoma is under discussion.

In TW(−) cases, when tumor emboli are found in the intrahepatic vasculature and bile ducts by means of pre- and intraoperative imaging diagnosis, removal of the tumor emboli is required.

4.4.10 Description of remained tumors in the remnant liver

In cases of reduction surgery, where remained tumors in the remnant liver are determined by macroscopically or by image diagnosis on liver resection, state of the tumors should be examined by using the ultrasonography and described according to (4.2).

4.4.11 Concomitant liver cirrhosis (Z)

1. Z_0. Normal liver
2. Z_1. Accompanying fibrosis but not defined as liver cirrhosis
3. Z_2. Liver cirrhosis

4.5 Clinical status of the host

4.5.1 Clinical stage (Table 1)

There are three clinical stages of hepatocellular carcinoma which are classified according to clinical and laboratory findings. The degree of progress is obtained by evaluating the patient's condition for each item, and when at least two items within any given stage are found to apply, that stage is then assigned.

Table 2. Macroscopic staging

Stage	Factor T	N	M
I	T1	N0	M0
II	T2	N0	M0
III	T3	N0	M0
	T1–3	N1	M0
IV-A	T4	N0–1	M0
IV-B	T1–4	N0–1	M1

4.5.2 Endoscopic findings of esophageal varices (EV)

1. EV(−). No concomitant esophageal varices
2. EV(+). Concomitant esophageal varices

4.6 Macroscopic staging (Table 2)

In macroscopic staging, the stage for each item is determined and the highest values selected.

The degree of macroscopic progress is classified into four stages, as follows:

1. T factor. This depends on three items: cancer size, whether it is single or multiple, and vascular invasion. Multiple tumors can be either multicentric tumors or intrahepatic metastatic tumors.
   a) T1. A single tumor of 2 cm or less in its greatest dimension without vascular invasion
   b) T2. A single tumor of 2 cm or less in its greatest dimension with vascular invasion
      i) Multiple tumors with a maximum tumor diameter of 2 cm or less confined to one lobe
      ii) A single tumor with a diameter exceeding 2 cm, without vascular invasion
   c) T3. A single tumor with a diameter exceeding 2 cm, with vascular invasion
      i) Multiple tumors with diameters exceeding 2 cm confined to one lobe
   d) T4. Multiple tumors in more than one lobe
      i) Associated vascular invasion in the first branch of the portal or hepatic veins
2. N factors.
   a) N0. No metastasis in the Group 1 lymph nodes
   b) N1. Metastasis in at least the Group 1 lymph nodes
3. M factors.
   a) M0. No distant metastasis
   b) M1. Distant metastasis

In the classification of lymph node metastasis (N) in section (4.1.2), $N_2(+)$ and $N_3(+)$ are included for convenience under M1 of M factors. For cases of ruptured liver cancer, there are no special items and the stage is decided from the above T, N and M classification.

The stage classification of liver cancer shows the degree of biological advance of the cancer and should also reflect the prognosis of the disease. For more accurate estimation, the histological findings should also be recorded and investigations should be performed in many cases. In the same stage, the resection rate, direct mortality and survival rates can be calculated, thus enabling a comparative study of the advantages and disadvantages of each therapeutic method. From this standpoint, it is recommended that the stage classification be based on a simultaneous consideration of the handling of concomitant liver cirrhosis, chronic hepatitis and esophageal varices even though they are not directly connected with the degree of progress of the liver cancer.

The degree of macroscopic advance is considered to be the same as the TNM classification of the UICC. In the same patient, the stage is almost the same as that given by the stage classification of the former general rules [1].

4.7 Types of hepatic resection (Hr)

4.7.1 Extent of resection
The methods are classified as follows according to the extent of resection.

1. Hr0. Resection of less than one subsegment
2. HrS. Resection of one subsegment
3. Hr1. Resection of one segment
4. Hr2. Resection of two segments
5. Hr3. Resection of three segments
6. Hr4. Resection of four segments

4.7.2 Resected segments
The names of the resected segments should be shown in parentheses. In cases where resections exceed the range concerned, the segment partially resected is should be added as + and small head letter of the segment.

In cases where concomitant resections or additional operations are performed, this fact should be noted. For example, when a splenectomy and a transabdominal esophageal transection are performed at the same time as a lateral segmentectomy, the entry should be: Hr1(L), splenectomy, transabdominal esophageal transection.

Abbreviations for common hepatic resection are as follows:

1. Left lobectomy: Hr2(L,M)
2. Right lobectomy: Hr2(P,A)
3. Lateral segmentectomy: Hr1(L)
4. Extended left lobectomy: Hr2+(L,M,a)
5. Left lobectomy with partial resection of caudate lobe:Hr2+(L,M,c)
6. Extended right lobectomy: Hr2+(P,A,m)
7. Posterior segmentectomy: Hr1(P)
8. Subsegmentectomy: for example of the anterior segment, HrS(A)
9. Subsegmentectomy in two areas: for example of the anterior and posterior segments; HrS(A)+HrS(P)
10. Trisegmentectomy: trisegmentectomy from the right, Hr3(P,A,M); trisegmentectomy from the left, Hr3(L,M,A); left lobectomy with simultaneous resection of caudal lobe, Hr3(L,M,C)
11. Wedge resection, enucleation, partial resection: for example wedge resection of the posterior segment, Hr0(P)

In the case of reduction surgery, for example, where tumors remain in the medial and lateral segments after right lobectomy: Red(L,M) Hr2(P,A)

4.7.3   Extent of lymph node dissection (R)

Resection according to the extent of lymph node dissection is classified in the following three stages:

1. R_0. Liver resection with no dissection or incomplete dissection of the Group 1 lymph nodes
2. R_1. Liver resection with dissection of the Group 1 lymph nodes
3. R_2. Liver resection with dissection of the Group 1 and confirmed Group 2 lymph nodes

4.8   Curative and non-curative resection

1. Curative resection
   a) Absolute curative resection.
      i) Liver resection TW(−) in Stage I
   b) Relative curative resection.
      i) Liver resection TW(+) but with tumor tissue removed in Stage I.
      ii) Liver resection Hr ≧ H, R ≧ N, TW(−) in Stage II or III

   iii) Liver resection Hr ≧ H, R ≧ N, TW(+) but with tumor tissue removed, and tumor diameter 5 cm or less in Stage II or III
   In either case, no tumor emboli must remain in the portal vein or bile duct in images of the remnant liver.
2. Non-curative resection
   a) Relative non-curative resection.
      Any liver resection other than a curative resection in which all the macroscopic tumor tissue is removed.
   b) Absolute non-curative resection.
      Liver resection with part of the macroscopic tumor tissue remaining

4.9   Record of Recurrent Tumor

In cases where patients underwent a liver resection other than absolute non-curative resection and no remnant tumors were identified by image diagnosis during operation, when recurrence of liver cancer is recognized, duration after the first operation, method of diagnosis of recurrence, and changes in tumor-markers as well as state of tumor according to (4.2) above should be described.

References

1. Liver Cancer Study Group of Japan (1983) The General Rules for the Clinical and Pathological Study of Primary Liver Cancer (in Japanese). (1st edn) Kanehara, Tokyo
2. Liver Cancer Study Group of Japan (1989) The General Rules for the Clinical and Pathological Study of Primary Liver Cancer. Jpn J Surg: 19:98–129
3. The Japanese Society of Gastroenterology (1987) New Trends in Gastroenterology, 1987. Sugahara K, (ed) International Committee of The Japanese Society of Gastroenterology, Tokyo pp 261–338
4. UICC: International Union Against Cancer (1987) TNM Classification of Malignant Tumor (4th edn). Hermanek P, Sobin LH, (eds) Springer-Verlag, Berlin pp 53–55
5. Liver Cancer Study Group of Japan (1991) The General Rules for the Clinical and Pathological Study of Primary Liver Cancer (in Japanese). (3rd edn) Kanehara, Tokyo

CHAPTER 39

Diagnosis of cholangiocellular carcinoma

Masahiko Tomimatsu and Hiroshi Obata[1]

1 Introduction

Cholangiocellular carcinoma, one of the primary liver cancers, is a malignant tumor which develops in the epithelium of the intrahepatic biliary system. This neoplasm is also called cholangioma, cholangiocarcinoma, or intrahepatic bile duct carcinoma. WHO [1] and the Liver Cancer Study Group of Japan [2] have adopted cholangiocarcinoma and cholangiocellular carcinoma, respectively.

Cholangiocellular carcinoma is classified into two groups, the peripheral type and the hilar type, according to its developmental site in the intrahepatic bile duct [3]. In this chapter, we will deal with the clinical characteristics and imaging which are useful for diagnosing cholangiocellular carcinoma. Special cases such as cystadenocarcinoma, and combined hepatocellular and cholangiocellular carcinoma are excluded from this study.

2 Pathogenesis

Most hepatocellular carcinomas are caused by hepatitis B and C viruses (HBV and HCV), but little is known about the pathogenesis of cholangiocellular carcinoma. There are several reports on diseases which might play causative roles in its development. In our experience between 1974 and 1990, 6 of 38 cases (15.8%) were complicated by hepatolithiasis. In Japan and other Asian countries, many studies have demonstrated an association with hepatolithiasis [3–6], while the association of cholangiocellular carcinoma with cystic duct anomalies has often been reported in Europe and the United States [7]. In addition, there are reports which cited the following as causes of cholangiocellular carcinoma: thorotrast, *Clonorchis sinensis* infection, liver cirrhosis, drugs such as oral contraceptives, inflammatory bowel diseases, primary sclerosing cholangitis, and others.

2.1 Hepatolithiasis

In Japan and Taiwan, cholangiocellular carcinomas associated with hepatolithiasis have been frequently reported [3–6]. In our study, 15.8% of the cases with cholangiocellular carcinoma also had hepatolithiasis (Fig. 1). The scarcity of reports on the association of these two clinical entities in Europe is probably due to a low incidence of hepatolithiasis [8, 9].

The mechanism by which hepatolithiasis and cholangiocellular carcinoma coexist has not been well established. Most authors have suggested that chronic infection and the stasis of hepatolithiasis can lead to the development of papillary or adenomatous epithelial hyperplasia and bile duct carcinoma [3–6, 8, 9]. They also found that hepatolithiasis does not provide the sole carcinogenic stimulus that results in malignancy. Bile duct carcinoma arising in association with hepatolithiasis is probably the cumulative result of several etiologic agents that might include nutritional, genetic, environmental, and immunologic factors.

Hepatolithiasis is one of the risk factors of cholangiocellular carcinoma. If it is discovered, the patient should be carefully evaluated and placed under close observation.

[1] Department of Gastroenterology, Tokyo Women's Medical College, 8-1 Kawada-cho, Shinjuku-ku, Tokyo, 162 Japan

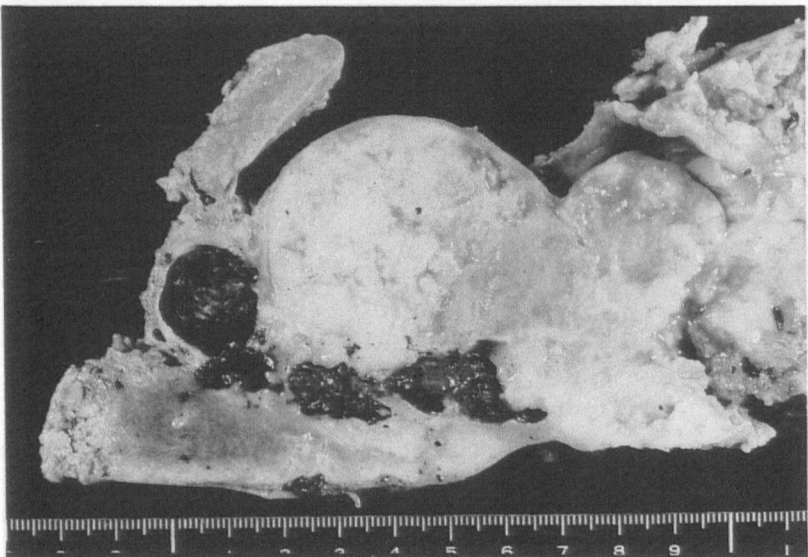

Fig. 1. Cholangiocellular carcinoma. Tumor is poorly demarcated and some intrahepatic calculi are seen in the bile duct adjacent to the tumor

2.2 Cystic duct anomalies

Cystic duct anomalies related to cholangiocellular carcinoma include von Meyenburg's complexes [10], congenital hepatic fibrosis [11, 12], congenial liver cysts [13], Caroli's disease [14–16], choledochal cysts [17], and others. The incidence of cholangiocellular carcinoma originating in cystic duct anomalies has been reported to be 2.5% to 15% [18].

2.3 Thorotrast

Thorotrast, a contrast medium for hepatosplenography which was used between 1930 and 1940, is deposited in the reticuloendothelial system and very frequently causes hepatic tumors because of damage from alpha ray exposure with $^{232}ThO_2$. Among hepatic tumors, cholangiocellular carcinoma and hemangiosarcoma develop with a high frequency [19].

2.4 Clonorchis sinensis

Clonorchis sinensis infestation, deemed responsible for development of cholangiocellular carcinoma in Hong Kong, accounts for 15% of primary hepatic carcinoma [20]. However, no reports have been published in Japan, Europe or the United States.

2.5 Cirrhosis

Over 60% of the hepatocellular carcinomas are accompanied by liver cirrhosis. In cholangiocellular carcinoma, on the other hand, cirrhosis is characteristically absent in the non-cancerous region. A survey by the Liver Cancer Study Group of Japan revealed complications with cirrhosis at a rate of about 17% [21], but detailed histological examination showed that most of them are sclerosing hepatic carcinomas or the combined type [7]. Therefore as a rule, the complication with cirrhosis is rarely seen. This was confirmed by the results of our study where only 1 of 38 cases was complicated by cirrhosis.

For hepatitis viruses associated with cirrhosis or hepatocellular carcinoma, 2 of 38 cases (5.3%) were HBsAg-positive. When samples obtained from 16 of these patients were tested for anti-HCV antibody (C-100.3, EIA kits; Ortho), 4 (25%) were found to be positive. In our study, over 70% of the patients with hepatocellular carcinoma or the combined type had seroconverted to anti-HCV, which suggests that HCV is directly

Table 1. Number, sex, and age of patients classified by location of the tumor in our study

Type	Number	Male:Female	Age (Mean ± S.D.)
Peripheral type	14	8:6	64.9 ± 10.2
Hilar type	24	14:10	59.1 ± 12.4
Total	38	22:16	61.2 ± 11.9

related to the pathogenesis of hepatocellular carcinoma.

In cholangiocellular carcinoma, the involvement of HCV was not as obvious. The positivity of anti-HCV has been found to be 25%. Further studies are necessary to elucidate the involvement of HCV in cholangiocellular carcinoma.

2.6 Other causative factors

The possible associations with drugs such as oral contraceptives [22], anabolic steroids [23], and methyldopa [24] have been reported. In addition, there are reports on cholangiocellular carcinoma associated with primary sclerosing cholangitis [25–27], ulcerative colitis [28–31], Crohn's disease [32–33], polycystic desease [34], *Salmonella* infection [35], and alpha-1-antitrypsin deficiency [36].

3 Incidence and patients

The incidence of cholangiocellular carcinoma among primary liver cancers ranges from about 0% to 26.8% [37]. According to the report of the Liver Cancer Study Group of Japan, cholangiocellular carcinoma numbered 256 among 4765 cases (5.4%) of primary liver cancer [21].

The male:female ratio in the incidence in Japan was as follows: Cholangiocellular carcinoma, 1.6:1; and hepatocellular carcinoma, 4.7:1. In women, cholangiocellular carcinoma was more prevalent than hepatocellular carcinoma [21]. In our data (Table 1), the ratios of men to women were 1.4:1 (22 men to 16 women) for cholangiocellular carcinoma and 4.7:1 for hepatocellular carcinoma, showing results similar to the abovementioned study.

In our study (Table 1), the age at the onset of the disease varies from 39 to 77 years, with a mean of 61.2 years, which is approximately equal to that for hepatocellular carcinoma (60.8 years). According to the study of the Liver Cancer Study Group of Japan, the mean age at the onset was 59.5 years in men and 62.4 years in women [21]. Cholangiocellular carcinomas with chronic inflammatory diseases such as Crohn's disease and ulcerative colitis, *Salmonella* infection, and alpha-1-antitrypsin deficiency, developed in patients who were still in their 20s [35, 36].

4 Symptoms

The clinical signs and symptoms of tumors vary according to the site of development in our study, 38 patients were categorized into the peripheral type (14 patients) and the hilar type (24 patients) to analyze their incipient symptoms.

The initial symptoms of the peripheral type were: Abdominal pain (6 patients, 42.9%), back pain (3, 21.4%), pyrexia (2, 14.3%), distention of the abdomen (1, 7.1%), and abdominal mass (1, 7.1%). Asymptomatic patients numbered 6 (42.9%). Abdominal pain was the most common initial symptom. Jaundice had not been present as an incipient symptom but was observed in 3 patients (21.4%) on admission.

For the hilar type, the initial symptoms were abdominal pain (10 patients, 41.7%), jaundice (6, 25%), general lassitude (4, 16.7%), back pain (2, 8.3%), and nausea, anorexia, or pyrexia (1 each, 4.2%). Six were asymptomatic carriers (25%). Jaundice was also noted from the early stage in a number of patients.

Asymptomatic cases of both types were discovered by imaging techniques during follow-ups for another disease or abnormal liver function detected at a health examination.

5 Laboratory data

Total serum bilirubin was elevated in approximately 30% of patients with either the peripheral or hilar type. Alkaline phosphatase levels were elevated in 42.9% of the peripheral type and 83.3% of the hilar type (Table 2). Approximately one-half of the cases in the peripheral type would escape detection if diagnosis is dependent on biochemical data alone. Therefore, additional procedures using image diagnosis and tumor markers are essential. Serum transaminase levels were elevated in approximately 50% of both types, however the increase was slight (less than 100 KU) in most cases.

Carcinoembryonic antigen (CEA), one of the tumor markers, was elevated in 9 of 31 cases (29%) in our study. By contrast, the positive reaction to CA 19-9, which is used as a tumor marker for pancreatic and biliary carcinomas, was noted in 80%. In the peripheral type, which exhibited less exaggerated increases in alkaline phosphatase levels, a positive reaction to CA 19-9

Table 2. Laboratory findings in 38 cases of cholangiocellular carcinoma

Laboratory data (normal range)	Peripheral type (n = 14)		Hilar type (n = 24)	
	Mean ± S.D.	No. of elevations (%)	Mean ± S.D.	No. of elevations (%)
Total bilirubin (0.1~1.0 mg/dl)	2.19 ± 3.32	4 (28.6)	2.32 ± 3.83	7 (29.2)
Alkaline phosphatase (70~260 IU)	385.9 ± 296.5	6 (42.9)	643.9 ± 727.5	20 (83.3)
Glutamic oxaloacetic transaminase (GOT) (6~25 KU)	42.1 ± 31.4	8 (57.1)	72.4 ± 109.9	15 (62.5)
Glutamic-pyruvic transaminase (GPT) (0~19 KU)	34.7 ± 36.0	7 (50.0)	51.0 ± 79.5	12 (50.0)
γ-GTP (0~40 mU/ml)	79.4 ± 62.2	7 (50.0)	157.5 ± 232.4	16 (66.7)

was noted in 72.3% (Fig. 2). Therefore, this marker is very useful for detection and diagnosis of cholangiocellular carcinoma. The positive reaction for alpha fetoprotein (AFP), and protein induced by vitamin K absence or antagonist II (PIVKA-II) were seen in 6.5% and 6.7%, respectively. CA 19-9 is the most reliable tumor marker for cholangiocellular carcinoma.

6 Imaging studies

Recent developments and popular use of imaging techniques, especially ultrasonography, greatly contribute to the early diagnosis of cholangiocellular and hepatocellular carcinomas. In our 38 cases, imaging studies identified tumors at the rate of 83.3%, 77.8%, and 85.3% by ultrasonography (US), computed tomography (CT), and hepatic angiography, respectively. When added with abnormal findings such as cholangiectasis, the tumor detection rates were raised to 91.7% by US, and 94.4% by CT. The rates of abnormal findings by the Liver Cancer Study Group of Japan were similar to those of our study (US, 92.0%; CT, 94.2%; and angiography, 82.8%) [21].

6.1 Ultrasonography

The rate of detection of the peripheral type by US did not differ much from that of the hilar type (76.9% for the former and 87% for the latter). Cholangiectasis was seen in less than half of the

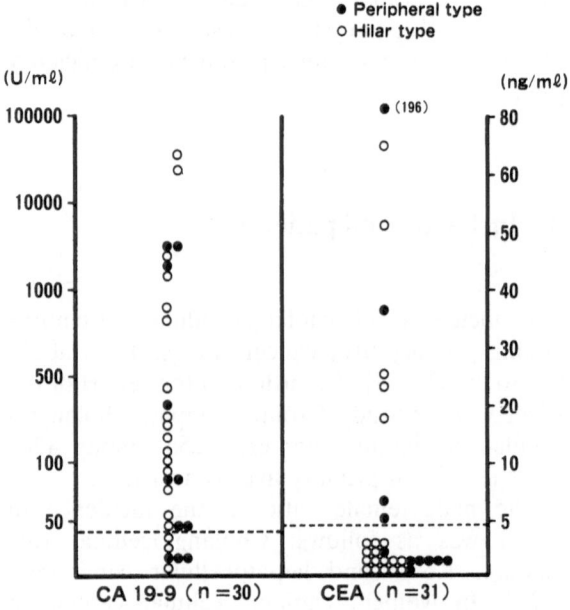

Fig. 2. Serum levels of CA 19-9 and carcinoembryonic antigen (CEA) in patient with cholangiocellular carcinoma (EIA)

peripheral type (46.2%), but 73.9% of the hilar type.

Cholangiocellular lesions are irregularly shaped or generally round. Most are poorly demarcated. Ultrasonograms of cholangiocellular carcinomas occasionally show echolucent zones, which are discrete around the periphery of tumors (Fig. 3). These zones are localized, indicate uneven thickness, and are different from those of hepatocellular carcinomas that showed circular lowechoic rings [38]. A tumor parenchymatous echograph may reveal a hyperechoic, hypoechoic, or mixed

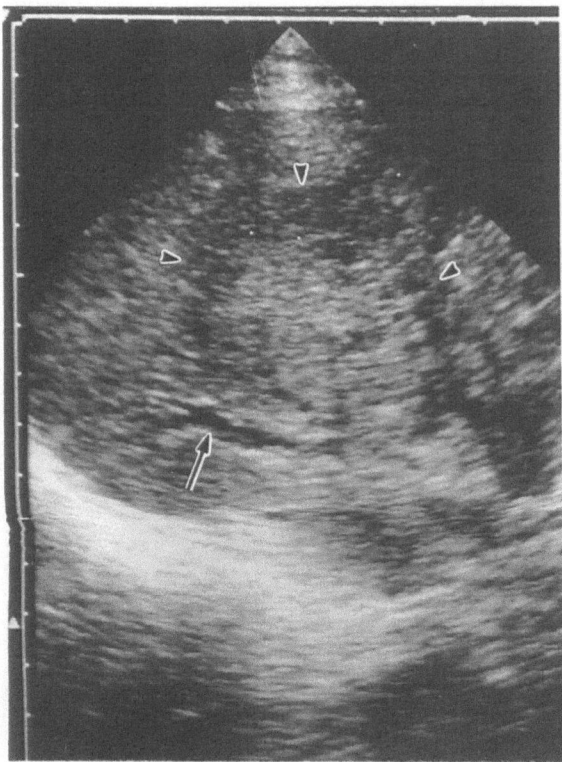

Fig. 3. Ultrasonogram of cholangiocellular carcinoma. Tumor is hypoechoic at the periphery (*arrowheads*) and hyperechoic in the interior. Peripheral bile duct is dilated (*arrow*)

pattern. Their frequency varies in each report [38].

In addition to peripheral bile duct dilatation (Fig. 3), findings characterizing cholangiocellular carcinoma include the internal architecture within the tumor, which is believed to be composed of the intrahepatic bile ducts or portal veins.

6.2 Computed tomography

The sensitivity of CT for tumors was 84.6% and 73.9% in the peripheral and hilar types, respectively. For cholangiectasis, the respective figures were 38.5% and 52.2%. For tumors detected by CT, the sensitivity is similar to that of US, however for cholangiectasis, it is lower than the rate of US. Smaller tumors are generally round. When the tumors are more than 3 cm in diameter, most are irregular in form and asociated with low density (Fig. 4). Contrast enhanced CT delineates more clearly about half the number of images; but unlike hepatocellular carcinoma, the high density ring around the rim of the tumor is not shown. Also unlike hepatocellular carcinoma, cholangiocellular carcinoma is not enhanced in the early stage of dynamic CT (20–30 seconds after bolus enhancement); and a less dense area appears at the periphery of the tumor when the interior is enhanced during the late stage (after 8–10 minutes) [39, 40]. It is relatively easy to distinguish cholangiocellular carcinoma from hepatocellular carcinoma, but differentiation from a single metastatic liver carcinoma is difficult.

6.3 Hepatic angiography

With hepatic angiography, tumors are seen at the rate of 76.9% and 90.5% for the peripheral and hilar types, respectively. The main findings

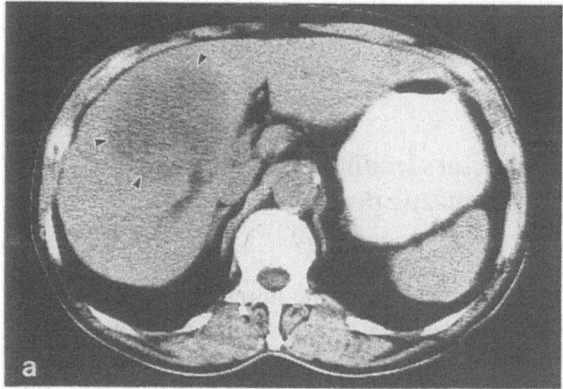
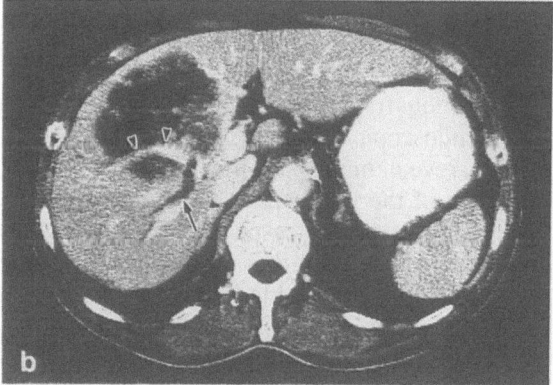

Fig. 4a,b. CT of cholangiocellular carcinoma. **a** Plain CT shows a poorly demarcated low density mass in left medial and right anterior segments of the liver (*arrow-heads*). **b** Postcontrast CT clearly demonstrates vessel-like structures in the tumor (*arrowheads*) and dilatation of the peripheral bile duct (*arrow*)

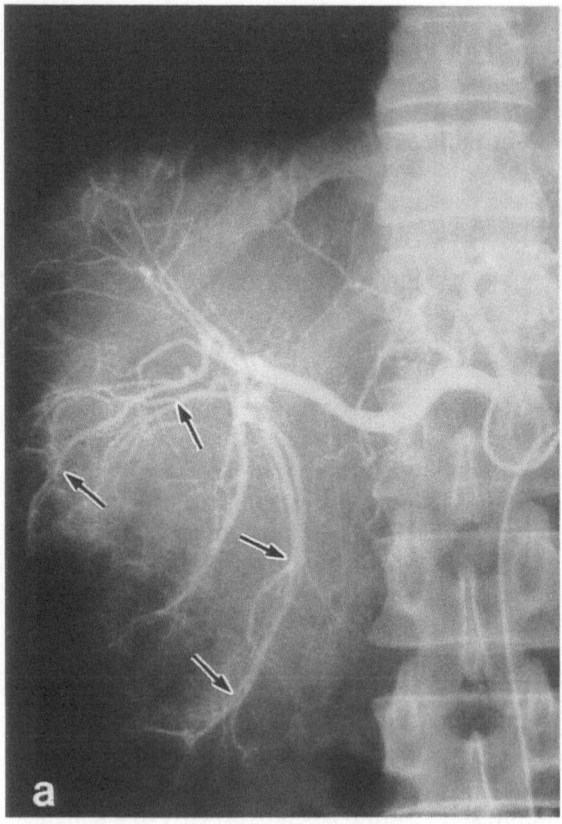
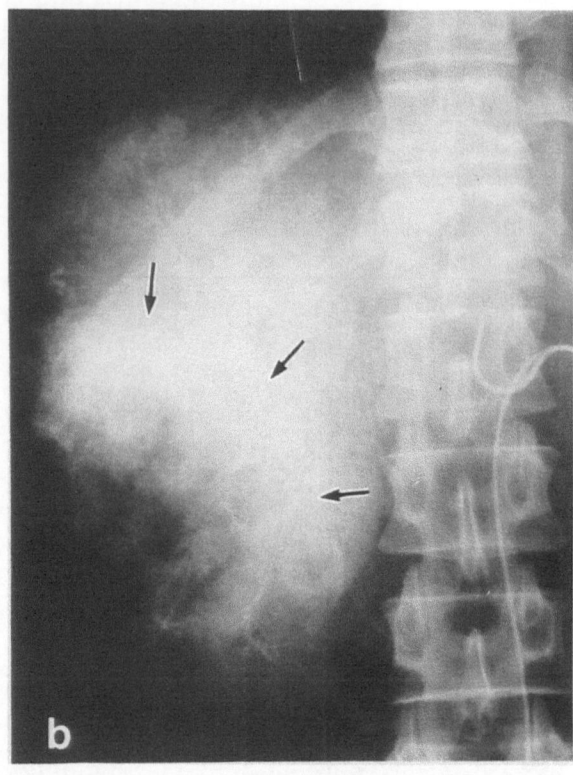

Fig. 5a,b. Hepatic angiogram of cholangiocellular carcinoma. **a** Arterial phase. Displacement of the right hepatic arteries is noted around a large mass in the right lobe (*arrows*). Subtle neovascularity is present. **b** Capillary phase. There is a hypervascular region in the periphery of the large mass (*arrows*)

include encasement and displacement of arteries (Fig. 5a) and occlusion of portal veins [41, 42]. Tumor stains are subtle, and their peripheral staining is a characteristic feature (Fig. 5b).

6.4 Other imaging studies

Percutaneous transhepatic cholangiography (PTC) and endoscopic retrograde cholangiography (ERC) reveal images of irregular stenosis and occlusion of the intrahepatic bile ducts.

Recently, magnetic resonance imaging (MRI) has been applied to the diagnosis of hepatic tumors. These T1-weighted images appear as a focal area of lower intensity as compared with the images of the liver parenchyma (Fig. 6a). T2-weighted images produce generally high intensity (Fig. 6b). A dilated intrahepatic bile duct, which is a characteristic finding of cholangiocellular carcinoma, displays a lower signal intensity than surrounding normal liver on T1-weighted images and a higher signal intensity on T2-weighted images, so it is possible to distinguish bile ducts from vessels in the liver.

Dilatation of the intrahepatic bile ducts is more clearly demonstrated by CT than MRI, but changes to vessels are more clearly demonstrated by MRI than CT [43].

7 Factors leading to detection and diagnostic procedures

In our study, one of the initial clues for detection of the peripheral type of cholangiocellular carcinoma was obtained from imaging techniques which were employed to find the causes for symptoms such as abdominal and back pain.

The peripheral type was detected in this manner in 8 out 14 patients (57.1%). Three cases

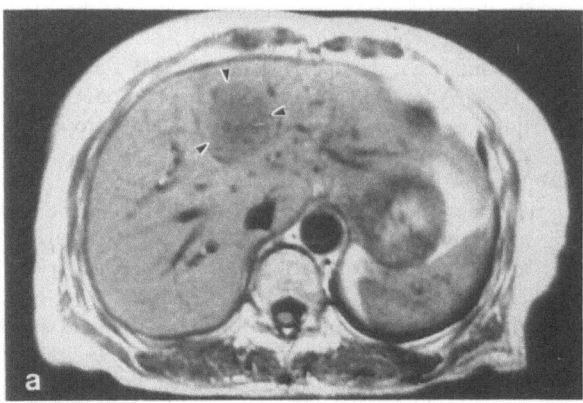 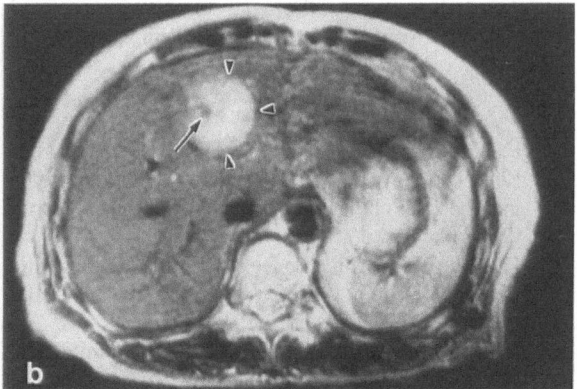

Fig. 6a,b. MR image of cholangiocellular carcinoma. **a** T1-weighted MR image. Tumor displays a lower signal intensity than the surrounding normal liver (*arrowheads*). **b** T2-weighted MR image. Tumor shows a high signal intensity (*arrowheads*) but contains a low signal intensity area suggestive of a vessel-like structure (*arrow*)

(21.4%) were diagnosed during follow-up of other diseases (1 case each of chronic hepatitis, liver cirrhosis, and diabetes mellitus). The remaining 3 (21.4%) were diagnosed as having hepatic dysfunction at a health examination: This included 2 with high alkaline phosphatase levels, and 1 with a high transaminase level.

The initial events leading to detection of 24 cases of the hilar type were 15 (62.5%) with symptoms such as abdominal pain and jaundice, 7 (29.2%) during follow-up for other diseases (3 with surgically treated digestive system diseases, 2 with liver diseases, 1 with a combination of hepatolithiasis and Caroli's disease, and 1 with gallbladder polyps), and 2 (8.3%) detected from a diagnosis of liver dysfunction (a high level of alkaline phosphatase).

In patients with either subjective symptoms or liver dysfunction, the test methods combining analysis of biliary enzymes (especially, alkaline phosphatase), isolation of tumor markers (CA 19-9 in particular), and imaging techniques (such as US and CT) are important to improve the diagnosis of cholangiocellular carcinoma. The diagnostic accuracy of combinations of various imaging techniques has been reported to be 60% to 80%. When the condition is complicated by hepatolithiasis in particular, it is conceivable that a definitive diagnosis may be difficult if only US or CT is employed. A comprehensive diagnosis employing an analysis of CA 19-9 and imaging techniques, and close follow-up are imperative. Regular follow-up examinations by analyses of biliary enzymes and CA 19-9, US, and other test modalities should be recommended for those in high risk groups, including patients with

cystic duct anomalies (such as Caroli's disease), hepatolithiasis, or with a history of exposure to thorotrast.

References

1. Gibson JB (1978) Histological typing of tumors of the livers, biliary tract and pancreas. International Histological Classification of Tumors. No. 20, WHO, Geneva
2. Japan Liver Cancer Study Group (1987) The general rules for the clinical and pathological study of primary liver cancer (in Japanese), 2nd edn. Kanehara, Tokyo
3. Okuda K, Kubo Y, Okazaki N, Arishima T, Hashimoto M, Jinnouchi S, Sawa Y, Shimokawa Y, Nakajima Y, Noguchi T, Nakano M, Kojiro M, Nakashima T (1977) Clinical aspect of intrahepatic bile duct carcinoma including hilar carcinoma: A study of 57 autopsy-proven cases. Cancer 39: 232–246
4. Chen M-F, Jan Y-Y, Wang C-S, Benjamin Jeng L-B, Hwang T-L, Chen S-C (1989) Intrahepatic stones associated with cholangiocarcinoma. Am J Gastroenterol 84:391–395
5. Nakanuma Y, Terada T, Tanaka Y, Ohta G (1985) Are hepatolithiasis and cholangiocarcinoma etiologically related? A morphological study of 12 cases of hepatolithiasis associated with cholangiocarcinoma. Virchows Archiv A 406:45–58
6. Koga A, Ichimiya H, Yamaguchi K, Miyazaki K, Nakayama F (1985) Hepatolithiasis associated with cholangiocarcinoma, possible etiologic significance. Cancer 55:2826–2829
7. Craig JR, Peters RL, Edmondson HE (1988) Tumors of the liver and intrahepatic bile ducts. In:

Atlas of tumor pathology, fascicle 26. Armed Forces Institute of Pathology, Washington DC

8. Sanes S, MacCallum JD (1942) Primary carcinoma of liver (cholangioma) in hepatolithiasis. Am J Pathol 18:675–687

9. Falchuk KR, Lesser PB, Galdabini JJ, Isselbacher KJ (1976) Cholangiocarcinoma as related to chronic intrahepatic cholangitis and hepatolithiasis. Am J Gastroenterol 66:57–61

10. Hormer LW, White HJ, Read RC (1968) Neoplastic transformation of von Meyenburg complexes of the liver. J Pathol Bacteriol 96:499–502

11. Daroca PJ, Jr Tuthill R, Read R (1975) Cholangiocarcinoma arising in congenital hepatic fibrosis. Arch Pathol 99:592–595

12. Parker RGF (1956) Fibrosis of the liver as a congenital anomaly. J Pathol 71:359–368

13. Azizah N, Paradinas FJ (1980) Cholangiocarcinoma coexisting with developmental liver cyst: A distinct entity different from liver cystadenocarcinoma. Histopathology 4:391–400

14. Jones AW, Shreeve DR (1970) Congenital dilatation of intrahepatic biliary ducts with cholangiocarcinoma. Br Med J 2:277–278

15. Gallagher PJ, Millis RR, Mitchinson MJ (1972) Congenital dilatation of the intrahepatic bile duct with cholangiocarcinoma. J Clin Pathol 25: 804–808

16. Phinney PR, Austin GE, Kadell BM (1981) Cholangiocarcinoma arising in Caroli's disease. Arch Pathol Lab Med 105:194–197

17. Alonso-Lej F, Rever WB, Cessangno DJ (1959) Congenital choledochal cyst with report of two and an analysis of 94 cases. Int Abstr Surg 108:1–30

18. Kawarada Y, Mizumoto R (1990) Diagnosis and treatment of cholangiocellular carcinoma of the liver. Hepatogastroenterol 37:176–181

19. Stole WE, Harrist TJ (1981) Defects in liver scans 29 years after injection of thorotrast. New Eng J Med 304:893–899

20. Hou PC (1956) The relationship between primary carcinoma of the liver and infestation with *Clonorchis sinensis*. J Pathol Bacteriol 72:239–246

21. The Liver Cancer Study Group of Japan (1990) Primary liver cancer in Japan. Ann Surg 211: 277–287

22. Ellis EF, Gordon PR, Gottlieb LS (1978) Oral contraceptives and cholangiocarcinoma. Lancet 1:207

23. Stromeyer FW, Smith DH, Ishak KG (1979) Anabolic steroid therapy and intrahepatic cholangiocarcinoma. Cancer 43:440–443

24. Broden G, Bengtsson L (1980) Biliary carcinoma associated with methyldopa therapy. Acta Chir Scand 500 (Suppl):7–12

25. Chapman BWG, Marborgh BA, Rhodes JM, Summerfield JA, Dick R, Scheuer PJ, Sherlock S (1980) Primary sclerosing cholangitis: A review of its clinical features, cholangiography, and hepatic histology. Gut 21:870–877

26. Qualman SJ, Haupt HM, Bauer TW, Taxy JB (1984) Adenocarcinoma of the hepatic duct junction: A reappraisal of the histologic criteria of malignancy. Cancer 53:1545–1551

27. Wee A, Ludwig J, Coffey RJ, LaRusso NF, Wiesner RH (1985) Hepatobiliary carcinoma associated with primary sclerosing cholangitis and chronic ulcerative colitis. Hum Pathol 16: 719–726

28. Ham JM (1968) Tumors of biliary epithelium and ulcerative colitis. Ann Surg 168:1088–1093

29. Akwari OE, Van Heerden JA, Foulle WT, Baggenstoss AH (1975) Cancer of the bile ducts associated with ulcerative colitis. Ann Surg 181: 303–309

30. Converse CF, Reagan JW, DeCosse JJ (1971) Ulcerative colitis and carcinoma of the bile ducts. Am J Surg 121:39–45

31. Ross AP, Braasch JW (1973) Ulcerative colitis and carcinoma of the proximal bile ducts. Gut 14: 94–97

32. Berman MD, Falchuk KR, Trey C (1980) Carcinoma of the biliary tree complicating Crohn's disease. Dig Dis Sci 25:795–797

33. Krause JR, Ayuyang HQ, Ellis LD (1985) Occurrence of three cases of carcinoma in individuals with Crohn's disease treated with metronidazole. Am J Gastroenterol 80:978–982

34. Landais P, Drunfeld J-P, Droz D, Drüeke T, Albouze G, Gogusev J, Chauveau D, Moynot A (1984) Cholangiocellular carcinoma in polycystic kidney and liver disease. Arch Intern Med 144: 2274–2276

35. Szilagri A, Mitmaker B, Lamoureux E (1990) Cholangiocarcinoma: A decade's experience at a community-based university hospital. Can J Gastroenterol 4:65–69

36. Parham DM, Paterson JR, Gunn A, Guthrie W (1989) Cholangiocarcinoma in two siblings with emphysema and alpha-1-antitrypsin deficiency. Q J Med, New Series 71:359–367

37. Mizumoto R, Kawarada (1987) Diagnosis and treatment of cholangiocarcinoma and cystic adenocarcinoma of the liver. In: Okuda K, Ishak K (eds) Neoplasms of the liver. Springer-Verlag, Tokyo, pp 381–396

38. Ohta H, Nakano S, Watahiki H, Takeda I, Sugiyama K, Hachisuka K, Yamaguchi A, Kondoh S, Kumada T (1983) Clinical study of cholangiocellular carcinoma—Mainly imaging diagnosis of cholangiocellular carcinoma (in Japanese). Jpn J Gastroenterol 80:1747–1753

39. Takayasu K, Ikeya S, Mukai K, Muramatsu Y, Makuuchi M, Hasegawa H (1990) CT of hilar cholangiocarcinoma: Late contrast enhancement in six patients. AJR 154:1203–1206

40. Itai Y (1987) Imaging diagnosis with computed tomography. In: Okuda K, Ishak K (eds) Neoplasm of the liver. Springer-Verlag, Tokyo, pp. 289–300

41. Reuter SR, Redman HC, Cho KJ (1986) Gastrointestinal angiography. WB Saunders, Philadelphia

42. Chuang VP (1987) Hepatic angiography. In: Okuda K, Ishak K (eds) Neoplasm of the liver. Springer-Verlag, Tokyo, pp 259–277

43. Dooms GC, Kerlan RK, Hricak H, Wall SD, Margulis AR (1986) Cholangiocarcinoma: Imaging by MR. Radiology 159:89–94

CHAPTER 40

Investigation of surgical treatment for cholangiocellular carcinoma

Toshimichi Nakayama, Hideki Saitsu, and Kazuharu Shigetomi[1]

1 Introduction

Cholangiocellular carcinoma (CCC), the malignant tumor arising from epithelial cells of the intrahepatic bile duct, has been classified as a primary liver cancer, although CCC has occurred less frequently than hepatocellular carcinoma (HCC) in Japan [1]. Most CCCs are advanced because a system for early diagnosis has not been established [2], and even though CCC is resectable, the prognosis is generally unfavorable [3–5]. We therefore studied clinically the 36 patients with CCC encountered at our hospital, and reported the current status of surgical treatment in Japan.

2 Patients and Methods

There were 36 patients with CCC encountered in our department as of the end of December, 1990. Twenty patients underwent hepatic resection and 16 patients were inoperable. The 20 resected cases were classified according to the Treatment Guidelines for Primary Liver Cancer [6], and a clinical study was conducted. Sixteen unresectable cases were also reviewed with the contraindications for resection (Table 1).

Table 1. Details of the primary liver cancer

Resected cases of primary liver cancer		
Hepatocellular carcinoma	266 cases	
Cholangiocellular carcinoma	20 cases	⎤ 36 cases
Unresectable cases of cholangiocellular carcinoma	16 cases	⎦

---

[1] The Second Department of Surgery, Kurume University School of Medicine, Kurume, Fukuoka, 830 Japan

3 Results

3.1 Age and Sex

The ages of the 36 patients with CCC ranged from 36 to 76 years old, and the mean age was 62.5 years old. Twenty five of these patients were men and 11 were women. The mean age of the HCC patients in our hospital for the same period was 57.9 years old, and the male to female ratio was 5.7:1. Thus the mean age of the CCC patients was 4.6 years older, and the proportion of women was higher.

3.2 Associated illnesses

In 6 cases, there was associated illnesses: Liver cirrhosis was present in 2 cases (10%), and hepatolithiasis in 4 cases (20%).

3.3 Size of the tumor

The smallest tumor was 11 mm, and the largest was 125 mm. The mean size of the tumor was 60.0 ± 31.6 mm (Table 2).

3.4 Gross classification of CCC

The twenty resected cases were divided into three types according to the gross classification on the cut surface of the liver. Eight cases were the nodular type (40%), 9 cases were the massive type (45%), and 3 cases were the diffuse type (15%). The massive and nodular types account for the majority of CCC.

Table 2. Age, sex, associated illnesses, and tumor size for 36 patients with CCC

Mean age (years)	Sex	Associated illnesses	Mean size of the tumor (mm)
62.5 ± 9.8	Men (25 cases) Women (11 cases)	Liver cirrhosis 2 cases Hepatolithiasis 4 cases	60.0 ± 31.6

Table 3. Classification in 20 resected CCC patients according to the treatment guidelines for primary liver cancer

Gross classification		Extent		Fibrinous encapsulation		Serosal infiltration	
Nodular	8 (40)	H_s	3 (15)	fc (+)	20 (100)	S_0	5 (25)
Massive	9 (45)	H_1	4 (20)			S_1	10 (50)
Diffuse	3 (15)	H_2 or more	13 (65)	fc (−)	0	S_2	5 (25)

Lymph node metastasis		Blood vessel invasion		Intrahepatic metastasis		Macroscopic progression	
n(−)	11 (55)	Vp_0	3 (15)	im_0	11 (55)	stage I	3 (15)
n_1(+)	1 (5)	Vp_1	10 (50)	im_1	2 (10)	stage II	1 (5)
n_2(+)	4 (20)	Vp_2	0	im_2	7 (35)	stage III	6 (30)
n_3(+)	4 (20)	Vp_3	7 (35)	im_3	0	stage IV	10 (50)

Methods of hepatic resection		Existence of cancer infiltration within 5 mm of the cut surface
Hr0	3 (15)	
Hr1	1 (5)	tw (+) 14 (70)
Hr2	10 (50)	
ext. Hr2	4 (20)	tw (−) 6 (30)
Hr3	1 (5)	

Percentage in parenthesis

3.5 Extent of the CCC (H)

Three cases (15%) occupied a hepatic subsegment (Hs), 4 cases (20%) occupied one segment (H1), and 13 cases (65%) occupied two or more segments (H2). Most CCCs occupied 2 segments or more.

3.6 Fibrinous encapsulation

Formation of a capsule at the boundary with nontumorous tissue was usually found in HCC in Japan, but capsule formation was not detected in any of the 20 resected cases of CCC.

3.7 Serosal infiltration (S)

The twenty patients were divided into three groups according to the degree of serosal infiltration (S0, S1 or S2) of the CCC. In S0, infiltration of the cancer is not quite exposed to the serosa; in S1, it is exposed to the serosa; and, in S2, it is exposed to the other organs. Five cases were S0 (25%), 10 were S1 (50%), and 5 were S2 (25%). The organs infiltrated in the 5 S2 cases were the greater omentum in 2 cases, and the diaphragm, gallbladder, and adrenal gland in one case each.

3.8 Lymph node metastasis (n)

The symbol n(−) indicates lymph node metastasis is not found, n1(+) shows there are metastasis in lymph nodes in group 1 (lymph nodes of the suprahepatic, subphrenic and hepatic hilus), n2(+) shows metastasis in lymph nodes in group 2 (lymph nodes of the hepatic artery, portal vein, bile duct and mediastinal), and n3(+) shows metastasis in lymph nodes in group 3 (posterior part of the pancreas, common hepatic artery, para-aortic). Eleven patients (55%) were n(−), 1 patient was n1(+), 4 patients (20%) were n2(+), and 4 patients (20%) were n3(+). Lymph node metastasis was detected in approximately half of the patients. This result was a higher proportion than the 2 (0.75%) cases of lymph node metastasis found out of 266 cases of HCC for the same period.

3.9 Blood vessel invasion (vp)

Only one case out of the 20 had associated tumor thrombus from the middle hepatic vein to the inferior vena cava (VCI). However, direct invasion was present in every case. In vp0, there is no vessel invasion; vp1 shows vessel invasion to the peripheral portal branch in the liver; vp2, the second portal branch is invaded; in vp3, trunks of the portal vein are invaded. There were only three cases (15%) which were vp0, 10 cases (50%) were vp1, and 7 cases (35%) were vp3. Vascular invasion was observed in 85% of the cases.

3.10 Intrahepatic metastasis (im)

In im0 there is no intrahepatic metastasis, im1 shows metastasis positive in the same segment as the main tumor, and im2 shows metastasis positive within 2 segments. Eleven patients (55%) were im0, 2 patients (10%) were im1, and 7 patients (35%) were im2.

3.11 Macroscopic progression (stages I–IV)

Three patients (15%) were stage I, 1 case (5%) was stage II, 6 cases (30%) were stage III, and 10 cases (50%) were stage IV. Thus, 80% of patients were stage III or higher.

3.12 Methods of the hepatic resection (Hr)

Hr0 represents partial hepatic resection, Hr1 represents one segmentectomy, Hr2 represents right or left lobectomy, Ext. Hr2 represents extended right or left lobectomy, and Hr3 represents trisegmentectomy. Three patients (15%) underwent Hr0, 1 patient (5%) Hr1, 10 patients (50%) Hr2, 4 patients (20%) Ext. Hr2, and 1 patient (5%) Hr3. Although those who underwent resection of 2 segments or more accounted for 75% of the total number of cases, there were only 4 cases in which the caudate lobe was resected in combination.

3.13 Existence of cancer infiltration (tw)

On less than 5 mm from the cut surface of the liver (tw).

Only 6 cases (30%) were tw(−), and the majority, 14 cases (70%), were tw(+) (Table 3).

3.14 Curative and non-curative resections

Only 6 cases (30%) of peripheral type CCC in which there was no hilar invasion consisted of curative resections, and the remaining 14 cases (70%) represented non-curative resections.

3.15 Prognosis

The survival rates of the 20 resected cases were: 1-year, 37.5%; and 3-year and 5-year, 18.5%. When broken down according to whether they were curative or non-curative resections, the curative 1-, 3-, 5-year rate was 50%, and the non-curative rates were: 1-year, 33.3%; and 3-year, 8.3%. The longest survival was 9 years 6 months in a patient who died of a recurrence (Fig. 1).

3.16 Reasons for non-resection

Peritoneal metastasis in 6 cases, im3 in 5, CCC in the whole liver (H4) in 2, and n3+H3+vp3, n3+ VCI invasion, and lung metastasis (M1) in one case each (Table 4).

4 Discussion

In Japan, the reported proportion of CCC in primary liver cancer, based on operative findings, accounted for 6.0% to 9.4% as it did in our result [3–5], and the incidence rates surveyed every two years over the past 10 years by the Japan Liver Cancer Research Society ranges from 3.9% to 6.4% [1, 7, 8]. CCC is a relatively rare disease, and it never accounts for more than 10% of primary liver cancer.

Even though there are a number of differences between CCC and HCC, CCC is in a similar classification as HCC in accordance with the Treatment Guidelines for the Primary Liver

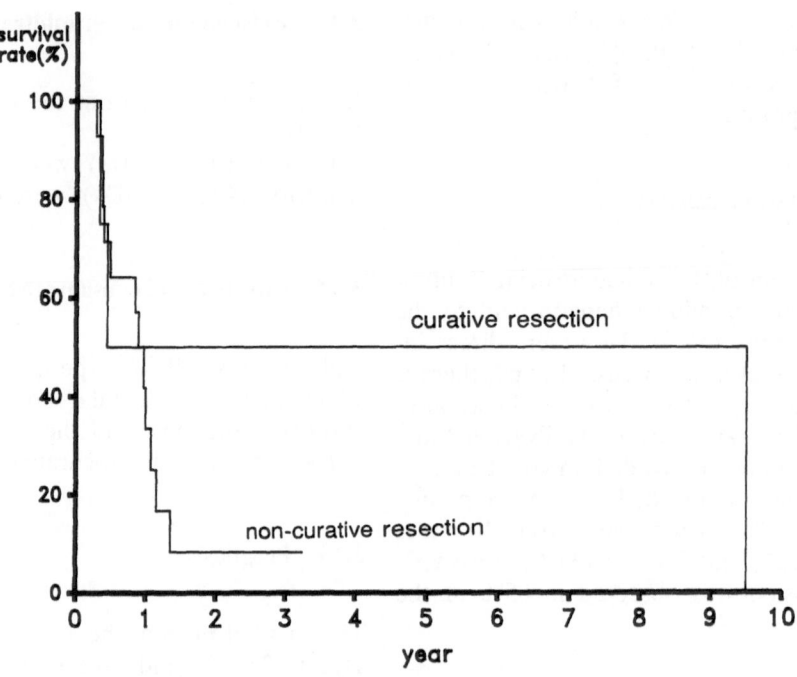

Fig. 1. The survival rates for curative and non-curative resection

Table 4. Reasons for unresectability in 16 CCC patients

P_2	im_3	H_4	$H_3 + vp_3$,	VCI invasion	M_1
				n_3	
6 (37.5)	5 (31.2)	2 (12.5)	1	1	1 (6.3)
			2 (12.5)		

Percentage in parenthesis

Cancer published by the Japan Liver Cancer Research Society [6], and treating these two groups in precisely the same way may produce many problems.

Nevertheless, there are no other suitable alternative guidelines, and so our study is conducted in accordance with the these guidelines.

Surgical treatment is the only possible method for treatment of CCC with long-term survival [3–5]. Unfortunately, satisfactory results have not been reported except according to the Liver Cancer Research Society's statistics [1], curative resections (86 cases) with 1-year survival rate of

70%, 3- and 5-year survival rates of 43% until the present time.

More favorable outcomes have been reported in surgical cases than in non-surgical ones with a mean survival of 2.2 years and maximum survival of more than 4 years [3]. Among 10 resected cases, 3 had one-year survival or more and the maximum survival was 3 years 2 months [4]. The 11 resected cases had an average survival of 9 months, and a maximum survival of 2 years 2 months were reported [5]. Although we have a patient who survived for 9 years 6 months after lateral segmentectomy for CCC 20 mm in diameter, the survival rate for 1, 3, and 5 years was 50% after curative resection (6 cases). The 1-year survival rate after non-curative resection (14 cases) was 33.3%, and the 3-year survival rate was 8.3%. Thus, it has been impossible to obtain satisfactory results even with curative resection, and it seemed to be more difficult to have long-term survival in non-resected cases.

The reasons for the poor prognosis of CCC patients were reportedly because 87.5% of the CCC were massive type, and 93.8% for extention more than T2. Additionally, the site of the tumor, located in the center of the medial segment in more than 70% of the cases [3], stage IV in all patients, tw(+) in spite of requiring R2 or more lymph node extirpation in 70%, and non-curative resections according to these guidelines in all cases [4] all contributed to the poor prognosis. In our cases, 80% of our own patients were in stage III or more (50% of which were stage IV), 70% were with tw(+), and only 6 cases receiving curative resection were so-called peripheral type of CCC without cancer infiltration into the hepatic hilus [9]. Not surprisingly, a major reason for unfavorable prognosis of the CCC appears to be tw(+) because of large tumor size. Thus, the surgical treatment for CCC is usually the only curative modality. Recently, Nimura et al. reported very favorable results with a 3-year survival rate of 55.1% and a 5-year rate of 40.5% by liver resection including the caudate lobe for curative resection without tw(+) in advanced bile duct carcinoma of the hepatic hilus [10]. Mimura et al. reported the double bypass technique in order to achieve curative resection [11], and Kumada et al. reported truncoumbilical bypass of the portal vein [12]. Therefore, an effort should be made to performed liver resection including the caudate lobe in hilar type CCC and peripheral type CCC which infiltrates the hepatic hilus. Since most CCC cases are advanced and unresectable because a system of early diagnosis has not been completed yet for CCC, unlike HCC [2].

In such inoperable cases, radiotherapy, chemotherapy and transarterial embolization (TAE) are alternative treatments. In CCC, TAE is not expected to be as efficacious as in HCC because CCC is generally hypovascular [13]. However, there have been reports that TAE has been efficacious in a few patients [3]. Hence, TAE seems to be a method of treatment that may be applied in patients with inoperable CCC because of H4 or im3.

The number of CCC cases treated by intra-operative irradiation is small, and the results have

not yet to be satisfactory [14]. However, there have been many reports of efficacy in the treatment of bile duct carcinoma of the hepatic hilus; and reports of efficacy are now occasionally seen in intraoperative radiation therapy with surgery [15, 16]. Intraoperative radiation therapy may also be efficacious in the treatment of CCC because the histology of CCC is similar to bile duct carcinoma.

Nevertheless, of the 16 patients inoperable CCC patients were judged to be so, 6 cases were P2, 5 cases were im3, 2 cases were H2, and there was one case each of n3+VCI invasion, n3+H3+vp3, and M1. In many of these cases these factors overlapped, and their general conditions were poor. It was impossible to carry out surgical treatment in such patients, and a system for early diagnosis should be established as soon as possible in order to improve the results of treatment in CCC.

References

1. Japan Liver Cancer Research Society, 9th National Primary Liver Cancer Follow-up Report (1987). Kyoto, Shinko Publishing pp 1–118
2. Motoo Y, Kobayashi K, Hatori S (1987) Diagnostic system for liver cancer. Liver, Bile, Pancreas 15:321–326
3. Igarashi K, Nakanishi M, Sano S, Konno T, Kasai Y, Morita Y (1984) Clinical aspect and therapy of Cholangiocarcinoma. Jpn J Gastroenterol Surg 17:2179–2184
4. Kobayashi T, Mimura H, Kim H, Takakura N, Hamazaki K, Tsuge K, Gouchi A, Takeuchi K, Funabiki S, Orita K (1987) Diagnosis and extension pattern of cholangiocellular carcinoma. Jpn J Gastroenterol Surg 20:2572–2578
5. Tsunoda T, Koga M, Tokunaga S, Eto T, Matsumoto T, Segawa T, Motoshima K, Izawa K, Tsuchiya R (1989) Diagnosis and surgical treatment of cholangiocarcinoma. Diagnostic imaging of the abdomen 9:1034–1041
6. Japan Liver Cancer Research Society: Treatment Guidelines for Primary Liver Cancer (1987) (Revised 2nd edition). Tokyo, Kanehara Publishing
7. Japan Liver Cancer Research Society: 5th National Primary Liver Cancer Follow-up Reports (1979). Kyoto, Shinko Publishing pp 1–42
8. Japan Liver Cancer Research Society: 6th National Primary Liver Cancer Follow-up Reports (1981). Kyoto, Skinko Publishing pp 1–100
9. Okuda K, Kubo Y, Okazaki N, Arishima T, Hashimoto M, Jinnouchi S, Sawa Y, Sjhimokawa Y, Nakajima Y, Noguchi T, Nakano M, Kojiro M,

Nakashima T (1977) Clinical aspects of intrahepatic bile duct including hilar carcinoma: A study of 57 autopsy-proven cases. Cancer 39:232–246

10. Nimura Y, Hayakawa N, Kamiya J, Kondo S, Shionoya S (1990) Hepatic segmentectomy with caudate lobe resection for bile duct carcinoma of the hepatic hilus. World J Surg 14:535–544

11. Mimura H, Kim H, Takakura K, Hamazaki K, Ochiai Y, Sakumoto S, Ozawa T, Orita K (1987) Radical block resection of complete hepatoduodenal ligament for bile duct carcinoma. Surgery 41:161–165

12. Kumada K, Ozawa K, Shimahara Y, Morikawa S, Okamoto R, Moriyasu F (1990) Truncoumbilical bypass of the portal vein in radical resection of biliary tract tumor involving the hepatic duct confluence. Br J Surg 77:749–751

13. Walter JF, Bookstein J, Bouford EV (1976) Newer angiographic obstructions in cholangiocarcinoma. Radiology 118:19–23

14. Kinami Y, Miyazaki I, Kurachi M, Takashima S, Shinmura K, Shinno B (1979) A study on operative results of carcinoma of the intrahepatic bile duct and the main hepatic bile duct junction and clinical features of patients with multiple carcinoma of the bile duct. Jpn J Gastroenterol Surg 12:908–913

15. Iwasaki Y, Todoroki K (1980) Intraoperative radiotherapy for carcinoma of the bile duct at the hepatic hilus. J Bil Panc 11:857–863

16. Tani M, Yahata K, Mikuriya S, Mamiya T, Asano M (1984) Radiotherapy for unresectable bile duct carcinoma at hepatic hilus. J Bil Panc 5: 1539–1549

CHAPTER 41

Hepatocellular carcinoma in taiwan

Chen-Guo Ker[1]

1 Introduction

Hepatocellular carcinoma (HCC) is the most common malignant tumor among males in Taiwan [1, 2]. In a prospective study, the risk of development of HCC for Taiwanese carriers of HBsAg antigen was found to be 200 to 300 times greater than that of non-carriers in 1981 [3]. In addition, the seroepidermiological study strongly supports the association of HBV infection with HCC. Chen [4] had an analysis of DNA extracted from HCC hepatocytes and found chromosomal integration of hepatitis B virus DNA sequences to prove their close relation.

Without question, surgical resection was the most common treatment modality for HCC, unfortunately, most of our patients were unresectable. Therefore, transcatheter hepatic arterial embolization, intra-tumorous ethanol injection and chemotherapy were utilized as non-surgical methods for those patients.

2 Patients and clinical characteristics

The incidence of HCC was relatively frequent and, out of a total of 2,865 cases, 2,530 male and 335 female patients were encountered in our hospital from 1981 to 1989, as shown in Fig. 1. The largest increase in cases was noted in the recent 3-year interval. The peak age of incidence was in the fourth and fifth decade. HCC associated with cirrhosis was approximately 70–80% in Taiwan. Portal vein thrombosis was an obstacle

---
[1] Division of Hepatobiliary Surgery, Department of Surgery, Kaohsiung Medical College Hospital, Kaohsiung, Taiwan

for tumor resection. The incidence of portal vein thrombosis was 27% (42/155) for single nodules, 43% (61/143) for multiple nodules, and 96% (110/115) for diffuse type HCC [5].

Diagnosis of HCC by echographic study is very reliable [6]. HCC patients can be found by periodically screening patients with elevated levels of alpha-fetoprotein from asymptomatic HBsAg carriers in Taiwan in 1975 [7]. Fine needle aspiration for histological diagnosis was not performed routinely and was not advisable because of seeding along the needle tract and spreading into the peritoneal cavity. Echographic study and serum alpha-fetoprotein determinatin was chosen as the primary aid for screening HCC. Subsequently, celiac angiography and computed tomography (CT) were applied for patients suspected of having HCC.

3 Resection of HCC

Hepatic resection has been accepted as a good choice of treatment for HCC due to the anatomy of the liver, advances in diagnostic imaging, and great improvement in the field of anesthesiology. A total of sixty-two patients with HCC were resected and the overall mortality rate (occuring one month postoperatively) was 4.8%. The causes of death were post-operative hepatic failure in two cases, and post-operative intra-abdominal bleeding in one case. It is not necessary to perform biliary drainage or to deal with the resected surface intra-operatively. Tumor resection was done mostly with the method of anatomic vascular isolation to prevent massive bleeding.

Extended lobectomy was performed on 7 patients, 5 on the right and 2 on the left, as shown in Fig. 2. The indication for extended hepatic

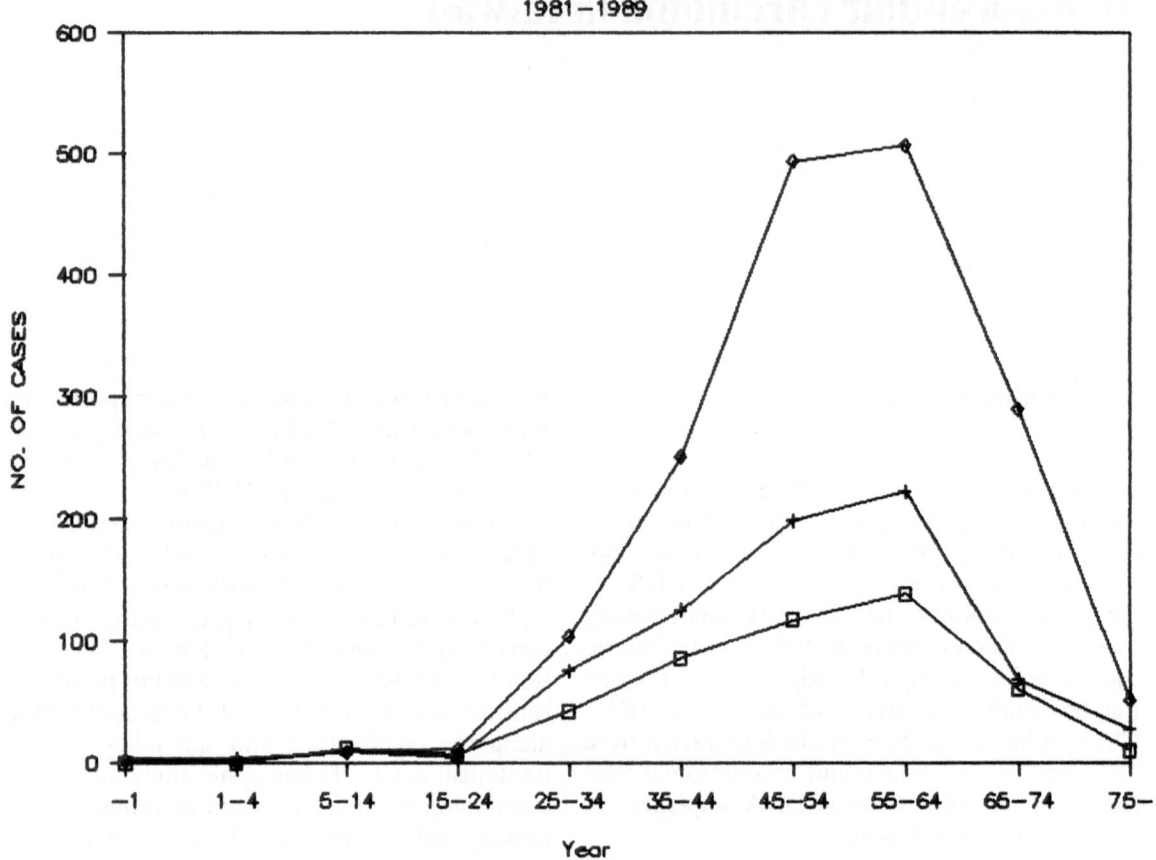

Fig. 1. The age distribution of hepatocellular carcinoma from 1981–1989 in Kaohsiung Medical College Hospital. *Open box*, 1981–3; *cross*, 1984–6; *open diamond*, 1987–1989

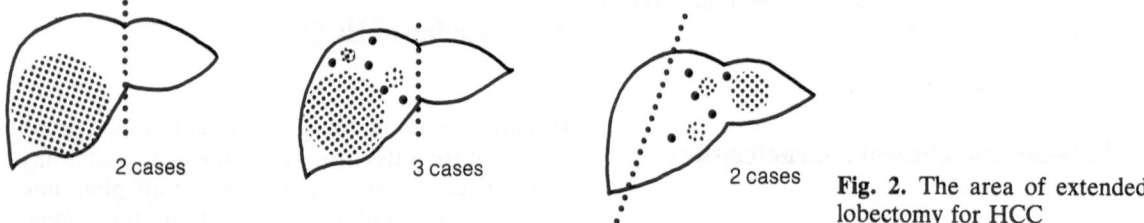

Fig. 2. The area of extended lobectomy for HCC

lobectomy should be more restricted than that of ordinary hepatic lobectomy. The morbidity was similar between extended and ordinary hepatic lobectomy. No operative mortality occurred in those 7 patients, and a good prognosis was achieved. Therefore, it is worthy to perform extended lobectomy of huge primary liver tumors without associated cirrhosis [8].

Out of all 62 patients, the median survival rate was 54 months for HCC patients without cirrhosis and 15.5 months for patients with cirrhosis. The

1-year, 2-year, 3-year, 4-year and 5-year survival rates were 40.6%, 29.0%, 21.1%, 18.0%, and 11.1% respectively. Of the patients who survived more than 5 years, their tumor size ranged from 4–12 cm in diameter, and there was no relation between the size of the tumor and survival time shown in Fig. 3. The prognosis for patients with big tumors was not always poor and that for patients with small tumors was not always good in our series. The poor prognostic factors included non-capsulated HCC with an irregular margin,

Fig. 3. Relationship between tumor size (cm) and survival (months). No correlation was observed

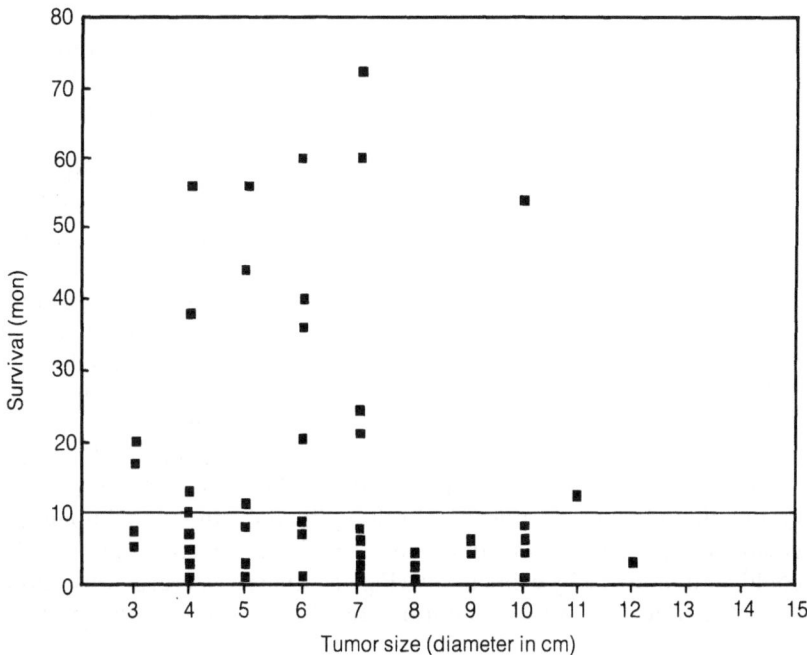

portal vein thrombosis, satellite nodules and vascular invasion. Overall, our surgical results were not comparable with other reports because of the small proportion of small HCC in our series.

4 Non-surgical treatment of HCC

4.1 Transcatheter hepatic arterial embolization

Transcatheter hepatic arterial embolization (TAE) has been frequently used for treating unresectable hepatic malignancy and appears to be an effective treatment for liver tumor [9, 10]. The follow-up study of HCC treated with TAE reported in our series showed that the 6-, 12-, 24- and 36- month survival rates were 81.0%, 57.0%, 30.6% and 21.6%, respectively [11]. There were four patients treated by TAE initially, followed by surgical resection 2–3 weeks later. The gross appearance of the resected specimen showed necrosis, but some clusters of cancer cells still remained microscopically. Therefore, HCC was not always curable with TAE alone, and a multi-disciplinary approach is necessary even in small HCC. In addition, TAE could be used to convert large unresectable HCC to resectable tumors.

In Taiwan, a pilot study of selective targeting treatment was done using lipiodol, a radioisotope

(I-131), which was infused into the HCC tumor via the hepatic artery was reported by Lui in 1990 [12]. The treatment results were encouraging. About 70% of the HCC cases had a good response to the treatment with a reduction of alpha-fetoprotein and a decease in tumor size. The overall median survival was 9 months, ranging from 2 to 17 months, from 10 patients. I-131 lipiodol treatment through the hepatic artery is simple, safe, inexpensive and effective.

4.2 Echo-guided intratumor ethanol injection

Our clinical experience with intratumor injection of absolute ethanol for the treatment of unresectable HCC began in 1988; and the size of the tumor was usually more than 3 cm in diameter [13]. Twenty-six patients, 22 male and 4 female, were recruited for treatment by echo-guided intratumor injection of absolute ethanol. All patients were diagnosed with primary HCC. Their ages ranged from 38 to 90 years, and the size of the tumor ranged from 3 to 11 cm in diameter. These patients were not subjected to surgical resection due to either liver cirrhosis or the failure of TAE. Before injection, the patients were temporarily anesthetized with Cytosol (5 mg/kg) and Succinyl-asta (1 mg/kg) without intratracheal intubation. A long guage 19 needle was used to percutaneously inject ethanol through

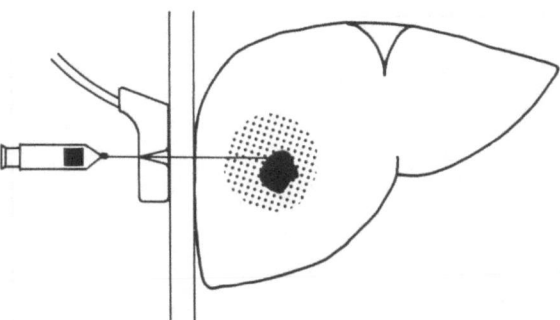

Fig. 4. Echo-guided intratumor injection of absolute ethanol for unresectable HCC

the puncture probe under the guidance of echography directly into the tumor. Absolute ethanol is slowly injected into the tumor itself and this could be monitored by echography (Fig. 4). Once ethanol is injected into the tumoral parenchyma, it becomes hyperechoic and is easily identified within the tumor. The procedure is repeated on the other side of the tumor whenever possible. The total amount of injected ethanol ranged from 15 to 278 ml for each patient and the maximal amount of injected ethanol was 65 ml in one session. On follow-up study, the 6-month, 12-month and 24-month survival rates were 61%, 38% and 11.5%, respectively. We believed and strongly suggested that echo-guided intratumor injection of absolute ethanol for the treatment of unresectable HCC is a simple and effective method. One example was a 55-year-old male with an HCC of 8.6×7.6 cm in the right posterior segment (Fig. 5a). Surgical resection was not possible due to associated cirrhosis and liver function impairment. Therefore, intratumor injection of 60 ml ethanol was performed and partial necrosis was shown, as seen in Fig. 5b. After 5 sessions of this procedure, the tumor mass

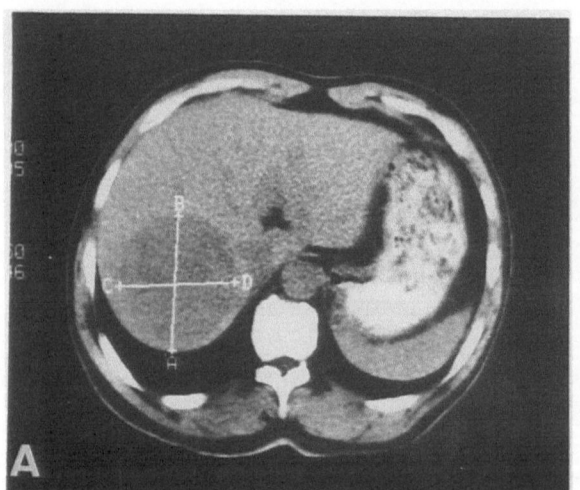

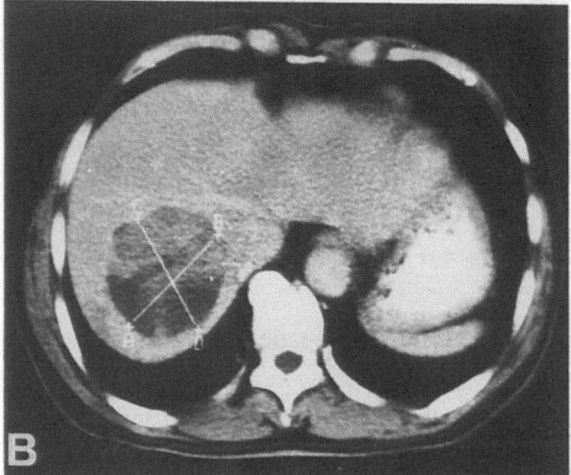

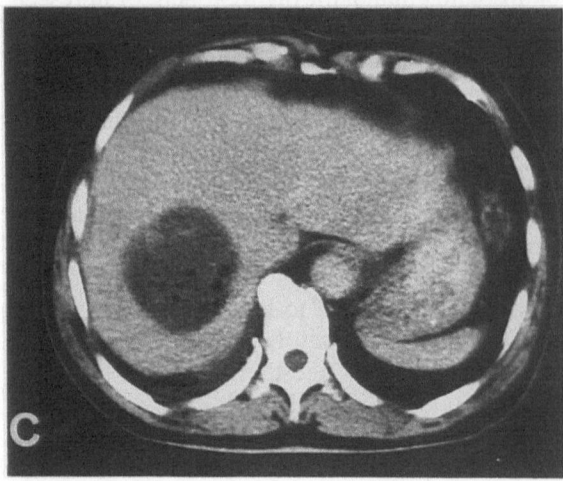

Fig. 5A–C. A A mass of 8.6×7.6 cm shown in the CT scan before intratumor injection. **B** Two weeks after injection of ethanol, necrosis was found in the partial portion of the tumor. **C** Two months later, the necrosis appeared complete after 5 sessions of this procedure

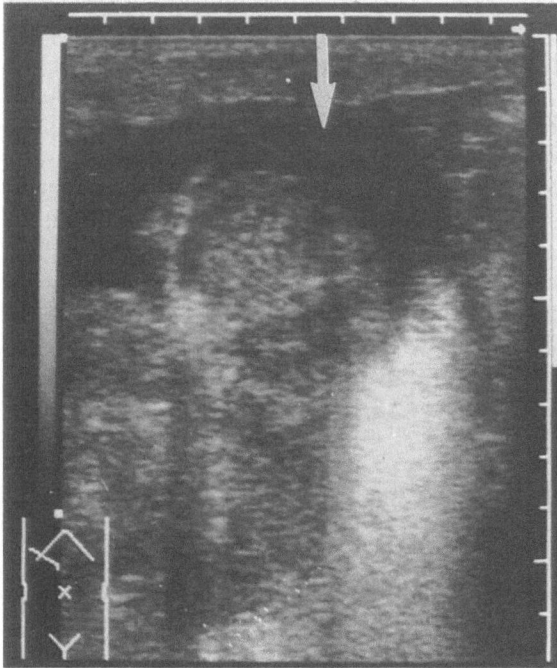

Fig. 6. Echography showed the ruptured nodule (*arrow*) of HCC

became wholly necrotic two months later (Fig. 5c). This patient was still in good health 24 months after treatment.

5 Spontaneous rupture of HCC

The incidence of spontaneous rupture of HCC was infrequent; there were 28 such patients encountered in our surgical department. The peak age of incidence was in the fourth decade and predominantly among males [14, 15]. The gross appearance in those patients was nodular in 5 cases (17.86%), massive in 4 (14.29%), diffuse in 11 (39.28%), and unknown in 8 (28.57%). The site of the tumor rupture was demonstrated by echographic study 33.3% of the time. The ruptured nodule located peripherally and fluid accumulation around this area as shown in Fig. 6. Extravasation from the ruptured tumor was demonstrated by celiac angiography only 11% of the time (Fig. 7). The mortality of spontaneous rupture is extremely high, and the prognoses were varied and were influenced by the choice of man-

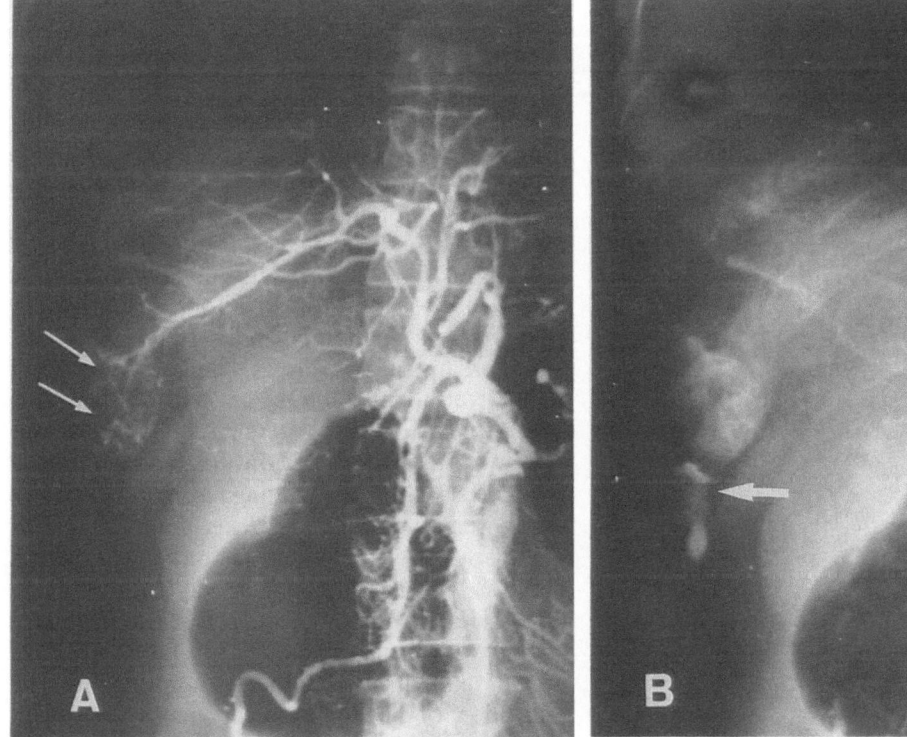
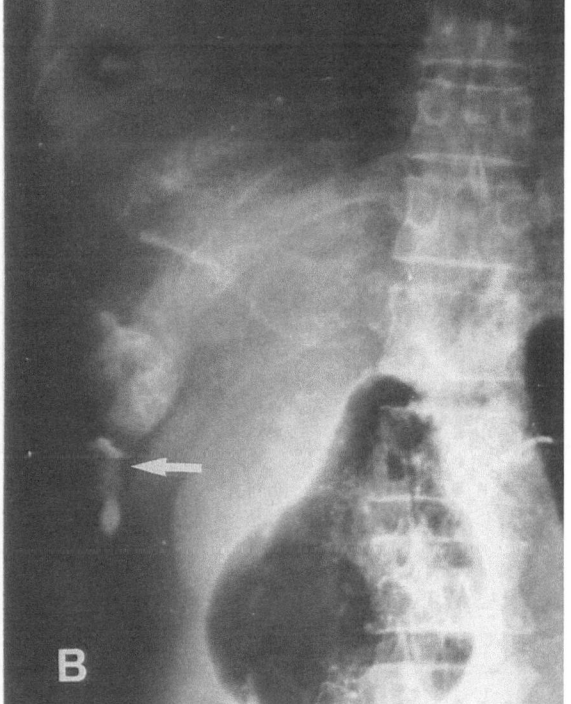

Fig. 7A,B. A Hypervascularity (*arrows*) was found in celiac angiography of HCC. **B** Extravasation of contrast media (*arrow*) was found in the tumor to identify the rupture side

416   C-G. Ker

agement. Treatment is aimed at controlling the hemorrhage first by TAE where possible [10]. Alternatively, resection of the tumor was possible if the echographic study showed the bleeding was located peripherally. We suggest that abdominal echo is a very effective and simple aid to help determine the best method of management. For single nodules, emergent laparotomy could be performed for resection of the ruptured nodule. For multiple nodules with associated cirrhosis, emergent TAE should be done first without delay to control the bleeding.

6 Functional reserve and operative mortality

Assessment of the functional reserve of the liver before resection is very important. Indocyanine green (ICG) and oral glucose tolerance (OGT) tests were useful for evaluation the risk of operation [16]. Post-operative infusion of branched chain amino acids for the resected liver tumor was strongly advised, especially for the cirrhotic patients in our series. [17].

We had conducted a retrospective study to determine the percentage of liver cell versus fibrous cells histologically. In liver cirrhosis, the percentage of parenchymal hepatocytes decreased and the fibrous tissue around the portal area increased. Therefore, the percentage of liver cells should be high in normal liver and decreased in cirrhotic liver.

The measurement was obtained from the histology of liver wedge biopsy, as shown in Fig. 8.

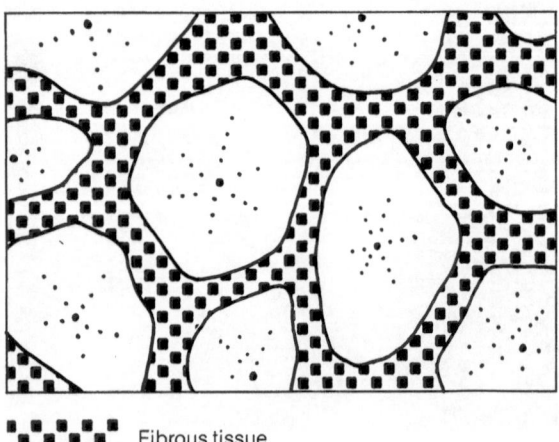

■■■■■ Fibrous tissue

Fig. 8. Histological measurement of the liver cells' area

The area (%) of liver cell unit was found to be 91.69 ± 2.40% in normal liver (n = 22). For post-hepatitis cirrhosis (n = 18), the percentage was 76 ± 7.59% and 82.12 ± 5.62% for resectable HCC (n = 17). There were three cases of post-operative mortality and their percentages were low, as shown in Fig. 9. Therefore, we strongly suggest that the tumor resection should be limited and conservative when the percentage of liver cells is lower than 80–85%. These results could provide us with a guide to assess the size of the liver tissue we have to resect by doing the frozen section intra-operatively where possible.

7 Discussion

The association between hepatitis B virus (HBV) infection and increased risk of developing hepatocellular carcinoma is well established [1, 2]. Studies in the mothers of adult HCC patients in Taiwan showed that the correlation between HCC and serum HBsAg was reported from 71% to 86% in Taiwan. The HBsAg positive rate in the mothers of HCC children was strikingly high, about 94% [18]. HBV transmission from the mother during perinatal period or early childhood is the most prevalent mode of HBV infection in HCC patients in Taiwan. The role of the father in HBV transmission is thought to be unimportant. The causal relation of vertical or perinatal transmission of HBV in the causation of adult and childhood HCC was also proven in Malaysia [19]. There were 6 patients with a family tendency towards HCC in our series, and there were 9 patients (11%) with a family tendency reported by Lee [7]. Therefore, the prophylactic role of childhood vaccination is emphasized.

The treatment modality is based on the location of the liver nodule, and the existence of cirrhosis, as shown in Fig. 10. Extended left or right lobectomy should be carried out for the main tumor as well as the surrounding daughter nodules which were overlooked on image diagnosis before the operation. From our series, there were 7 cases (11.3%) with extended lobectomy with uneventful results. From other reports, extended lobectomy was performed on 5.7% [20] and 3.3% [21] of patients who underwent resection. The indication of hepatic resection in patients with cirrhosis was demonstrated by Lin and Lee [20] in Taiwan under the following conditions: (1) Hepatic lobectomy is indicated for the right or

Fig. 9. The percentage of liver cells of control, post-hepatitis necrosis and HCC resected liver. *Closed circle*, death

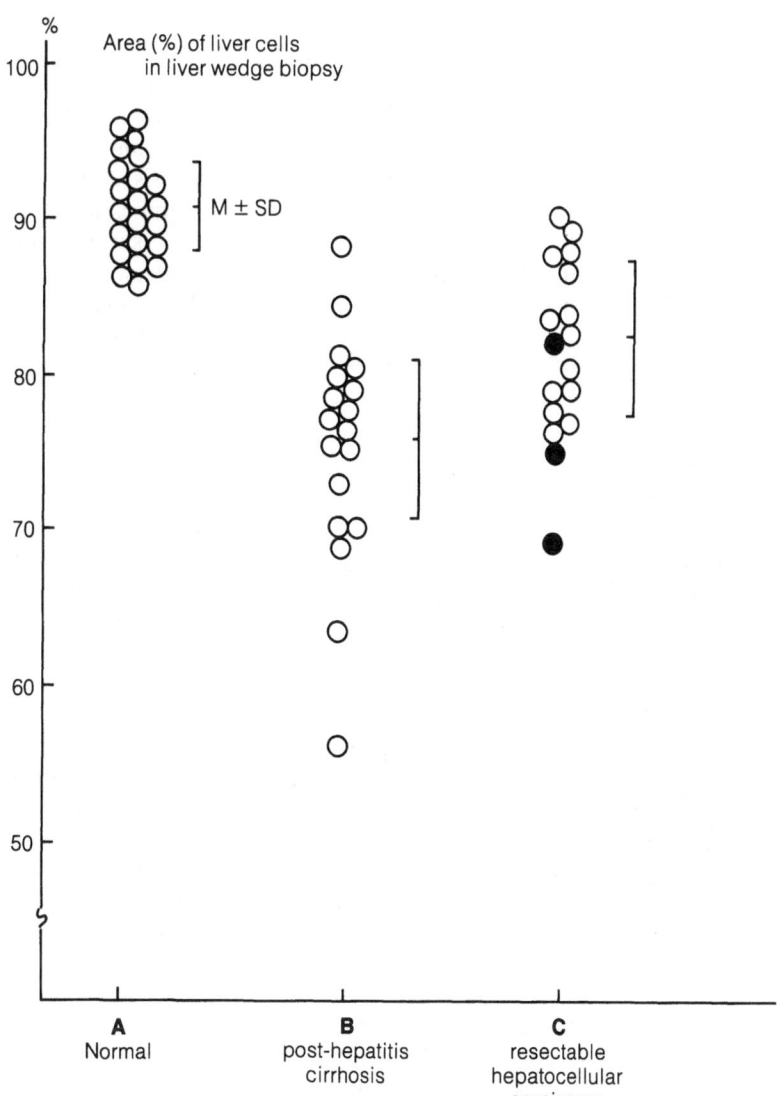

the left lobe if the cancer free lobe is macroscopically normal, and (2) In the presence of moderately advanced cirrhosis with a coarse nodular liver surface, hepatic lobectomy of the left, but not the right lobe, can be performed. It should be noted that in cases with advanced cirrhosis, hepatic lobectomy for either lobe is contraindicated. Limited partial liver resection should be followed even in the case of asymptomatic small HCC with cirrhosis. Additionally, Lin and Lee [20] had suggested that partial resection may induce hepatic failure if a nodule larger than 5 cm in diameter close to the hilary area in the right lobe is removed. In Taiwan, the operative mortality of HCC ranged from 3% to 5.6% [17, 10, 21] and 4.8% in our series. Post-operative rupture bleeding of esophageal varicies is a challenge to

surgeon. In cases with HCC, portal hypertension, and a past history of esophageal bleeding, it is better to perform limited liver resection and esophageal blocking procedure to prevent postoperative esophageal varices from rupturing.

In our series, neither the tumor size, the tumor location nor the patient's sex and age affected the patient's survival. In symptomatic HCC, adequate resection margins were closely related to good survival [7]. However, in asymptomatic small HCC, the presence of multifocal lesions, and hence adequate safety margins did not prevent tumor recurrence [22]. In our experience, poor prognostic factors included non-capsulated tumors with an irregular margin, positive portal vein thrombosis, presence of satellite nodules, and direct vascular invasion. Overall, post-

418   C-G. Ker

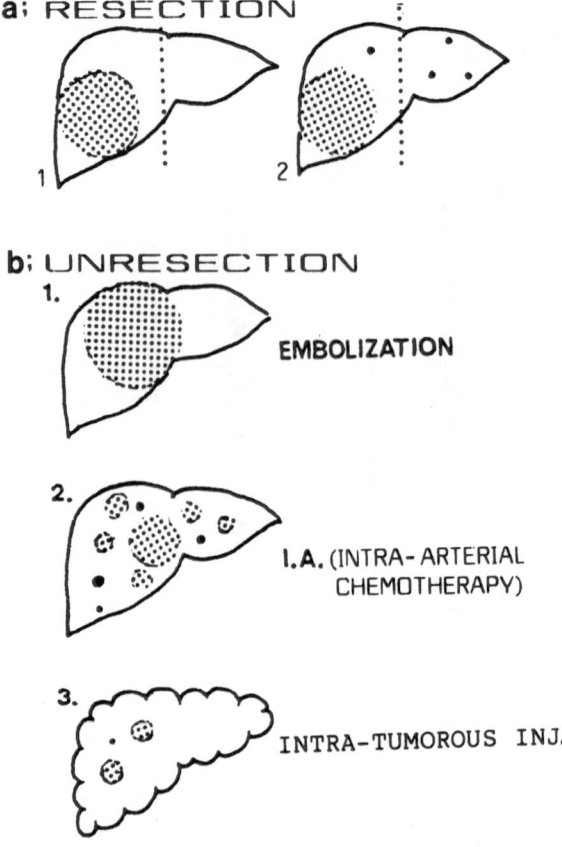

a; RESECTION

b; UNRESECTION

1. EMBOLIZATION

2. I.A. (INTRA-ARTERIAL CHEMOTHERAPY)

3. INTRA-TUMOROUS INJ.

Fig. 10a,b. Treatment of modalities of HCC

common DNA patterns among HCC patients proved to be aneuploid (78%) and diploid (22%) reported by Chen [24]. There was no correlation between DNA distribution and hepatitis B surface antigen positivity, the presence of liver cirrhosis or tumor size. In addition, there was no significant correlation between the DNA pattern and survival rates in patients with HCC who underwent hepatic resection in Taiwan. In Mainland China, Cong and Wu [25] studied DNA stemline and well correlated with small HCC and large HCC. Small HCC were diploid in 22 cases (73.3%) and aneuploid in 8 cases (26.7%) but large HCC were diploid in 4 cases (15.4%) and aneuploid in 22 cases (84.6%). The post-operative 5-year survival rate of patients with small HCC was 62.1% which was higher than the rate of 27.7% of patients with large HCC ($P < 0.05$).

In conclusion, HCC is a common disease in Taiwan and is difficult to treat. Although arriving at the diagnosis is not difficult, the results of treatment are not at all satisfactory. Surgical resection is considered the treatment of choice, however, the recurrence rate is high. Tumor clonality of primary or daughter nodules should be determined by the technique of integrated HBV DNA analysis. Hopefully, the choice of treatment will be decided based on the underlying etiology of the disease and good results will be achieved in the future.

operative follow-up of resected HCC cases showed a 5-year survival rate of less than 25% in Taiwan [7, 20, 21]. The surgical results were not satisfactory compared with other countries. The variation resulted from the difference in the biologic characteristics of liver cancer. The results of chemotherapy for HCC was not satisfied at all. But the rational for the treatment with prolonged continuous intra-arterial chemotherapy using a low-volume chronometric portable pump is based on the fact that it can deliver a high concentration of anticancer agent to the organ over a fairly long period of time through arterial blood supply, and producing a constant bombardment of anti-metabolities to the reproducing neoplastic cell. Sheen [23] reported that of 62 HCC patients treated by intra-arterial infusion chemotherapy, 32 (48%) showed a response to the treatment. The survival time for the those who responded varied from 3.3 to 24.5 months with a median of 6.9 months.

Flow cytometric DNA pattern was classified into two types: Diploid and aneuploid. The most

1. Sung JL, Wang TH, Yu JY (1967) Clinical study on primary carcinoma of the liver in Taiwan. Am J Dig Dis 12:1036–1049
2. Lin TM, Chang LC, Chen, KP (1977) A statistical analysis on mortality of malignant neoplasms in Taiwan. J Formosan Med Assoc 76:656–668
3. Beasley PR, Hwang LY, Lin CC (1981) Hepatocellular carcinoma and hepatitis B virus: A prospective study of 22,707 men in Taiwan. Lancet 2:1129–1133
4. Chen JY, Harrison JT, Lee CS, Chen DS, Zuckerman A (1988) Detection of hepatitis B virus DNA in hepatocellular carcinoma: Analysis by hybridization with subgenomic DNA fragments. Hepatology 8:518–523
5. Chen SC, Chang WY, Wang LY, Lin ZY, Chuang WL, Hsieh MY, Jan CM, Chen CY (1987) Sonographic study of portal vein thrombosis in hepatocellular carcinoma. Kaohsiung J Med Sci 3:49–55
6. Ker CG, Hsieh JS, Huang TJ, Sheen PC, Wu CC, Tasi JF, Jan CM, Chen CY (1982) Echographic

pattern of hepatocellular carcinoma. J Formosan Med Assoc 81:1396–1403

7. Lee CS, Sung JL, Huang LY, Sheu JC, Chen DS, Lin TY, Beasley RP (1986) Surgical treatment of 109 patients with symptomatic and asymptomatic hepatocellular carcinoma. Surgery 99:481–490

8. Ker CG, Lee KT, Hsieh JS, Huang TJ, Sheen PC (1985) Extended hepatic lobectomy for treatment of liver tumor. Kaohsiung J Med Sci 1:289–296

9. Yamada R, Sato M, Kawabata M (1983) Hepatic artery embolization in 120 patients with unresectable hepatoma. Radiology 148:397–401

10. Chen MF, Jan YY, Lee TY (1986) Transcatheter hepatic arterial embolization followed by hepatic resection for the spontaneous rupture of hepatocellular carcinoma. Cancer 58:332–335

11. Hsieh MY, Wu DK, Lu SN, Wang LY, Chang WY (1989) The outcome of hepatocellular carcinoma treated with transcatheter arterial chemoembolization. Kaohsiung J Med Sci 6:628–635

12. Lui WY, Liu RS, Chiang JH, Lo JG, Lai KH, King KL, Chang HC, Wei YY, Chi CW, Peng FK, Chen WK (1990) Report of a pilot study of intra-arterial injection of I-131 Lipiodol for the treatment of hepatoma. Chinese Med J (Taipei) 46:125–133

13. Ker CG, Chen JS, Lee KT, Sheen PC (1990) Echoguided intratumor ethanol injection for treatment of unresectable HCC. In: Viral hepatitis and hepatocellular carcinoma. Sung JL and Chen DS (eds) Excerpta Medica. Current Clinical Practice Series 57:R651–656

14. Ker CG, Hou MF, Lee KT, Hsieh JS, Huang TJ, Sheen PC (1986) Echographic assessment of spontaneous rupture of hepatocellular carcinoma. J Ultrasound Med ROC 3:1–4

15. Wang JR, Ker CG, Hou MF, Lee KT, Hsieh JS, Huang TJ, Sheen PC (1986) A clinical review of hemoperitoneum due to spontaneous rupture of hepatocellular carcinoma. Kaohsiung J Med Sci 2:179–183

16. Mizumota R, Noguchi T (1983) Indication of hepato-biliary surgery and risk of operation for primary liver malignancy (in Japanese). Kan Tan Sui 6:13–20

17. Ker CG, Sheen PC (1986) Clinical evalutation of branched chain amino acids for treatment of hepatic encephalopathy. Kaohsiung J Med Sci 2: 228–233

18. Chang MH, Chen DS, Hsu HC, Hsu HY, Lee CY (1989) Maternal transmission of hepatitis B virus in childhood hepatocellular carcinoma. Cancer 64: 2377–2380

19. Cheah PL, Looi LM, Lin HP, Yap SF (1990) Childhood primary hepatocellular carcinoma and hepatitis B virus infection. Cancer 65:174–176

20. Lin TY, Lee CS, Chen KM, Chen CC (1987) Role of surgery in the treatment of primary carcinoma of the liver: A 31-year experience. Br J Surg 74: 839–842

21. Chen MF, Hwang TL, Jeng LB Benjamin, Jan YY, Wang CS, Chen FF (1989) Hepatic resection in 120 patients with hepatocellular carcinoma. Arch Surg 124:1025–1028

22. Lee CS, Hwang LY, Beasley RP, Hsu HC, Lee HS, Lin TY (1988) Prognostic significance of histologic findings in resected small hepatocellular carcinoma. Acta Chir Scand 154:199–203

23. Sheen MC, Huang TJ, Sheen PC, Ho YH, Chang WY, Chen CY (1984) Intra-arterial infusion chemotherapy of primary liver cancer. J Formosan Med Assoc 83:800–806

24. Chen MF, Hwang TL, Tsao KC, Sung CF, Chen TJ (1991) Flow cytometric DNA analysis of hepatocellular carcinoma: Preliminary report. Surg 109:455–458

25. Cong W, Wu M (1990) The biopathologic characteristics of DNA content of hepatocellular carcinoma. Cancer 66:498–501

CHAPTER 42

Prognostic factors in surgical patients with hepatocellular carcinoma

Soo Tae Kim, K. P. Kim, and D. Y. Noh[1]

1 Introduction

Primary hepatocellular carcinoma is one of the most prevalent fatal tumors in Korea. Without surgical resection or other forms of treatment, patients usually die within 6 months after the appearance of symptoms, but if the tumor is completely resected, the 5-year survival rate is almost 30%. Complete surgical resection plays a leading role in current treatment.

Not all patients survive equally well, and research is now focusing on prognostic factors which might be valuable in the long-term prognosis. Factors evaluated so far include age, preoperative liver function, cirrhosis, intraoperative bleeding, and size or pathological characteristics of the tumor. Despite the large number of studies being carried out, there have been differing reports from many investigators.

2 Patients and methods

This 10-year study was carried out between October 1978 and September 1988, using data on 239 patients who underwent hepatic resection to treat histologically proven hepatocellular carcinoma. Follow-up was possible with 217 patients out of the total 239, and we were able to confirm survival or death by medical records, personal communication, or telephone calls.

The male to female ratio of the patients was 5:1. The patients were predominantly in the fifth and sixth decades (75.2%), and the mean age was

51 years (Fig. 1). The patients were divided into two groups, one with curative, the other with palliative resection (Table 1). Palliative resections were carried out on 62 patients. Adjacent organ invasion was seen in 13 of these patients, gross angioinvasion in 5 patients, and distant metastasis in 2 patients; only primary tumors were resected in these cases. Postoperative pathologic examinations revealed positive resection margins in 37 of these patients. Postoperative examinations with ultrasonography (US) and computed tomography (CT) demonstrated residual tumors in the liver remnants in 5 patients.

We analyzed the prognostic importance of 12 variables, using univariate and multivariate regression models on data from 167 patients who underwent curative resections, to search for factors which might be valuable in the long-term prognosis. To compute the survival rate and survival curve, cases of operative mortality (deaths within 30 postoperative days) were excluded. The overall operative mortality rate was 7.5%.

Twelve variables were subject to univariate analysis and survivals according to these variables were calculated using the actuarial method of Kaplan and Meier [1]. The significant level of difference between curves was assessed with the Log-rank test. Factors with a P value below 0.05 in the univariate analysis were submitted to multivariate analysis using Cox's regression model [2].

3 Results

Of 239 patients, major resections were done on 91 patients (38%), and minor resections on 148 patients (62%). Curative resections were performed on 177 patients (74.1%) and palliative

[1] Department of Surgery, College of Medicine, Seoul National University Hospital, Chongno-Ku, Seoul, 110-744, Korea

Table 1. Operations performed

	Type	CR	PR	Total
Major resection	Right trisegmentectomy	6	3	9
	Right lobectomy	39	18	57
	Left lobectomy	20	5	25
Minor resection	Right segmentectomy	31	7	38
	Left segmentectomy	15	7	22
	Bisegmentectomy	1	0	1
	Subsegmentectomy and tumor exision	65	22	87
Total		177	62	239

CR, curative resection; PR, palliative resection

No. of patients

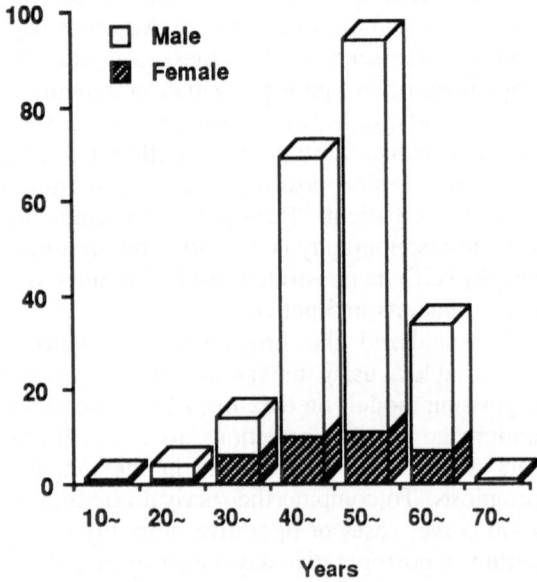

Fig. 1. Age and sex distribution of 217 patients with primary hepatocellular carcinoma

Table 2. Survival rates of patients with curative and palliative resection (excluding operative and hospital mortality)

	CR	PR
1YSR	69.1%	39.1%
2	47.1%	32.4%
3	41.3%	24.3%
4	36.7%	0.0%
5	33.3%	0.0%

YSR, year survival rate; CR, curative resection; PR, palliative resection

Survival rate (%)

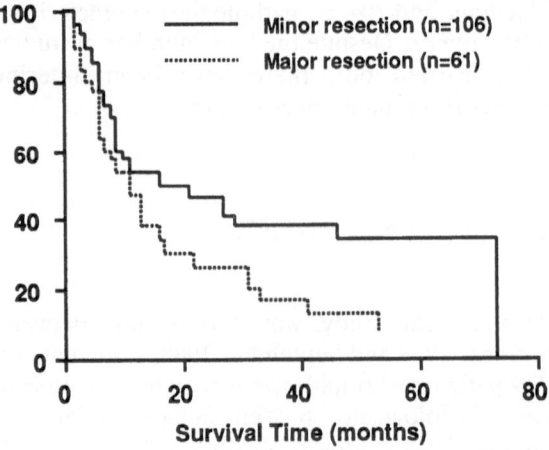

Fig. 2. Survival curves according to the type of resection in curative resection ($P < 0.05$)

resections on 62 patients (25.9%) (Table 1). The survival rates (including actuarial analysis) of curatively resected patients surviving operation at 1, 3, and 5 years were 61.1%, 41.3%, and 33.3%, respectively (Table 2). There was a significant difference in the survival rate between the patients with curative and palliative resections ($P < 0.05$).

The survival rates of curatively resected patients according to the 12 variables tested were as follows:

1. Among curatively resected patients, *major resections* were performed on 61 patients and minor resections on 106 patients, and there was a significant difference in the survival rate of the two groups ($P = 0.05$) (Fig. 2).

2. The reserved liver function according to *Child's classification* influenced the long-term prognosis (A > B > C, $P = 0.01$) (Fig. 3). In the case of group C, mean survival was 2.3 months and all patients died within 7 months. The positive hepatitis B surface antigen (HBsAg) rate

Survival rate (%)

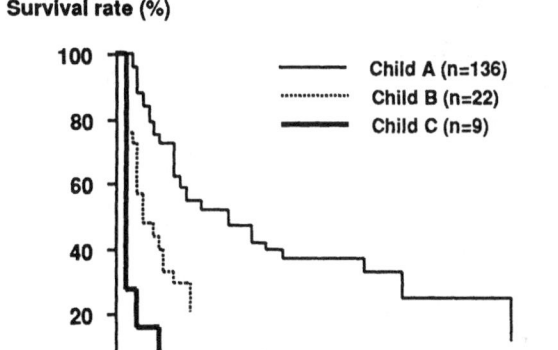

Fig. 3. Survival curves according to Child's classification in curative resection ($P < 0.05$)

Survival Rate (%)

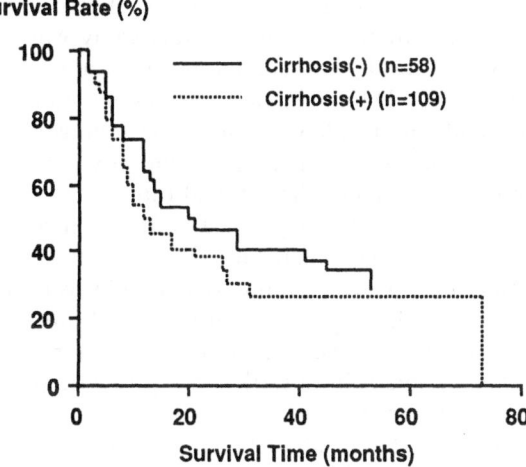

Fig. 4. Survival curves according to cirrhosis in curative resection ($P > 0.05$)

Survival rate (%)

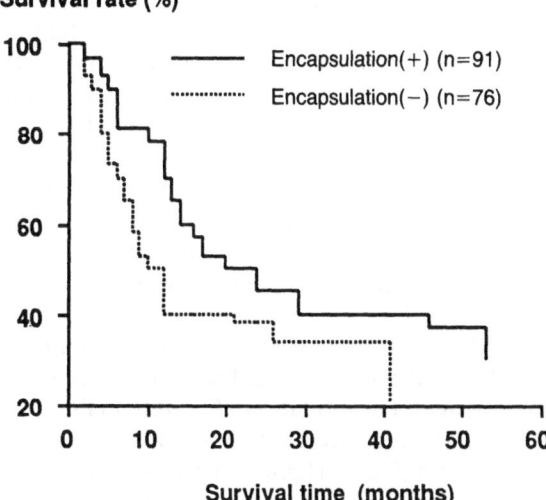

Fig. 5. Survival curves according to encapsulation in curative resection ($P < 0.05$)

Survival Rate (%)

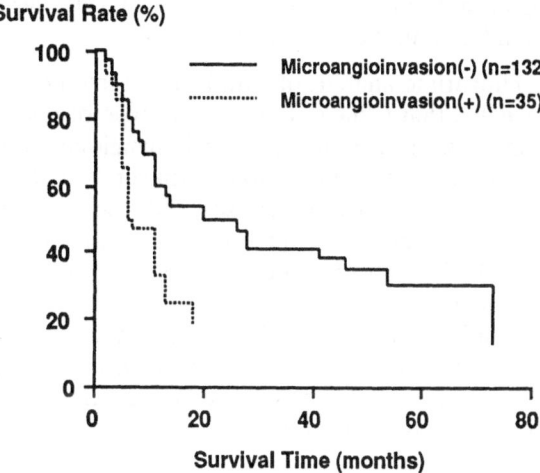

Fig. 6. Survival curves according to microangioinvasion in curative resection ($P < 0.05$)

was 74.8%. The positive HBsAg rate was higher in the group with cirrhosis than in the group without cirrhosis ($P < 0.05$).

3. *Alpha-fetoprotein (AFP) levels* of over 20 ng/ml were recorded in 72% of the patients. The level of AFP and the size of the tumor were not related, and preoperative levels did not influence the survival rate ($P = 0.16$).

4. The survival rates of *male and female* patients were not significantly different ($P = 0.98$).

5. Groups above and below 50 years of *age* did not show differences in the survival rate ($P = 0.28$).

6. Patients were divided into two groups according to the *volume of blood transfusion*

during hepatic resection, one with more than ten pints of blood transfused and the other with less then ten pints. The volume of blood transfusion did not influence the survival rate ($P = 0.25$).

7. Classification by *gross type* revealed single nodular, single nodular with perinodal extension, multinodular discrete, multinodular confluent, and massive types. No significant difference in the survival rates was found ($P = 0.89$).

Histologic findings were examined in relation to the prognosis. The histologic characteristics included the largest diameter of the tumor, presence of associated disease, encapsulation, microangioinvasion, and histologic types of the tumor.

8. According to the *size* of the tumor, patients were divided into two groups, one with tumors greater than 5 cm (n = 118) and the other with tumors less than 5 cm (n = 49). The size of the tumor did not influence the survival rate (P = 0.15).

9. *Liver cirrhosis* was seen in 109 patients (65%), whereas normal liver function was found in 58 patients (35%). The presence or absence of the cirrhosis did not influence the survival rate (P = 0.42) (Fig. 4).

10. *Encapsulation* was found in 91 patients (54.8%) and higher survival rates were found in patients with encapsulation (P = 0.02) (Fig. 5).

11. *Microangioinvasion* was found in 35 patients (20.9%). Higher survival rates were seen in those without microangioinvasion (P = 0.001) (Fig. 6).

12. Classification by *histologic type* revealed macrotrabecular, microtrabecular, acinar, solid, scirrhous, pelioid, and fibrolamellar types. No significant difference of the survival rates was found among these types (P = 0.84).

Univariate analysis of curatively resected cases revealed that Child's classification, type of resection, encapsulation, and microangioinvasion significantly affected the long-term survival (P < 0.05), but sex, age, tumor size, AFP levels, cirrhosis, volume of blood transfusion, and histopathologic subtype did not have statistical meaning.

Multivariate analysis showed that microangioinvasion, Child's classification, and encapsulation were significant factors in predicting survival in decreasing order (Table 3).

4 Discussion

Primary hepatocellular carcinoma is one of the most fatal tumors in Korea. Patients with this disease usually die within six months after appearance of symptoms. However, among patients who undergo surgical resection, the mean survival is 10–20 months and the 5-year survival rate is about 30% [3, 4].

It is estimated that annual mortality of patients with hepatocellular carcinoma is 250,000 worldwide and 100,000 in China. Hepatocellular carcinoma is much more common in sub-Saharan Africa, Southeast Asia, and the Pacific Islands than in North and Central America, most parts of Europe, the Middle East, and the Soviet Union

Table 3. Univariate and multivariate analysis of prognostic factors: Influence on survival

Factors	Univariate	Multivariate
Microangioinvasion	P = 0.001	P = 0.0008
Child's classification	P = 0.01	P = 0.036
Encapsulation	P = 0.02	P = 0.039
Type of resection	P = 0.05	P = 0.38
Sex (M:F)	P = 0.98	
Age (under, over 50)	P = 0.28	
Size (under, over 5 cm)	P = 0.15	
AFP (<20, 20–200, >200 ng/ml)	P = 0.16	
Cirrhosis (yes, no)	P = 0.42	
Transfusion (under, over 10 pints)	P = 0.25	
Gross type	P = 0.89	
Histologic type	P = 0.84	

[5]. Recently, its incidence has been increasing in Korea and it is now the second leading cause of death by cancer in males and the fifth in females. The annual incidence rate is 10.1% of all cancers. The male to female ratio of this study was 5:1, and this result was similar to the report from Japan (4.7:1) [6]. The mean age in our study was 51, and this result was somewhat younger than the report from Japan. Age and sex were not found to influence the survival rate.

The positive HBsAg rate was 74.8%; including positive anti-HBs and anti-HBc, it was 91.8%. Therefore, we can assume that HCC was closely related to the hepatitis B virus or viral infection. This feature was similar to the report from China (65.4%) and Taiwan (80%) [5, 7]. Liver cirrhosis was seen in 65% of the patients. The Liver Cancer Study Group of Japan reported a positive HBsAg rate of 26% with 73% of patients having liver cirrhosis [6]. They said that it seemed to be related with non-A non-B virus infection at the time of blood transfusion or activation of cirrhosis with alcoholism. Although in Western countries hepatocellular carcinoma develops in cirrhosis due to alcoholism [8–12], hepatitis B virus is important in the pathogenesis of cirrhosis in areas like Korea where the disease is endemic. As well as the hepatitis B virus, the non-A non-B virus should be cautiously followed.

Many prognostic factors of hepatocellular carcinoma have been investigated in the past: curative resection, tumor size, nodule number, encapsulation, capsule infiltration, venous invasion, grade of anaplasia, androgen receptors, blood transfusion, resection margin, and maximal removal rate of indocyanine green. Among these factors, encapsulation and tumor size have been discussed most frequently. In addition, because of the predominance of hepatocellular carcinoma in male patients, the study of androgen receptors gained attention. Patients with the presence of androgen receptors showed worse prognosis than those with no detectable amount of androgen receptors. It is likely that testosterones enhance the growth and invasiveness of hepatocellular carcinoma which is mediated by androgen receptors in the tumor [13, 14].

In this study, the prognostic importance of variables including age, sex, tumor size, AFP levels, cirrhosis, volume of blood transfusion, type of resection, Child's classification, histopathologic subtype, encapsulation, and microangioinvasion were analyzed. The size of the tumor did not influence the survival rate in this study. With regards to the small hepatocellular carcinoma, better survival rates of 67.9% and 53.4% at 5 and 10 years, respectively, have been reported [5, 15].

AFP levels are absolutely necessary for screening or monitoring. Tang et al. also emphasized early detection by monitoring and performance of limited resection at subclinical recurrence [5]. The presence or absence of the cirrhosis did not influence the survival rate. The importance of cirrhosis as a prognostic factor seems to decrease in other countries.

The volume of blood transfusion during hepatic resection did not influence the survival rate. Several methods of saving blood during hepatic resection made less blood transfusion required. These methods include vascular isolation techniques (total, unilobar, or segmental), use of new instruments (ultrasonic dissector, microwave, infrared coagulator, argon beam coagulator), and new local hemostatic agents (Avitene, Tisseel). It seems that the volume of blood transfusion influences the short-term prognosis but not the long-term prognosis [16–19].

Gross types of HCC have been classified into single nodular, single nodular with perinodal extension, multinodular discrete, multinodular confluent, and massive types. Growth patterns have been classified into expanding (I), spreading (II), multinodular (IIIa), and diffuse (IIIb) types. Histologic patterns have been classified into trabecular (macro and micro), acinar, solid, scirrhous, pelioid, and fibrolamellar types. Cytologic patterns have been classified into cirrhotomimetic, clear cell, pleomorphic, and spindle cell types [20–25]. There was no significant difference in the survival rate among these subtypes. However, patients with the fibrolamellar type may have a better prognosis than other types, as the one patient with this type survived more than 25 months [15, 26–28].

In terms of the extent of resection, three types of major resection and four types of minor resection were employed. There was a significant difference in the survival rate between these two groups. Although the size of tumor did not influence survival, it seems that smaller excisions achieved better survival through minor resection.

Encapsulation was found in 91 patients (54.8%) and frequently seen with the expanding tumor type. Patients with encapsulation showed higher survival than patients without encapsulation. There are some reports about the difference of survival according to capsule invasion [6, 29]. Microangioinvasion is also a characteristic of the spreading type which may have a poor prognosis, and patients with microangioinvasion showed low survival in this study.

Child's classification as a guide to reserved liver function can be used in the long-term prognosis. The survival was better in Child Class A > B > C in decreasing order. In addition, maximal removal rate of indocyanine green has been employed in some patients [30].

Through univariate analysis four factors appeared to be significant indicators in the prognosis of hepatocellular carcinoma. However, multivariate analysis showed that microangioinvasion, Child's classification, and encapsulation were the most valuable factors in predicting survival after surgical treatment of hepatocellular carcinoma.

References

1. Kaplan EL, Meier P (1958) Nonparametric estimation from incomplete observation. J Am Stat Assoc 53:457
2. Cox DR, Oakes D (1984) Analysis of survival data. Chapman and Hall
3. Nagassue N, Yutaya H, Hamada T, Hirose S, Kanashima R, Inoituchi K (1984) The natural history of hepatocellular carcinoma. Cancer 54:1461
4. Okuda K, Ohtsuki T, Obata H, Tomimatsu M, Okazaki N, Hasegawa H, Nakajima Y, Ohnishi K (1985) Natural history of hepatocellular carcinoma and prognosis in relation to treatment: Study of 850 patients. Cancer 56:918
5. Tang ZY, Yu YQ, Zhou XP, Ma ZC, Yang R, Lu JZ, Lim ZY, Yang BH (1989) Surgery of small hepatocellular carcinoma: Analysis of 144 cases. Cancer 64:536

6. The Liver Cancer Study Group of Japan (1990) Primary liver cancer in Japan: Clinicopathologic features and results of surgical treatment. Ann Surg 211:277

7. Tong MJ, Sun SC, Schaeffier BT, Cheng NK et al. (1971) Hepatitis associated antigen and hepatocellular carcinoma in Taiwan. Ann Int Med 75:689

8. Bassendine MF, Dellaseta L, Salmeron J, Thanas HC, Sherlock A (1983) Incidence of hepatitis B virus infection in alcoholic liver disease, HBsAg negative chronic active liver disease and primary liver cell carcinoma in Britain. Liver 3:65

9. Brechoch C, Nalpas B, Courouce AM, Dwhamel G et al. (1982) Evidence that hepatitis B virus has a role in liver cell carcinoma in alcoholic liver disease. N Eng J Med 306:1384

10. Omata M, Ashcavat M, Liew CT, Peters RL (1979) Hepatocellular carcinoma in the USA: Etiologic consideration. Gastroenterology 76: 279

11. Scudamore CH, Ragaz J, Kluflinger AM, Owen DA (1988) Hepatocellular carcinoma: Comparison of oriental and caucasian patients. Am J Surg'155: 659

12. Smalley SR, Moertel CG, Hilton JF, Weiland LH, Weiand HS, Adson MA, Melton LJ 3rd, Batts C (1988) Hepatoma in the non-cirrhotic liver. Cancer 62:1414

13. Nagasue N, Chang YC, Hayashi T, Galizia G et al. (1989) Androgen receptor in hepatocellular carcinoma as a prognostic factor after hepatic resection. Ann Surg 209:424

14. Johnson LF et al. (1972) Association of anabolic androgenic steroid therapy with development of hepatocellular carcinoma. Lancet 1:123

15. Lee CS, Hwang LY, Beasley P, Hsu HC, Lee HS (1988) Prognostic significance of histologic findings in resected small hepatocellular carcinoma. Acta Chir Scand 154:199

16. Attali P, Prod'homme S, Pelletier G, Papoz L, Ink O et al. (1987) Prognostic factors in patients with hepatocellular carcinoma. Cancer 59:2108

17. John A, Ryan JF 2nd (1989) Liver resection without blood transfusion. Am J Surg 157:472

18. Garrison RN, Cryer HM, Howard DA, Polk HC (1984) Clarification of risk factors for abdominal operations in patients with hepatic cirrhosis. Ann Surg 199:648

19. Nagao T, Goto S, Kawno N et al. (1987) Hepatic resection for hepatocellular carcinoma. Ann Surg 205:33

20. Okuda K, Musha H, Nakajima Y, Kubo Y, Shimokawa Y et al. (1977) Clinicopathologic features of encapsulated hepatocellular carcinoma: A study of 26 cases. Cancer 40:1240

21. Wood WJ, Rawlings M, Evans H, Lim CNH (1988) Hepatocellular carcinoma: Importance of histologic classification as a prognostic factor. Am J Surg 155:663

22. Edmonson HA, Steiner PE (1954) Primary carcinoma of the liver: A study of 100 cases among 48,900 necropsies. Cancer 7:462

23. Gibson JG (1978) International histologic classification of tumors, No 20. Histological types of tumors of the liver, biliary tracts, and pancreas. World Health Organization, Geneva

24. Nakashima T, Okuda D, Kojiro M et al. (1983) Pathology of hepatocellular carcinoma in Japan: 232 consecutive cases autopsied in ten years. Cancer 51:863

25. Okuda K, Peters RL, Simson IW (1984) Gross anatomic features of hepatocellular carcinoma from three disparate geographic areas: Proposal of a new classification. Cancer 54:2165

26. Berman MA, Burnham JA, Sheahan DG (1988) Fibrolamellar carcinoma of the liver: An immunohistochemical study of nineteen cases and a review of the literature. Hum Pathol 19:784

27. Craig JR, Peters RL, Edmondson HA, Omata M (1980) Fibrolamellar carcinoma of the liver: A tumor of adolescents and young adults with distinctive clinicopathologic features. Cancer 46:372

28. Vecchio FM (1988) Fibrolamellar carcinoma of the liver: A distinct entity within hepatocellular tumors. A review. Appl Pathol 6:139

29. Hsu HC, Wu TT, Wu MZ, Sheu JC, Lee CS, Chen DS (1988) Tumor invasiveness and prognosis in resected hepatocellular carcinoma: Clinical and pathogenetic implications. Cancer 61:2095

30. Kawano N et al. (1988) Long-term prognosis of surgical patients with hepatocellular carcinoma. Cancer Chemother Pharmacol 23:129

CHAPTER 43

Management of hepatocellular carcinoma in Hong Kong: The Queen Mary Hospital experience

Edward C.S. Lai and John Wong[1]

1 Introduction

Primary hepatocellular carcinoma (HCC) is prevalent in various parts of Asia including Hong Kong which has a predominant Chinese population. Even in China, the incidence varies according to the place of birth and permanent residence. In Qi-dong county of Kiangsu province in China, an incidence of 54 per 100,000 has been noted [1]. On the other hand, a high incidence of 1,158 per 100,000 was reported by Beasley and associates in Taipei among male carriers of the hepatitis B surface antigen (HB_sAg) [2].

A close examination of the population in Hong Kong revealed that residents who were born locally had a much lower risk of developing HCC (0.5 per 10,000 population) when compared to immigrants from different parts of the Kwangdong province, despite the geographic proximity between the two areas in Southern China [3]. Nevertheless, primary liver cancer, including lesions in the intrahepatic bile ducts, has been the second leading cause of death from cancers in Hong Kong in the last decade. In 1989 and 1990, the mortality rate relating to these hepatic tumors was 29.1 and 7.8 per 100,000 population for males and females respectively, with the peak incidence at the age of 55–65 years [4]. Between January 1972 and the end of May 1991, a total of 1,646 patients had their HCC managed primarily in the Department of Surgery, University of Hong Kong at Queen Mary Hospital. The present report summarizes our experience in the management of these patients over the past 19 years and its current status.

2 Management of patients with unresectable HCC

During the past two decades, the resection rate for HCC has been low since more than 85% of our patients present late with advanced disease. The prognosis of patients with unresectable disease is poor, with a median survival of 3.5 weeks reported from our hospital [5]. In order to improve the outlook for these unfortunate people, different means have been explored over the years to identify better palliative measures.

Interruption of the arterial supply to the hepatic tumor attracted enthusiastic support in the early seventies. Extension of the concept of hepatic artery ligation included the use of hepatic dearterialization [6, 7] and hepatic artery ligation followed by regional chemotherapy either via the stump of the divided artery or the portal vein [8–11]. The potential values derived from these palliative surgical procedures were examined prospectively in 1981 in a randomized control trial. A total of 166 patients with unresectable disease were randomized and were treated with hepatic dearterialization, hepatic artery ligation followed by regional chemotherapy delivered either via the hepatic artery or the portal vein, or external radiotherapy. In addition to the high postoperative mortality rates encountered following these palliative surgical interventions, there was no improvement in survival rates when compared to patients in the control group [12]. In view of the already limited life expectancy of these patients with unresectable disease, the routine use of hepatic artery ligation and its modification could not be recommended.

Over the years, intravenous systemic chemotherapy with various chemotherapeutic agents has been the mainstay treatment for our patients with unresectable tumors. Among different agents tried elsewhere, intravenous doxorubicin has

---

[1]Department of Surgery, University of Hong Kong, Queen Mary Hospital, Hong Kong

shown the most encouraging results [13–17]. Based on a randomized control study at our hospital, a median survival of 10.6 weeks was achieved with the use of doxorubicin, and this was significantly better than the 7.5 weeks observed among patients who received no specific therapy for their neoplasms [18]. Our results with doxorubicin showed that when given alone, it was superior to the results obtained by using a combination of 5-fluorouracil, methotrexate, cyclophosphamide and vincristine [19]. Nonetheless, the response rate was still limited to 24% observed among our 45 patients.

In order to improve the efficacy of doxorubicin, a combination of other agents was explored. In vivo and in vitro experimental data suggested that the addition of verapamil, a calcium-channel blocker, could potentiate the efficacy of doxorubicin, especially on chemo-resistant tumors [20–22]. Furthermore, in vivo clinical and experimental evidence showed that the function of the cirrhotic liver could also be improved by chronic verapamil intake [23, 24]. A prospective analysis of 28 patients in our department, however, did not show any apparent potentiation of the tumoricidal effect of systemic doxorubicin on HCC by the addition of verapamil. Instead, there was an escalation in both the incidence and severity of the side-effects [25].

Currently, epirubicin, as a single agent, is the drug of choice for patients with advanced HCC if systemic chemotherapy is indicated. When the portal venous system is patent, transcatheter arterial embolization with gelfoam after selective injection of an emulsion of lipiodol and cisplatinum at 6- to 8-week intervals can be considered if the disease is confined to the liver. Our experience with the use of interventional angiography has been limited as the program has only been available in the past three and a half years.

3 Hepatic resection for patients with HCC

3.1 Patients and Methods

Among the 1,646 patients treated in our department, 250 (15.2%) of them had liver resection for their tumor, and these patients form the basis of the present review. There were 217 males and 33 females with a mean age of 53.9 ± 12.3 years (range: 21–79 years). When patients were stratified according to the size of the lesions, 201

patients had large HCC measuring more than 5 cm in diameter (mean diameter ±S.D., 11.3 ± 4.1 cm). The remaining 49 patients had small tumors of less than 5 cm in size (mean diameter ±S.D., 3.6 ± 1.3 cm).

3.1.1 Preoperative evaluation
A complete preoperative diagnostic work-up aims to provide information on the localization of the tumor, detection of occult disease elsewhere in the body and assessment of the severity of concomitant cirrhosis. Quantitative measurement of the serum alpha-fetoprotein (AFP) level before surgery is considered mandatory for subsequent reference after successful resection.

Investigations on patients undergoing surgery included percutaneous ultrasonography, hepatic and superior mesenteric angiography, and computed tomography. When the diagnosis of HCC was uncertain, lipiodol, an oily contrast medium, was given after the hepatic artery had been selectively cannulated, followed by computed tomography 10–14 days later. The use of scintigraphy, frequently performed in the past, has been abandoned since the introduction of more sensitive imaging studies. Similarly, the practise of using peritoneoscopy as a routine examination before surgical exploration has ceased in recent years. While the procedure was safe in our experience, information gathered from other investigations was sufficient to decide to use laparotomy.

Although the use of computed tomography and ultrasonography provided a reasonable estimate of the physical volume of the hepatic remnant after the proposed hepatectomy, the functional reserve was determined through the percentage of indocyanine green retention measured at 15 minutes after an intravenous injection [26]. A major hepatic resection, either a right or left trisegmentectomy, was considered contraindicated when the retention exceeded 15%.

3.1.2 Techniques of hepatic resection
Before 1987, all hepatic resections were conducted using vertical abdominal incisions at different sites depending on the lateralization of the hepatic neoplasm. A left lobe tumor would be approached through an upper midline incision whereas a right thoraco-abdominal incision would be used when the lesion resided in the right hepatic lobe. In the past four years, all explorations were performed through a bilateral subcostal incision with or without sternal extension. Under exceptionally difficult situations, a thoracotomy was added to facilitate mobilization.

Intraoperative ultrasonography has been routinely performed for exploration since June 1987. When patients are elected for anatomical lobectomy, complete interruption of the portal vein and hepatic artery was first secured. When non-anatomical hepatic resection was decided on, the outline of the tumor and the proposed line of parenchymal transection were initially marked on the Glisson's capsule with diathermy under ultrasound guidance. Whenever possible, the ipsilateral branch of the hepatic vein was divided extrahepatically for patients undergoing anatomical resection. However, temporary control by the application of small vascular clamps were used for those who were subjected to limited hepatectomy such as wedge excision, subsegmentectomy, or segmentectomy. During parenchymal transection, temporary cessation of blood supply to the liver was carried out by the application of vascular clamps on the hepatic pedicle (Pringle's maneuver) for all patients, irrespective of the extent of hepatectomy.

Transection was accomplished by fracturing the hepatic parenchyma using a pair of artery forceps, especially in patients with a cirrhotic liver. After the Glisson's capsule was divided by diathermy, the intervening hepatic tissue was crushed between the blades following closely the intended transection line. On the other hand, in anatomical segmentectomy or resection in non-cirrhotic livers, the use of an ultrasonic dissector is an option. With all the intact branches of vascular and biliary systems exposed, these structures were individually divided between titanium clips for small branches and ligatures for larger ones. Vascular occlusion was applied in cycles of a warm ischemic period of about 20 minutes followed by a 3-minute reperfusion of the liver with release of all the vascular clamps. Clamps would then be reapplied to continue the hepatic transection in repeated cycles until the completion of resection. Hemostasis was secured by sutures where necessary, followed by the application of hemostatic sponges to the raw surface of the hepatic remnant before closure. Drains were routinely inserted in all cases irrespective of the magnitude of hepatic resection.

In the past $2\frac{1}{2}$ years, the common hepatic artery was cannulated via the gastroduodenal artery whenever the vascular anatomy allowed. The other end of the catheter was connected to a subcutaneous port. Besides providing an easy access to the hepatic vasculature for repeated angiographic studies of the hepatic remnants at follow-up, additional regional chemotherapy could also be given via the same route when necessary. The entire procedure usually takes 30 minutes.

3.1.3 Follow-up

Follow-up after surgery was scheduled at monthly intervals for the first postoperative year and every 2–4 months thereafter. Before 1984, monitoring depended on clinical examination, chest radiographs, and hepatic angiograms when intrahepatic recurrence was suspected. In the last 7 years, routine AFP assay and percutaneous ultrasound examination of the hepatic remnants at regular intervals were added. For patients who had successful cannulation of the hepatic artery, angiographic studies were performed at 6-weekly intervals by puncturing the subcutaneous port using a special needle for contrast medium injection.

All diseases discovered after operation were considered as recurrences. A diagnosis of recurrent disease was established histologically whenever possible or, in the absence of histologic confirmation, on a combination of raised AFP titer and characteristic imaging findings.

4 Results

4.1 Clinical features

A majority (93.6%) of the 250 patients were symptomatic at the time of their initial presentation. Among the 16 patients whose lesions were diagnosed during the asymptomatic stage, 12 had small HCC. Epigastric pain with palpable liver was the most frequent presentation. Spontaneous rupture of the tumor was encountered in 39 patients and 17 of them had hypovolemic shock at presentation; this was significantly more frequently seen among patients with small HCC (7 of 49 patients versus 10 of 201 patients; $P < 0.02$). Other symptoms, such as anorexia and weight loss of over 10 pounds, were less common when compared with patients suffering from large HCC ($P < 0.002$).

In the past 4 years, significantly more small HCC and asymptomatic tumors were successfully diagnosed and resected. Among the 101 patients resected since 1987, 29 had lesions which measured 5 cm or less ($P < 0.003$) and 15 of them had asymptomatic tumors ($P < 0.001$). Serologically, 162 of the 225 patients (72%) with known hepatitis

Table 1. Clinical features and laboratory data of 250 patients who had hepatectomy for hepatocellular carcinoma

	Large HCC (n = 201)	Small HCC (n = 49)
Age (years)	54.5 ± 12.0	52.7 ± 11.4
Tumor size (cm)	11.3 ± 4.1	3.6 ± 1.3
HB$_s$Ag positive (%)	69.4	85.0
AFP > 200 ng/ml (%)	61.7	57.5
Asymptomatic lesions (%)*	2.0	24.5
Hemoglobin (gm/l)	13.1 ± 2.3	13.0 ± 2.1
Platelets (10^9/ml)*	205.0 ± 83.0	138.0 ± 62.0
Creatinine (mmol/l)	0.097 ± 0.027	0.105 ± 0.075
Total bilirubin (mmol/l)	20.0 ± 30.0	23.0 ± 35.2
Albumin (gm/l)	39.6 ± 5.5	39.8 ± 6.9
Prothrombin time (seconds over control)	1.2 ± 1.2	1.2 ± 1.1
ICG retention (%)[a]	14.1 ± 8.4	16.8 ± 12.5

All continuous variables were expressed as mean ±S.D.
* $P < 0.0001$
[a] Indocyanine green retention measured at 15 minutes was available in 66 patients with large HCC and 24 patients with small HCC only

B antigen (HB$_s$Ag) status were positive. A raised AFP titer of over 400 ng/ml was found in 89 of the 175 patients with quantitative results available. As for the remaining 86 patients, 26 had AFP titers between 200 and 400 ng/ml, and 29 had titers between 20 and 200 ng/ml. Twenty-five of the 31 patients with normal AFP titers (less than 20 ng/ml) had large HCC. Details of the different clinical features and other laboratory data of patients with resected HCC are listed in Table 1.

4.2 Operative procedures and results

No patient with HCC in the present series underwent attempts at preoperative embolization. Major hepatic resection, either as hemihepatectomy (137 patients) or extended hemihepatectomy (45 patients) constituted the core of our experience with liver resection and most of these procedures were performed for lesions that resided in the right hepatic lobe (136 patients). None of the 68 patients who had limited hepatectomy had their portal vein injected with dye or starch microspheres, nor balloon occlusion at the time of surgery under intraoperative ultrasound guidance.

Among the 39 patients who were diagnosed as having spontaneous rupture of primary tumor, initial hemostasis was achieved surgically in 19

Table 2. Postoperative complications in 250 patients who had hepatectomy for hepatocellular carcinoma

Complications	Large HCC (n = 201)	Small HCC (n = 49)
Wound infection	14	2
Wound dehiscence	1	1
Abdominal sepsis	8	2
Intra-abdominal hemorrhage	16	2
Gastrointestinal bleeding	2	0
Bronchopneumonia	17	3
Pleural effusion	67	11
Variceal bleeding	3	1
Biliary fistula	4	0
Infected ascites	1	0
Total	106	18

Table 3. Mortality rates of 250 patients who had hepatectomy for hepatocellular carcinoma

	No. of patients	No. of Operative deaths	No. of Hospital death
Small HCC	49	3	5
Large HCC	201	27	43
Total	250	30	48

by interrupting the arterial supply to the lesion followed by elective hepatic resection. Seven of the 20 patients who had emergency hepatectomy continued bleeding despite the use of hepatic artery ligation, and the remaining 13 patients had their diagnoses made at the time of laparotomy. None of these patients underwent therapeutic arterial embolization radiologically.

4.3 Morbidity and mortality

Postoperative complications of different magnitudes developed in 124 patients (49.6%) and these are listed in Table 2. Ten of the 49 patients (20.4%) with small HCC required reexploration; three died (6.1%) within 30 days and, with two additional patients, a total of five patients (10.2%) succumbed within the same hospitalization following hepatic resection. There was no statistical difference in the mortality rates with regard to the size of the primary liver cancer (Table 3). A significant reduction in the number of reexplorations was observed from 1987 (46 of 149 patients versus 11 of 101 patients; $P < 0.001$). However, although the postoperative mortality figures were lowered in recent years (8.9% and

Table 4. Causes of death among the 250 patients who had hepatectomy for hepatocellular carcinoma

Causes	Large HCC (n = 201)	Small HCC (n = 49)
Malignant cachexia	89	20
Multiorgan failure	19	5
Hepatic failure	11	0
Postoperative bleeding	11	1
Bronchopneumonia	3	0
Heart failure	2	0
Tension pneumothorax	0	1
Ruptured recurrence	0	1
Intra-abdominal sepsis	6	2
Total	141	30

Table 5. Pathologic features of 250 patients with resected hepatocellular carcinoma (HCC) according to tumor size

Pathologic features	Large HCC (n = 201)	Small HCC (n = 49)
Eggel's nodular* type (%)	56.0	79.4
No. of nodules* >2 (%)	64.2	47.0
Edmondson's grade I & II (%)	24.1	30.8
Encapsulation (%)*	40.8	66.7
Capsular invasion (%)	29.5	32.0
Liver invasion (%)	65.9	52.4
Microsatellite formation (%)	52.9	39.3
Venous permeation*	75.8	50.0
Clear cell >30% (%)	15.5	30.4
Moderate/severe mononuclear cell infiltration (%)	25.0	40.0
Cellular architecture trabecular type (%)	87.0	87.1
Bile production (%)	35.2	36.0
Cirrhosis in adjacent* liver (%)	69.5	87.5

* $P < 0.05$ using chi-squared test

15.8% for 30-day and hospital mortality rates respectively), statistically it was not significant when compared with past results. Seven of the 20 patients (35%) who had undergone emergency resection succumbed within the same hospitalization following surgery. The causes of death of patients who had hepatic resection for HCC are outlined in Table 4.

4.4 Pathologic data and resection margin

Among the 163 patients with information on their cirrhotic status in their non-tumorous liver, 119 patients (73%) had cirrhosis. Based on the classification described by Edmondson and Steiner [27], well differentiated lesions of grades I and II were encountered in 35 of the 138 patients with available pathological information (25.4%). The majority of patients had clear cells (78 of 126 patients with information available) as part of their cellular composition but these made up 30% or less of the total in all patients. Tumor capsule was present in 60 of the 130 patients with available information and evident capsular invasion was seen in 36 of them. Microsatellite formation was demonstrated in half of the patients in the present series. Venous permeation was noted in 113 of 160 patients with information available. While the incidence of venous permeation ($P < 0.005$) and incomplete histologic disease clearance ($P < 0.02$) were significantly higher among patients with large HCC, tumor capsule was more frequently encountered in small HCC ($P < 0.02$). Details of different pathologic features studied and comparisons with that of large HCC are listed in Table 5.

Macroscopic distance of the resection margin, which was taken as the shortest distance between the edge of the lesion to the line of liver transection, was available in 167 patients with details as follows: 0.5 cm or less, 50 patients; 0.5–1 cm, 32 patients; 1–2 cm, 56 patients; over 2 cm, 29 patients. Additional documentation of the histologic disease clearance at the line of parenchymal transection was available in 103 patients, 30 of them (29.1%) had residual histologic disease at the resection margin. Among the 24 patients with small HCC with complete information, two patients (8.3%) whose macroscopic margin was negligible in one and measured between 0.5 and 1 cm in the other, had residual disease at the resection margin verified on pathologic examination.

4.5 Results of follow-up

Information on 14 patients in the present series was not available for follow-up. With the exclusion of the 30 patients who died within 30 days after surgery, 146 of the remaining 206 patients (66.4%) developed recurrent tumor within a median follow-up of 10.1 months. Intrahepatic disease was detected in 115 patients, 85 of whom had their recurrences confined to the hepatic remnant and 30 had disease detected also elsewhere. The remaining 31 patients had extrahepatic recurrences alone. Forty patients presented with advanced recurrent disease and no specific treatment could be offered. Systemic chemotherapy with doxorubicin was given in 54 patients. Twenty-two patients underwent attempts at re-resection for localized recurrences and two had radiotherapy for spinal and pelvic secondaries. Since 1987, nine patients had either transcatheter arterial embolization, with or without the addition of an emulsion of lipiodol and cisplatinum; eight had intra-lesional injection of absolute alcohol under percutaneous ultrasound guidance; and four had a combination of the above-mentioned nonoperative measures for recurrent lesions. A significantly better survival was observed among patients with confirmed recurrences who were managed after 1987. The median survival estimated from the date of diagnosis of the recurrent disease was 4 months before 1987 and 7.5 months in recent years ($P < 0.03$).

The disease-free survival rates of the 49 patients with small HCC at 1 year, 3 years, and 5 years were 41%, 20.7%, and 13.8%, and the survival rates for the same periods were 55%, 28%, and 22%, respectively. The corresponding figures for patients with large HCC were 27.3%, 13.8%, and 7.7% for disease-free survival and 44%, 20.6%, and 15.8% for survival, respectively. When the long-term outlook of patients who had hepatic resection for HCC were studied according to sizes, superior results of both the disease-free survival (9.6 months versus 4.8 months; $P < 0.02$) and survival (median survival: 17 months versus 9.9 months; $P < 0.05$) were observed among patients with tumors less than 5 cm in diameter.

5 Comments

When a patient presents with primary HCC, hepatic resection provides the only chance of long-term survival and possibly a cure [28]. Over the years, the dramatic reduction in operative morbidity and mortality have made hepatectomy a safe and viable option for the management of patients with HCC. Among the various factors which could have contributed to the unsatisfactory results observed in Queen Mary Hospital, we consider the advanced stage of disease important. In contrast to reports from elsewhere in Asia where patients with small asymptomatic lesions accounted for over 60% of patients undergoing liver resection [29–33], patients who had major

liver resection for large HCC dominated our series. Even when our patients with small HCC had significantly fewer symptoms compared with their counterparts with large HCC, less than one-fourth of the 49 patients had their tumor detected at the asymptomatic stage by screening. Although a superior prognosis was observed in the present analysis in contrast to our previous communication in surgery for small HCC [34], our results have remained poor when compared with other series from this part of the world [30, 35, 36]. The presence of symptoms has been identified as a poor prognostic determinant affecting survival of patients with HCC. According to Lee and associates [32], symptomatic patients fared significantly worse than asymptomatic ones when lesions of all sizes were considered together. Even when patients were subjected to liver transplantation, patients with clinically occult neoplasms also fared better [37]. Clearly, aggressive surgery for HCC when they are diagnosed at the small asymptomatic stage could improve the long-term outlook of these patients.

Based on our recent analysis, spontaneous ruptured tumor has become less frequent than in the past. The incidence has dropped from 14.5% before 1972 [38] to 4.5% [39] in the recent 15 years up to 1987. In view of the poor immediate postoperative outcome, even with the present improved results, and the uncertain benefits of the long-term prognosis, routine urgent hepatectomy is not advisable. Furthermore, as the overall mortality from surgical exploration, irrespective of the procedure elected, has been in the order of about 75% [39], radiological intervention should be tried for initial hemostasis [40]. In the absence of radiological support for embolization, hepatic artery ligation together with other local measures, such as plication or packing, could provide satisfactory hemostasis before deciding on the appropriate definitive measure for these patients.

The improved survival for patients with proven recurrent disease in recent times could be attributed to either an earlier diagnosis with a more vigilant follow-up program, more effective remedial measures, or a combination of both factors. When compared with the use of systemic chemotherapy for patients with unresectable recurrences, the improvement of the quality of survival provided by the use of interventional angiography or intra-lesional injection of alcohol was remarkable in our experience.

From the current analysis, the importance of prevention and early diagnosis of hepatocellular carcinoma cannot be over-emphasized. The close association between hepatitis B infection and the risk of developing primary liver cancer is well recognised. Indeed, hepatitis B had been incriminated for 66.3% of patients with cirrhosis and 90%–98% of patients with HCC in Hong Kong. The overall prevalence of serological markers of hepatitis B was 47.7%, with HB$_s$Ag being detected in 9.6% in the population of our locality [41]. Although the policy of routine immunization against hepatitis B virus for all new-born infants was introduced in 1988 [42], we are pessimistic about the possibility of improving our results in Hong Kong over the next few decades unless a screening program for early cancer detection becomes available in the near future.

References

1. Gibson JB (1983) Primary cancers of the liver. J R Coll Surg Edinb 28:275–281
2. Beasley RP, Hwang LY, Lin CC, Chien CS (1981) Hepatocellular carcinoma and hepatitis B virus. A prospective study of 22,707 men in Taiwan. Lancet 2:1129–1133
3. Ong GB, Chan PKW (1976) Primary carcinoma of the liver. Surg Gynecol Obstet 143:31–38
4. "Hong Kong Annual Department Report 1989–1990" (1990) Ed: Director of Health Services. Government Information Service, Hong Kong, Tables 18, 19
5. Lai CL, Lam KC, Wong KP, Wu PC, Todd D (1981) Clinical features of hepatocellular carcinoma: Review of 211 patients in Hong Kong. Cancer 47:2746–2755
6. Balasegaram M (1972) Complete hepatic dearterialization for primary carcinoma of the liver. Report of twenty-four patients. Am J Surg 124:340–345
7. Almersjo O, Bengmark S, Rudenstam CM, Hafstrom L, Nilsson LAV (1972) Evaluation of hepatic dearterialization in primary and secondary cancer of the liver. Am J Surg 124:5–9
8. Ansfield FJ, Ramirez G, Skibba JL, Bryan GT, Davis HL Jr., Wirtanen GW (1971) Intrahepatic arterial infusion with 5-fluorouracil. Cancer 28:1147–1151
9. Gulesserian HP, Lawton RL, Condon RE (1972) Hepatic artery ligation and cytotoxic infusion in treatment of liver metastases. Arch Surg 105:280–285
10. Fortner JG, Mulcare RJ, Solis A, Watson RC, Golbey RB (1973) Treatment of primary and secondary liver cancer by hepatic artery ligation and infusion chemotherapy. Ann Surg 178:162–172
11. Murray-Lyon IM, Parsons VA, Blendis LM, Dawson JL, Rake MO, Laws JW, Williams R (1970) Treatment of secondary hepatic tumours by ligation of hepatic artery and infusion of cytotoxic drugs. Lancet 2:172–175
12. Lai ECS, Choi TK, Tong SW, Ong GB, Wong J (1986) Treatment of unresectable hepatocellular carcinoma: Results of a randomized controlled trial. World J Surg 10:501–509
13. Olweny CL, Toya T, Katongole-Mbidde E, Mugerwa J, Kyalwazi SK, Cohen H (1975) Treatment of hepatocellular carcinoma with Adriamycin. Preliminary communication. Cancer 36:1250–1257
14. Olweny CL, Katongole-Mbidde E, Bahendeka S, Otim D, Mugerwa J, Kyalwazi SK (1980) Further experience in treating patients with hepatocellular carcinoma in Uganda. Cancer 46:2717–2722
15. Johnson PJ, Williams R, Thomas H, Sherlock S, Murray-Lyon IM (1978) Induction of remission in hepatocellular carcinoma with doxorubicin. Lancet 1:1006–1009
16. Vogel CL, Bayley AZ, Brooker RJ, Anthony PP, Ziegler JL (1977) A phase II study of adriamycin (NSC 123127) in patients with hepatocellular carcinoma from Zambia and the United States. Cancer 39:1923–1929
17. Falkson G, Moertel CG, Lavin P, Pretorius FJ, Carbone PP (1978) Chemotherapy studies in primary liver cancer: A prospective randomized clinical trial. Cancer 42:2149–2156
18. Lai CL, Wu PC, Chan GCB, Lok ASF, Lin HJ (1988) Doxorubicin versus no antitumor therapy in inoperable hepatocellular carcinoma. A prospective randomized trial. Cancer 62:479–483
19. Choi TK, Lee NW, Wong J (1984) Chemotherapy for advanced hepatocellular carcinoma. Adriamycin versus quadruple chemotherapy. Cancer 53:401–405
20. Tsuruo T (1983) Reversal of acquired resistance to vinca alkaloids and anthracycline antibiotics. Cancer Treat Rep 67:889–894
21. Rogan AM, Hamilton TC, Young RC, Klecker RW Jr, Ozols RF (1984) Reversal of adriamycin resistance by verapamil in human ovarian cancer. Science 224:994–996
22. Pradhan SG, Basrur VS, Chitnis MP, Adwani SH (1984) In vitro enchancement of adriamycin cytotoxicity in human myeloid leukemia cells exposed to verapamil. Oncology 41:406–408
23. Reichen J, Hirlinger A, Ha HR, Sagesser S (1986) Chronic verapamil administration lowers portal pressure and improves hepatic function in rats with liver cirrhosis. J Hepatol 3:49–58
24. Kong CW, Lay CS, Tsai YT, Yeh CL, Lai KH, Lee SD, Lo KJ, Chiang BN (1986) The hemodynamic effect of verapamil on portal hypertension in patients with postnecrotic cirrhosis. Hepatology 6:423–426
25. Lai ECS, Choi TK, Cheng CH, Mok FPT, Fan ST, Tan ESY, Wong J (1990) Doxorubicin for un-

resectable hepatocellular carcinoma. A prospective study on the addition of verapamil. Cancer 66: 1685–1687

26. Okamoto E, Kyo A, Yamanaka N, Tanaka N, Kuwata K (1984) Prediction of the safe limits of hepatectomy by combined volumetric and functional measurements in patients with impaired hepatic function. Surgery 95:586–592

27. Edmondson HA, Steiner PE (1954) Primary carcinoma of the liver: A study of 100 cases among 48,900 necropsies. Cancer 7:462–503

28. Lee NW, Wong J, Ong GB (1982) The surgical management of primary carcinoma of the liver. World J Surg 6:66–75

29. Nagasue N, Yukaya H, Ogawa Y, Sasaki Y, Chang YC, Niimi K (1986) Clinical experience with 118 hepatic resections for hepatocellular carcinoma. Surgery 99:694–701

30. Nagao T, Inoue S, Goto S, Mizuta T, Omori Y, Kawano N, Morioka Y (1987) Hepatic resection for hepatocellular carcinoma. Clinical features and long-term prognosis. Ann Surg 205:33–40

31. Yamanaka N, Okamoto E, Toyosaka A, Mitunobu M, Fujihara S, Kato T, Fujimoto J, Oriyama T, Furukawa K, Kawamura E (1990) Prognostic factors after hepatectomy for hepatocellular carcinoma. A univariate and multivariate analysis. Cancer 65:1104–1110

32. Lee CS, Sung JL, Hwang LY, Sheu JC, Chen DS, Lin TY, Beasley RP (1986) Surgical treatment of 109 patients with symptomatic and asymptomatic hepatocellular carcinoma. Surgery 99:481–490

33. Chen MF, Hwang TL, Jeng LBB, Jan YY, Wang CS, Chou FF (1989) Hepatic resection in 120 patients with hepatocellular carcinoma. Arch Surg 124:1025–1028

34. Lai ECS, Ng IOL, You KT, Fan ST, Mok FPT, Tan ESY, Wong J (1991) Hepatic resection for small hepatocellular carcinoma: The Queen Mary Hospital experience. World J Surg 15:654–659

35. Tang ZY, Yu YQ, Zhou XD, Ma ZC, Yang R, Lue JZ, Lin ZY, Yang BH (1989) Surgery of small hepatocellular carcinoma. Analysis of 144 cases. Cancer 64:536–541

36. Hsu HC, Wu TT, Wu MZ, Sheu JC, Lee CS, Chen DS (1988) Tumor invasiveness and prognosis in resected hepatocellular carcinoma. Clinical and pathogenetic implications. Cancer 61:2095–2099

37. Iwatsuki S, Gordon RD, Shaw BW Jr, Starzl TE (1985) Role of liver transplantation in cancer therapy. Ann Surg 202:401–407

38. Ong GB, Chu EPH, Yu FYK, Lee TC (1965) Spontaneous rupture of hepatocellular carcinoma. Br J Surg 52:123–129

39. Lai ECS, Wu KM, Choi TK, Fan ST, Wong J (1989) Spontaneous ruptured hepatocellular carcinoma. An appraisal of surgical treatment. Ann Surg 210:24–28

40. Chen MF, Jan YY, Lee TY (1986) Transcatheter hepatic arterial embolization followed by hepatic resection for the spontaneous rupture of hepatocellular carcinoma. Cancer 58:332–335

41. Yeoh EK, Chang WK, Kwan JPW (1984) Epidemiology of viral hepatitis B infection in Hong Kong. In: Lam SK, Lai CL, Yeoh EK (eds) Viral hepatitis B infection in the Western Pacific region: Vaccine and control. World Scientific, Singapore, pp 33–41

42. Hong Kong 1991 (1991) Roberts D (ed). Government Information Services, Hong Kong, p 162

CHAPTER 44

Treatment of hepatocellular carcinoma: A summary of 33 years' experience

Zhao-You Tang, Ye-Qin Yu, Xin-Da Zhou, Bing-Hui Yang, Ji-Zhen Lu, Zhi-Ying Lin, Zeng-Chen Ma, Sheng-Long Ye, Kang-Da Liu, and Zhu-Yuan Yu[1]

1 Introduction

Hepatocellular carcinoma (HCC), the most common type (90–95%) of primary liver cancer (PLC), causes 100,000 deaths every year in China. However, based on various strategies aimed at controlling this neoplasm, HCC has become "partly curable" instead of "incurable." In China, hepatectomy for HCC started in the 1950s, liver cancer cell lines were established in the 1960s, field work in high risk areas, including epidemiology, etiology, and screening, have been conducted from the 1970s [1, 2], and small HCC resection became an important clinical feature in the 1970s and 1980s [3–7]. During the past ten years, substantial progress has been made in the field of basic liver cancer research, studies have focused on the relation between hepatitis B virus (HBV) and HCC, a set of protooncogenes and HCC-related genes have been studied, and cytoreduction and sequential resection for unresectable HCC have become new trends [8].

2 Patients and methods

From January 1958 to December 1990, 1,450 patients with pathologically proven HCC were treated at our institute. The median age was 48 (13–82 years). The HBV background was more predominant than hepatitis C virus (HCV) infection. Positivity of serum HBsAg was 69.1% (685/992), anti-HBc was 72.1% (80/111). However, positivity of serum anti-HCV was only 8.3%

(31/376). Associated cirrhosis was found in 86.8% of patients, and macronodular cirrhosis amounted to 60.7%.

Of the entire series, 28.8% of patients were diagnosed as having HCC by alpha fetoprotein and/or ultrasonography (US) screening or by monitoring of high risk populations. Subclinical HCC amounted to 22.4% of the entire series. Small HCC (less than 5 cm) was found in 314 patients (28.9%). The median diameter of the HCC nodule in the entire series was 8 cm. AFP was abnormal (more than 20 ng/ml) in 73.5% of patients. Resection was done in 741 patients (51.1%), palliative surgery other than resection was performed in 480 patients (33.1%), and conservative treatment was given in 229 patients (15.8%).

Re-operation (including re-resection or other palliative surgery) for recurrence or metastases was done in 96 patients. Thirty four patients received second stage resection after marked shrinkage of tumor.

Survival rates were calculated by the life table method. All of the data were treated by microcomputer.

3 Comparison of results from three decades

The entire series was divided into 3 groups: 1958–1968 (n = 113), 1969–1979 (n = 404), 1980–1990 (n = 933). As shown in Table 1, the marked increase in the 5-year survival rate (2.8%, 10.5%, and 36.6%, respectively) and 10-year survival rate (2.8%, 7.8%, and 23.1%) coincided with the increased proportion of small HCC in the series (0.9%, 9.9%, and 25.2%), increased number of patients who underwent re-resection for subclinical recurrence (0, 14, 59), and in-

[1] Liver Cancer Institute, Shanghai Medical University, Shanghai 200032, People's Republic of China

Table 1. Comparison of the three decades

	1958–1968 (n = 113)	1969–1979 (n = 404)	1980–1990 (n = 933)
Small HCC	1 (0.9%)	40 (9.9%)	235 (25.2%)
Re-resection	—	14	59
Second stage resection	—	1	33
Resection (%)	25.7	32.9	62.1
Operative mortality (%)	20.7	11.3	1.9
Survival 5-year (%)	2.8	10.5	36.6
10-year (%)	2.8	7.8	23.1

creased number of patients who underwent cyto-reduction and sequential resection (second stage resection) (0, 1, 33). Moreover, the increasing proportion of small HCC in the series has resulted in marked increases in the rate of resection (25.7%, 32.9%, and 62.1%) and decreases in operative mortality (20.7%, 11.3%, and 1.9%). This all indicates that the role of surgery has become greater with the progress of early detection and more effective multimodal treatment [9].

4 Analysis of patients surviving more than five years

Large series of PLC patients with 5-year survival have rarely been reported in the literature. When Curutchet reviewed the worldwide literature for the period 1905–1970, only 45 patients had survived 5 years [10]. However, based on the rapid progress in early detection and multimodal treatment, we recently reported large series of long-term survivors [11–13].

Over the period 1958–1986 (followed up in August 1991), 125 patients with PLC surviving more than 5 years gathered at our institute. All were proved pathologically to be HCC. Thirty seven of them had survived more than 10 years, the longest being 30 years. Of these 125 patients, 55.2% were discovered by screening, 48.0% of the patients were subclinical HCC, 80.7% of the patients had solitary tumors, and 52.8% of patients had tumors smaller than 5 cm in size. Pathological findings revealed that 78.3% of tumors were grade II according to Edmondson's grading, and all patients associated with cirrhosis. The serum HBsAg was positive in 63% and anti-HBc in 80% of the patients who were checked with HBV markers.

The therapeutic pattern of the series indicated that 108 patients received resection; 65 patients were small HCC resection and 43 patients were non-small HCC resection. Re-resection for subclinical recurrence or solitary lung metastasis was done in 26 patients with resection. Limited resection amounted to 54.6% of patients with resection. Of the total 125 patients, 17 received palliative surgery other than resection, including hepatic artery ligation, cannulation, cryosurgery, or a combination of these. Eight of the 17 patients received second stage resection due to marked shrinkage of the tumor. It could be seen that early resection remained the major approach for long-term survival, and re-resection for subclinical recurrence was also of proved merit. Resection of large tumors was still useful but less effective. Cytoreduction and sequential resection was a new trend.

5 Small HCC resection

During the past two decades, we have published a good number of papers concerning small HCC or subclinical HCC [3–7, 14–18]. In the 1970s, we mainly carried out mass screening in the natural population by AFP serosurveys [19]. In the 1980s, two changes in early detection happened: instead of natural population screening, we mainly carried out high risk population screening (people who had a history of hepatitis and/or positive serum HBsAg, and were in the 40–65 age group). Recently, we emphasized that regular health checkups should include AFP tests and US. Furthermore, AFP and/or US should be used for early detection instead of AFP serosurveys alone.

AFP and US remained the best for early diagnosis. Many tumor markers were tried, but none proved superior to AFP [20].

For localization, US was non-invasive, less expensive, and sensitive enough to detect 1-cm HCC. Lipiodol computed tomography (CT) was of value to detect 0.5-cm HCC. Tc-99 m PMT delayed imaging was of value to detect small HCC with 50.0% positivity, but high specificity [21].

For early treatment, resection remained the best. Limited resection was the method of choice to increase resectability and decrease operative mortality [22]. With a good retractor and right subcostal incision, it was not necessary to enter the chest to resect small HCC located in all regions. Using a careful step-by-step resection technique, hilum occlusion was only used in individual patients with deep sited lesions.

The results of subclinical HCC or small HCC resection were encouraging [23]. Between 1967 and 1990, 250 patients with small HCC received resection, the operative mortality was 1.6%, 5-year survival 66.3%, and 10-year survival 48.9%. Limited resection was not inferior to that of lobectomy.

In recent years, transcatheter arterial embolization (TAE) or ultrasound-guided intralesional injection have also been employed to treat patients with small HCC who are contraindicated to surgery. However, the long-term results were not as good as resection. Based on a study of subclinical or small HCC, a new concept of the natural history of HCC was also established [24].

6   Non-small HCC resection

Although the progress of non-small HCC resection was not as encouraging as that of small HCC resection, some advances were achieved as a result of early diagnosis and improved surgical techniques as well as multimodal treatment. Ten years ago when we reported on 153 PLC resections (1958–1978), the operative mortality was 12.4%, and 5-year survival 23.6% [25]. However, of the 491 patients with non-small HCC resection

Table 2. Survival of unresectable HCC (surgically verified) (n = 709)

	1958–1968 (n = 53)	1969–1979 (n = 124)	1980–1990 (n = 303)
Second stage resection (number of patients)	—	1	33
Survival: (%)			
1 year	3.8	31.4	53.6
3 years	—	6.7	29.7
5 years	—	0.5	21.4
10 years	—	—	12.8

during the period 1958–1990, the operative mortality was only 5.7% and 5-year survival 31.2%. Resection of PLC of the hepatic hilus was also studied; 5-year survival after resection of hepatic hilus PLC in 65 patients was 39.2%, which was lower than that of resection in the non-hilus area with a similar tumor size [26].

7   Re-resection for subclinical recurrence

In 1984, we reported on re-resection for subclinical recurrence and found that it was an important approach to prolong survival further after radical resection of HCC [27]. Over the period 1958–1990, 73 patients with liver recurrence (n = 66) or solitary lung metastasis (n = 7) received re-resection. No operative mortality was found. The 5-year survival and 10-year survival calculated from the first operation was 52.5% and 26.0%, respectively, and were 40.6% and 30.3% from the time of re-resection. Therefore, re-resection can not only prolong survival but can also provide another curative outcome. This is emphasized to follow-up patients after curative HCC resection every 2–3 months using AFP determination and US. Limited resection is the method of choice for re-resection. Cryosurgery, TAE, ethanol injection, hapatic artery ligation, and/or cannulation with chemotherapy are suggested for patients contraindicated to resection.

In further research, the structure of the integrated HBV DNA was analyzed to determine the origin of recurrent and multinodular HCC. The results indicated that both unicentric and multicentric origins existed [28].

8   Cytoreduction and sequential resection for unresectable HCC

As shown in Table 2, 5-year survival of surgically verified unresectable HCC increased from 0% in 1958–1968 (n = 53), to 0.5% in 1969–1979 (n = 124), and 21.4% in 1980–1990 (n = 303). This improvement coincided with the increased number of patients with cytoreduction and sequential resection (second stage resection) (0, 1, and 33, respectively). Therefore, cytoreduction and sequential resection might be important approaches to prolonging survival in patients with unresectable HCC.

In recent years, several papers from our institute have been published concerning this aspect [29–32], and some key points will be delineated below.

8.1 Approach to cytoreduction

In the past, marked shrinkage of the tumor was rarely encountered after non-resectional therapy, mainly because the therapeutic effect of different treatment modalities was not effective enough, and combination with different modalities was rarely employed. However, in the past ten years, different kinds of regional therapy appeared, such as cryosurgery [33], ultrasound-guided intralesional ethanol injection, microwave therapy, TAE, fractionated regional radiotherapy, targeting therapy, and so on. Moreover, improved combinations of treatment have been tried, particularly the integration of biological response modifiers.

At our institute, experimental studies using nude mice bearing human HCC xenografts demonstrated that the best response rate was in the triple combination group; fractionated radiotherapy (or radioimmunotherapy, RIT), plus cisplatin, plus mixed bacterial vaccine (MBV) immunotherapy. The double combination group, with radiotherapy (or RIT), plus cisplatin, or radiotherapy (or RIT), plus MBV, was superior to single modality treatment [34].

Retrospective clinical studies also revealed that multiple combination treatment with hepatic artery ligation (HAL), plus hepatic artery infusion (HAI), plus radiotherapy (and/or RIT) yielded the highest second stage resection rate (30.6%) and the highest 5-year survival (28.0%), whereas in the double combination groups (HAL + HAI, or HAL + cryosurgery), the second stage resection rate was 10.9%–18.8% and 5-year survival 9.4%–18.1%. Single treatment was disappointing; no patient received second stage resection and 5-year survival was only 7.2%. These results show that new and effective regional therapy and multiple combination might be key links for cytoreduction [32].

8.2 Sequential resection

Limited resection was done in all of the patients with sequential resection. Pathological examination revealed that residual cancer cells were

Table 3. Survival of different surgical treatment groups (1958–1990)

	No. of patients	Survival (%)		
		3 years	5 years	10 years
Small HCC resection	250	78.7	66.3	48.9
Cytoreduction and sequential resection	34	76.6	62.0	49.6
Non-small HCC resection	491	39.1	31.2	22.5
Palliative surgery other than resection	346	17.1	9.0	4.6

found in 70.6% (24/34) of surgical specimens after second stage resection, indicating the importance of sequential resection in the eradication of residual cancer.

The time for sequential resection is suggested as follows: a) when the tumor has shrunk to 50% of the original diameter and with a decline in serum AFP levels, b) when there is normalization of the albumin/globulin ratio, c) when US or CT indicate that curative resection is technically feasible. In this study, the median time from the first operation to sequential resection was 5 months.

8.3 Outcome of sequential resection

Of the 34 patients receiving sequential resection, the 5-year survival was as high as 62.0%, which was similar to that of small HCC resection (66.3%, n = 250), double that of non-small HCC resection (31.2%, n = 491), and much higher than that of palliative surgery other than resection only (9.0%, n = 346) (Table 3). The favorable 5-year survival coincided with the relatively small median tumor size (4 cm) at the time of sequential resection.

8.4 Candidates for cytoreduction and sequential resection

It is clear that only a small number of patients with unresectable HCC can be candidates for cytoreduction and sequential resection. Patients with solitary encapsulated unresectable HCC in right cirrhostic liver were the best candidates. However, right lobe unresectable HCC with few nearby daughter nodules can also be tried.

9 Regional therapy

Regional therapy is a new trend in the field of solid tumor therapy. At our institute, cryosurgery has been employed since 1974 to treat unresectable but superficially located HCC with acceptable results [33]. TAE was acknowledged to be the treatment of choice for unresectable HCC. In our hospital, 345 patients received TAE from July 1986 to December 1989; 30 of them gained the chance of second stage resection, and chemoembolization was considered much better than that of hepatic arterial infusion chemotherapy alone [35]. Percutaneous portal vein (branch) embolization and chemotherapy was also tried alone or in combination with TAE to control the peripheral zone of the HCC nodule [36]. Percutaneous intralesional ethanol injection was also performed in patients with primary or recurrent small HCC but contraindicated to surgery. However, incomplete necrosis was found in many patients. Alternating fractionated regional radiotherapy and chemotherapy was another attractive approach, and of 30 patients so treated, 11 received second stage resection and the overall 3-year survival was 61% [37].

10 Targeting therapy

Targeting therapy using antibodies (Abs) or monoclonal Abs as carriers has become an attractive field in the past 10 years. Although, RIT has not yet been well established clinically, the preliminary results were encouraging.

From 1983 to 1990, in vitro and in vivo comparisons were made among 12 carriers: anti-HCC ferritin Ab (FtAb), L subunit ferritin MAb, H subunit ferritin MAb, anti-human HCC MAb, AFP-Ab, AFP-MAb, pyridoxyl-5-methyl tryptophan (PMT), Cholylglycyl tyrosine (CGT), EDDA, Rhodamine 6GDN, Lipiodol, Iophendylatum. Six cytotoxic agents (I-131, I-125, Y-90, Adriamycin, Methotrexate, Vincristine) conjugated to Abs were also studied. Great difference was found among the immunohistochemistry, nude mice bearing human HCC, and clinical studies [38–40].

10.1 Clinical results of radioimmunotherapy using I-131 anti-HCC ferritin antibody

As a part of multimodal therapy, 41 patients with unresectable HCC were treated; 13 of them obtained second stage resection due to marked shrinkage of tumor, and 3-year survival of the 41 patients was 25.9%. Radioimmunoimaging demonstrated good targeting to the tumor area. Hepatic arterial administration was superior to intravenous administration, the sensitivity in day 7 was 100% in the former and 76.5% in the latter, with the tumor/liver ratio 1.74 ± 0.57 and 1.34 ± 0.39, respectively. In addition, with hepatic arterial administration there was an unexpectedly low anti-antibody detection rate compared to that with the intravenous method (0/14 versus 4/11) [41, 42].

10.2 Clinical results of targeting therapy using I-131 lipiodol

Transhepatic arterial injection of I-131 Lipiodol was carried out in 34 patients with unresectable HCC. The tumor/liver ratio was even higher than that of I-131 FtAb. AFP levels declined in 69% (18/26) of the patients. Tumor shrinkage was observed in 74% (25/34) of the patients. Eleven patients (32%) obtained second stage resection. The 1-, 2- and 3-year survivals were 82%, 55%, and 55% respectively [43].

11 Conclusion

In the 1950s and 1960s, the understanding of intrahepatic anatomy resulted in a marked improvement of prognosis by lobectomy of HCC and benefits to 5%–10% of all patients. In the 1970s and 1980s, the use of AFP serosurveys and US monitoring in high risk populations opened a new era of small HCC resection, and this has benefited another 5%–10% of HCC patients. With the advances of regional therapy and biological response modifiers since the 1980s, cytoreduction and sequential resection have also become attractive methods, and this will also benefit a further 5%–10% of HCC patients, particularly those with unresectable HCC.

References

1. Tang ZY (1986) Progress in liver cancer research in China. In: Editorial Committee of Current Medicine in China (eds) Current Medicine in China. People's Medical Publishing House, Beijing, pp 353–360
2. Tang ZY, Wu MC, Xia SS (eds) (1989) Primary liver cancer. China Acad Publishers, Beijing; Springer, Berlin, pp 1–495
3. Tang ZY, Yu YQ, Lin ZY, Zhou XD, Yang BH, Cao YZ, Lu JZ, Tang CL (1979) Small hepatocellular carcinoma: Clinical analysis of 30 cases. Chin Med J 59:35–40
4. Shanghai Coordinating Group for Research on Liver Cancer (Tang ZY, Yu EX, Wu CE, Gu XY) (1979) Diagnosis and treatment of primary hepatocellular carcinoma in the early stages: A report of 134 cases. Chin Med J 92:801–806
5. Tang ZY (1980) Screening and early treatment of primary liver cancer with special reference to eastern China. Ann Acad Med Singapore 9: 234–239
6. Tang ZY, Ying YY, Gu TJ (1982) Hepatocellular carcinoma: Changing concepts in recent years. In: Popper H, Schaffner F (eds) Progress in liver diseases, vol VII. Grune and Stratton, New York, pp 637–647
7. Tang ZY (ed) (1985) Subclinical hepatocellular carcinoma. China Acad Publishers, Beijing; Springer, Berlin, pp 1–366
8. Tang ZY (ed) (1991) Advances in liver cancer and hepatitis research: 1991 Shanghai International Symposium on liver cancer and hepatitis. Shanghai Medical University Press, Shanghai, pp 1–162
9. Tang ZY, Yu YQ, Zhou XD (1986) The changing role of surgery in the treatment of primary liver cancer. Semin Surg Oncol 2:103–112
10. Curutchet HP, Terz JJ, Kay S, Lawrence W (1971) Primary liver cancer. Surgery 70:467–479
11. Zhou XD, Tang ZY, Yu YQ, Yang BH, Lin ZY, Lu JZ, Ma ZC, Tang CL (1989) Long-term survivors after resection for primary liver cancer. Clinical analysis of 19 patients surviving more than ten years. Cancer 63:2201–2206
12. Zhou XD, Tang ZY, Yu YQ, Ma ZC, Yang BH, Lu JZ, Lin ZY (1989) Hepatocellular carcinoma: Some aspects to improve long-term survival. J Surg Oncol 41:256–262
13. Zhou XD, Tang ZY, Yu YQ, Ma ZC, Yang BH, Lu JZ, Lin ZY, Tang CL (1991) Prognostic factors of primary liver cancer: A report of 83 patients surviving 5 years or more compared with 811 patients surviving less than 5 years. J Exp Clin Cancer Res 10:81–86
14. Tang ZY, Yu YQ, Yang BH (1987) Subclinical hepatocellular carcinoma. In: Wagner G, Zhang YH (eds) Cancer of the liver, esophagus, and nasopharynx. Springer, Berlin, pp 64–72
15. Tang ZY (1987) Recent advances in the study of small hepatocellular carcinoma. In: Editorial committee of Current Medicine in China (ed) Current Medicine in China. People's Medical Publishing House, Beijing, pp 136–146
16. Tang ZY (1987) Surgical treatment of subclinical cases of hepatocellular carcinoma. In: Okuda K, Ishak KG (eds) Neoplasms of the liver. Springer, Tokyo, pp 367–373
17. Tang ZY (1989) Small hepatocellular carcinoma. In: Tang ZY, Wu MC, Xia SS (eds) Primary liver cancer. China Acad Publishers, Beijing; Springer, Berlin, pp 191–203
18. Tang ZY, Yu YQ, Zhou XD, Ma ZC, Yang R, Lu JZ, Lin ZY, Yang BH (1989) Surgery of small hepatocellular carcinoma: Analysis of 144 cases. Cancer 64:536–541
19. Tang ZY, Yang BH, Tang CL, Yu YQ, Lin ZY, Weng HZ (1980) Evaluation of population screening for hepatocellular carcinoma. Chin Med J 93: 795–799
20. Tang ZY, Yang BH (1989) Further evaluation of alpha fetoprotein as tumor marker for hepatocellular carcinoma with special reference to subclinical cancer. In: Tang ZY, Wu MC, Xia SS (eds) Primary liver cancer. China Acad Publishers, Beijing; Springer, Berlin, pp 172–179
21. Chen SL, Zhao HY, Yuan AN, Tang ZY, Ma ZC (1991) Diagnostic value of Tc-99m PMT delayed hepatobiliary imaging in small hepatocellular carcinoma: An analysis of 62 cases (in Chinese). Chin J Oncol 13:30–32
22. Yu YQ, Tang ZY, Zhou XD (1980) Experience in resection of small hepatocellular carcinoma. Chin Med J 93:491–494
23. Tang ZY, Yu YQ, Zhou XD (1983) Surgical treatment of subclinical hepatocellular carcinoma (HCC) and its ultimate outcome: A comparative study of 74 cases of subclinical HCC and 229 cases of clinical HCC undergone surgery. J Exp Clin Cancer Res 3:261–268
24. Tang ZY (1981) A new concept on the natural course of hepatocellular carcinoma. Chin Med J 94:585–588
25. Tang ZY, Yu YQ, Zhou XD, Chen QM (1981) Factors influencing primary liver cancer resection survival rate. Chin Med J 94:749–754
26. Yu YQ, Tang ZY, Ma ZC, Zhou XD, Lu JZ (1991) Resection of the primary liver cancer of the hepatic hilus. Cancer 67:1322–1325
27. Tang ZY (1984) An important approach to prolonging survival further after radical resection of AFP positive hepatocellular carcinoma. J Exp Clin Cancer Res 3:359–366
28. Liang XH, Loncarevic IF, Tang ZY, Yu YQ, Zentgraf H, Schroder CH (1991) Resection of hepatocellular carcinoma: Oligocentric origin of recurrent and multinodular tumours. J Gastroenterol Hepatol 6:77–88
29. Tang ZY, Yu YQ (1986) Long-term survival of hepatocellular carcinoma with reference to the role

of early resection, multioperation, and multi-modality treatment. Gann Monogr Cancer Res 31:185–190

30. Tang ZY, Yu YQ, Ma ZC, Yang R, Zhou XD, Liu KD, Lu JZ, Bao YM, Lin ZY, Yang BH (1989) Conversion of surgically verified unresectable to resectable hepatocellular carcinoma: A report of 26 patients with subsequent resection. Chin J Cancer Res 1:41–47

31. Tang ZY (1989) Conversion of nonresectable to resectable hepatocellular carcinoma. In: Editorial Committee of Current Medicine in China (ed) Current medicine in China. People's Medical Publishing House, Beijing, pp 215–221

32. Tang ZY, Yu YQ, Zhou XD, Ma ZC, Lu JZ, Liu KD, Lin ZY, Yang BH, Fan Z, Hou Z, Zhang M (1991) Cytoreduction and sequential resection: A hope for unresectable primary liver cancer. J Surg Oncol 47:27–31

33. Zhou XD, Tang ZY, Yu YQ, Ma ZC (1988) Clinical evaluation of cryosurgery in the treatment of primary liver cancer: A report of 60 cases. Cancer 16:1–4

34. Bao YM, Tang ZY, Liu KD, Ma ZC, Xue Q, Qin WL (1989) Radioimmunotherapy combined with chemotherapy and immunotherapy for nude mice bearing human hepatocellular carcinoma. Chin J Oncol 11:245–247

35. Lin G, Wang JH, Gu ZM (1991) Hepatic arterial infusion chemotherapy and embolization for the treatment of liver cancer: Effects and some influential factors. In: Tang ZY (ed) Advances in liver cancer and hepatitis research. Shanghai Medical University Press, Shanghai, p 126

36. Xu DB, Zhou M, Yu YQ, Xu ZZ, Sheng L (1991) Preliminary results of percutaneous portal vein embolization and chemotherapy in the treatment of primary liver cancer. In: Tang ZY (ed) Advances in liver cancer and hepatitis research: 1991 Shanghai International Symposium on Liver Cancer and Hepatitis. Shanghai Medical University Press, Shanghai, p 129

37. Lu JZ, Tang ZY, Yu YQ (1991) Alternating chemotherapy and fractionated radiotherapy in the treatment of primary liver cancer. In: Tang ZY (ed) Advances in liver cancer and hepatitis research: 1991 Shanghai International Symposium on Liver Cancer and Hepatitis. Shanghai Medical University Press, Shanghai, p 142

38. Tang ZY, Liu KD, Guo YD, Ma ZC, Yu D, Yu ZY, Bao YM, Lu JZ, Lin ZY, Yu YQ, Zhou HY, Chen KJ, Qian F, Yuan AN, Wu ZM (1986) Tumor imaging and targeting therapy for hepatocellular carcinoma: Preliminary results of experimental and clinical studies. Chin Med J 99:855–860

39. Tang ZY, Ma ZC (1989) Establishment of transplantable human hepatocellular carcinoma in nude mice and their use in studies of tumor markers and radioimmunodetection. In: Tang ZY, Wu MC, Xia SS (eds) Primary liver cancer. China Acad Publishers, Beijing; Springer, Berlin, pp 172–179

40. Tang ZY, Liu KD, Fan Z, Lu JZ, Hou Z, Zhang YJ, Bao YM, Yu ZY, Zhou D, Xia XL, Tang WY, Ma ZC, Lin ZY, Zhou XD, Yu YQ, Yang BH, Zhao HY, Yuan AN, Zhou YG (1991) Eight years' studies on tumor imaging and targeting therapy for hepatocellular carcinoma. In: Tang ZY (ed) Advances in liver cancer and hepatitis research: 1991 Shanghai International Symposium on Liver Cancer and Hepatitis. Shanghai Medical University Press, Shanghai, pp 148–149

41. Liu KD, Tang ZY, Bao YM, Lu JZ, Qian F, Yuan AN, Zhao HY (1989) Radioimmunotherapy for hepatocellular carcinoma (HCC) using I-131 anti HCC isoferritin IgG: Preliminary results of experimental and clinical studies. Int J Radiat Oncol Biol Phys 16:319–323

42. Tang ZY, Liu KD, Bao YM, Lu JZ, Yu YQ, Ma ZC, Zhou XD, Yang R, Gan YH, Lin ZY, Fan Z, Hou Z (1990) Radioimmunotherapy in the multimodality treatment of hepatocellular carcinoma with reference to second look resection. Cancer 65:211–215

43. Lu JZ, Tang ZY, Zhao HY (1991) Transhepatic artery injection of I-131 (or I-125) labeled Lipiodol for treatment of primary liver cancer. In: Tang ZY (ed) Advances in liver cancer and hepatitis research. Shanghai Medical University Press, Shanghai. p 149–150

Addendum (3)

CHAPTER 45

Summary of the data from a follow-up study by the Liver Cancer Study Group of Japan

The Liver Cancer Study Group of Japan has collected enormous amounts of data from more than 30,000 cases of primary liver cancer throughout the country since 1965. The data includes epidemiology, past medical history, diagnostics, pathology, surgical treatment, and so on. Here, the characteristics and the changing trends with regard to HCC in Japan will be demonstrated.

Table 1. Total number of histologically-proven patients in the 4th–9th surveys

	Male	Female	Total
Hepatocellular carcinoma	10,587	2,209	12,796
Cholangiocellular carcinoma	571	363	934
Mixed type	130	44	174
Hepatoblastoma	102	54	156
Sarcoma	15	9	24
Others	—	—	219

Total number of patients: 38,225

Table 2. Age distribution in histologically-proven patients from the 5th–9th surveys

Age (years)	HCC	CCC
1–9	27	1
10–19	43	0
20–29	91	12
30–39	420	37
40–49	1,365	104
50–59	4,183	191
60–69	3,628	276
70–79	1,423	163
80–	125	18
Total	11,305	802

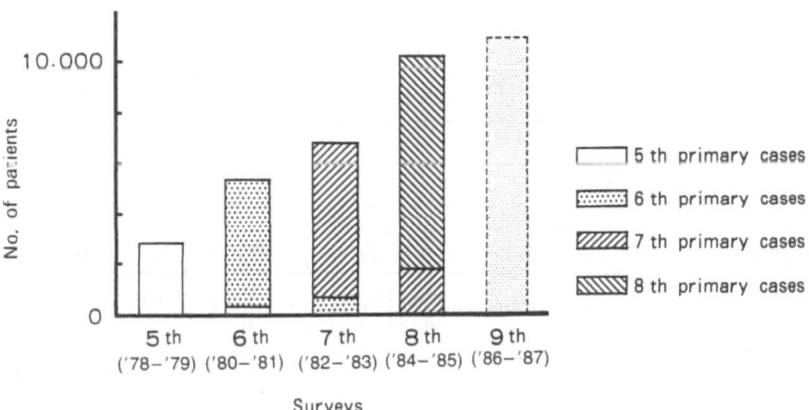

Fig. 1. Number of patients registered in each survey

Table 3. Past medical history

	6th (1980–1981)	7th (1982–1983)	8th (1984–1985)	9th (1986–1987)
Blood transfusion	313/1,568 (20.0%)	373/1,623 (23.0%)	404/1,754 (23.0%)	539/2,319 (23.2%)
Alcohol intake (86 g of alcohol per day for more than 10 years)	538/1,668 (32.3%)	510/1,749 (29.2%)	626/1,927 (32.5%)	792/2,545 (31.1%)

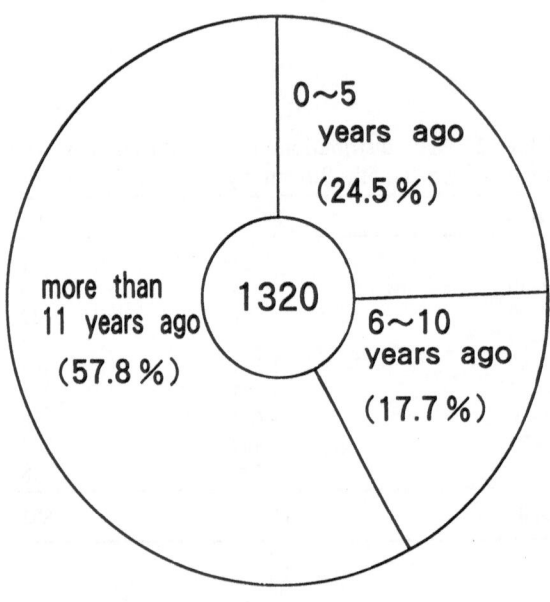

Fig. 2. Past history of blood transfusion. Data from the 6th–9th surveys

Table 4. Past history of liver disease. Data from the 5th–9th surveys

Acute hepatitis	Chronic hepatitis	Liver cirrhosis
2,658/20,960 (12.7%)	9,705/20,862 (46.5%)	13,158/23,020 (57.2%)

Table 5. Positivity of HBsAg in relation to age. Data from the 6th–9th surveys

Age (years)	Positive	Negative	Total
0–9	7 (35.0%)	13	20
10–19	13 (43.3%)	17	30
20–29	22 (42.3%)	30	52
30–39	209 (71.8%)	83	291
40–49	557 (43.8%)	714	1,271
50–59	851 (22.8%)	2,869	3,720
60–69	506 (20.7%)	2,443	2,949
70–79	145 (13.8%)	1,050	1,195
80–	9 (11.5%)	78	87

Table 6. Positivity of HBV-associated antigen and antibody of HCC patients

	4th (1968–1977)	5th (1978–1979)	6th (1980–1981)	7th (1982–1983)	8th (1984–1985)	9th (1986–1987)
HBsAg	266/654 (40.7%)	325/954 (34.0%)	517/1,645 (31.4%)	489/1,779 (27.5%)	476/1,933 (24.6%)	556/2,480 (22.4%)
HBsAb	87/499 (17.4%)	132/618 (21.3%)	315/1,215 (25.9%)	408/1,525 (26.8%)	456/1,688 (27.0%)	481/2,086 (23.1%)
HBcAb	—	30/49 (61.2%)	165/227 (72.7%)	365/523 (69.8%)	549/800 (68.6%)	715/1,116 (64.1%)
HBeAg	—	9/95 (9.4%)	34/258 (13.2%)	110/623 (17.7%)	129/871 (14.8%)	160/1,150 (13.9%)
HBeAb	—	23/89 (25.8%)	78/238 (32.8%)	186/563 (33.0%)	272/781 (34.6%)	349/1,055 (33.1%)

Table 7. AFP levels

AFP level (ng/ml)	4th (1968–1977)	5th (1978–1979)	6th (1980–1981)	7th (1982–1983)	8th (1984–1985)	9th (1986–1987)
≤20	} 150 (22.0%)	146 (16.2%)	328 (18.9%)	386 (20.8%)	474 (23.2%)	716 (27.6%)
21–200		149 (16.5%)	314 (18.1%)	387 (20.8%)	506 (24.8%)	710 (27.4%)
201–1,000	} 287 (42.0%)	370 (41.0%)	1,738 (17.5%)	393 (21.1%)	368 (18.0%)	438 (16.9%)
1,001–10,000			355 (20.4%)	373 (20.1%)	399 (19.5%)	418 (16.1%)
10,000–100,000	} 246 (36.0%)	} 238 (26.4%)	278 (16.0%)	214 (11.5%)	198 (9.7%)	221 (8.5%)
100,001–			158 (9.1%)	107 (5.8%)	97 (4.8%)	89 (3.4%)

Table 8. Changes in the modality of diagnostic imagings

		5th	6th	7th	8th	9th
Scintigraphy	Ratio performed	2,169/2,520 (86.1%)	3.404/4,269 (79.7%)	3,615/5,326 (67.9%)	3,643/7,012 (52.0%)	3,211/8,893 (36.1%)
	Positivity	2,008/2,169 (92.6%)	3,045/3,404 (89.5%)	3,121/3.615 (86.3%)	3.026/3.643 (83.1%)	2,513/3,211 (78.3%)
Angiography	Ratio performed	1,627/2,518 (64.6%)	3,028/4,276 (70.8%)	4,260/5,345 (79.7%)	5,749/6,985 (82.3%)	7,650/8,982 (85.2%)
	Positivity	1,415/1,627 (87.0%)	2,659/3,028 (87.8%)	3,747/4,260 (88.0%)	5,133/5,749 (89.3%)	6,650/7,650 (86.9%)
Ultrasound	Ratio performed	851/2,394 (35.5%)	2,749/4,169 (66.0%)	4,586/5,217 (87.9%)	8,142/8,582 (94.9%)	13,466/13,881 (97.0%)
	Positivity	—	2,517/2,749 (91.6%)	4.320/4,586 (74.2%)	7,833/8,142 (96.2%)	13,135/13,466 (97.5%)
Computed Tomography	Ratio performed	739/2,519 (29.3%)	2,907/4,232 (68.7%)	4,422/5,245 (84.3%)	6,285/6,879 (91.4%)	8,003/8,736 (91.6%)
	Positivity	672/739 (90.9%)	2,728/2,907 (93.8%)	4,184/4,422 (94.6%)	5,944/6,285 (94.6%)	7,565/8,003 (94.5%)

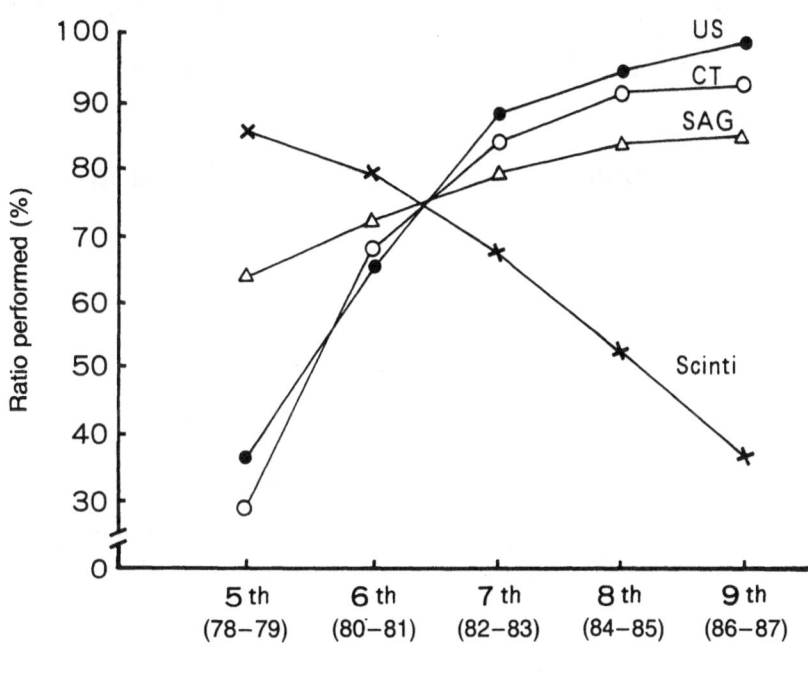

Fig. 3. Changes in diagnostic modality. *US*, ultrasound; *CT*, computed tomography; *SAG*, selective angiography; *Scinti*, scintigraphy

Table 9. Histology of HCC. Data from the 5th–9th surveys

Trabecular	Pseudoglandular	Solid	Sclerosing	Total
2,695 (78.0%)	267 (7.7%)	437 (12.6%)	57 (1.6%)	3,456

Table 10. Edmondson-Steiner classification. Data from the 5th–9th surveys

I	I–II	II	II–III	III	III–IV	IV	Total
109	290	1,900	589	729	55	57	3,729
(2.9%)	(7.8%)	(51.0%)	(15.8%)	(19.5%)	(1.5%)	(1.5%)	

trabecular

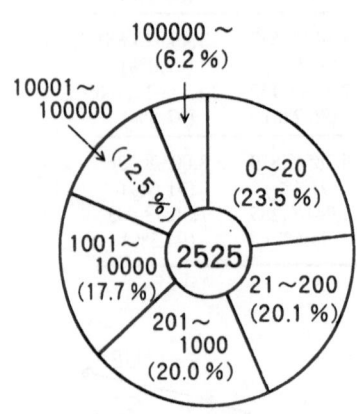

pseudoglandular

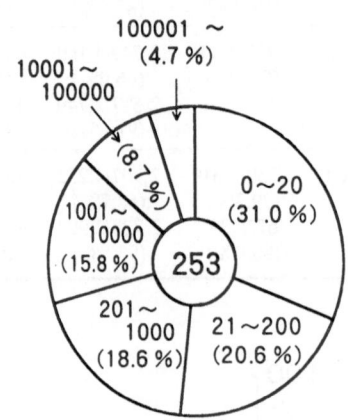

solid

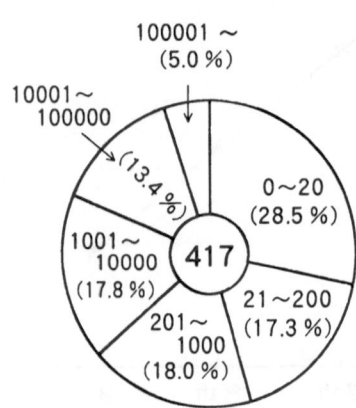

sclerosing

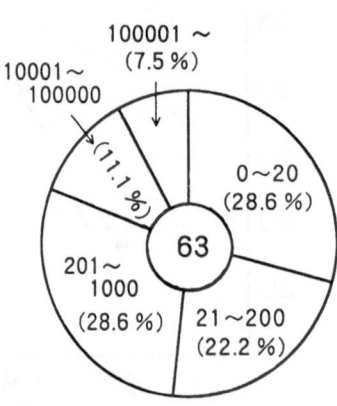

Fig. 4. Serum level of alpha-fetoprotein (AFP) in relation to histological type of HCC. Data from the 6th–9th surveys

Fig. 5. Serum level of AFP in relation to the Edmondson-Steiner classification. Data from the 6th–9th surveys

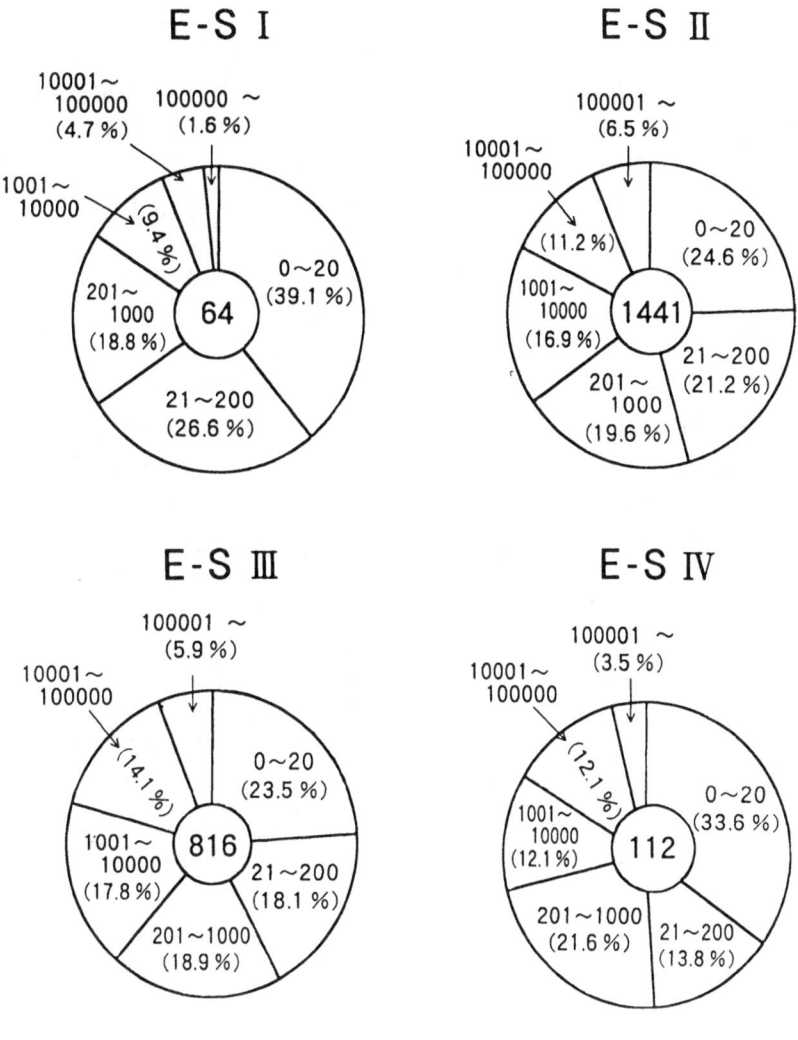

Table 11. Pathology of HCC: Surgical specimen and operative findings

	7th	8th	9th
Growth pattern			
Expansive growth	717/854 (84.0%)	1,052/1,158 (90.8%)	1,571/1,687 (93.1%)
Infiltrative growth	137/854 (16.0%)	106/1,158 (9.2%)	116/1,687 (6.9%)
Capsule formation (Fc)	638/819 (77.9%)	953/1,168 (81.6%)	1,410/1,732 (81.4%)
Capsule infiltration (Fc-inf)	266/660 (40.3%)	377/1,023 (36.9%)	514/1,532 (33.6%)
Septum formation (Sf)	262/641 (40.9%)	472/1,060 (44.5%)	697/1,602 (43.5%)
Serosal infiltration	398/917 (43.4%)	538/1,254 (42.9%)	705/1,785 (39.5%)
Distant metastasis	19/966 (2.0%)	24/1,264 (1.9%)	41/1,526 (2.7%)
Accompanying liver disease	869/1,002 (86.7%)	1,111/1,261 (88.1%)	1,522/1,747 (87.1%)
Peritoneal metastasis	27/1,016 (2.7%)	14/1,285 (1.1%)	15/1,816 (0.8%)
Lymphnode metastasis	51/835 (6.1%)	37/1,153 (3.2%)	41/1,689 (2.4%)
Tumor thrombus			
Portal vein	140/679 (20.6%)	173/1,117 (15.5%)	244/1,697 (14.4%)
Hepatic vein	38/662 (5.7%)	52/1,082 (4.8%)	79/1,592 (5.0%)
Intraductal growth	24/678 (3.5%)	29/1,158 (2.5%)	48/1,672 (2.9%)

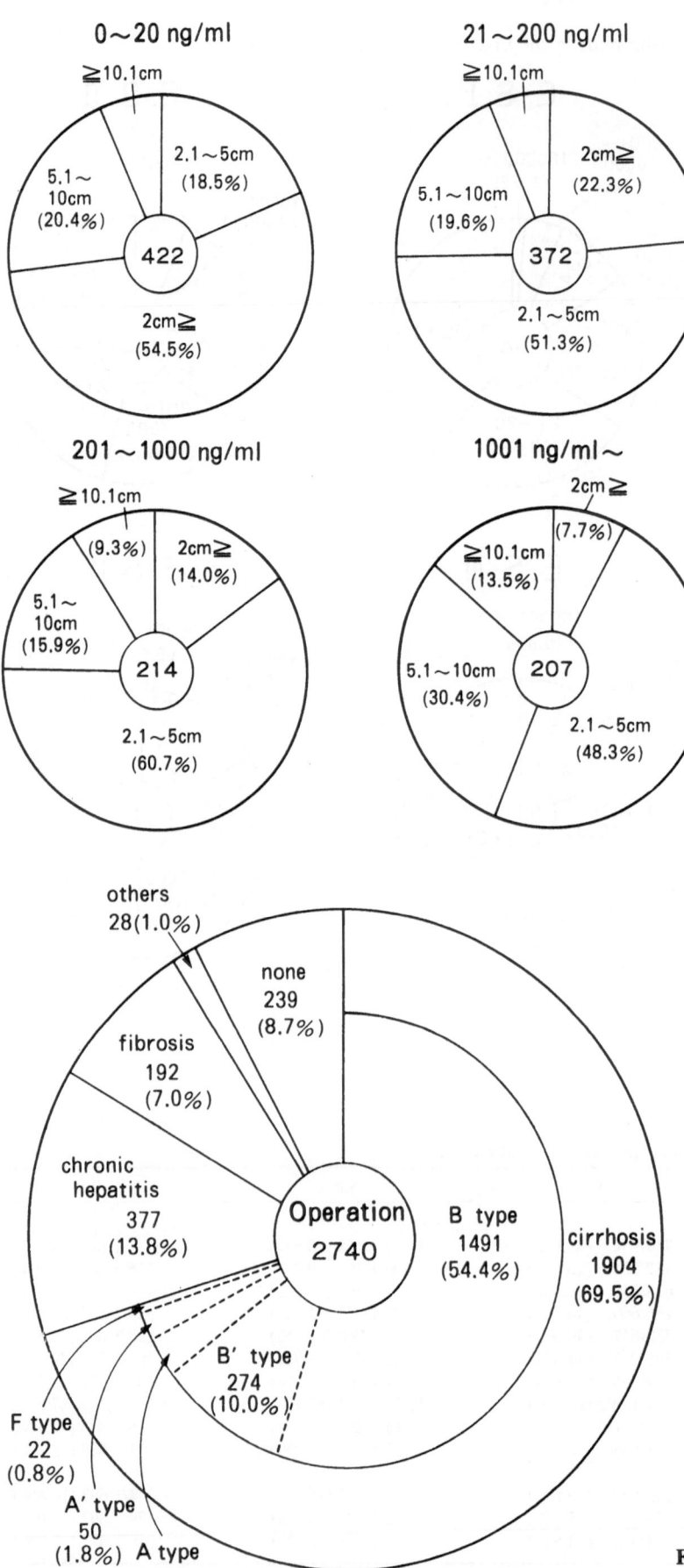

0∼20 ng/ml

≥10.1cm

2.1∼5cm
(18.5%)

5.1∼
10cm
(20.4%)

422

2cm≧
(54.5%)

21∼200 ng/ml

≥10.1cm

2cm≧
(22.3%)

5.1∼10cm
(19.6%)

372

2.1∼5cm
(51.3%)

Fig. 6. Serum level of AFP in relation to tumor size. Data from the 6th–9th surveys

201∼1000 ng/ml

≥10.1cm

(9.3%)

2cm≧
(14.0%)

5.1∼
10cm
(15.9%)

214

2.1∼5cm
(60.7%)

1001 ng/ml∼

2cm≧

(7.7%)

≥10.1cm
(13.5%)

5.1∼10cm
(30.4%)

207

2.1∼5cm
(48.3%)

others
28(1.0%)

none
239
(8.7%)

fibrosis
192
(7.0%)

chronic
hepatitis
377
(13.8%)

Operation
2740

B type
1491
(54.4%)

cirrhosis
1904
(69.5%)

B′ type
274
(10.0%)

F type
22
(0.8%)

A′ type
50
(1.8%)

A type
67
(2.4%)

Fig. 7. Accompanying liver disease at operation. Data from the 8th and 9th surveys

450

Fig. 8. Accompanying liver disease at autopsy. Data from the 8th and 9th surveys

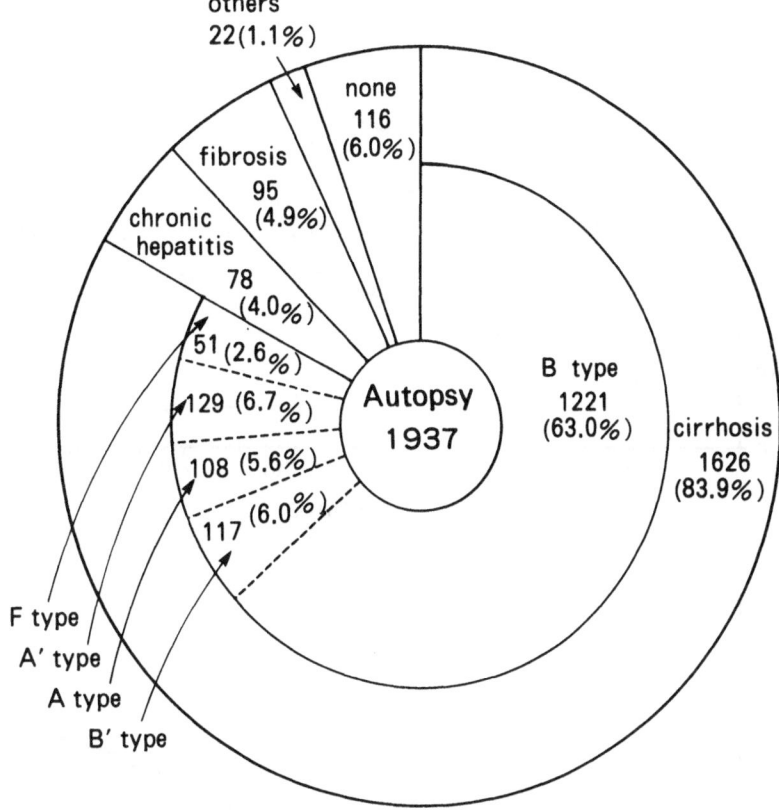

Table 12. Distant metastasis of HCC at autopsy

	5th	6th	7th	8th	9th
Lung	248 (45.1%)	574 (48.0%)	444 (46.0%)	444 (46.7%)	511 (47.4%)
Bone	53 (9.7%)	113 (10.1%)	92 (10.3%)	107 (12.1%)	118 (11.9%)
Brain	7 (1.3%)	13 (1.7%)	11 (1.8%)	11 (1.9%)	9 (1.3%)
Peritoneum	78 (16.0%)	172 (15.1%)	164 (17.8%)	148 (16.6%)	161 (15.9%)
Intraperitoneal organ	92 (16.7%)	187 (16.3%)	189 (20.2%)	153 (16.8%)	193 (18.7%)
Adrenal gland	58 (10.5%)	124 (10.7%)	112 (12.0%)	117 (12.9%)	155 (15.0%)
Skin	8 (1.5%)	11 (1.0%)	10 (1.1%)	14 (1.6%)	8 (0.8%)
Lymphnode	192 (34.9%)	—	204 (30.2%)	213 (30.5%)	252 (32.4%)
Others	65 (11.8%)	122 (13.1%)	119 (15.6%)	138 (17.0%)	172 (19.2%)

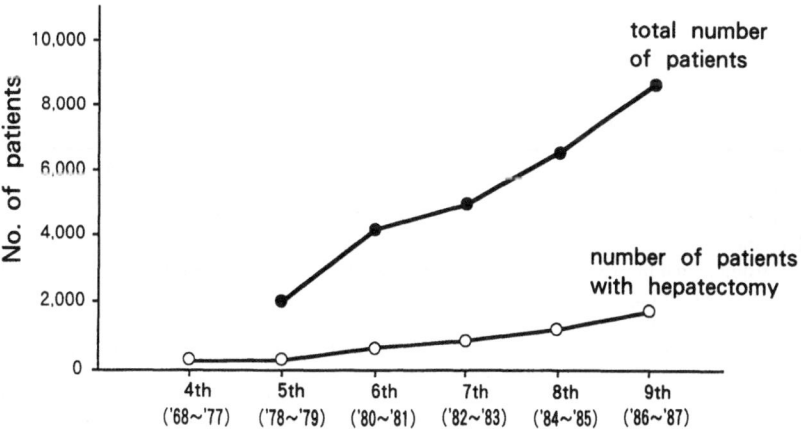

Fig. 9. Changes in resectability

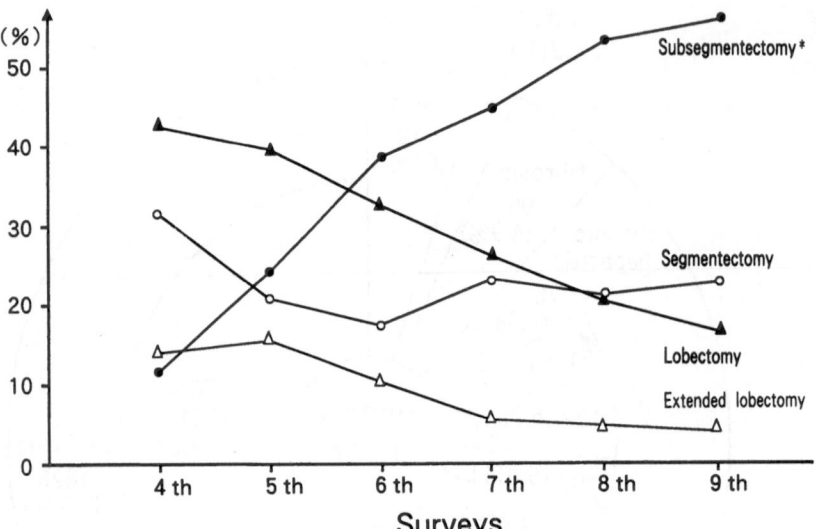

Fig. 10. Changes in operative methods. Subsegmentectomy includes partial hepatic resection of smaller part than a subsegment. Subsegment is defined as Couinaud's segment

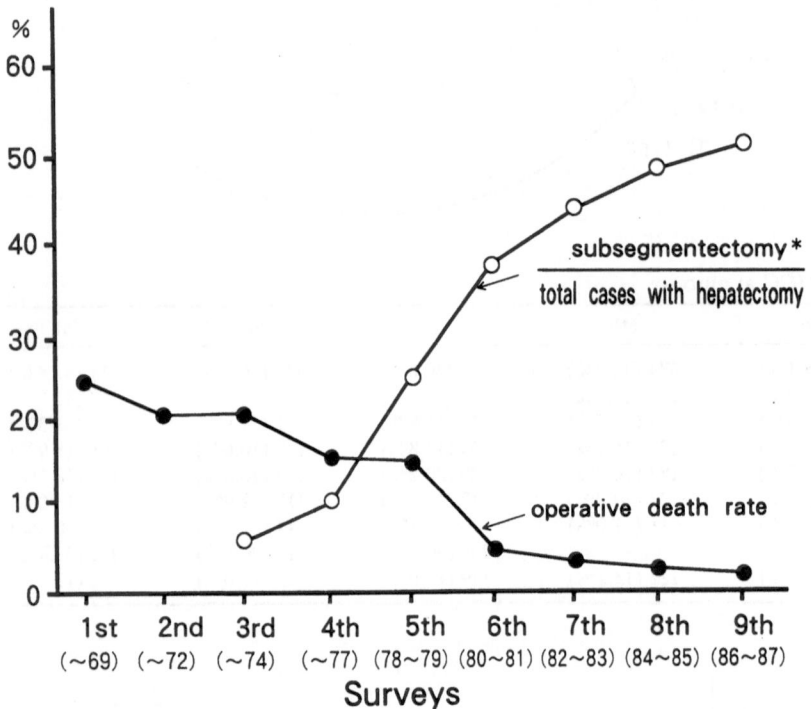

Fig. 11. Relationship between operative death rate and increased proportion of subsegmentectomy in operative method

Table 13. Cause of death of HCC patients

	6th (n = 1,464)	7th (n = 1,270)	8th (n = 1,217)	9th (n = 1,375)
Cancer	453 (30.9%)	438 (34.5%)	402 (33.0%)	505 (36.2%)
Hepatic failure	451 (30.8%)	416 (32.8%)	442 (36.3%)	510 (36.6%)
Gastrointestinal bleeding	185 (12.6%)	119 (9.4%)	105 (8.6%)	70 (5.0%)
Rupture of esophageal varices	151 (10.3%)	121 (9.5%)	102 (8.4%)	110 (7.9%)
Rupture of tumor	163 (11.1%)	127 (10.0%)	125 (10.3%)	157 (11.3%)
Operative death	61 (4.2%)	49 (3.9%)	41 (3.4%)	43 (3.1%)
Others	146	121	111	123
Unknown	69	77	105	153

Fig. 12. Summary of causes of death in the 6th–9th surveys

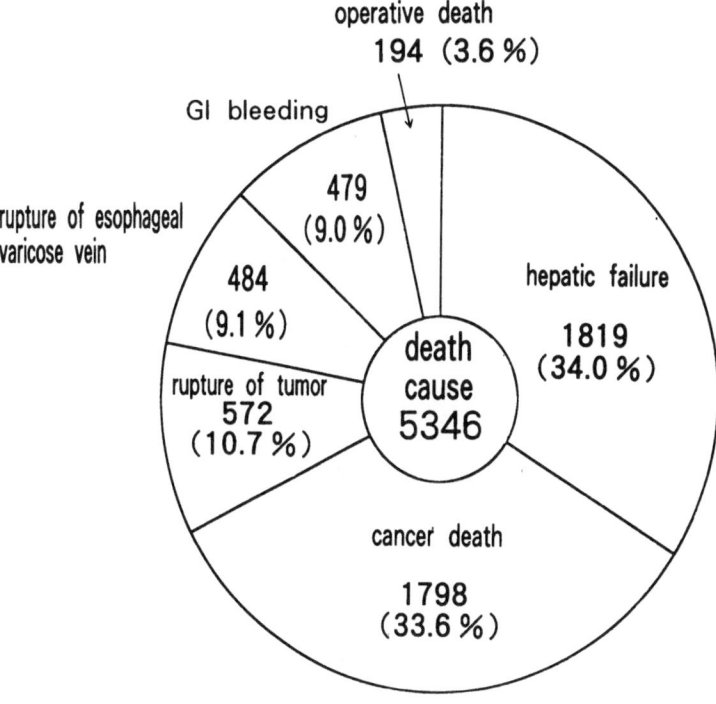